Temporomandibular Disorders
An Evidence-Based Approach to Diagnosis and Treatment

Temporomandibular Disorders

An Evidence-Based Approach to Diagnosis and Treatment

Edited by

Daniel M. Laskin, DDS, MS
Professor and Chairman Emeritus
Department of Oral and Maxillofacial Surgery
School of Dentistry
Division of Oral and Maxillofacial Surgery
Department of Surgery
School of Medicine
Virginia Commonwealth University
Richmond, Virginia

Charles S. Greene, DDS
Clinical Professor
Director of Orofacial Pain Studies
Department of Oral Medicine and Diagnostic Sciences
College of Dentistry
University of Illinois
Chicago, Illinois

William L. Hylander, DDS, PhD
Professor
Department of Biological Anthropology and Anatomy
Director
Duke University Primate Center
Duke University
Durham, North Carolina

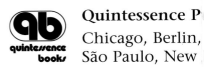
Quintessence Publishing Co, Inc
Chicago, Berlin, ~~Tokyo, London, Paris, Milan,~~ arcelona, Istanbul,
São Paulo, New ~~Delhi, Moscow, Prague, and W~~ rsaw

TMData Resources
formerly MyoData
TMD & Snoring Materials/Services
(800) 533-5121

Library of Congress Cataloging-in-Publication Data

Temporomandibular disorders : an evidence-based approach to diagnosis
  and treatment / edited by Daniel M. Laskin, Charles S. Greene, William
  L. Hylander.
      p. ; cm.
  Includes bibliographical references and index.
  ISBN 0-86715-447-0 (hardcover)
  1. Temporomandibular joint—Diseases. 2. Evidence-based medicine.
I. Laskin, Daniel M. II. Greene, Charles S. III. Hylander,
William L.
  [DNLM: 1. Temporomandibular Joint Disorders--diagnosis. 2. Temporo-
mandibular Joint Disorders--therapy.   WU 140.5 T287 2006]
RK470.T42 2006
617.5'22--dc22

                                                         2005026903

© 2006 Quintessence Publishing Co, Inc

Quintessence Publishing Co, Inc
4350 Chandler Drive
Hanover Park, IL 60133
www.quintpub.com

Editor: Kathryn Funk
Design: Dawn Hartman
Production: Patrick Penney and Dawn Hartman

Printed in Singapore

This book is dedicated to our friend and colleague Bernard G. Sarnat, MD, MS, DDS—teacher, mentor, researcher, and clinician—whose pioneering efforts in the field led the way to the establishment of a more scientific approach to the diagnosis and treatment of temporomandibular disorders.

TABLE OF CONTENTS

PREFACE

This book continues the tradition established more than 50 years ago with the publication of Dr Bernard G. Sarnat's monograph on the TMJ (*The Temporomandibular Joint*, Thomas, 1951). That volume was based on a series of symposia and lectures held at the University of Illinois College of Dentistry in Chicago involving some of the pioneers in the field. It was the first to deal comprehensively with this emerging field, clarifying some of the existing controversies, but it was relatively brief because of the limited information available at that time. Subsequently, three more extensive editions were published in 1964, 1980, and 1992, with the last two co-edited by the senior editor of this book (DML). The basic premise of all four editions was to integrate the expertise of multiple basic scientists and clinicians in order to address the biologic complexity of the temporomandibular system as well as the clinical challenges of diagnosis and treatment.

In this new book we have maintained that collaborative process but have made significant changes in the organization and manner of presentation of the latest information. As in the past, many of the most eminent researchers and clinicians in the world were invited to summarize the current status of their particular field of expertise. In keeping with the current thrust in both medicine and dentistry, these authors were asked to use evidence-based knowledge rather than opinion as the fundamental standard for arriving at the conclusions and recommendations in their particular chapter. However, when this was not possible because of a lack of supporting data or rapid changes in the field, they were asked to highlight the areas of agreement and disagreement within their discipline. As a result, the reader can see where there are deficiencies in our present knowledge base, which in itself is valuable information. More importantly, however, the reader can see which cur-

rent practices of diagnosis and treatment are strongly supported by scientific research and which are supported only by practical experience and/or anecdotal evidence.

Although once again divided into two parts, the first addressing the biologic basis of TMDs and the second covering clinical management of these disorders, this book features an otherwise unique and innovative organization. The two sections in the first part of the book separate normal TMJ anatomy and function from the various pathologies, injuries, and dysfunctional conditions that can affect the TMJ complex. In the second part, a section on diagnostic modalities in current use, with a critical review of the evidence supporting their sensitivity, specificity, and clinical value, precedes the section on the diagnosis of specific clinical conditions. Likewise, chapters on the various therapeutic modalities that have been recommended in the literature, with each method subjected to critical scrutiny, precede the section on specific treatment protocols. This final section emphasizes the actual clinical management of patients with various TMDs based on the combination of scientific and clinical information discussed in the earlier sections.

The challenge for editors of a book with multiple authors is to weave all the parts together into a whole cloth. With 42 authors writing 36 chapters, we did not expect this to be easy, nor did we expect unanimity of opinion on every subject. Readers will certainly notice some different viewpoints among the authors as they read this book, which reflects the current reality of this complex and often controversial field. The pace of new developments in certain aspects of TMD-related pain has been so fast that, to keep the book current, some chapters were being modified up to the final publication deadline. This was especially true in such areas as the pathophysiology of myofascial pain and osteoarthritis, sensory and motor neurophysiology, fibromyalgia, and pharmacologic approaches to patient management. In addition, recent advances in the biobehavioral dimensions of diagnosing TMDs, as well as managing them, have significantly changed the current landscape for understanding the affected patients—especially those with chronic pain conditions.

Another difficulty in having multiple authors writing about a complex subject such as TMDs is to maintain consistency in terminology. For example, in the United States degenerative joint disease is usually referred to as *osteoarthritis*, whereas in Europe it is termed *osteoarthrosis*. In this text we have chosen to use the former designation. The term *condyle* is also often used when *condylar process* is meant. The latter consists of both the condyle (the uppermost part, also referred to as the *condylar head*) and a condylar neck. An even more difficult situation is found in the use of the term *temporomandibular disorder* (TMD). When used correctly, it is a singular term referring to a particular arthrogenous or myogenous condition, and therefore it requires a modifying term in order to be specific (eg, a patient has a myofascial TMD). However, in the literature authors often use *TMD* as an all-inclusive label so that it is impossible to determine which conditions are being included (eg, TMD is a biopsychosocial condition). To avoid such confusion, we have used the term *TMD* with a modifier when referring to a specific disorder and *TMDs* when the group of conditions is being discussed.

In an area with so much misinformation and confusion, it is a significant challenge to put aside personal bias and opinion and base one's conclusions only on what has been substantiated in the scientific literature. The contributors to this book are to be congratulated for accepting this challenge and fulfilling it most admirably. In doing so, they have not only lent clarity to the subject of TMDs but also made a significant contribution to improved patient care.

A. Omar Abubaker, DMD, PhD
Professor and Chairman
Department of Oral and Maxillofacial Surgery
School of Dentistry
Division of Oral and Maxillofacial Surgery
Department of Surgery
School of Medicine
Virginia Commonwealth University
Richmond, Virginia

Leon A. Assael, DMD
Professor and Chairman
Department of Oral and Maxillofacial Surgery
School of Dentistry

Professor
Department of Surgery
School of Medicine
Oregon Health & Science University
Portland, Oregon

Radhika Chigurupati, DMD, BDS
Assistant Clinical Professor
Department of Oral and Maxillofacial Surgery
School of Dentistry
University of California
San Francisco, California

Glenn T. Clark, DDS, MS
Professor of Diagnostic Sciences and Director
Center for Orofacial Pain and Oral Medicine
School of Dentistry
University of Southern California
Los Angeles, California

Lewis Clayman, DMD, MD
Clinical Professor
Department of Oral and Maxillofacial Surgery
School of Dentistry
University of Michigan
Ann Arbor, Michigan

Clinical Associate Professor
Department of Otolaryngology/Head and
    Neck Surgery
Wayne State University School of Medicine
Detroit, Michigan

Chief
Oral and Maxillofacial Surgery Services
Sinai-Grace Hospital
Detroit Medical Center
Detroit, Michigan

Lambert G. M. de Bont, DDS, PhD
Professor and Head
Department of Oral and Maxillofacial Surgery
University Medical Center
University of Groningen
Groningen, The Netherlands

Raymond A. Dionne, DDS, PhD
Chief
Pain and Neurosurgery Mechanisms Branch
National Institute of Dental and Craniofacial
    Research
National Institutes of Health
Bethesda, Maryland

Ronald Dubner, DDS, PhD
Professor and Chairman
Department of Biomedical Sciences
Baltimore College of Dental Surgery
University of Maryland Dental School
Baltimore, Maryland

Samuel F. Dworkin, DDS, PhD
Professor Emeritus
Department of Oral Medicine
School of Dentistry
Department of Psychiatry and Behavioral
    Sciences
School of Medicine
University of Washington
Seattle, Washington

Jocelyne S. Feine, DDS, MS, HDR
Professor and Graduate Program Director
Faculty of Dentistry
McGill University
Montreal, Québec, Canada

Luigi M. Gallo, PD, PhD, MEng
Senior Research Associate and Director of the
    Experimental Laboratory
Clinic for Masticatory Disorders and Complete
    Dentures
Center for Dental and Oral Medicine and
    Maxillofacial Surgery
University of Zurich
Zurich, Switzerland

Stuart A. Gansky, MS, DrPH
Associate Professor
Department of Preventive and Restorative
    Dental Sciences
Division of Oral Epidemiology and Dental
    Public Health
School of Dentistry
University of California
San Francisco, California

Yoly M. Gonzalez, DDS, MS
Assistant Professor
Department of Oral Diagnostic Sciences
School of Dental Medicine
State University of New York at Buffalo
Buffalo, New York

Charles S. Greene, DDS
Clinical Professor and Director of Orofacial
    Pain Studies
Department of Oral Medicine and Diagnostic
    Sciences
College of Dentistry
University of Illinois
Chicago, Illinois

Frank I. Hohn, DDS, FRCD(C)
Clinical Professor
College of Dentistry
University of Saskatchewan
Saskatoon, Saskatchewan, Canada

Head
Department of Dentistry/Oral and
    Maxillofacial Surgery
Saskatoon Health Region
Saskatoon, Saskatchewan, Canada

Linda L. Huang, DDS, MD
Chief Resident
Division of Oral and Maxillofacial Surgery
School of Dental and Oral Surgery
Columbia University
New York, New York

William L. Hylander, DDS, PhD
Professor and Director of the Duke University
    Primate Center
Department of Biological Anthropology and
    Anatomy
Duke University
Durham, North Carolina

Leonard B. Kaban, DMD, MD
Walter Guralnick Professor
Department of Oral and Maxillofacial Surgery
Harvard School of Dental Medicine
Massachusetts General Hospital
Boston, Massachusetts

**Dean A. Kolbinson, DMD, MSD,
    FRCD(C)**
Professor and Associate Dean
College of Dentistry
University of Saskatchewan
Saskatoon, Saskatchewan, Canada

Mauno Könönen, DDS, Odont Dr
Professor
Institute of Dentistry
Department of Oral and Maxillofacial Diseases
University of Helsinki
Helsinki Central Hospital
Helsinki, Finland

Sigvard Kopp, DDS, PhD
Professor and Chairman
Department of Clinical Oral Physiology
Institute of Odontology
Karolinska Institutet
Huddinge, Sweden

Regina Landesberg, DMD, PhD
Associate Professor
Division of Oral and Maxillofacial Surgery
School of Dental and Oral Surgery
Columbia University
New York, New York

Tore A. Larheim, DDS, PhD
Professor
Department of Maxillofacial Radiology
Institute of Clinical Dentistry
Faculty of Dentistry
University of Oslo
Oslo, Norway

Daniel M. Laskin, DDS, MS
Professor and Chairman Emeritus
Department of Oral and Maxillofacial Surgery
School of Dentistry
Division of Oral and Maxillofacial Surgery
Department of Surgery
School of Medicine
Virginia Commonwealth University
Richmond, Virginia

James P. Lund, BDS, PhD
Professor and Dean
Faculty of Dentistry
McGill University
Montreal, Quebec, Canada

Member
Center of Research in Neurological Sciences
University of Montreal
Montreal, Quebec, Canada

Louis G. Mercuri, DDS, MS
Professor
Department of Surgery
Division of Oral and Maxillofacial Surgery and
    Dental Medicine
Stritch School of Medicine
Loyola University Medical Center
Maywood, Illinois

Robert L. Merrill, DDS, MS
Adjunct Professor and Director
Graduate Orofacial Pain Program
School of Dentistry
University of California
Los Angeles, California

Stephen B. Milam, DDS, PhD
Professor and Hugh B. Tilson Endowed Chair
Department of Oral and Maxillofacial Surgery
University of Texas Health Science Center
San Antonio, Texas

Hajime Minakuchi, DDS, PhD
Visiting Research Scholar
Center for Orofacial Pain and Oral Medicine
School of Dentistry
University of Southern California
Los Angeles, California

Norman D. Mohl, DDS, PhD
SUNY Distinguished Service Professor Emeritus
Department of Oral Diagnostic Sciences
School of Dental Medicine
State University of New York at Buffalo
Buffalo, New York

Ales Obrez, DMD, PhD
Associate Professor
Department of Restorative Dentistry
College of Dentistry
University of Illinois
Chicago, Illinois

Richard Ohrbach, DDS, PhD
Associate Professor
Department of Oral Diagnostic Sciences
School of Dental Medicine
State University of New York at Buffalo
Buffalo, New York

Octavia Plesh, DDS, MS
Professor
Department of Preventive and Restorative
    Dental Sciences
School of Dentistry
University of California
San Francisco, California

M. Anthony Pogrel, DDS, MD, FRCS(E)
Professor and Chairman
Department of Oral and Maxillofacial Surgery
School of Dentistry
University of California
San Francisco, California

Ke Ren, MD, PhD
Associate Professor
Department of Biomedical Sciences
Baltimore College of Dental Surgery
University of Maryland Dental School
Baltimore, Maryland

Barry J. Sessle, BDS, MDS, PhD
Professor
Faculty of Dentistry
Center for the Study of Pain
University of Toronto
Toronto, Ontario, Canada

Boudewijn Stegenga, DDS, PhD
Professor and Director of Clinical Research
Department of Oral and Maxillofacial Surgery
University Medical Center
University of Groningen
Groningen, The Netherlands

Diane Stern, DDS
Clinical Professor
Division of Oral and Maxillofacial Surgery
Miller School of Medicine
Department of Surgery
University of Miami
Miami, Florida

Professor
Department of Oral Diagnostic Sciences
College of Dental Medicine
Nova Southeastern University
Fort Lauderdale, Florida

Christian S. Stohler, DDS, Dr Med Dent
Professor and Dean
Baltimore College of Dental Surgery
University of Maryland Dental School
Baltimore, Maryland

J. Mark Thomason, BDS, PhD, FDS, RCS(Ed)
Professor
Department of Prosthodontics and Oral Rehabilitation
School of Dental Sciences
University of Newcastle
Newcastle upon Tyne, United Kingdom

Adjunct Professor
Faculty of Dentistry
McGill University
Montreal, Quebec, Canada

Maria J. Troulis, DDS, MSc
Associate Professor
Department of Oral and Maxillofacial Surgery
Harvard School of Dental Medicine
Massachusetts General Hospital
Boston, Massachusetts

Bengt Wenneberg, DDS, Odont Dr
Associate Professor
Faculty of Odontology
University of Göteborg
Göteborg, Sweden

Per-Lennart Westesson, MD, PhD, DDS
Professor and Director of Division of Diagnostic and Interventional Neuroradiology
Department of Radiology
School of Medicine and Dentistry
University of Rochester
Rochester, New York

Professor
Department of Oral Diagnostic Sciences
School of Dental Medicine
State University of New York at Buffalo
Buffalo, New York

PART I

Biologic Basis

SECTION A

Anatomy and Function

Chapters 1–4

SECTION B

Pathophysiology of TMDs

Chapters 5–9

Functional Anatomy and Biomechanics of the Masticatory Apparatus

William L. Hylander

Temporomandibular Joint

Articulating Bodies

The temporomandibular or craniomandibular articulation is the articulation between the mandible and the cranium. The bony elements of this articulation are the mandibular condyles below and the squamous temporal bones above. This articulation consists of two synovial joints: left and right temporomandibular joints (TMJs).

The TMJ is a complex joint both morphologically and functionally. An articular disc made up of dense fibrous connective tissue with varying amounts of fibrocartilage is interposed between the temporal bone and the mandible, dividing the articular space into upper and lower compartments. Gliding or translatory movements occur primarily in the upper compartment, while the lower compartment functions primarily as a hinge or rotary joint. Therefore, the TMJ is often classified as a hinge joint with a movable socket.

Most synovial joints have hyaline cartilage lining their articulating surfaces. In contrast, the articulating surfaces of the TMJ are lined by dense, avascular, fibrous connective tissue. The presence of this type of tissue has often been interpreted as indicating that the TMJ must not bear any stress because known load-bearing synovial joints are lined by hyaline cartilage. Over the last 25 to 30 years, however, a considerable amount of evidence has accumulated indicating that the TMJ is indeed a load-bearing

joint.[1] If so, then why does this joint have such peculiar articular tissues? The answer to this question is directly related to the evolutionary history of this joint, which in turn is reflected in its early ontogeny.[2]

The bones of a typical synovial joint are cartilage-replacement bones that are initially preformed in hyaline cartilage. Most of this cartilage is eventually calcified and then replaced by bone during ontogeny, although the cartilage lining the articular surfaces persists in a modified form. In contrast, the bones of the TMJ are dermal or membrane bones. Rather than being preformed in cartilage, they are formed directly from intramembranous centers of ossification. These developing bones become completely surrounded by periosteum, including the areas that eventually form the articular surfaces of the TMJ. The periosteum lining these articular surfaces is gradually transformed during its early development into the dense fibrous articular tissues of the TMJ. Articular forces acting through the TMJ play an important role in this gradual transformation. Articular forces also continue to play a major role in the development of these tissues well into adult life[3] (see chapter 3).

Thus, the lack of hyaline cartilage on the articular surfaces of the TMJ simply reflects its unique ontogenetic and phylogenetic development, rather than indicating that this joint is incapable of bearing reaction force. Although there is a secondary cartilage in the condyle of the growing mandible, this cartilage does not form part of the articular surface because the periosteum-derived articular tissues cover it.[4,5]

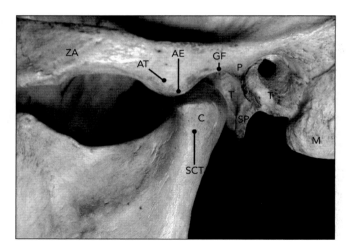

Fig 1-1 Lateral view of a robust adult male human skull. The mandibular condyle is pulled slightly out of the glenoid fossa. The bony TMJ and surrounding areas include the following structures: (ZA) posterior root of zygomatic arch; (AT) location of articular tubercle; (AE) crest of the articular eminence; (GF) roof of the glenoid fossa; (P) postglenoid process; (T) tympanic portion of the temporal bone; (C) mandibular condyle; (SCT) location of subcondylar tubercle; (SP) styloid process (tip broken); (M) mastoid process.

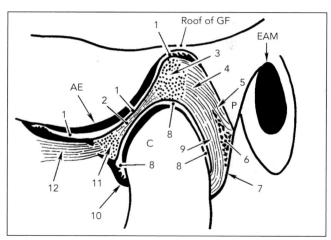

Fig 1-2 Parasagittal section of the TMJ. (C) Mandibular condyle; (AE) articular surface of articular eminence; (P) postglenoid process; (EAM) external auditory meatus; (1) upper joint compartment; (2) intermediate zone; (3) posterior band; (4) bilaminar zone; (5) upper portion of bilaminar zone; (6) spongy tissue with a profuse nerve and blood supply; (7) posterior portion of joint capsule; (8) lower joint compartment; (9) lower portion of bilaminar zone; (10) anterior portion of joint capsule; (11) anterior band; (12) small portion of the superior head of the lateral pterygoid muscle. Note the thick dense fibrous avascular tissues covering the articular eminence and the mandibular condyle, as well as the thin roof of the glenoid fossa (GF). (Modified from Hylander[2] with permission.)

Mandibular condyle

The articular surface of the mandible is the upper and anterior surface of the condyle (Fig 1-1). The adult human condyle is about 15 to 20 mm from side to side and 8 to 10 mm from front to back. Its long axis is at right angles to the plane of the mandibular ramus. Because of the flare of the ramus, however, the long axes of the left and right condyles cross approximately at the anterior margin of the foramen magnum, forming an obtuse angle varying from 145 to 160 degrees.

The articular surface of the condyle is strongly convex when viewed from the side and less so when viewed from the front. The articular surface faces upward and forward so that in side view the condylar neck is bent forward. As seen from in front, the articular convexity often resembles a tentlike configuration that is divided into medial and lateral slopes by a variably prominent crest. The lateral pole of the condyle extends slightly beyond the outer surface of the ramus and is roughened for the attachment of the articular disc and the temporomandibular ligament (TML). Furthermore, there often is a well-developed lateral subcondylar tubercle, an attachment site for the

TML.[6,7] The medial pole of the condyle juts considerably beyond the inner surface of the ramus, and is also slightly roughened for the attachment of the articular disc.

Variations in the shape of the condyle are common. Moreover, some of the irregularities of the bony articular surface are apparently obscured and smoothed by the thick covering of fibrous tissue that is derived from and directly continuous with the periosteum of the mandible.

Glenoid (mandibular) fossa and articular eminence

The terms *glenoid fossa*, *mandibular fossa*, and *articular fossa* are often used interchangeably, but only the glenoid and mandibular fossa are synonymous. The glenoid fossa is the concavity within the temporal bone that houses the mandibular condyle. Its anterior wall is formed by the articular eminence of the squamous temporal bone and its posterior wall by the tympanic plate, which also forms the anterior wall of the external acoustic meatus. The bony roof of the glenoid fossa is paper thin and often appears translucent when held against the light (Fig 1-2). This is but one indication that the roof of this fossa is not the major load-bearing portion of the temporal component of the TMJ.

The articular fossa is that portion of the glenoid fossa that is lined by articular tissues. It is formed entirely by the squamous portion of the temporal bone (Figs 1-1 and 1-3). The posterior part of the articular fossa is elevated to a ridge called the *posterior articular lip*. In most individuals, the posterior articular lip is higher and thicker at its lateral end and thus is visible from the side as a cone-shaped process between the articular fossa and the tympanic plate (see Figs 1-1 and 1-2). This structure is the postglenoid process. The lateral border of the articular fossa is sometimes marked by a narrow, low ridge or crest (see Fig 1-3). Medially, the articular fossa is bounded by a bony plate that leans against the spine of the sphenoid bone. This medial plate is sometimes drawn out into a triangular process, the temporal spine.

In the back and lateral part of the glenoid fossa, a fissure separates the tympanic portion from the squamous portion of the temporal bone. This fissure, called the *tympanosquamosal fissure*, separates the articular and the nonarticular portions of the glenoid fossa (see Fig 1-3). Medial to this fissure, a bony plate of the petrous portion of the temporal bone, the tegmen tympani, protrudes between the tympanic and squamous portions. Therefore, instead of a tympanosquamosal fissure, along the medial aspect of the glenoid fossa there are an anterior petrosquamosal fissure and a posterior petrotympanic fissure. The petrotympanic fissure is slightly widened laterally to permit the passage of the chorda tympani nerve and the anterior tympanic blood vessels. These neurovascular structures are located within the glenoid fossa, but not within the articular fossa.

It is important to make a distinction between the *articular eminence* and the *articular tubercle*. The articular eminence is the transverse bar of dense bone that forms the posterior root of the zygomatic arch and the anterior wall of the articular fossa. It has a large articular surface. In contrast, the articular tubercle is the small bony projection situated lateral to the articular eminence. Unlike the articular eminence, the articular tubercle is not an articular surface. Instead, it serves as the attachment area for portions of the TML.

The articular eminence is somewhat saddle shaped. It is strongly convex in a side view and moderately concave when viewed from the front or back. The degree of this convexity and concavity is highly variable. Fine bony ridges often outline the medial and lateral borders of the articular eminence (see Fig 1-3). The anterior slope of the eminence, the preglenoid plane, rises gently from the infratemporal surface of the squamous temporal bone; its precise anterior boundary is often indistinct. The condyle and disc move anterior to the summit of the eminence and

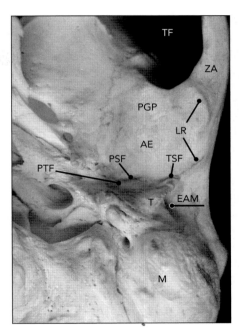

Fig 1-3 Basal view of the left side of a human cranium. The bony TMJ and surrounding areas include the following structures: (TF) temporal foramen; (ZA) posterior root of zygomatic arch; (PGP) preglenoid plane; (LR) lateral ridges of preglenoid plane, articular eminence, and glenoid fossa; (AE) articular eminence; (PTF) petrotympanic fissure; (PSF) petrosquamosal fissure; (TSF) tympanosquamosal fissure; (T) tympanic portion of the temporal bone; (EAM) external auditory meatus; (M) mastoid process.

onto the preglenoid plane during wide opening. The gentle anterior slope facilitates posterior movements of the mandibular condyle and disc from this anterior position.

Although a thin layer of fibrous tissue covers the roof of the articular fossa, the fibrous tissue covering the articular eminence is thick and quite firm (see Fig 1-2). Moreover, unlike the roof, the articular eminence is made up of a fairly thick layer of dense bone. These morphologic characteristics reinforce the hypothesis that the articular eminence, but not the fossa, is loaded by routine joint reaction forces developed among the articular surfaces of the mandibular condyle, the articular disc, and the squamous temporal bone.

Articular disc

The articular disc is derived ontogenetically from a mesenchymal block of tissue that also gives rise to the capsule of the TMJ and the lateral pterygoid muscle.[8] This tissue mass is positioned between the developing squamous temporal bone and mandibular condyle. In adults the uppermost part (or superior head) of the lateral pterygoid muscle often retains its original connection to the capsule and articular disc of the TMJ.[9]

The articular disc is a firm, oval, fibrous plate positioned between the mandibular condyle and the articular fossa and eminence (see Fig 1-2). Its central part, the intermediate zone, is considerably thinner than its periphery, the anterior and posterior bands. Anteriorly the disc continues as the anterior attachment and is fused to the capsule of the TMJ. Posteriorly the disc continues as the posterior attachment or bilaminar zone, a thick double layer of vascularized connective tissue. The bilaminar zone splits into two parts: (1) an upper fibroelastic layer that attaches to the postglenoid process, posterior articular lip, and tympanosquamosal fissure; and (2) a lower fibrous layer that attaches to the posterior portion of the condylar neck immediately below the articular tissues. Posteriorly these two layers are separated by the intermediate layer, which contains loose connective tissue that attaches to the posterior wall of the joint capsule. The posterior attachment has a profuse supply of nerves and blood vessels.[10,11]

Unlike its anterior and posterior attachments, the disc is not attached to the capsule laterally or medially. Instead, it is tightly bound directly to the medial and lateral poles of the mandibular condyle. It is these attachments of the disc that cause it to move along with the mandibular condyle. It is often stated that the position of the disc relative to the condyle is influenced by the pull of the superior head of the lateral pterygoid muscle, because a small portion of this muscle often attaches to the disc (see Fig 1-2). Thus, contraction of the superior head of the lateral pterygoid is thought to protract the disc anteromedially or limit posterolateral retraction movements of the disc. The influence of this muscle on the articular disc, however, is not a settled issue. As the superior head of the lateral pterygoid also attaches to the mandibular condyle and the disc is tightly bound to the medial and lateral poles of the condyle, this muscle arguably may have no special influence on movements of the articular disc relative to the condyle.[12,13]

Blood vessels and nerves are absent in the intermediate zone, that is, the firm central region of the articular disc, as well as in the avascular fibrous layers covering both the mandibular and temporal articular surfaces of the joint. The lack of these neurovascular structures is compatible with the hypothesis that there is considerable reaction force along this portion of the joint. Finally, over the years, it has been suggested that one main function of the articular disc is to reduce stress concentrations between the articular surfaces of the mandibular condyle

and squamous temporal bone; that is, the compliant nature of the disc helps to distribute reaction force more evenly along these joint surfaces.[14]

Articular Capsule and Ligaments

The fibrous capsule of the TMJ attaches to the squamous portion of the temporal bone along the outer limits of the articular surface of the articular eminence, fossa, and preglenoid plane. Posteriorly, the capsule arises from the postglenoid process, posterior articular lip, and tympanosquamosal fissure. The articular capsule is quite thin anteromedially, medially, and posteriorly, but it is thick anterolaterally and laterally where it attaches to the articular tubercle.[15] This reinforced lateral portion of the capsule is the temporomandibular ligament (Fig 1-4).

The anatomy of the capsule and the TML are somewhat controversial, and this is likely due to their considerable variability.[2,16,17] DuBrul[15] described the TML as being divided into two layers: a wide, fan-shaped superficial portion and a narrow deep portion. The broad origin of the superficial portion along the articular tubercle and its narrower insertion along the condylar neck accounts for its somewhat fan-shaped morphology. Its anterior fibers run from the articular tubercle obliquely down and back, while the posterior fibers have a more vertical orientation. Fibers of the deep portion are said to run horizontally (anteroposteriorly), and this portion is described as a ligamentous band that attaches along the lateral pole of the mandibular condyle and extends to a crest situated along the articular tubercle.[15] Based on Scapino's excellent description[6] of the anatomy of the TMJ, it appears that the deep horizontal band described by DuBrul[15] is likely part of the lateral aspect of the joint capsule and disc.[13] Scapino[6p28] refers to this lateral band as the *lateral polar ligament*.

The joint capsule and its TML function to limit movements of the mandible (Figs 1-4 and 1-5). The vertical fibers limit distraction movements of the condyle from the articular eminence and fossa, the horizontal fibers (polar ligaments) prevent excessive retrusive movements of the condyle, and the posterior portion of the capsule limits protrusive movements (see Fig 1-5). Finally, it has been suggested that the anterior part of the capsule and the anterolateral part of the TML may limit the amount of condylar rotation during jaw opening, although most of this limitation is imposed by the stretched jaw-closing muscles.[2] Finally, modeling procedures suggest that the only limitations to maximum jaw opening are those linked to the jaw-closing muscles.[18]

The synovial membrane, a highly vascularized layer of connective tissue, lines all structures of the articulation that

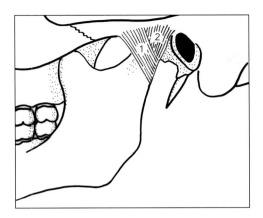

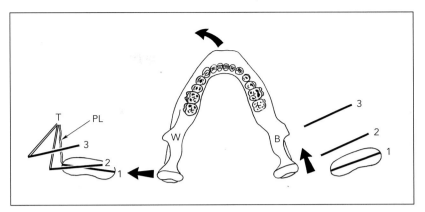

Fig 1-4 Lateral view of the (1) temporomandibular and (2) capsular ligaments. Most of the fibers of these ligaments are aligned either vertically or in a combined vertical and oblique direction. Some of the deepest fibers are aligned horizontally. (Modified from Hylander[2] with permission.)

Fig 1-5 Mandible during left lateral movement. (W) Working side; (B) balancing side; (PL) polar ligament that attaches to the lateral pole of the mandibular condyle and the (T) articular tubercle and disc (see Scapino[6]). Position 1: The working-side (w-s) and balancing-side (b-s) condyles just prior to left lateral movement. Position 2: The left lateral movement is initiated. The w-s condyle first rotates about a vertical axis that passes through its center. Then, the lateral polar ligament becomes taut and prevents the lateral pole of the w-s condyle from moving any further posteriorly. This condyle now shifts slightly laterally. The b-s condyle translates medially, anteriorly, and downward along the articular eminence. Position 3: With continued movement, the w-s condyle has shifted further laterally and slightly anteriorly. The lateral polar ligament guides this movement. The b-s condyle continues to translate medially, anteriorly, and downward along the eminence. The relative amount of rotation of the w-s condyle has been exaggerated. (arrows) Direction of movement of the chin and the w-s and b-s mandibular condyles. (Modified from Hylander[2] with permission.)

do not experience compressive reaction force. The largest area of synovial lining covers the upper and lower surfaces of the posterior attachment, including the loose connective tissue binding the posterior border of the disc to the capsule. Synovial tissue also lines the inner aspect of the fibrous capsule. When the condyle is positioned in the glenoid fossa, the synovial membrane forms rather heavy folds posteriorly. When the condyle is protruded toward the summit of the articular eminence, the folds disappear as the synovial tissues are stretched.

The blood supply to the capsule and disc is provided mainly by branches from a maxillary artery. The sensory nerves for proprioception and pain are branches of the auriculotemporal, deep temporal, and masseteric nerves. Blood vessels and nerves are numerous in the posterior portions of the articular disc and fibrous capsule.

Accessory Ligaments

Two structures have been described as accessory ligaments of the temporomandibular articulation: the sphenomandibular and the stylomandibular ligaments.

Sphenomandibular ligament

The sphenomandibular ligament is derived from Meckel's cartilage. It arises from the spine of the sphenoid bone and is directed downward and outward (Fig 1-6). It inserts on the mandible at the mandibular lingula, which is located along the upper border of the mandibular foramen. In most individuals, the sphenomandibular ligament is a thin layer of connective tissue with indistinct anterior and posterior borders.

It has been suggested that this ligament protects the blood vessels and nerves passing through the mandibular foramen from additional tensile stress during jaw opening and closing.[19] It has no influence on mandibular movements.

Stylomandibular ligament

The stylomandibular ligament is a reinforced sheet of cervical fascia that extends from the styloid process and stylohyoid ligament to the region of the mandibular angle (see Fig 1-6). Many of its fibers are attached to the back edge of the lower part of the mandibular ramus; others

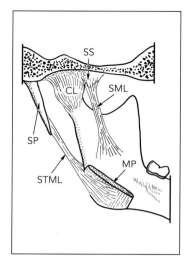

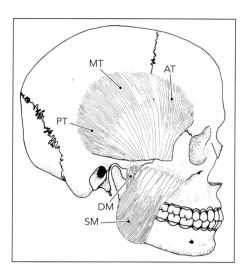

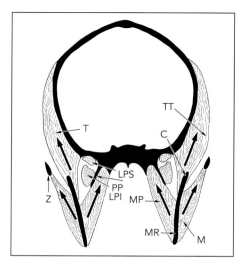

Fig 1-6 Medial view of the mandible and the sphenomandibular and stylomandibular ligaments. (SP) Styloid process; (CL) capsular ligament; (SS) sphenoidal spine; (SML) sphenomandibular ligament; (STML) stylomandibular ligament; (MP) medial pterygoid muscle. (Modified from Hylander[2] with permission.)

Fig 1-7 Masseter and temporalis muscles. (PT) Posterior temporal; (MT) middle temporal; (AT) anterior temporal; (DM) deep masseter; (SM) superficial masseter. (Modified from Hylander[2] with permission.)

Fig 1-8 Coronal section of the muscles of mastication. (T) Temporalis; (TT) central tendon of temporalis muscle; (Z) zygomatic arch; (C) coronoid process; (LPS) lateral pterygoid, superior head; (PP) pterygoid process (lateral); (LPI) lateral pterygoid, inferior head; (MP) medial pterygoid; (MR) mandibular ramus; (M) masseter. *(heavy arrows)* General direction of pull of the anterior temporalis, superficial masseter, and medial pterygoid muscles. (Modified from Hylander[2] with permission.)

continue onto the deep fascia along the medial surface of the medial pterygoid muscle. The upper border of the stylomandibular ligament is a thickened cordlike structure.

This ligament is relatively loose when the jaws are both closed and wide open; it is tensed only when the mandible is maximally protruded. Thus, apparently this ligament can limit excessive protrusive movements.

Muscles of the Mandible

Four powerful muscles, the masseter, the temporalis, the medial pterygoid, and the lateral pterygoid, are often referred to as the *muscles of mastication*. This label is quite misleading because these muscles act in conjunction with various muscle groups of the face, tongue, palate, and hyoid bone, during mastication. This chapter does not attempt to describe all of these muscle groups, although it does consider the morphology and function of the most important muscles that play a role in mandibular movements.

Masseter Muscle

The masseter muscle stretches as a rectangular plate from the zygomatic arch to the lateral surface of the mandibular ramus (Figs 1-7 and 1-8). It is divided into a superficial masseter and a smaller deep masseter. The superficial masseter arises from the lower border of the zygomatic arch as strong tendinous fibers. The most anterior fibers may arise from the outer corner of the zygomatic process of the maxilla. Posteriorly the origin of the superficial portion ends along the zygomaticotemporal suture.

In side view, the muscle fibers of the superficial masseter are directed downward and backward to insert along the angle of the mandible. In a frontal view, it can be seen that these fibers are directed downward and medially (see Fig 1-8). The mandibular attachment of the superficial masseter extends along the lower one third of the posterior border of the ramus and along the lower border of the mandible anterior to the third molar; it covers, more or less, the lower half of the lateral surface of the ramus. The field of insertion has ridges into which the tendons insert and grooves between the ridges into which the fleshy fibers insert.

The superficial masseter is covered on its outer surface by a strong tendinous layer that extends down from the zygomatic arch over the upper third or half of the muscle. Superficially, the tendon appears to end with a downwardly convex border or in a zigzag line. However, the tendon does not actually end along this line. Instead, it continues a short distance into the muscle mass. If the overlying tissues are not too thick, the border of this tendon can be viewed during mastication as it contrasts with the bulging muscle bundles below the tendon. Alternating tendinous and fleshy bundles are present within the superficial portion. Thus, the structure of this muscle is rather intricate, and it is often referred to as a *multipinnate muscle.*

If the superficial masseter muscle is strongly developed, the area of its insertion is slightly widened, giving the anterior border of the muscle a concave appearance when viewed from the side. Posteriorly the fibers of the superficial masseter wrap around the posterior and inferior aspects of the angle of the mandible, joining fibers of the medial pterygoid muscle in a tendinous raphe. This muscular arrangement is called the *pterygomasseteric sling.*

The deep and superficial portions of the masseter fuse anteriorly, but posteriorly the two can be separated. The fibers of the deep masseter arise from the entire length of the zygomatic arch up to the anterior slope of the articular eminence. Some of its fibers may also arise from the lateral wall of the TMJ capsule.[12,20]

The deep masseter inserts above the superficial masseter along the mandibular ramus as a triangular-shaped insertion field. The base of this triangle faces posteriorly while the apex faces anteriorly. In side view the fibers of the deep masseter, which have a near vertical alignment, pass downward at an angle of about 30 to 40 degrees to the fibers of the more obliquely aligned superficial masseter.

The masseter muscle is a powerful elevator of the mandible. A lateral view reveals that the deep masseter exerts primarily a vertical force on the mandible. In contrast, the superficial masseter exerts a vertical and slightly anteriorly directed force on the mandible that is approximately perpendicular to the occlusal plane of the molars (see Fig 1-7). The entire masseter also exerts a lateral component of force on the mandible (see Fig 1-8).

The masseter muscle is derived from the first branchial arch and therefore is innervated by the trigeminal nerve (cranial nerve V). More specifically, the masseteric nerve, a small branch from the mandibular or third division of the trigeminal nerve (V_3), innervates the masseter muscle. This nerve passes above the lateral pterygoid muscle and then, after passing through the mandibular notch behind the tendon of the temporalis muscle, enters the

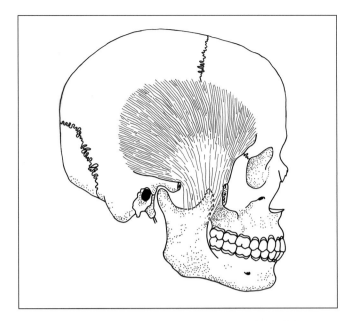

Fig 1-9 Temporalis muscle. The masseter muscle and the zygomatic arch have been removed. (Modified from Hylander[2] with permission.)

medial surface of the deep masseter muscle. The masseteric nerve supplies the deep masseter, perforates it, and then enters the superficial masseter.

Temporalis Muscle

The fan-shaped temporalis muscle has its origin along the lateral surface of the skull and the dense fascia overlying this muscle (Figs 1-7 and 1-9). The bony attachment field, the temporal fossa, is encircled above by the inferior temporal line. This attachment field includes a narrow strip of the parietal bone, the greater part of the temporal squama, the temporal surface of the frontal bone, and the temporal surface of the greater wing of the sphenoid bone. Muscle fibers and tendons also arise from the postorbital septum, which is the bony partition separating the temporal fossa from the orbit. Both the zygomatic and frontal bones and the greater wing of the sphenoid contribute to the formation of the postorbital septum. The bony field of origin of the temporalis muscle reaches downward to include the infratemporal crest of the sphenoid.

Many of the temporalis muscle fibers originate from the medial surface of the temporalis fascia. The temporalis fascia attaches to the superior temporal line and the upper border of the zygomatic arch. Passing downward from the superior temporal line, the temporalis fascia thickens considerably and then splits into two layers; the superficial layer continues into the periosteum of the zygomatic arch along its lateral surface, and the deep layer extends into the periosteum of the zygomatic arch along its medial surface. The superficial and deep layers are joined together by irregular bands of connective tissue. The outer layer is thickened and, when palpated, gives the impression of bone.

The bundles of the temporalis muscle converge toward the opening located between the zygomatic arch and the lateral surface of the skull (temporal foramen) (see Fig 1-3). The tip of the coronoid process projects into this opening. The anterior fibers of the temporalis muscle, which form the major bulk of the muscle, are largely vertical; the fibers in the middle part of the muscle are increasingly oblique. The most posterior fibers run forward almost horizontally, bend around the posterior root of the zygomatic arch in front of the articular eminence, and pass downward vertically to the mandible (see Fig 1-9).

The flesh of the temporalis muscle is divided unequally by the central tendon, a tendinous plate that is partially visible along the lateral aspect of this muscle (see Fig 1-9). Most of the fibers of the temporalis muscle are situated medial to this plate. This is unlike the condition in monkeys and apes, in which the central tendon is not visible because it is covered by the superficial "head" of the temporalis muscle.[21,22] As part of an overall evolutionary reduction of the masticatory apparatus, this lateral portion of the temporalis muscle was apparently lost. In humans, the tendon of the superficial masseter is also visible superficially (see Fig 1-7), whereas in monkeys and apes this tendon is covered by muscle tissue. As with the temporalis muscle, humans seem to have lost the most superficial portion of the superficial masseter.

Temporalis muscle fibers arise from the temporalis fascia laterally and the skull medially and insert into this tendinous plate. Therefore, this muscle is often characterized as being bipinnate. The fibers of the temporalis muscle are actually much shorter than most illustrations indicate, although they are longer than those of the masseter muscle. These longer fibers are to be expected because during wide opening the temporalis is, of necessity, stretched much more than the masseter and medial pterygoid muscles. This differential stretching is linked to the location of the instantaneous (or helical) axis of mandibular rotation[2] (see chapter 2).

The middle and posterior portions of the temporalis muscle, respectively, are attached along the apex of the coronoid process and along its posterior slope to the deepest point of the mandibular notch. The more superficial fibers of the anterior temporalis muscle insert along the apex of the coronoid process, the anterior surface of the coronoid process, and the mandibular ramus. The

deeper fibers of the anterior temporalis attach along the medial anterior surface of the mandibular ramus.

These two groups of fibers send tendons down toward the posterior end of the alveolar process and are separated from each other by a downwardly widening cleft. The inner or deep tendon, which juts medially from the mandibular ramus and reaches downward into the region of the lower third molar, is stronger and longer than the superficial tendon, which is attached to the anterior border of the coronoid process and mandibular ramus. The space or area of the mandible between the superficial and deep tendons is the retromolar fossa.

Similar to the masseter muscle, the temporalis muscle mainly elevates the mandible. Its fan-shaped morphology indicates that its direction of pull varies considerably, depending on which portions are mechanically active. Superfically it appears that its most posterior fibers retract the mandible because of their horizontal orientation along the side of the skull; however, as previously noted, when the condyle is situated in the mandibular fossa the fibers of the posterior temporalis are bent around the posterior root of the zygomatic arch at a sharp angle and thus are oriented vertically. Therefore, this portion of the temporalis muscle exerts primarily an upward force on the mandible during normal closure.

On the other hand, when the condyle is translated anteriorly into a more protruded position, these posterior fibers likely retrude the mandible because in this instance the posterior temporalis is aligned more horizontally. As its most posterior fibers pass very close to the condyle, the posterior temporalis probably also functions as a stabilizer of the TMJ.

The middle and obliquely aligned portion of the temporalis muscle is capable of exerting a vertical and retracting force on the mandible. Most of the anterior portion is capable of a vertical pull on the mandible. That portion of the anterior temporalis originating from the postorbital septum, however, likely pulls the mandible upward and forward. Finally, the deep fibers of the anterior temporalis that originate along and just above the infratemporal crest pull the mandible upward and somewhat medially. Thus, the morphology of the entire temporalis muscle indicates that its fibers are capable of considerable variability in their direction of pull.

The temporalis muscle is innervated by the deep temporal branches of the anterior trunk of V_3. Of the three deep temporal nerves ordinarily present, the posterior and middle branches arise as separate filaments from the anterior trunk immediately after the trigeminal nerve emerges through the foramen ovale. The anterior branch is initially united with the buccal nerve; this common trunk, which lies in a sulcus adjacent to the foramen ovale, runs anteriorly and laterally, close to the base of the skull. It is held in place by a ligament that bridges the sulcus. If this ligament ossifies, it contributes to the formation of the temporobuccal foramen.

The anterior temporal nerve usually separates from the buccal nerve after the latter has passed between the two heads of the lateral pterygoid muscle. Its most anterior portion, however, is not positioned nearly as far forward as the anterior portion of the superficial masseter.

Medial Pterygoid Muscle

The medial pterygoid muscle is situated on the medial side of the mandibular ramus (Fig 1-10; see also Fig 1-8). When viewed from the side, it appears to be the anatomic counterpart of the masseter muscle. It is a powerful rectangular muscle, although smaller than the masseter. Its main origin is in the pterygoid fossa, a depression located between the back edges of the medial and lateral pterygoid plates of the sphenoid bone. The deepest fibers arise by strong tendons, while others arise directly from the medial surface of the lateral pterygoid plate. A flat tendon covers the medial surface of the muscle at its origin, and it is as wide as the tensor veli palatini, with which it is in contact.

The most anterior fibers of the medial pterygoid arise from the outer and inferior surface of the pyramidal process of the palatine bone and from the adjacent parts of the maxillary tuberosity. These fibers, which are referred to as the *superficial head* of the medial pterygoid, are positioned lateral to the lateral pterygoid muscle. The remaining and largest portion of this muscle, the deep head, is positioned medial or deep to the lateral pterygoid muscle (see Fig 1-8).

The fibers of the medial pterygoid muscle run downward, backward, and laterally and are inserted along the medial surface of the angle of the mandible. The field of insertion is approximately triangular and is located between the mandibular angle and the mylohyoid groove. As noted earlier, the fibers of the medial pterygoid muscle often meet fibers of the masseter in a tendinous raphe behind and below the mandibular angle (the pterygomasseteric sling).

From its field of origin, the internal structure of the medial pterygoid muscle is a complicated alternation of fleshy and tendinous parts, similar to the temporalis and masseter muscles. The muscle fibers, arising from one tendon (attaching to the cranium) and ending on another (attaching to the mandible), are arranged at an angle to the general orientation of the muscle. This bipinnate or multipinnate arrangement gives the muscle fibers of the medial pterygoid (and masseter) a braided appearance and increases its capability for generating large forces.

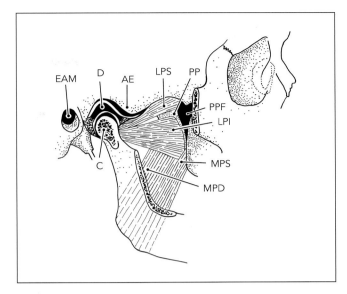

Fig 1-10 Medial and lateral pterygoid muscles. (EAM) External auditory meatus; (D) articular disc; (C) mandibular condyle; (AE) articular eminence; (LPS) lateral pterygoid, superior head; (PP) pterygoid plate (lateral); (PPF) pterygopalatine fossa; (LPI) lateral pterygoid, inferior head; (MPS) medial pterygoid, superficial portion; (MPD) medial pterygoid, deep portion. The zygomatic arch and coronoid process have been removed, and the TMJ has been sectioned parasagittally. (Modified from Hylander[2] with permission.)

The overall fiber orientation of the medial pterygoid muscle in side view is similar to that of the superficial portion of the masseter muscle, and therefore it is primarily an elevator of the mandible. However, unlike the masseter, which exerts a lateral component of force on the mandible, the medial pterygoid exerts a medial component of force on the mandible. Furthermore, unlike in most nonhuman primates, in humans the medial component of the medial pterygoid muscle is relatively larger than the lateral component of the superficial masseter (see Fig 1-8).

The nerve to the medial pterygoid arises from V_3 immediately before it divides into its anterior and posterior trunks. The medial pterygoid nerve, which also innervates the tensor tympani and tensor veli palatini muscles, reaches the medial pterygoid muscle at its upper posterior border.

Lateral Pterygoid Muscle

The lateral pterygoid muscle arises from two heads (see Figs 1-8 and 1-10). The inferior head is about three times larger than the superior head.[23,24] The superior head (sometimes called the *superior pterygoid*)[25] originates from the infratemporal surface of the greater wing of the sphenoid medial to the infratemporal crest. From its origin, the fibers of the superior head run almost horizontally backward and laterally in close relation to the external surface of the cranial base. The inferior head originates from the outer surface of the lateral pterygoid plate. Although the fibers of the inferior head also run backward and laterally, they pass upward at an angle of about 45 degrees relative to the superior head.

The two heads of the lateral pterygoid muscle are separated at their origins by a wide gap but fuse in front of the TMJ. The fibers of the superior head are attached primarily to a roughened fossa on the anteromedial surface of the condylar neck. This fossa is called the *pterygoid fovea*. In addition, a small portion of the superior head is frequently attached directly to the anteromedial part of the TMJ capsule and extends into the anteromedial part of the articular disc. All of the fibers of the inferior head insert into or along the periphery of the pterygoid fovea. This description of the lateral pterygoid is based on the work of numerous authors.[2,12,13,15,20,26–28]

Disputing the previous description of the lateral pterygoid, Griffith and Sharpe[10] and Honée[23] have stated that the two heads do not fuse in front of the TMJ and that the entire superior head is attached to the capsule and disc. However, Meyenberg et al[12] dissected 25 TMJs and found that, although the two heads of the lateral pterygoid always fuse in front of the TMJ, the superior head of the lateral pterygoid did not attach to the articular disc in 40% of their dissections. In these instances the lateral pterygoid attached entirely to the pterygoid fovea. In the remaining 60%, a small portion of the superior head of the lateral pterygoid attached to the anteromedial aspect of the articular capsule and disc, while the remainder of the muscle attached to the pterygoid fovea. Similarly, the work of Wilkinson[13] confirms the results of Meyenberg et al.[12]

There is some EMG evidence indicating that, arguably, the lateral pterygoid muscle is made up of two functionally distinct parts. The superior head is said to contract during jaw closing while the inferior head contracts during protraction, opening, and shifting of the jaw to one side.[29–32] For this reason, the probable different functions of each head have to be discussed separately.

Some researchers prefer to consider the two heads of the lateral pterygoid as two separate muscles, the superior pterygoid (superior head) and the inferior pterygoid (inferior head).[18,25] If this rationale were followed, many other muscles throughout the mammalian body should be renamed (eg, the deltoid). It is preferable not to do so because named muscles are anatomic, not functional, entities. Moreover, and perhaps most importantly, changing of anatomic names often causes needless confusion.

The resultant force of the superior head of the lateral pterygoid on the condyle is directed forward and medially. In side view it passes nearly perpendicular (70 to 90 degrees) to the posterior slope of the articular eminence and to the articular surface of the condyle that faces this slope. Therefore, this part of the lateral pterygoid stabilizes the mandibular condyle against the articular eminence during biting and mastication.[2,33]

The resultant force of the inferior head on the condyle is also directed forward and medially. Its direction of pull is more tangential to the articular surfaces of the TMJ than is that of the superior head. Bilateral contraction of the lower head of the lateral pterygoid muscle pulls the mandibular condyles and articular discs down, along, and over the articular eminence. This movement is mandibular protrusion. Unilateral action of the inferior head shifts the midline of the mandible to the opposite side (lateral excursion).

Finally, if either or both heads of the lateral pterygoid muscle are actively recruited during mandibular closure, this muscle must experience an eccentric or lengthening contraction.[13,34] Under these conditions the lateral pterygoid muscle exhibits considerable stiffness[35]; this also facilitates joint stability by controlling or limiting condylar movements.

The nerve to the lateral pterygoid muscle is usually a branch of the buccal nerve, which is a branch of the anterior trunk of V_3.

Digastric Muscle

As the name implies, the digastric (two-bellied) muscle consists of an anterior belly and a posterior belly (Fig 1-11). A strong, round, intermediate tendon connects these two straight, nearly parallel-fibered muscle bellies. The posterior belly arises from the mastoid notch medial to the mastoid process; the intermediate tendon is held to the body of the hyoid bone by a fascial loop. The anterior belly attaches to the digastric fossa of the mandible. This fossa is located along the lingual surface of the lower border of the mandible slightly lateral to the midline.

In side view, the two bellies of the muscle form an obtuse angle. The posterior belly is much longer than the anterior belly and is only slightly flattened in the mediolateral direction. Gradually tapering anteriorly, the posterior belly continues into the round intermediate tendon. The shorter anterior belly, which arises from the intermediate tendon, generally comprises a thick lateral part and a thin medial part. It is flattened dorsoventrally. Its insertion into the digastric fossa is partly fleshy and partly tendinous.

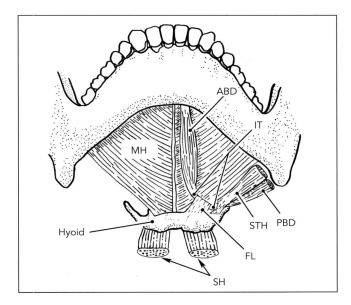

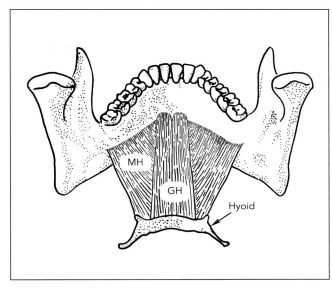

Fig 1-11 Hyoid muscles. (MH) Mylohyoid; (ABD) anterior belly of the digastric; (SH) sternohyoid; (STH) stylohyoid; (PBD) posterior belly of the digastric. Note the fascial loop (FL) surrounding the intermediate tendon (IT) of the digastric. (Modified from Hylander[2] with permission.)

Fig 1-12 Geniohyoid (GH) and mylohyoid muscles (MH). (Modified from Hylander[2] with permission.)

The intermediate tendon is attached to the hyoid bone by a condensation of deep cervical fascia, which forms a loop around the tendon and is sometimes separated from it by a synovial bursa. The fibers of this fascial loop are attached to the greater horn and the lateral part of the body of the hyoid. The length of the fascial loop varies, as does the distance of the tendon from the hyoid and the angle between the posterior and anterior bellies of the muscle. The longer the loop and the greater the distance between the hyoid bone and the intermediate tendon, the more obtuse the angle between the two bellies.

Variations in the digastric muscle are frequent and are almost entirely confined to its anterior belly. The most common deviation from its typical shape consists of midline connections between the two parts of the anterior belly. Also, accessory muscle bundles may occupy some or all of the space between the right and left segments of the anterior digastric belly.

It is usually stated that if the hyoid is fixed by the action of the infrahyoid muscles, contraction of the digastric muscles pulls the front of the mandible back and down and thus facilitates retrusive and opening movements of the mandible. Although a study of hyoid movements during opening and closing of the jaws suggests that the hyoid bone is never completely fixed during mastication,[36,37] the digastric muscle generally appears to function as stated. If the teeth are held firmly

in occlusion (by the jaw-closing muscles), then contraction of the entire digastric elevates the hyoid as long as the infrahyoid muscles are relatively relaxed.

The bellies of the digastric muscle are derived from the first and second branchial arches and are innervated by the mandibular division of the trigeminal (V_3) and the facial nerve (cranial nerve VII), respectively. The mylohyoid nerve, which is a branch of the inferior alveolar nerve, innervates the anterior belly, a first-arch derivative. A branch of the facial nerve supplies the posterior belly, a second-arch derivative.

Mylohyoid Muscle

The mylohyoid muscle forms a muscular diaphragm or floor for most of the oral cavity (Figs 1-11 and 1-12). It is a flat, continuous, pentagonal sheet of muscle located deep to the anterior belly of the digastric. The base of this pentagon attaches to the body of the hyoid bone, and the two adjacent sides of the base have a free edge. The remaining two sides attach to the medial or lingual aspect of the left and right mandibular corpora along the mylohyoid line. The apex of this pentagon attaches to the midline lingual surface of the mandible.

The most posterior fibers along the mandibular corpus, which originate at the level of the third molar, pass medially, downward, and posteriorly to insert along the ventral aspect of the body of the hyoid (see Fig 1-11). The middle and anterior fibers along the corpus have a similar orientation, although they do not attach directly to the hyoid. Instead, they attach to a midline mylohyoid raphe connecting the body of the hyoid with the lingual midline surface of the mandible. This raphe divides the mylohyoid into left and right sides.

Occasionally the anterior belly of the digastric is fused to the ventral surface of the mylohyoid. This fusion reflects the embryologic origin of these two muscles from a common muscle mass derived from the first branchial arch. V_3 innervates the mylohyoid muscle via the mylohyoid nerve.

The anatomy of the mylohyoid suggests that it can slightly raise the hyoid (and tongue) and floor of the mouth. Moreover, if the mandible is stabilized, it can also pull the hyoid forward. In the event that the hyoid is stabilized or being pulled down and/or backward, this muscle can also depress the mandible.

Geniohyoid Muscle

The geniohyoid muscle is a strap-shaped muscle that runs from the ventral surface of the body of the hyoid to the lingual aspect of the mandible immediately lateral to the midline (see Fig 1-12). It is located superficial to the mylohyoid. The muscle is made up of nearly parallel muscle fibers that run straight from origin to insertion. The anatomy of the geniohyoid indicates that if the mandible is stabilized in occlusion, these muscles can slightly raise the hyoid (and tongue) during contraction, and it can pull these structures forward. Conversely, in the event that the hyoid is pulled downward and/or backward, the geniohyoids can depress the mandible.

The geniohyoid muscles are not branchial arch derivatives. These muscles are the serial homologs of the musculi rectus abdominis, and this is why they are often described as belonging to the "rectus cervicis" group, the straight muscles of the neck.[38] The geniohyoids are innervated by ventral rami of the first and second cervical nerves. These nerve fibers connect to the left and right hypoglossal nerves (cranial nerve XII) to reach the floor of the mouth.

Stylohyoid and Infrahyoid Muscles

The stylohyoid muscle is a thin, round muscle with fibers that run between the styloid process of the temporal bone and the greater horn and body of the hyoid (see Fig 1-11). Prior to its insertion in the hyoid, it is split by, and therefore surrounds, the intermediate tendon of the digastric muscle. The stylohyoid is a derivative of the second branchial arch and therefore is innervated by the facial nerve (VII). It presumably functions as a stabilizer, retractor, and elevator of the hyoid bone. Little is known about activity patterns of this muscle, but it is unlikely to have much influence on mandibular movements.

There are four longitudinally arranged, strap-shaped muscles in the so-called infrahyoid muscle group. These straight, parallel-fibered muscles, which contribute to the ventral body wall of the neck, are the remaining members of the rectus cervicis group.[38] Two of these muscles form a deep layer, and two form a superficial layer. The two muscles in the deep layer attach to the outer surface of the thyroid cartilage. The fibers of the thyrohyoid pass upward from the thyroid cartilage to attach to the ventral surface of the body of the hyoid; the fibers of the sternothyroid pass downward from the thyroid cartilage to attach to the deep surface of the manubrium of the sternum. The two muscles of the superficial layer both attach to the ventral surface of the body of the hyoid. The sternohyoid attaches to the manubrium of the sternum and the omohyoid attaches to the upper border of the clavicle (see Fig 1-11).

The infrahyoid muscles presumably have an important role in both stabilizing and lowering of the hyoid. Moreover, they may also function to control or limit upward movement of the hyoid. Therefore, these muscles, working in conjunction with the so-called suprahyoid muscle group (ie, the stylohyoid, mylohyoid, geniohyoid, and digastric muscles), function to control hyoid, tongue, and mandibular positions. Although the omohyoid attaches to the clavicle, its small size precludes the possibility that it has an important influence on shoulder movements.

The infrahyoid muscles are innervated by the cervical ventral rami (first, second, and third cervical nerves) via a delicate loop of motor fibers known as the *ansa cervicalis*.

Functional and Biomechanical Analysis of the TMJ

In a discussion of the mechanics of the TMJ, the masticatory movements can often be more easily understood if the free (or empty) movements of the mandible are considered first. *Free* or *empty movements* are defined as those occurring without food in the oral cavity. These movements are contrasted with the biting and masticatory movements of the jaw, which are those associated with the incising and chewing of food.

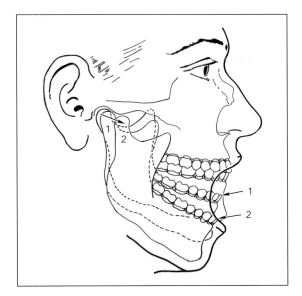

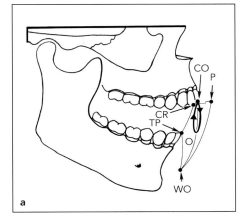

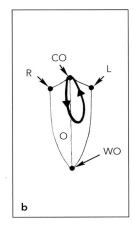

Fig 1-13 Rotation and translation of the mandibular condyle during opening. *(arrow through the condyle)* Direction of condylar translation during opening; (1) moderate jaw opening; (2) near wide opening. (Modified from Hylander[2] with permission.)

Fig 1-14 *(a)* Border movements of the mandible in the sagittal plane. The thin dark lines indicate the movement of the tip of the mandibular central incisors relative to the maxillary teeth. (CR) Centric relation; (CO) centric occlusion; (P) maximum protrusion; the border movement lines drawn between the aforementioned points are tooth-determined positions. (WO) Wide-open position; (TP) transitional point at which continued opening involves anterior translation of the condyle. The arc CR-TP involves pure rotation of the condyle with the condyle in the retruded position. The arc TP-WO combines condylar rotation and translation. The arc P-WO reflects opening in the maximum protruded position. The arc O reflects habitual opening and closing empty movements. The heavy lines with the arrows indicate mandibular incisor movements during chewing on the left side. *(b)* Border movements of the mandible in the frontal plane. Maximum lateral positions along the left (L) and right (R) sides are shown. The points R, CO, and L and the arcs R-CO and CO-L are tooth-determined positions. (Modified from Hylander[2] with permission.)

Free Movements of the Mandible

Two basic movements of the mandible can be distinguished: *(1)* the rotary or hinge movement, which is a rotation of the mandible around a transverse axis passing through the centers of the mandibular condyles, and *(2)* the translatory or sliding movement, which is a bodily movement of the mandible in the anteroposterior and/or mediolateral direction (Fig 1-13). The rotating movement occurs mainly between the disc and condyle in the lower joint compartment, while anteroposterior and mediolateral translatory movements occur mainly between the articular eminence and disc (and mandible) in the upper compartment of the temporomandibular articulation. The translation movements need not be symmetric between the left and right joints. Finally, because translation occurs simultaneously with rotation (in most or all instances), during normal rotary movements the center of rotation is not located within the mandible or condyle.[39]

The free movements of the mandible, combining rotation and translation, include opening and closing; protrusion and retrusion (symmetric forward and backward movements); and lateral shifts of the mandible. The extreme or outer limits of the various combinations of these movements define what has been called the *border movements of the mandible* (Fig 1-14; see chapter 2 for further discussion).[40,41]

Opening and closing

Although highly variable, on average a nearly equal or linear combination of translation and rotation is observable in the opening and closing movements of the mandible (see Fig 1-13).[39] Translation brings the disc and condyle forward and downward along the posterior slope of the articular eminence. The condyle and disc may even move anterior to the greatest height of the articular eminence onto the pre-glenoid plane (see Fig 1-13). The opening movement is so extensive that normally the opening between the maxillary and mandibular incisors easily accommodates three fingers (40 to 60 mm).

If a finger is placed just in front of the tragus of the ear, the forward and downward sliding of the mandibular condyle can be felt. The soft tissues behind the moving condyle sink in slightly and a shallow groove often becomes visible during jaw opening. The movement of the mandibular condyle also influences the width of the cartilaginous part of the external acoustic meatus to a slight degree. If a finger is introduced into the external acoustic meatus, it is easy to feel the prominence of the lateral pole of the mandibular condyle on the cartilaginous anterior wall of the meatus and the widening of this passage when the mouth is opened.

Protrusion and retrusion

The forward and backward movements of the mandible are mainly, but not exclusively, translatory. The mandible can be pulled forward extensively, with the mandibular teeth slightly separated from or in light contact with the maxillary teeth (protrusion). The mandibular condyles are pulled forward together with the articular discs at this time. Therefore, the movement occurs primarily in the upper compartment of the TMJ, and it is symmetric. The reversal of the forward movement, retrusion, is also mainly translatory. These forward condylar movements, which can be confirmed easily by palpation, are limited by the posterior portion of the joint capsule.[18]

Most people with a relatively normal masticatory apparatus can retrude the mandible 1 to 2 mm from the full occlusal position or centric occlusion (see Fig 1-14). The capsular and polar ligaments of the TMJ limit retrusion from this position. This retruded position beyond centric occlusion (referred to as *centric relation*) is not reached during normal jaw movements in humans, although by definition it falls along the border movements of the mandible. It is quite clear that, with the exception of occlusal contacts between the maxillary and mandibular teeth, most routine movements of the incisor point of the mandible do not occur along the border movements (see chapter 2) for a further discussion of the functional significance of centric relation as well as the border movements of the mandible.

Lateral shift

A lateral shift of the mandible (eg, a shift to the right) results if the condyle and disc on the opposite or left side are pulled forward, downward, and medially along the articular eminence (see Fig 1-5). In this instance, the left side is often called the *balancing side (b-s) condyle*, whereas the right side is called the *working-side (w-s) condyle*. The w-s condyle, sometimes called the *resting condyle*, executes a very limited movement at this time. This movement consists primarily of a rotation of the mandible around a nearly vertical axis located within or immediately behind the w-s condyle. This movement also results in a slight transverse translation of the two condyles toward the working side (see Fig 1-5).

As already noted, during the lateral shift of the mandible, the w-s condyle rotates about a vertical axis and moves slightly laterally. This rotational movement is influenced by the same limitations that are placed on the retrusive movement of the mandible from centric occlusion. That is, the lateral pole of the condyle can move backward only about 1 to 2 mm until restricted by the polar ligaments of the capsule and disc. Continued rotation of the w-s condyle is prevented as the lateral polar ligament becomes taut. Under guidance of this ligament, the center of the w-s condyle is forced to move slightly forward and laterally (see Fig 1-5). The lateral component of this movement is often called the *Bennett movement*. As noted, the different movements of the w-s and b-s condyles can be easily palpated.

Action of Muscles in Free Mandibular Movements

Descriptions of muscle function in this and later sections are based primarily on electromyographic (EMG) data and on a muscle's presumed mechanical capabilities. The EMG data provide information as to when (and in restricted situations a relative sense of how much) a muscle is generating tension; the presumed mechanical capabilities of a muscle are based on its overall morphology. Because the EMG literature is extensive, the interested reader is referred to earlier works.[29,32,34,37,42–55]

The mandibular muscles combine in various patterns to execute movements of the mandible. It is especially important to realize that one muscle may act synergistically with different muscles at different times. Moreover, antagonistic muscles may act simultaneously so as to control jaw movements. In no instance does a single muscle act independently; instead, muscles act in groups and almost always in surprisingly large groups. In addition, a single muscle may have portions that can function differentially.

For heuristic purposes, the most important muscles that affect the movements of the mandible can be divided into three groups. These include *(1)* elevators: the temporalis, masseter, and medial pterygoid muscles; *(2)* depressors: the digastric, mylohyoid, and geniohyoid muscles; and *(3)* protractors: the lateral pterygoid muscles.

The retractors of the mandible do not constitute an independent group; they are the digastric muscles and the obliquely aligned fibers of the temporalis muscles. When the stylohyoid and infrahyoid muscles fix the hyoid, the mylohyoid and geniohyoid may also help retract the protruded mandible. The fibers of the deep portion of the masseter also help retract the protruded mandible. Thus, both elevators and depressors can function as retractors of the mandible. The infrahyoid muscles function to control hyoid movements, and therefore their action is important during both jaw opening and jaw closing.

Protrusion

Protrusion of the mandible is primarily the result of contraction of the inferior heads of the lateral pterygoid muscles, although there is also slight activity of the masseter and medial pterygoid muscles at this time. The temporalis muscle is not usually active during this movement, and the depressors are only slightly active. The lateral pterygoid muscles pull the mandibular condyles (and discs) forward and downward along the articular eminences, while the elevators and depressors apparently stabilize the position of the mandible relative to the maxilla. The contraction of the elevators and the depressors in an unresisted forward thrust is often not noticeable on palpation. However, if the mandible is moved to the extreme forward position, contraction of the superficial masseters can be felt.

Retrusion

When the condyles are situated in the mandibular fossa, the obliquely aligned middle fibers of the temporalis muscle combine forces with the depressors so as to retrude the mandible, while the remaining elevators exhibit varying amounts of activity. The depressing component of force from the suprahyoid muscles is apparently neutralized by the activity of the elevator muscles. From the maximum protruded position, the posterior temporalis assists the middle temporalis during mandibular retrusion.

Opening

The opening movement is caused by gravity, relaxation of the elevator muscles, and a combined action of the lateral pterygoid, geniohyoid, mylohyoid, and digastric muscles. The role of the infrahyoid muscles during opening is unclear. Presumably they are active so as to depress the hyoid during wide opening.

If the opening movement occurs without resistance, the depressors act without any great force. If the amount of opening is only slight, relaxation of the elevators and the force of gravity can accomplish this movement. When wide opening occurs, the protracting force of the inferior head of the lateral pterygoid muscles acting on the condyles and discs combines with the depressing and retracting force of the geniohyoid, digastric, and mylohyoid muscles acting on the chin and body of the mandible. These combined forces produce extensive rotatory and translatory opening jaw movements.

Closing

The elevators of the mandible execute the closing movement. If the mouth is opened to its maximal extent, the timing of the activation and relaxation of the different parts of these muscles may be important for proper closure.[27] During maximum opening, each disc and condyle glides anterior to the summit of the articular eminence onto the preglenoid plane. At the beginning of mouth closure, the discs and condyles are moved back from this anterior position. The elevators execute this phase of the closing movement. This action returns the jaw to the rest or occlusal position.

Lateral shift

Lateral shift of the mandible results from an asymmetric variation of protrusion; that is, the b-s lateral pterygoid muscle combines forces with the slightly active elevators. The middle portion of the w-s temporalis muscle must assist in this movement by holding the w-s condyle and preventing it from deviating anteriorly to any great extent.

Masticatory Movements of the Mandible

Movements of the mandible during chewing frequently involve the application of considerable force. In addition, although there is a general overall pattern of movement of the mandible during mastication, the actual movements vary in detail both in and between individuals. Moreover, in a given individual, these movements are in part dependent on the shape and proportions of the jaws and teeth, the type of food masticated, and the stage of bolus formation.

Of course, all masticatory movements of the mandible occur within or along its border movements. As noted earlier, with the exception of during occlusal contact between the maxillary and mandibular teeth, these movements are actually well within the border movements. Thus, with the exception of occlusal movements, knowing the extent of the border movements provides little information for inferring actual jaw movements during chewing.

The chewing movements are combinations of rotation and translation, the two basic mandibular movements previously described. Moreover, the masticatory jaw movements are of two general kinds: a cutting movement, as in biting off a piece of food, and a crushing and grinding movement that comminutes a piece of food. The cutting of food into bite-sized pieces, often referred to as *incision*, is carried out mainly by the incisors, although the canines and premolars are often used for these purposes. The rhythmic and repetitive crushing and grinding of food, termed *mastication*, is carried out almost exclusively along the premolars and molars. Finally, when eating mechanically resistant foods, chewing usually occurs unilaterally; ie, chewing takes place on only one side of the dental arch.

Incision

Unlike movements during mastication, jaw movements during incision have received little attention over the years. The following account is based primarily on the early work of Jankelson et al[56] and Sheppard.[57]

Starting from the rest or occlusal position, incision can be divided into three parts. First, depression of the mandible opens the mouth, and the extent of the opening is primarily dependent on the size of the food object. Second, the mandible is elevated or closed. There is an upward and forward movement of the mandibular incisors and an upward and backward movement of the mandibular condyles during jaw closure, and this part of incision continues until the maxillary and mandibular incisors contact the food object. Third, following food contact, the jaw continues to close with the simultaneous application of force on the food object.

These three parts of incision can be referred to as the *opening*, *closing*, and *power strokes*, respectively. In many instances, the closing stroke does not exist simply because, when the food object is large (eg, a whole apple), the amount of jaw opening is just enough to accommodate this object between the maxillary and mandibular incisors.

Mandibular movements during the opening and closing strokes of incision are presumably very similar to the free mandibular opening and closing movements. Jaw movements during the power stroke of incision, however, differ from simple jaw-closing movements, particularly in the presence of an incisor overbite. That is, as the anterior

teeth approach the edge-to-edge position during incision, the entire mandible moves backward and upward as the edges of the mandibular incisors and canines glide along the lingual surfaces of the maxillary incisors and canines until full molar occlusion is reached. The food item is cut and sheared prior to or at initial tooth contact. Once initial tooth contact has been attained, the morphology of the anterior teeth and TMJ influences mandibular movements to a large extent.

Patterns of jaw movement during incision are also influenced by use of the hands. In some instances food is vigorously pulled or rotated away from the mouth, while in other instances the hands play a less active role by simply positioning the food object between the maxillary and mandibular anterior teeth during incision.

Mastication

Similar to incision, mastication or chewing can also be conveniently described as consisting of three basic parts: opening, closing, and power strokes (Fig 1-15).[45] These three strokes combine to make up a single chewing cycle, and all chewing cycles associated with the mastication of a single piece of food are referred to as a *chewing sequence*.

A chewing cycle begins with opening of the mouth; as the mandible is depressed, the midline incisal point is ordinarily swung slightly to the nonchewing or balancing side and then back to the chewing or working side (Fig 1-16). This movement is the opening stroke. The amount of opening varies from one chewing cycle to the next, and it depends partly on the size and consistency of the food object. From the position of maximum opening, the mandibular incisors are then moved upward, forward, and away from the midline toward the working side. This portion of the upward jaw movement is the closing stroke. Completion of the closing stroke leads to the power stroke, which is the forceful contact on the food between the occlusal surfaces of the molar and premolar teeth. The w-s teeth posterior to the canine are moved back toward the midline during the power stroke. With the exception of those movements associated with contact between the maxillary and mandibular teeth, the mandibular incisor movements during mastication are well within the border movements (see Fig 1-14).

When tough, mechanically resistant foods are chewed, the power stroke of mastication often ends before the maxillary and mandibular teeth make contact. This type of power stroke is called *puncture crushing*. However, a power stroke often does involve direct contact between the maxillary and mandibular teeth; this type of power stroke is called *tooth-tooth contact*. Generally, more transverse movement of the mandible occurs during a tooth-

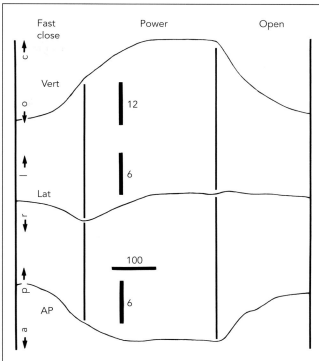

Fig 1-15 Movements of the tip of the mandibular central incisor during unilateral mastication of tough food along the right side. (Vert) Tracing of vertical jaw movements; *(arrows)* direction of (c) closing and (o) opening movements. (Lat) Tracing of lateral movements; *(arrows)* direction of (l) left and (r) right movements. (AP) Tracing of anteroposterior movements; *(arrows)* direction of (p) posterior and (a) anterior movements. The tracing of vertical jaw movements indicates the fast close, power, and opening strokes of mastication. The horizontal bar indicates 100 milliseconds. The thick vertical bars labeled 12 and 6 indicate 12 and 6 mm of incisor movement, respectively. These jaw movements were recorded with a magnet-sensing jaw-tracking system. (Modified from Hylander[2] with permission.)

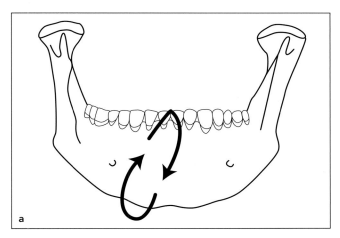

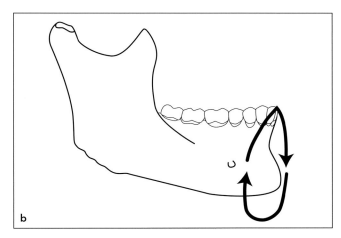

Fig 1-16 *(a)* Frontal and *(b)* lateral views of the mandible. *(arrows)* Movement of the incisal tip of the mandibular central incisors during unilateral mastication on the right side. The relative amount of movement has been exaggerated. (Modified from Hylander[2] with permission.)

tooth contact power stroke than during a puncture-crushing power stroke.

In a power stroke involving tooth-tooth contact there is an upward, slightly anterior, and medial movement of the mandibular molars (relative to the maxillary molars) on the working or chewing side and an upward, lateral, and slightly backward movement of the mandibular molars on the balancing or nonchewing side.[58,59] The teeth either continue to be moved into centric occlusion, or these occlusal movements are abruptly terminated and the opening stroke is initiated. When viewed in the transverse or occlusal plane, the mandible at this time rotates around a vertical axis positioned in or somewhat behind the w-s mandibular condyle.

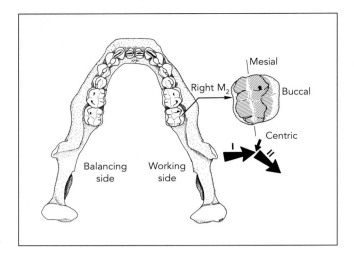

Fig 1-17 Occlusal view of the mandible demonstrating the direction of tooth movement during phase I and phase II movements. The mandibular right second molar (M₂) has been enlarged, and the hatched lines along its occlusal surface are aligned parallel to the orientation of movement of its occluding antagonists. The arrows demonstrate the direction of movement of the maxillary right second molar relative to the mandibular right second molar. The movement of the mandibular second molar, relative to the maxillary molar, is opposite to the direction indicated by the *arrows*. Phase I movements begin at the initiation of tooth-tooth contact and terminate when the working-side (w-s) mandibular molars have moved upward and medially into centric occlusion. The mandible is rotating about a variably located vertical axis in the region of the w-s mandibular condyle during phase I. Phase II starts when the w-s mandibular molars are moved slightly downward, medially, and anteriorly out of centric occlusion; this phase terminates when molar tooth contact is broken. (Modified from Hylander[2] with permission.)

The previously described tooth contact movements posterior to the canines are often called *phase I* (or *buccal phase*) movements[60,61] (Fig 1-17). Following phase I, one of two things happens. Either the power stroke ends and tooth contact is lost as the jaws open, or the power stroke continues into *phase II* (or *lingual phase*) movements.[60,61] Prior to the phase II movement, however, the teeth and jaws are held stationary in centric occlusion during what has been referred to as the *motionless period* of mastication.[62] This period is said to last about 200 milliseconds,[62] although data in Fig 1-15 indicate that in this particular subject it lasted only about 50 to 75 milliseconds.

Phase II movements occur when the w-s mandibular teeth, which are positioned in centric occlusion, are moved

slightly downward, forward, and toward the nonchewing side of the jaw while still maintaining occlusal contact. The phase II movement then glides directly into the opening stroke of mastication as tooth contact is lost.[60,63]

Action of Muscles During Masticatory Movements

Incision

The EMG activity of the jaw muscles has not been systematically analyzed throughout entire episodes of incision. It is assumed that the muscle activity patterns during the opening and closing strokes of incision are very similar to those during the free opening and closing movements.[2,64] If so, the opening stroke is initiated by activity of the depressor group of muscles, followed by contraction of the inferior heads of the lateral pterygoid muscles. At this time the mandible is rotated open and the condyles are translated forward. The closing stroke is initiated by the jaw-closing or elevator muscles.

During the power stroke of incision, the elevator muscles contract more or less synchronously, which is unlike the situation during unilateral mastication. It was once thought that most of the muscle force during incision was due to bilateral contraction of the medial pterygoid and masseter muscles, while the temporalis muscle contributed little or nothing.[2,65] However, EMG experiments demonstrate that during incision all of the jaw-closing muscles are important for generating bite force, including the temporalis muscle.[46] In contrast, only the medial pterygoid and masseter muscles exert much force during isometric incisor clenching.[48,52,66-68]

The lateral pterygoid muscle is also thought to be active during the power stroke of incision. This suggestion is based on several factors: *(1)* the observation that both heads of the lateral pterygoid muscle are active during incisor clenching,[29] *(2)* the assumption that the TMJ must be stabilized during incision, and *(3)* the fact that this muscle is ideally positioned to perform the stabilizing function. Presumably the mandibular condyles must be stabilized because the power stroke of incision occurs when reaction and muscle forces are often large and rapidly changing both in direction and amount. For example, when a large food object suddenly breaks during incision, the holding force and stiffness of each lateral pterygoid muscle prevents an uncontrolled posterior and upward displacement of the mandibular condyles as the condyles and discs are situated precariously near the summit or along the posterior slope of the articular eminence.

Mastication

Much of what follows are typical jaw muscle activity patterns and jaw movements. The reader should bear in mind that these patterns and movements often exhibit considerable variability both in and between individual subjects. In the description of the muscle activity patterns, as noted earlier, the side on which the food bolus is located is referred to as the *working side*. Many writers also refer to this side as the *ipsilateral* or *active side*. The side opposite to the location of the bolus is referred to as the *balancing side*. This side is also referred to as the *contralateral*, *nonworking*, or *supporting side*.

Muscle activity patterns of the jaw elevators during mastication are fairly well known, although some details have yet to be worked out. Less is known about the activity patterns for the lateral pterygoid and depressor muscles, and little is known about the stylohyoid and infrahyoid muscles. Much of the following description is based on the pioneering and classic work of Møller,[48,49] as well as the research of others.[32,42,44,53]

The opening stroke is initiated by activity of the depressor group; the mylohyoid usually contracts somewhat earlier than the digastric muscles (Fig 1-18). Initial activity of the depressor group slightly overlaps activity of the relaxing elevator muscles.[48,49,51,69,70] Shortly (about 80 milliseconds) thereafter, the inferior heads of the lateral pterygoid muscles begin to contract; activity on the working side frequently precedes activity on the balancing side. The mandible is slightly depressed when the opening moments of the depressor group exceed the closing moments of the relaxing elevator group. The mandible continues to open, and often the w-s corpus moves toward the balancing side as both condyles and discs translate forward. The w-s corpus moves back toward the midline during opening when the level of activity in the b-s lateral pterygoid muscle (inferior head) exceeds that of the w-s muscle. EMG data indicate that the jaw elevators are often weakly active during jaw opening.[51,69]

In some instances, actual jaw-closing movement appears to precede electrical activity of the elevator muscles.[45] This observation, however, is probably due to inadequate amplification of the EMGs of the elevator muscles during low levels of activation.[50] During the initial phase of closing, the depressor group continues to exhibit EMG activity. Presumably the simultaneous activation of the elevators and depressors facilitates well-controlled and precise jaw movements during mastication.

The closing stroke is often initiated by contraction of the b-s superficial masseter and medial pterygoid muscles. The chewing side of the mandible continues to be moved laterally at this time, largely because of the activity of these muscles. Studies in both humans and nonhu-

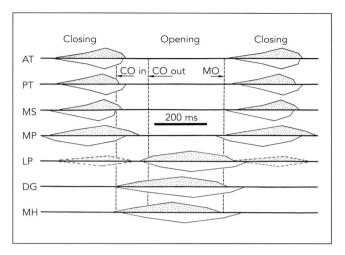

Fig 1-18 Electromyographic (EMG) activity of jaw muscles during unilateral mastication of chewing gum. (AT) Anterior temporalis; (PT) posterior temporalis; (MS) masseter (superficial portion); (MP) medial pterygoid; (LP) lateral pterygoid; (DG) digastric; (MH) mylohyoid. The working-side muscle (stippled) is above the solid black line and the balancing-side muscle (not stippled) is below this line. This figure presents mean normalized EMG values and therefore does not indicate the considerable amount of EMG variability within and between subjects during mastication. Both the *(solid lines)* "primary" (lower head?) and *(dashed lines)* "secondary" (upper head?) activity patterns of the lateral pterygoid muscle have been included (from Møller[48]). *(vertical dashed lines)* Movement of the teeth (CO in) into centric occlusion, (CO out) out of centric occlusion, and when the jaws are (MO) maximally open. Note the coactivation of elevator and depressor muscles during occlusion and at maximum opening.

man primates indicate that this lateral movement is also assisted by the w-s temporalis.[48,71] Collectively, this group of three muscles (w-s temporalis muscle and b-s masseter and medial pterygoid muscles) is frequently referred to as *triplet I* or *diagonal I*.[71–77]

Following activation of the triplet I muscles, the b-s anterior temporalis muscle and the w-s superficial masseter and medial pterygoid muscles are activated, followed closely by the b-s posterior temporalis muscle. This causes the chewing side of the mandible to be moved back toward the midline. The combined effect of this second group of elevators, often referred to as *triplet II* or *diagonal II*, is closing of the jaws, during which the working side of the mandible eventually moves back toward the midline.[71–77]

When the maxillary and mandibular teeth are in forcible contact with food or with one another, the EMG activity of the elevators reaches a maximum.[42,48,49] The period of maximum occlusal force is often about 40 to 80 milliseconds after the peak EMG activity, and this period of maximum force occurs prior to and during the initial period of centric occlusion.[34,78] The teeth and jaws are then rapidly unloaded as the jaw elevators relax and the jaw depressors begin to develop tension. The entire cycle is repeated with the activation of the depressor muscles late in the terminal portion of the power stroke.[32,54,79,80]

Activity of the superior head of the lateral pterygoid muscle during the chewing cycle is said to occur during closing and/or the early part of the power stroke,[29–31] although this idea continues to be controversial. The behavior of this part of the lateral pterygoid remains unclear because of difficulties involving verification of electrode position and the possibility of EMG cross-talk from adjacent muscles.[20,32,54,79,80]

There are some interesting and important details of muscle behavior during the power stroke that have not yet been discussed. As previously noted, peak muscle activity in the b-s superficial masseter and medial pterygoid muscles frequently precedes peak activity in their w-s counterparts during tooth-tooth contact power strokes. Moreover, the temporalis muscles exhibit the reverse pattern; peak activity of the w-s temporalis precedes that of the b-s temporalis. Thus, peak activity of the w-s temporalis and b-s medial pterygoid and superficial masseter (triplet I or diagonal I) frequently precedes peak activity of the b-s temporalis and w-s medial pterygoid and superficial masseter (triplet or diagonal II).[71–77] Furthermore, as a group, overall levels of activity tend to be larger in the triplet II muscles. In contrast, all of these muscles reach peak activity almost simultaneously during puncture-crushing power strokes.

These different timing patterns relate directly to different mandibular movements. Puncture crushing is often associated with little or no mediolateral components of jaw movement, unlike the jaw movements during tooth-tooth contacts. Because puncture crushing is primarily a series of up-and-down vertical strokes,[42] jaw muscle activity tends to be rather synchronous at this time. In contrast, tooth-tooth contact power strokes are often associated with extensive mediolateral movement of the mandible, and this movement is accomplished by asynchronous jaw muscle activity.

Another interesting aspect of jaw muscle activity during mastication has to do with the relative amount of muscle force recruitment from the w-s and b-s muscles. EMG data suggest that the w-s and b-s temporalis and deep masseter muscles exhibit similar amounts of activity in humans during unilateral mastication,[48,49,64] but the w-s superficial masseter and medial pterygoid muscles are often much more active than their b-s counterparts.[48,49]

The actual pattern of force recruitment for the superficial masseter and medial pterygoid muscles, however, is variable and largely related to the mechanical properties of the chewed food.[34,81] EMG data on humans indicate that chewing soft foods results in about 3.0 times more relative force from the w-s masseter than from the b-s masseter, whereas during the mastication of tough foods the contribution of force from the w-s masseter is about 1.5 times greater than that from the b-s masseter.[34] This is important because the relative amount of muscle force from the working and balancing sides has an important influence on the TMJ reaction forces. This point will be developed in a later section.

Finally, although there are two distinctive phases (phase I and II) of occlusal contact during chewing, considerable evidence in nonhuman primates demonstrates that maximum occlusal force occurs prior to or during phase I, and that negligible occlusal force occurs during phase II movements.[82–84]

Functional Significance of Condylar Translation

One of the most interesting characteristics of the human TMJ is the frequent occurrence of considerable anteroposterior or fore-aft translation. TMJ stability during biting is likely influenced by this situation. Presumably the direction and magnitude of the various muscular and reaction forces acting on the mandible are adjusted continuously so as to minimize any instability. Nevertheless, if condylar translation contributes to TMJ instability, as it must, what is the functional significance of condylar translation, particularly anteroposterior translation? That is, what are the benefits of extensive condylar translation?

As repeatedly noted, the mandibular condyles of humans are capable of translation both mediolaterally and anteroposteriorly. Mediolateral condylar translation occurs in all mammals, even in those species that experience little or no anteroposterior condylar translation. Apparently the main function of mediolateral condylar translation in mammals is to enhance occlusal function, ie, to facilitate movements of the mandibular teeth in the transverse or occlusal plane relative to the opposing maxillary teeth during the power stroke of mastication. Moreover, many mammals are unable to bring their maxillary and mandibular teeth into occlusion without mediolateral translation simply because, unlike humans, their maxillary dental arch is much wider mediolaterally than is their mandible.[2]

Unlike mediolateral condylar translation, anteroposterior translation of the condyle does not occur in all mammals. For example, it does not occur in carnivorans (members of the order Carnivora, such as dogs, cats, bears, and raccoons). The apparent explanation for why carnivorans have little or no anteroposterior translation is that their TMJs are designed to ensure condylar stability so as to pre-

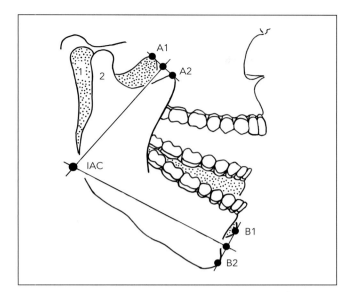

Fig 1-19a Approximate location of the instantaneous axis of rotation: Two arbitrary positions of the mandible during symmetric opening from position 1 (stippled mandible) to position 2 (unstippled mandible). A line tangent to the tip of the coronoid process (A1 and A2) and another to the tip of the chin (B1 and B2) have been constructed for positions 1 and 2 during opening. Two perpendicular lines have been constructed to lines A1–A2 and B1–B2. These two perpendicular lines cross at the approximate location of the instantaneous axis of mandibular rotation (IAC) in the moderately open position.

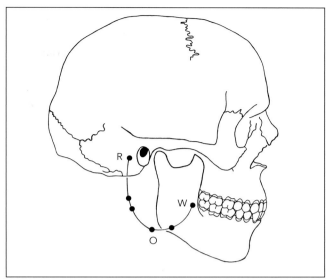

Fig 1-19b Path of the instantaneous axis of rotation of the mandible during simple opening according to Grant.[89] The instantaneous axes of rotation in the (R) rest, (O) moderately open, and (W) wide-open positions are shown. However, work by Merlini and Palla[39] indicates that the rest and wide-open positions are in reality located much lower (see Gallo et al[90] and Gibbs et al[59] for the various locations of the instantaneous axis of rotation of the mandible during mastication; also see chapter 2 of this book). (Modified from Hylander[2] with permission.)

vent dislocation of the mandible due to the erratic, unpredictable nature of the forces applied to their jaws when subduing struggling prey.[85] One way to prevent jaw dislocation is by having a tightly fitted TMJ that cannot translate anteroposteriorly because of its interlocking bony and ligamentous configuration. Although not all modern carnivorans subdue struggling prey, it is assumed that this behavior characterized the earliest members of this order, and that is why even the entirely herbivorous giant panda has a TMJ incapable of anteroposterior translation.[86]

This brings us back to the question of why humans and many other mammals have a TMJ that is able to translate extensively in an anteroposterior direction. As noted, condylar translation enhances occlusal function, and this likely explains the origin of mammalian anteroposterior translation. This explanation, however, is inadequate to explain the full range of anteroposterior translation. In humans and in many other mammals, the amount of anteroposterior translation of the condyles during the power stroke of mastication is much less than their actual capability. Moreover, most anteroposterior condylar translation occurs during wide jaw opening and

closing from this wide-open position, well before the occlusal phase of chewing. Thus, although anteroposterior translation evolved to enhance occlusal events, extensive anteroposterior translatory movements of the condyles must have evolved for a different reason.

There are a number of hypotheses to explain the functional significance of extensive anteroposterior condylar translation in humans and other noncarnivoran mammals.[87] One of these can be referred to as the *airway impingement hypothesis*. This hypothesis states that in mammals with mandibular condyles positioned high above the occlusal plane (eg, humans, gorillas, horses, and cattle), forward translation of the condyle during wide jaw opening prevents the tongue and angle of the mandible from rotating backward and pressing against the cervical airway and thereby disrupting its integrity.[87,88] There is only a small amount of backward movement of the angle of the human mandible (and tongue) during wide jaw opening because the condyles translate forward at that time (Figs 1-13, 1-19a, and 1-19b).

There are two major problems with the airway impingement hypothesis. One is that it only attempts to explain condylar translation in mammals whose mandibular condyles lie well above the occlusal plane. It cannot account for the extensive anteroposterior condylar translation found in many mammals whose mandibular condyles are positioned low at the level of the occlusal plane (eg, insectivorans and many strepsirrhine primates and marsupials), which presumably is the primitive condition for mammals. Because it is extremely doubtful that the tongue or mandible of these latter mammals would impinge on their airway even if they did not translate their condyles forward during jaw opening,[87] it is more reasonable to believe that extensive anteroposterior condylar translation evolved for some other reason.

The second problem with the airway impingement hypothesis is that there is simply no convincing evidence to indicate that the integrity of the human airway would be compromised by the mandible and tongue if condylar translation failed to occur during jaw opening.

DuBrul[15] has proposed a similar hypothesis to explain the extensive anteroposterior condylar translation in humans. He suggested that extensive readjustments of the human skull to upright bipedal locomotion resulted in a "greatly narrowed space between jaw and mastoid process" and thus "A wide opening of the jaw in a pure, back-swinging hinge is therefore now impossible."[15(p122)] The main problem with this explanation is that the capability for anteroposterior translation of the mandibular condyles is not confined to humans, and therefore the explanation for its presence cannot be plausibly linked solely to upright posture in humans.

Another hypothesis, referred to as the *sarcomere length hypothesis*, states that anteroposterior condylar translation is a mechanism to minimize the sarcomere length changes in the masseter and medial pterygoid muscles throughout a wide range of jaw gapes.[91,92] In humans (and also in macaques and rabbits) the instantaneous axis (or helical axis or screw axis) of rotation during jaw opening is in the region of the masseter–medial pterygoid complex (see Figs 1-19a and 1-19b).[89,91,93] This indicates that the origin and insertion of the masseter and medial pterygoid muscles are stretched much less during wide jaw opening than they would be if the mandible were simply hinged open. In contrast, the origin and insertion areas of the posterior and middle portions of the temporalis are separated more when forward condylar translation is combined with jaw opening, whereas those of the anterior temporalis are more or less unaffected. Thus, because the masseter–medial pterygoid complex is larger than the combined middle and posterior portions of the temporalis, it indicates that the overall elevator muscle mass in humans (also, eg, monkeys and rabbits) is stretched less than it would be if the condyles did not

translate forward during wide opening. Or conversely, most of the elevator muscle mass is compressed less than it would be if the condyles did not translate backward during jaw closing from the wide-open position.

It is important to minimize muscle stretch (or compression) during jaw opening (and closing) because the amount of force a muscle fiber can generate is inversely proportional to how much it is stretched (or compressed) beyond its resting sarcomere length.[94] Minimizing the amount of sarcomere length change beyond its resting length allows the masseter–medial pterygoid complex to function at a wide variety of gapes without causing a major reduction in the amount of force it can generate. Several investigators[85,91,93] have concluded that the amount of masseter stretch (in humans, macaques, and rabbits) during jaw opening would indeed greatly affect the ability of this muscle to generate force if the condyles did not translate forward.

However, it has been suggested that the sarcomere length hypothesis must be false because it is based on the incorrect assumption that the mandibular elevators are capable of generating maximum force when the teeth are in or near occlusion.[87,88,91] Actually, the sarcomere length hypothesis need not be based on this admittedly erroneous assumption. The sarcomere length hypothesis simply states that stretching and compressing of the masseter–medial pterygoid complex is minimized during extensive anteroposterior translatory movement of the condyles so that this powerful muscle mass is able to generate high levels of force at a wide variety of gapes. Although the jaw muscles do not generate maximum force during occlusion, the exact point at which the jaw muscles are capable of generating maximum force is irrelevant to the argument.

In summary, although mediolateral and anteroposterior condylar translation in mammals may have initially evolved to enhance occlusal function, this explanation does not account for the extensive anteroposterior movements experienced by many mammals. The two major hypotheses that attempt to explain the functional significance of these extensive movements, the airway impingement and sarcomere length hypotheses, are arguably inadequate to varying degrees. Nevertheless, unlike simple hinge movements, anterior condylar translation clearly results in a reduction of sarcomere length change in the masseter and medial pterygoid muscles during wide jaw opening in humans. In contrast, it is not clear whether failure of the condyles to translate forward during jaw opening would have any effect whatsoever on respiratory function.

Finally, a third hypothesis has been advanced to explain the functional significance of condylar translation.[93] This hypothesis suggests that condylar translation (and the associated inferior shifting of the instantaneous center of

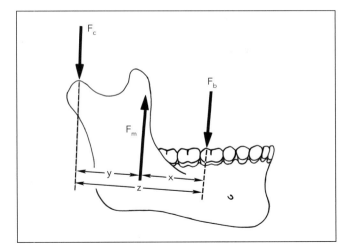

Fig 1-20 Human mandible functioning as a lever during biting along the mandibular first molar. Only the vertical components of the muscle and reaction forces are included in this figure. The (F_m) resultant muscle force of the jaw elevators is located posterior to the bite point (mandibular first molar). To maintain static equilibrium under these conditions, the muscle force is divided into (F_b) a reaction force along the bite point and (F_c) a reaction force along the two mandibular condyles. For a given amount of muscle force, F_b can be determined by analyzing moments about F_c: $F_b = (F_m)(y)/z$. F_c can be determined by analyzing moments about F_m or F_b: $F_c = (F_b)(x)/y$ or $F_c = (F_m)(x)/z$. (Modified from Hylander[2] with permission.)

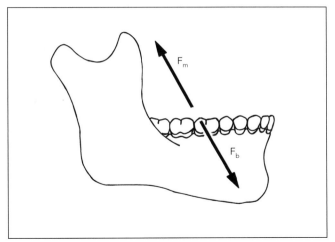

Fig 1-21 Nonlever action of the mandible. The (F_m) resultant muscle force of the jaw elevators passes through the bite point. All of the muscle forces acting on the mandible result in an equal and opposite (F_b) reaction force along the bite point. To maintain static equilibrium under these conditions, it is unnecessary to have any reaction force acting along the condyles. (Modified from Hylander[2] with permission.)

rotation) is due to the differential passive elastic components of the jaw adductors. Although the passive elastic components of the jaw adductors most likely explain much of the path taken by the instantaneous or helical axis of rotation during jaw opening, this hypothesis is more of a proximate rather than an ultimate explanation. That is, it does not explain why the passive elastic components in the jaw muscles are distributed in such a manner as to reduce muscle stretch of the masseter and medial pterygoid muscles.

Mandibular Biomechanics

Lever versus nonlever action of the mandible

For more than 100 years, most researchers have assumed that the mandible functions as a lever during both biting and the power stroke of mastication, while the mandibular condyle acts as a fulcrum[95–97] (Fig 1-20). However, this hypothesis has been and continues to be challenged by those who have suggested, either directly or indirectly, that there is little or no reaction force at either mandibu-

lar condyle and, therefore, that the condyles do not act as fulcrums during biting or mastication.[78,98–109]

Several lines of argument have been presented in support of the proposition that the condyles do not function as fulcrums, and they have usually been based on one of two assertions: First, the resultant masticatory muscle force always passes through the bite point during biting or chewing (Fig 1-21); therefore, it is unnecessary to have force acting along the mandibular condyle to satisfy conditions of static equilibrium. Second, the tissues of the TMJ are unsuited to withstand reaction force; therefore, the mandibular condyles cannot act as fulcrums if their tissues are incapable of bearing stress.

However, many studies have indicated that the resultant masticatory muscle force does not always pass through the bite point.[65,92,110] Moreover, other studies have demonstrated morphologically and experimentally that the tissues of the TMJ are capable of dissipating joint reaction force.[65] Therefore, there is little evidence to support either of the above assertions regarding the nonlever action of the mandible.[65,96]

Although most researchers agree that the mandible functions as a lever, there have been a number of disagree-

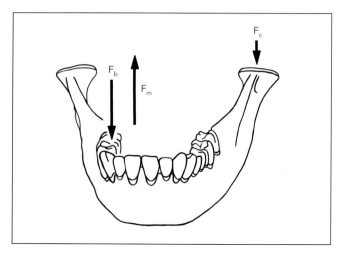

Fig 1-22 Forces acting along the mandible in the frontal projection. Only the vertical components of the muscle and reaction forces are included in this figure. Frequently the jaw elevators on the working side generate slightly more force than the elevators on the balancing side. Under these conditions, the resultant muscle force (F_m) is located to the working side of the midline. (F_b) Bite force; (F_c) condylar reaction force along the balancing side.[65] Under conditions of static equilibrium, only the balancing-side condyle need be unloaded. (Modified from Hylander[2] with permission.)

ments over methods of analysis and the modeling of external muscle and reaction forces during mandibular function. Until recent years these disagreements fell within the context of the following three questions:

1. How does one go about analyzing moments acting on the mandible?
2. What type of lever best describes the way the mandible functions?
3. In what projection is the mandible best analyzed?

Most researchers, when attempting a biomechanical analysis of the mammalian mandible, have analyzed moments about the load-bearing portion (or center) of the mandibular condyle in the lateral projection.[85,111–113] This is a useful procedure when analyzing muscle and bite force moments because it eliminates the need to consider moments associated with condylar reaction forces. Alternatively, moments can also be analyzed about the bite point or the resultant muscle force. This would eliminate the need to consider moments associated with the bite force or the resultant muscle force, respectively.

Over the years, various researchers have insisted that moments should be analyzed about the instantaneous axis

of rotation of the mandible.[19,89] However, this procedure makes the analysis slightly more complicated because none of the muscle force or reaction force moments can be ignored.[65,114] Of course moments can be analyzed about any point, because by definition the summation of moments about any point is equal to zero under conditions of static equilibrium. Ordinarily it is simply more convenient to analyze moments about the bite, muscle, or condylar reaction forces. The choice of which points to use is directly linked to the nature of the problem.

In an attempt to model mandibular function, many researchers have argued about whether the mammalian jaw functions as a class III, class II, or as a modified class I bent lever.[112,113] Most textbooks describe the mandible of humans as a class III lever,[15] but this concept is overly simplistic because it implies that the various external forces acting on the mandible lie within the same plane. Moreover, an analysis of moments acting on the mandible is not dependent on making this distinction, and such a classification gives little, if any, insight into how mammalian jaws work.[2,115]

The mammalian mandible has often been analyzed solely in the lateral projection. Although this procedure is particularly appropriate for an analysis of incisal biting or bilateral molar biting, it does not allow a separate analysis of reaction force along each TMJ during unilateral mastication or biting. For example, if the muscles on the working side of the human jaw are assumed to be slightly more active than those on the balancing side during the power stroke of mastication, as most or all studies have suggested,[48,49] the resultant muscle force must be located between the midline and the w-s condyle (Fig 1-22). For this system to be in static equilibrium under these conditions, a compressive reaction force must be acting on the b-s condyle. Based on this simple model, it was suggested that the b-s condyle likely experiences more reaction force than does the w-s condyle in humans.[65]

A better approach to modeling the biomechanics of the mandible is to perform a three-dimensional analysis of the magnitude and direction of all muscle and reaction forces.[116–118] This, however, is beyond the scope of this chapter. Following a landmark and important study by Smith,[110] a simplified analysis of forces and moments in both the lateral and frontal projections can be performed based on the assumption that all muscle and reaction forces are essentially vertical and parallel to one another. Although it is doubtful whether such conditions ever exist, particularly during unilateral mastication, this analysis provides interesting insights into patterns of reaction force along the working and balancing TMJs.

To analyze TMJ reaction force during unilateral biting, moments are first taken about the bite force in the lateral

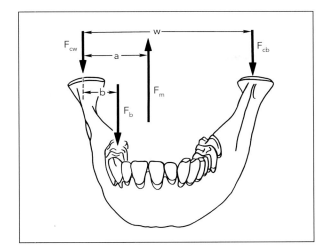

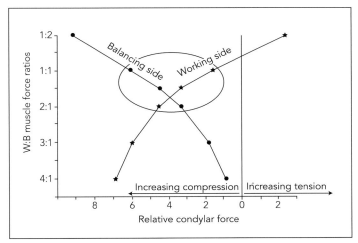

Fig 1-23 Forces acting along the mandible in the frontal projection (after Smith[110]). Only the vertical components of the muscle and reaction forces are included in this figure. (F_m) Resultant muscle force; (F_b) bite force; (F_{cw}) condylar reaction force along the working-side condyle; (F_{cb}) condylar reaction force along the balancing-side condyle. F_{cw} can be determined by taking moments about F_{cb} (ie, $F_{cw} = [(F_m)(a) - (F_b)(b)]/w$). For a given amount of F_m, the values of F_b and F_c (total condylar reaction force) are determined by analyzing moments in the lateral projection (see Fig 1-20). F_{cb} can then be determined by analyzing moments about F_{cw} or F_b or F_m. The easiest way, however, is to simply subtract F_{cw} from F_c (ie, $F_{cb} = F_c - F_{cw}$). (Modified from Hylander[2] with permission.)

Fig 1-24 Plot of relative working-side (w-s) condylar reaction force values *(stars)* and balancing-side (b-s) condylar reaction force values *(circles)* during isometric biting along the mandibular first molar for various working-balancing (W:B) muscle force ratios. The total muscle force is held constant, although the W:B muscle force ratio varies. The ratio 4:1 indicates that the w-s muscle force is 4.0 times larger than the b-s muscle force. The ratio 1:1 indicates that the w-s and b-s muscle force values are identical. Under most conditions, the actual muscle force ratios fall within the oval-shaped region. (Modified from Hylander[2] with permission.)

projection in order to solve for total condylar reaction force (see Fig 1-20). Prior to doing so, it is necessary to assign a relative value to the total muscle force applied (the combined w-s and b-s muscle force). After calculating the relative total condylar reaction force, this force is subtracted from the total muscle force to solve for the magnitude of the bite force (see Fig 1-20).

The next step involves analyzing moments in the frontal projection. First, moments are taken about the w-s condyle to solve for the amount of force along the b-s condyle or vice versa (Fig 1-23). Although the total relative bite and muscle force are already known from the analysis of moments in the lateral projection, in order to proceed with the frontal-projection analysis, the ratio of the w-s to b-s muscle forces must be estimated, so that the resultant muscle force can be positioned. If this ratio is 1.0 (forces from both working and balancing sides are equal), the resultant muscle force is in the midline. If the ratio is greater than 1.0 (if the w-s muscle force is greater), the resultant muscle force lies to the left of the midline for bit-

ing on the left side. If appreciably less than 1.0, which is highly unlikely, it lies to the right of the midline. Once its position is determined and the calculation of the b-s condylar reaction force is made, the w-s condylar reaction force is solved by simply subtracting the b-s condylar reaction force from the total condylar reaction force.

When this method of analysis is used, a calculation of human TMJ reaction force with a constant total amount of muscle and bite force during isometric biting along the mandibular first molar indicates that, although the total condylar reaction force does not vary, the amount of w-s and b-s condylar forces varies as a function of the relative amount of muscle force from the working and balancing sides (Fig 1-24). If the w-s muscle force is 4.0 times larger than the b-s muscle force (an unlikely occurrence), the w-s condyle experiences about 7.0 times more force than does the b-s condyle. If the w-s muscle force is 2.0 times larger than the b-s muscle force (a more likely occurrence), the w-s condylar force is about 1.4 times larger than the b-s condylar reaction force. If the w-s muscle force is 1.5

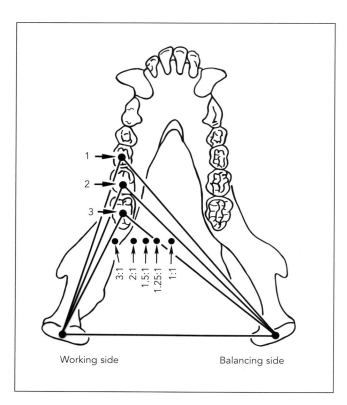

Fig 1-25 Occlusal view of a macaque monkey mandible: Triangles 1, 2, and 3 are "triangles of support" during biting[126] along the mandibular left first, second, and third molars, respectively. The position of the resultant muscle force is indicated by the solid circles for various working-balancing recruitment patterns. For example, when the working-side muscle force is 2.0 times larger than the balancing-side muscle force, the resultant muscle force is located at 2:1 (see text for discussion). (Modified from Hylander[2] with permission.)

indicates that the ratio of w-s to b-s muscle force often varies as a function of the mechanical properties of the food, magnitude of the bite force, and location of the bite point. For example, as nonhuman primates and humans engage in more powerful masticatory power strokes, most subjects tend to recruit relatively greater amounts of b-s muscle force. That is, when macaque monkeys chew pieces of apple with no attached skin, the w-s masseter tends to generate about 3.0 times more force than the b-s masseter. When they chew primarily tough wads of apple skin, the w-s elevator muscle force is about 1.5 times greater than that of the b-s elevators.[47,81]

These results, coupled with the theoretical analysis presented in Fig 1-24, suggest that differential loading along the w-s and b-s TMJs during the power stroke of mastication likely varies according to the mechanical properties of the food eaten. Moreover, a slight shift in the ratio of the w-s to the b-s muscle force results in marked differences in TMJ loading patterns. The b-s TMJ may be loaded more than the w-s TMJ under some conditions, while the reverse may prevail under other conditions.

Experiments on macaques also indicate that under very limited and restricted conditions (eg, powerful isometric biting along the mandibular third molar, the w-s TMJ can either be negligibly loaded or loaded in tension.[33] Although this can be demonstrated mathematically from a three-dimensional analysis or from an analysis in both the lateral and frontal projections, it is more easily visualized if the muscle and reaction forces acting along the mandible are analyzed in the occlusal projection.[125,126] In this model, the macaque mandible is supported on three points during unilateral biting along the left first molar: the left and right mandibular condyles and the left first molar. These three points form what Greaves[126] refers to as the triangle of support (triangle 1 in Fig 1-25). Triangles of support during biting along the left second and third molars are triangles 2 and 3, respectively.

The point 1:1 in Fig 1-25 is the position of the resultant elevator muscle force when equal amounts are contributed by both the working and balancing sides. The direction of this force along this point is toward the reader and, as a first approximation, is perpendicular to the plane of the page. When the w-s muscle force is either 2.0 or 3.0 times greater than the b-s muscle force, the resultant muscle force is located at points 2:1 or 3:1, respectively. When the position of the resultant adductor muscle force lies at 1:1 during biting along the left first molar, all points within triangle 1 experience compression, ie, a force directed away from the reader and into the plane of the page. If the resultant muscle force is positioned at 2:1 or 3:1 during biting along the first, second, or third molar, a similar situation prevails. In contrast, when the muscle force is positioned at 1.25:1 dur-

times larger than the b-s muscle force (another likely occurrence), the condylar forces are reversed, so that now the force on the b-s condyle is about 1.4 times larger than the force on the w-s condyle. When the w-s muscle force is equal to the b-s muscle force (a somewhat unlikely occurrence), the b-s condylar force is about 4.0 times larger than the w-s condylar force. Finally, when the b-s muscle force becomes larger than the w-s muscle force (an even more unlikely occurrence), the w-s condyle becomes unloaded or actually experiences tension.

This analysis demonstrates that differential loading of the mandibular condyles during isometric biting (and mastication) is highly dependent on slight shifts in muscle recruitment patterns (see Picq[119] for a similar analysis). Work in nonhuman primates[47,77,120,121] and humans[122–124]

ing biting along the third molar, the w-s (left) condyle is unloaded. Only the third molar and the b-s condyle need be loaded in compression to achieve static equilibrium at this time.

Finally, a very different situation prevails when the position of the resultant muscle force lies outside the triangle of support during biting along the third molar, ie, at 1:1. Under these conditions of equal muscle force on the working and balancing sides, the b-s condyle and the third molar are loaded in compression, but there is a tendency for the condyle (and disc) on the working side to lift off the articular eminence because the resultant muscle force causes the mandible to rotate about an axis defined by the triangle connecting the third molar and the b-s condyle (3). If this were to actually occur, presumably this would be countered by the TML. This is an unlikely occurrence simply because during third molar biting the w-s and b-s muscle forces are not equal. Instead, the usual occurrence is that w-s muscle force exceeds the b-s muscle force.[122,123]

When humans have unilateral TMJ pain, they often prefer to chew on the same side as the painful joint.[41] This has led some to suggest that it occurs because the b-s condylar forces normally exceed the w-s condylar forces.[127] That is, these subjects are attempting to avoid the larger reaction forces that normally occur along their b-s condyle. It is more likely, however, that patients prefer to chew on the painful side to minimize condylar movements during the power stroke of mastication, because the b-s condyle has a much larger excursive movement during chewing.[2,65,128]

Differential loading within the TMJ

In humans, the load-bearing portion of the TMJ is located along the articular surfaces of the articular eminence and the mandibular condyle. There is considerable evidence, however, that reaction forces within this articular region are not always equally distributed. The evidence for differential loading in the human TMJ initially came from studies on patterns of surface modeling and pathologic changes in the TMJ. For example, Moffett and coworkers[129] have shown that the lateral aspect of the human TMJ models differently than the medial aspect. Although these modeling patterns do not necessarily indicate the nature of the loading pattern, they do suggest possible differences in mechanical loading patterns within the TMJ.

A number of studies on degenerative changes in the human TMJ also suggest differential loading in the joint. For example, Oberg and coworkers[130] noted that the majority of articular disc perforations occur along the lateral aspect of the TMJ. Because pathologic changes in joints are

often related to local mechanical factors, these data indicate that the lateral aspect of the human TMJ experiences more stress (stress equals force per unit area), more "wear and tear," than the medial aspect. The distribution of glycosaminoglycans in the articular tissues of the human TMJ also indicates that the lateral aspect of the joint may experience more stress than the medial aspect.[131,132]

There are several possible reasons why the lateral aspect of the TMJ experiences more stress than its medial aspect.[2,133,134] One is related to mandibular distortions or strains that occur due to relatively large muscle and reaction forces.[33,115,135] Experiments on nonhuman primates indicate that the mandibular corpus is twisted during the power stroke of mastication and during isometric biting. This twisting, which results in eversion of the lower border of the mandible and inversion of the coronoid process, causes the lateral part of the mandibular condyle to be pressed more vigorously against the articular eminence than its medial part (Fig 1-26a). This presumably occurs to varying degrees on both the w-s and b-s condyles. The routine presence of these distortions is a reminder of the limitations associated with analyses that model the mandible as a perfectly rigid structure (see chapter 2). Instead, during forceful biting and chewing behavior, the mandible experiences a certain amount of distortion or deformation.

Perhaps the most important reason for differential loading in the TMJ during unilateral mastication is related to the mediolateral translation of the condyle relative to the articular eminence. As noted earlier, the w-s condyle experiences a lateral shift (Bennett shift or movement) during the opening stroke of mastication. This is followed by a medial shift of the same condyle from this lateral position during the closing and power strokes. The medial shift is not only correlated with the occurrence of maximum masticatory force (and therefore maximum condylar reaction force), but it is also associated with the w-s condyle's being positioned somewhat more laterally relative to the articular eminence. This causes the more lateral part of the condyle (and disc) to be pressed against the more lateral portion of the articular eminence (Fig 1-26b), while contact is reduced or lost between the medial half of the condyle, disc, and articular eminence.

Thus, throughout the early part of the power stroke, and into the phase I movement, the lateral aspect of the w-s TMJ may experience more force per unit area (stress) than its medial aspect because of the position of the condyle and disc relative to the articular eminence. When centric occlusion has been reached, the load-bearing portion of the condyle and eminence no longer has a steep medial-to-lateral gradient of increasing joint reaction force. Instead, the TMJ reaction force is more evenly distributed along the condyle, disc, and eminence. Phase II movement probably

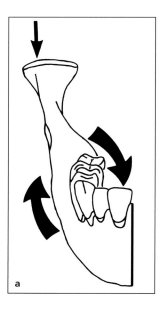
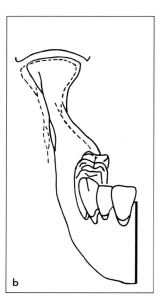

Fig 1-26 *(a)* Differential loading of the TMJ. The mandibular corpus during mastication and biting is twisted about its long axis. *(curved arrows)* Direction of twisting of the posterior half of the mandible. This pattern of twisting about the long axis of the mandibular corpus causes the *(straight arrow)* lateral aspect of the TMJ to receive a greater load than the medial aspect of the TMJ. *(b)* Mandibular condyle and articular eminence on the working-side (w-s) TMJ during mastication. The disc is not shown. *(dashed lines)* The w-s condyle is shifted laterally during the opening stroke of mastication. This movement causes the medial aspect of the mandibular condyle and the articular eminence to lose forceful contact with one another. This in turn causes the lateral aspect of the TMJ to receive a greater load than the medial aspect during jaw closing as the w-s condyle is moved back to its central position along the articular eminence (see text for discussion). (Modified from Hylander[2] with permission.)

does not result in significant differential loading in the TMJ simply because masticatory forces, and therefore condylar reaction forces, have declined considerably or are absent at this time.[82–84]

Although the b-s TMJ may frequently experience more overall force than the w-s TMJ during powerful chewing, as indicated earlier, presumably its articular surfaces will be more evenly loaded because the b-s condyle does not experience a mediolateral type of movement that modifies the position of the articular components and thereby causes large stress concentrations. Instead, the b-s condyle mainly translates posteriorly along the articular eminence (see chapter 2).

Summary

Descriptions of the morphology of the bony elements, disc, and fibrous capsule of the TMJ, as well as the attachment patterns and morphology of the muscles of the mandible, have provided the background for an analysis of mandibular movements, jaw muscle function, and mandibular biomechanics. These discussions served as the basis for an analysis of the nature of TMJ reaction forces during chewing and biting. This analysis demonstrates that TMJ reaction forces during unilateral mastication often vary between the balancing and working sides. In some instances, the w-s TMJ is loaded more than the b-s TMJ. However, the b-s TMJ is probably loaded more than the w-s TMJ during forceful unilateral chewing and biting. Differential loading likely occurs in the TMJ, with

the lateral portion of this joint being loaded more than the medial portion.

Acknowledgments

The author is indebted to the National Science Foundation and the National Institutes of Dental and Craniofacial Research for their more than 25 years of support for his work on the biomechanics of the primate masticatory apparatus.

References

1. Hylander WL. Mandibular function and temporomandibular joint loading. In: Carlson DS, McNamara JA, Ribbens KA (eds). Developmental Aspects of Temporomandibular Joint Disorder. Ann Arbor, MI: University of Michigan, 1985:19–35.
2. Hylander WL. Functional anatomy of the temporomandibular joint. In: Sarnat BG, Laskin DM (eds). The Temporomandibular Joint: A Biological Basis for Clinical Practice, ed 4. Philadelphia: Saunders, 1992:60–92.
3. Bouvier M, Hylander WL. The effect of dietary consistency on morphology of the mandibular condylar cartilage in young macaques (*Macaca mulatta*). In: Dixon AD, Sarnat BG (eds). Factors and Mechanisms Influencing Bone Growth. New York: Liss, 1982:569–579.
4. Duterloo HS, Jansen HW. Chondrogenesis and osteogenesis in the mandibular condylar blastema. Rep Congr Eur Orthod Soc 1969;109–118.

5. Dechow PC, Carlson DS. Development of mandibular form: Phylogeny, ontogeny, and function. In: McNeill C (ed). Science and Practice of Occlusion. Chicago: Quintessence, 1997:3–22.

6. Scapino RP. Morphology and mechanism of the jaw joint. In: McNeill C (ed). Science and Practice of Occlusion. Chicago: Quintessence, 1997:23–40.

7. Griffin CJ. The prevalence of the lateral subcondylar tubercle of the mandible in fossil and recent man with particular reference to Anglo-Saxons. Arch Oral Biol 1977;22:633–639.

8. Van der Linden EJ, Burdi AR, de Jongh HJ. Critical periods in the prenatal morphogenesis of the human lateral pterygoid muscle, the mandibular condyle, the articular disk, and medial articular capsule. Am J Orthod Dentofacial Orthop 1987;91:22–28.

9. Harpman JA, Woollard HA. The tendon of the lateral pterygoid muscle. J Anat 1938;73:112–115.

10. Griffin CJ, Sharpe CJ. The structure of the adult human temporomandibular meniscus. Aust Dent J 1960;5:190–195.

11. Rees L. The structure and function of the mandibular joint. Br Dent J 1954;96:125–133.

12. Meyenberg K, Kubik S, Palla S. Relationships of the muscles of mastication to the articular disc of the temporomandibular joint. Schweiz Monatsschr Zahnmed 1986;96:815–834.

13. Wilkinson TM. The relationship between the disk and the lateral pterygoid muscle in the human temporomandibular joint. J Prosthet Dent 1988;60:715–724.

14. Nickel JC, Iwasaki LR, McLachlan KR. Effect of the physical environment on growth of the temporomandibular joint. In: McNeill C (ed). Science and Practice of Occlusion. Chicago: Quintessence, 1997:115–124.

15. DuBrul EL. Oral Anatomy. St Louis: Ishiyaku-EuroAmerica, 1988.

16. Savalle WP. Some aspects of the morphology of the human temporomandibular joint capsule. Acta Anat 1988;131:292–296.

17. Nell A, Niebauer G, Sperr W, Firbas W. Special variations of the lateral ligament of the human TMJ. Clin Anat 1994;7:267–270.

18. Koolstra JH, Naeije M, van Eijden TMGJ. The three-dimensional active envelope of jaw border movements and its determinants. J Dent Res 2001;80:1908–1912.

19. Moss M. Functional anatomy of the temporomandibular joint. In: Schwartz L (ed). Disorders of the Temporomandibular Joint: Diagnosis, Management, Relation to Occlusion of Teeth. Philadelphia: Saunders, 1959.

20. Widmalm SE, Lillie JH, Ash MM Jr. Anatomical and electromyographic studies of the lateral pterygoid muscle. J Oral Rehabil 1987;14:429–446.

21. Oxnard CE. Contribution of the analysis of form. Am Zool 1980;20:695–705.

22. Oxnard CE. The Order of Man: A Biomathematical Anatomy of the Primates. New Haven, CT: Yale University Press, 1984.

23. Honée GL. The anatomy of the lateral pterygoid muscle. Acta Morphol Neerl Scand 1972;10:331–340.

24. Schumacher GH. Funktionelle Morphologie der Kaumuskulatur. Jena, Germany: Fischer, 1961.

25. Stern JT Jr. Essentials of Gross Anatomy. Philadelphia: Davis, 1988.

26. Moritz T, Ewer R. Der ansatz des musculus pterygoideus lateralis am kiefergelenk des menschen. Dtsch Zahnarztl Z 1987;42:680–685.

27. Sicher H. Functional anatomy of the temporomandibular joint. In: Sarnat BG (ed). The Temporomandibular Joint, ed 2. Springfield, IL: Thomas, 1964:28–57.

28. Wilkinson TM, Maryniuk GA. Sequential sagittal dissections of the temporomandibular joint. J Dent Res 1983;62:655.

29. Gibbs CH, Mahan PE, Wilkinson TM, Mauderli A. EMG activity of the superior belly of the lateral pterygoid muscle in relation to other jaw muscles. J Prosthet Dent 1984;51:691–702.

30. Lipke DP, Gay T, Gross BD, Yaeger JA. An electromyographic study of the human lateral pterygoid muscle [abstract]. J Dent Res 1977;56B:230.

31. McNamara JA Jr. The independent functions of the two heads of the lateral pterygoid muscle. Am J Anat 1973;138:197–205.

32. Wood WW, Takada K, Hannam AG. The electromyographic activity of the inferior part of the human lateral pterygoid muscle during clenching and chewing. Arch Oral Biol 1986;31:245–253.

33. Hylander WL. An experimental analysis of temporomandibular joint reaction force in macaques. Am J Phys Anthropol 1979;51:433–456.

34. Hylander WL, Johnson KR, Crompton AW. Loading patterns and jaw movements during mastication in *Macaca fascicularis*: A bone-strain, electromyographic, and cineradiographic analysis. Am J Phys Anthropol 1987;72:287–314.

35. Rack PM, Westbury DR. The short range stiffness of active mammalian muscle and its effect on mechanical properties. J Physiol (Lond) 1974;240:331–350.

36. Crompton AW, Cook P, Hiiemae K, Thexton AJ. Movement of the hyoid apparatus during chewing. Nature 1975;258:69–70.

37. Palmer JB, Rudin NJ, Lara G, Crompton AW. Coordination of mastication and swallowing. Dysphagia 1992;7:187–200.

38. Cartmill M, Hylander WL, Shafland J. Human Structure. Cambridge, MA: Harvard University Press, 1990.

39. Merlini L, Palla S. The relationship between condylar rotation and anterior translation in healthy and clicking temporomandibular joints. Schweiz Monatsschr Zahnmed 1988;98:1191–1199.

40. Posselt U. Physiology of Occlusion and Rehabilitation. Oxford: Blackwell Scientific, 1968.

41. Ramfjord SP, Ash MM Jr. Occlusion. Philadelphia: Saunders, 1971.

42. Ahlgren J. Mechanism of mastication: A quantitative cinematographic and electromyographic study of masticatory movements in children, with special reference to occlusion of the teeth. Acta Odontol Scand 1966;24(suppl 44):1–109.

43. Carlsöö S. Nervous coordination and mechanical function of the mandibular elevators. Acta Odontol Scand 1952;10(suppl 2):1–132.

44. Hannam AG, Wood WW. Medial pterygoid muscle activity during the closing and compressive phases of human mastication. Am J Phys Anthropol 1981;55:359–367.

45. Hiiemae KM. Mammalian mastication: A review of the activity of the jaw muscles and movements they produce in chewing. In: Butler PM, Joysey KA (eds). Development, Function and Evolution of Teeth. New York: Academic Press, 1978:359–398.

46. Hylander WL, Johnson KR. Temporalis and masseter muscle function during incision in macaques and humans. Int J Primatol 1985;6:289–322.

47. Hylander WL, Johnson KR, Crompton AW. Muscle force recruitment and biomechanical modeling: An analysis of masseter muscle function in *Macaca fascicularis*. Am J Phys Anthropol 1992;88:365–387.

48. Møller E. The chewing apparatus: An electromyographic study of the action of the muscles of mastication and its correlation to facial morphology. Acta Physiol Scand 1966;69(suppl 280):1–229.

49. Møller E. Action of the muscles of mastication. In: Kawamura Y (ed). Frontiers of Oral Physiology. Basel: Karger, 1974:121–158.

50. Stohler CS, Yamada Y, Ash MM Jr. Non-linear amplification of electromyographic signals with particular application to human chewing. Arch Oral Biol 1985;30:217–219.

51. Stohler CS, Yamada Y, Ash MM Jr. Antagonistic muscle stiffness and associated reflex behavior in the pain-dysfunctional state. Helv Odontol Acta 1985;29:13–20.

52. Vitti M, Basmajian JV. Integrated actions of masticatory muscles: Simultaneous EMG from eight intramuscular electrodes. Anat Rec 1977;187:173–189.

53. Wood WW. Medial pterygoid muscle activity during chewing and clenching. J Prosthet Dent 1986;55:615–621.

54. Phanachet I, Whittle T, Wanigaratne K, Klineberg IJ, Sessle BJ, Murray GM. Functional heterogeneity in the superior head of the human lateral pterygoid. J Dent Res 2003; 82:106–111.

55. van Eijden TMGJ, Koolstra JH. A model for mylohyoid muscle mechanics. J Biomech 1998;31:1017–1024.

56. Jankelson B, Hoffman GM, Hendron JA. Physiology of the stomatognathic system. J Am Dent Assoc 1953;46:375–386.

57. Sheppard IM. Incisive and related movements of the mandible. J Prosthet Dent 1964;14:898–906.

58. Gibbs CH, Messerman T, Reswick JB, Derda HJ. Functional movements of the mandible. J Prosthet Dent 1971;26: 604–620.

59. Gibbs CH, Reswick JB, Messerman T. Functional movements of the mandible. In: Engineering Design Center Report No. EDC 4-69-24. Cleveland: Case Western Reserve University, 1969:159–184.

60. Kay RF, Hiiemae KM. Jaw movement and tooth use in recent and fossil primates. Am J Phys Anthropol 1974;40:227–256.

61. Mills JRE. The relationship between tooth patterns and jaw movements in the Hominoidea. In: Butler PM, Joysey KA (eds). Development, Function and Evolution of Teeth. New York: Academic Press, 1978:341–353.

62. Gibbs CH. Electromyographic activity during the motionless period in chewing. J Prosthet Dent 1975;34:35–40.

63. Yeager JA. Mandibular path in the grinding phase of mastication—A review. J Prosthet Dent 1978;39:569–573.

64. Belser UC, Hannam AG. The contribution of the deep fibers of the masseter muscle to selected tooth-clenching and chewing tasks. J Prosthet Dent 1986;56:629–638.

65. Hylander WL. The human mandible: Lever or link? Am J Phys Anthropol 1975;43:227–242.

66. Greenfield BE, Wyke BD. Electromyographic studies of some of the muscles of mastication. Br Dent J 1956;100:129–143.

67. Latif A. An electromyographic study of the temporalis muscle in normal persons during selected positions and movements of the mandible. Am J Orthod 1957;43:577–591.

68. Pruzansky S. The application of electromyography to dental research. J Am Dent Assoc 1952;44:49–68.

69. Stohler CS, Ashton-Miller JA, Carlson DS. The effects of pain from the mandibular joint and muscles on masticatory motor behaviour in man. Arch Oral Biol 1988;33:175–182.

70. Winnberg A, Pancherz H. Head posture and masticatory muscle function. An EMG investigation. Eur J Orthod 1983;5:209–217.

71. Hylander WL, Wall CE, Vinyard CJ, et al. Temporalis function in anthropoids and strepsirrhines: An EMG study. Am J Phys Anthropol 2005;(in press).

72. Weijs WA. Evolutionary approach of masticatory motor patterns in mammals. In: Bels VL, Chardon M, Vandewalle P (eds). Biomechanics of Feeding in Vertebrates. Berlin: Springer-Verlag, 1994:282–320.

73. Herring SW. The dynamics of mastication in pigs. Arch Oral Biol 1976;21:473–480.

74. Herring SW. Morphological correlates of masticatory patterns in peccaries and pigs. J Mamm 1985;66:603–617.

75. Herring SW. The ontogeny of mammalian mastication. Am Zool 1985;25:339–349.

76. Herring SW. Muscles of mastication: Architecture and functional organization. In: Davidovitch Z (ed). Biological Mechanisms of Tooth Movement and Craniofacial Adaptation. Columbus, OH: Ohio State University, College of Dentistry, 1992:541–548.

77. Herring SW. Epigenetic and functional influences on skull growth. In: Hanken J, Hall BK (eds). The Skull, vol 1. Development. Chicago: University of Chicago, 1993:153–206.

78. Graf H. Occlusal forces during function. In: Rowe NH (ed). Occlusion: Research in Form and Function. Ann Arbor, MI: University of Michigan School of Dentistry, 1975:90–109.

79. Phanachet I, Wanigaratne K, Whittle T, Uchida S, Peeceeyen S, Murray GM. A method for standardizing jaw displacements in the horizontal plane while recording single motor unit activity in the human lateral pterygoid muscle. J Neurosci Meth 2001;105:201–210.

80. Phanachet I, Whittle T, Wanigaratne K, Murray GM. Functional properties of single motor units in inferior head of human lateral pterygoid muscle: Task relations and thresholds. J Neurophysiol 2001;86:2204–2218.

81. Hylander WL. Mechanical properties of food and recruitment of masseter force [abstract]. J Dent Res 1983;62:297.

82. Hylander WL, Crompton AW. Loading patterns and jaw movements during the masticatory power stroke in macaques. Am J Phys Anthropol 1980;52:239.

83. Hylander WL, Picq PG, Johnson KR. A preliminary stress analysis of the circumorbital region in *Macaca fascicularis*. Am J Phys Anthropol 1987;72:214.

84. Wall CE, Vinyard CJ, Johnson KR, Williams SH, Hylander WL. A preliminary study of the phase II occlusal movements during chewing in *Papio*. Am J Phys Anthropol 2005;(in press).

85. Smith JM, Savage RJG. The mechanics of mammalian jaws. School Sci Rev 1959;141:289–301.

86. Davis DD. The giant panda: A morphological study of evolutionary mechanisms. Fieldiana: Zool Memoirs 1964;3:1–339.

87. Smith RJ. Functions of condylar translation in human mandibular movement. Am J Orthod 1985;88:191–202.

88. Smith RJ. Comparative functional morphology of maximum mandibular opening (gape) in primates. In: Chivers DJ, Wood BA, Bilsborough A (eds). Food Acquisition and Processing in Primates. New York: Plenum Press, 1984:231–255.

89. Grant PG. Biomechanical significance of the instantaneous center of rotation: The human temporomandibular joint. J Biomech 1973;6:109–113.

90. Gallo LM, Fushima K, Palla S. Mandibular helical axis pathways during mastication. J Dent Res 2000;79:1566–1572.

91. Carlson DS. Condylar translation and the function of the superficial masseter muscle in the rhesus monkey (*M mulatta*). Am J Phys Anthropol 1977;47:53–63.

92. Hylander WL. Incisal bite force direction in humans and the functional significance of mammalian mandibular translation. Am J Phys Anthropol 1978;48:1–8.

93. Weijs WA, Korfage JAM, Langenbach GEJ. The functional significance of the position of the centre of rotation for jaw opening and closing in the rabbit. J Anat 1989;162:133–148.

94. Carlson FD, Wilkie DR. Muscle Physiology. Englewood Cliffs, NJ: Prentice-Hall, 1974.

95. Gysi A. Studies on the leverage problem of the mandible. Dent Dig 1921;27:74–84, 144–150, 203–208.

96. Picq PG, Plavcan JM, Hylander WL. Nonlever action of the mandible: The return of the hydra. Am J Phys Anthropol 1987;74:305–307.

97. Ryder SA. On the mechanical genesis of tooth forms. Proc Acad Nat Sci Philadelphia 1878;79:45–80.

98. Frank L. Muscular influence on occlusion as shown by x-rays of the condyle. Dent Dig 1950;56:484–488.

99. Frankel VH, Burstein AH. Orthopaedic Biomechanics. Philadelphia: Lea & Febiger, 1970.

100. Roberts D. The etiology of the temporomandibular joint dysfunction syndrome. Am J Orthod 1974;66:498–515.

101. Roberts D, Tattersall I. Skull form and the mechanics of mandibular elevation in mammals. Am Mus Nat Hist Novitates 1974;2536:1–9.

102. Robinson M. The temporomandibular joint: Theory of reflex controlled nonlever action of the mandible. J Am Dent Assoc 1946;33:1260–1271.

103. Scott JH. A contribution to the study of mandibular joint function. Br Dent J 1955;98:345–349.

104. Steinhardt G. Anatomy and function of the temporomandibular joint. Int Dent J 1958;8:155–156.

105. Tattersall I. Cranial anatomy of the Archaeolemurinae (Lemuroidea, Primates). Anthropol Pap Am Mus Nat Hist 1973;52:1–110.

106. Taylor RMS. Nonlever action of the mandible. Am J Phys Anthropol 1986;70:417–421.

107. Wilson GH. The anatomy and physics of the temporomandibular joint. 2. J Natl Dent Assoc 1921;8:236–241.

108. Wilson GH. The anatomy and physics of the temporomandibular joint. 1. J Natl Dent Assoc 1920;7:414–420.

109. Kubein-Meesenburg D, Nagerl H, Schwestka-Polly R, Fanghanel J. Principles of general joint mechanics: Occlusal and articular morphology and mandibular movements. In: Proceedings of the 10th International Symposium on Dental Morphology. Berlin: M Marketing-Services, 1995:406–410.

110. Smith RJ. Mandibular biomechanics and temporomandibular joint function in primates. Am J Phys Anthropol 1978;49:341–350.

111. Crompton AW, Hiiemae K. How mammalian molar teeth work. Discovery 1969;5:23–34.

112. Davis DD. Masticatory apparatus in the spectacled bear *Tremarctos ornatus*. Fieldiana: Zoology 1955;37:25–46.

113. Turnbull WD. Mammalian masticatory apparatus. Fieldiana: Geology 1970;18:149–356.

114. Stern JT Jr. Biomechanical significance of the instantaneous center of rotation: the human temporomandibular joint. J Biomech 1974;7:109–110.

115. Hylander WL. Mandibular function in *Galago crassicaudatus* and *Macaca fascicularis*: An in vivo approach to stress analysis of the mandible. J Morphol 1979;159:253–296.

116. Nelson GJ. Three Dimensional Computer Modeling of Human Mandibular Biomechanics [thesis]. Vancouver: University of British Columbia, 1986:149–262.

117. Osborn JW, Baragar FA. Predicted pattern of human muscle activity during clenching derived from a computer assisted model: Symmetric vertical bite forces. J Biomech 1985;18:599–612.

118. Smith DM, McLachlan KR, McCall WD Jr. A numerical model of temporomandibular joint loading. J Dent Res 1986;65:1046–1052.

119. Picq PG. L'articulation temporo-mandibulaire des hominidés fossiles: Anatomie comparée, biomécanique, évolution, biométrie. Mem Sci Terre 1983;83-17:1–183.

120. Vinyard CJ, Williams SH, Wall CE, Johnson KR, Hylander WL. Jaw-muscle electromyography during chewing in Belanger's treeshrews (*Tupaia belangeri*). Am J Phys Anthropol 2005:(in press).

121. Hylander WL, Ravosa MJ, Ross CF, Wall CE, Johnson KR. Symphyseal fusion and jaw-adductor muscle force: An EMG study. Am J Phys Anthropol 2000;112:469–492.

122. Spencer M. Force production in the primate masticatory system: Electromyographic tests of biomechanical hypotheses. J Hum Evol 1998;34:25–54.

123. Spencer M. Constraints on masticatory system evolution in anthropoid primates. Am J Phys Anthropol 1999;108:483–506.

124. Blanksma NG, van Eijden TMGJ. Electromyographic heterogeneity in the human temporalis and masseter muscles during static biting, open/close excursions, and chewing. J Dent Res 1995;74:1318–1327.

125. Druzinsky RE, Greaves WS. A model to explain the posterior limit of the bite point in reptiles. J 1979;160:165–168.

126. Greaves WS. The jaw lever system in ungulates: A new model. J Zool Lond 1978;184:271–285.

127. Naeije M, Hofman N. Biomechanics of the human temporomandibular joint during chewing. J Dent Res 2003;82:528–531.

128. Hylander WL. Functional anatomy. In: Sarnat BG, Laskin DM (eds). The Temporomandibular Joint: A Biological Basis for Clinical Practice, ed 3. Springfield, IL: Thomas, 1980:85–113.

129. Moffett BC, Johnson LC, McCabe JB, Askew HC. Articular remodeling in the adult human temporomandibular joint. Am J Anat 1964;115:119–142.

130. Oberg T, Carlsson GE, Fajers CM. The temporomandibular joint. A morphologic study on a human autopsy material. Acta Odontol Scand 1971;29:349–384.

131. Kopp S. Topographical distribution of sulphated glycosaminoglycans in human temporomandibular joint disks. A histochemical study of an autopsy material. J Oral Pathol 1976;5:265–276.

132. Kopp S. Topographical distribution of sulfated glycosaminoglycans in the surface layers of the human temporomandibular joint. A histochemical study of an autopsy material. J Oral Pathol 1978;7:283–294.

133. Beek M, Koolstra JH, van Ruijven LJ, van Eijden TMGJ. Three-dimensional finite element analysis of the human temporomandibular joint disc. J Biomech 2000;33:307–316.

134. Werner JA, Tillmann B, Schleicher A. Functional anatomy of the temporomandibular joint. Anat Embryol 1991;183:89–95.

135. Korioth TWP. Simulated physics of the human mandible. In: McNeill C (ed). Science and Practice of Occlusion. Chicago: Quintessence, 1997:179–186.

Anatomy and Function of the TMJ

Ales Obrez and Luigi M. Gallo

Mandibular anatomy and function have long been of great interest to biomedical scientists and clinicians. One major objective has been to understand and record the mandibular border movements in order to design and fabricate an articulator that in theory represents the mechanical equivalent of the maxillomandibular complex in vivo. Thus, the properly designed articulator essentially allows the clinician to replicate the patient's mandibular border movements and simulate mandibular function. The use of an accurately designed articulator is often seen as an essential prerequisite for those patients who require more extensive dental rehabilitation. In these cases, the majority of the prosthesis fabrication process is accomplished indirectly in the laboratory setting, away from the patient.

Most articulators are based on the concept of "ideal dental occlusion" and "ideal maxillomandibular articulation." This in turn has been based on empirical and/or scientific evidence about dental and temporomandibular joint (TMJ) morphology, mandibular movements, and mandibular function. Studies on mandibular movements range from simple extraoral observations of the mandible to more sophisticated tracings of the condyle itself during the mandibular border and functional movements. Because of the complexity of the TMJ, as well as inaccuracies in extraoral observations, progress toward a full understanding of mandibular movement has been slow.

Depending on its design, articulators may have adjustable articular analogs. The "articular fossa" of the articulator is the mechanical equivalent of the articular fossa of the mandible, while the "condylar ball" is the equivalent of the mandibular condyle. Clinical dentistry has accepted the theory that each individual adjustment of the articular complex is possible if mandibular border movements are correctly recorded on the patient and then transferred to the articulator. The transfer of the condylar path during mandibular border movements for the purpose of articulator adjustment is advocated because such movements are much less variable than are functional movements (eg, chewing). Mandibular border movements are extreme movements and, by definition, constrained by the anatomic features of the skeletal, ligamentous, dental, and muscular components of the masticatory system. Functional movements, in contrast, are primarily influenced by the neuromuscular system and by the nature of the food that is being masticated (eg, consistency and size of the bolus).

Based on the presumed intraindividual reproducibility and stability of the TMJ morphology and the mandibular border movements, several underlying concepts have maintained their prominence in clinical dentistry throughout the years:

1. Properly functioning condyles normally rotate more than translate during the initial portion of simple mandibular opening.
2. There is only one stationary axis of condylar rotation during the initial stage of assisted opening and closing.
3. The position of the transverse axis of rotation during initial mandibular opening determines a repeatable mandibular position.
4. This defined reference position of the mandible is fixed in relation to the cranium throughout life.

5. By definition, this position coincides with the centric relation (CR) position of the condyle.

6. In the sagittal plane, this transverse axis of rotation is invariably located within or in close proximity to the condylar head.

7. This axis of rotation is readily transferable to an articulator.

With the advancement of science and technology, however, it is now possible to analyze the TMJ in three dimensions during mandibular function with a high degree of precision. Based on these types of analyses, information has emerged that now challenges traditional understanding of TMJ function and its interpretations. The concept of one stationary transverse axis, as well as the concept that TMJ function and morphology remain stable throughout life, have been questioned as a result of extensive jaw-tracking, biometric, and morphologic studies. Consequently, it is now generally accepted that there are significant intraindividual and interindividual variations in human TMJ morphology and function, including significant variation in the various spatial relationships of the TMJ components, irrespective of the instantaneous position of the mandible during its movement.

This variation is a result of a continuous and often changing relationship between the morphology and the function of the TMJ. As mandibular function influences long-term processes such as growth, development, and modeling or remodeling of the joint, it also causes immediate reversible changes in morphology of the TMJ components as a result of their unique structural properties. In turn, morphology of the joint components in part influences the biomechanics of the TMJ.

To present this relationship in a comprehensive way, this chapter starts with a review of the essential background knowledge of the TMJ morphology as it relates to condylar function. It is followed by a description of the evolution of the kinematic studies related to mandibular function. The chapter concludes with a synthesis of the current understanding of TMJ morphology as it relates to TMJ function based on studies using the latest kinematic methods.

Morphology

To establish a reproducible maxillomandibular position in patients without occlusal support or stable interocclusal relationships, clinicians have generally relied on the concept of mandibular CR. Historically, this mandibular position has been described in terms of the anatomic relationships among the condylar head, the articulating disc, and the articulating fossa and is thus independent of tooth contact.[1,2] Although defined strictly within the context of anatomic relationships of the various components of the TMJ, clinical use of CR has been based on the assumptions that (1) the normal reference condylar position coincides with the position of the condyles as they rotate around their stationary transverse axis and (2) this condylar axis is readily recordable and transferable to the articulator. To relate this definition to current understanding of mandibular biomechanics, a brief review of pertinent TMJ morphology is necessary (also see chapter 1).

The TMJ is anatomically classified as a synovial diarthrosis, an articulation between the condylar head and squamous portion of the temporal bone (see Fig 1-1). The condylar process of the mandible forms the mandibular part of the TMJ. The condylar head is not a perfect geometric shape. In frontal view, the condylar head appears more like a tent-shaped structure.[3] Two distinctive surfaces can be observed to slope divergently, medially and laterally, from the crest of the condylar convexity. The lateral part of the disc and the temporomandibular ligament attach to the lateral pole of the condyle. The medial pole provides an attachment only for the disc.

In a lateral view, the condylar head shows an irregular convex structure. Two distinctive surfaces can also be observed to slope divergently, anteriorly and posteriorly, from the crest of the condylar convexity (see Fig 1-2). When viewed in the horizontal plane, the long axis of the condyle is positioned in both the mediolateral and anteroposterior directions. Thus, in this plane, the long axes of both left and right condylar heads are not directly aligned with each other. Instead, these axes cross each other anterior to the foramen magnum, forming an angle that ranges from 140 to 160 degrees.

Condylar Head

The superior and anterior surfaces of the condylar head are the articulating areas. There is significant variation in form and size of the condylar head as well as in the outline of the articular fossa and the articular eminence.[4-9] In both males and females, condylar asymmetry between the left and right sides is often significant.[4] The shape of the condylar head varies from rounded to flattened on its superior surface.[10-12] In approximately 5% of individuals, changes in the general form of the condylar head occur during development.[10] In addition, the condylar head is rounder in younger individuals than in adults.

The actual form of the condylar head depends on the thickness of the connective tissue layers covering it.[13,14]

For example, on the anterior slope of the condylar head, the layers are thicker than on the posterior slope. The thickness of the articular layers is thought to correlate with the amount of load exerted on the condylar surface.[15] Thus, thicker layers are thought to be associated with higher loads.

Glenoid Fossa

The glenoid (or mandibular) fossa is the temporal component of the TMJ. It is a concave area on the inferior part of the squama of the temporal bone (see Fig 1-2). The functional part of the glenoid fossa, ie, the region that is covered by the articular tissue, is called the *articular fossa*.[16] The general shape of the articular fossa is irregular and does not uniformly conform to the shape of the condylar head. Although concave both mediolaterally and anteroposteriorly, it is larger mediolaterally than anteroposteriorly.[7] Similar to the condylar head, the articular fossa can vary significantly in form.[5] These variations in form appear to be independent of the shape of the condylar head.[17]

The articular fossa is bordered anteriorly by the posterior slope of the articular eminence, medially and superiorly by the wall of the temporal bone, and posteriorly by the postglenoid process or tubercle (see Figs 1-1 and 1-3). Posteriorly, the postglenoid process borders the tympanic plate. This process separates the external acoustic meatus from the area of the TMJ. Between these two structures are the squamotympanic fissure (which does not always exist as a separate entity), separating medially into the petrosquamosal fissure (medioanteriorly), and the petrotympanic fissure (medioposteriorly).[18] The chorda tympani nerve (providing taste sensation to the anterior two thirds of the tongue) and minor blood vessels pass through the petrotympanic fissure. Because the petrotympanic fissure is located posterior to the area of the condylar movements, impingement of the condyle on these structures is not likely.[3,19] The three fissures divide the articular fossa into a larger anterior portion and a smaller posterior portion (see Fig 1-3).

The posterior part supports loose retroarticular tissue composed of connective tissue, fat, veins, and nerves.[18,20] Between the posterior wall of the articular fossa and the tympanic plate of the external auditory meatus is the postglenoid tubercle or postglenoid (retroarticular) process, a bony ridge (posterior articular lip) that extends inferiorly. This is the site of attachment for the articular capsule. In many individuals, this ridge is wider on its lateral part.[3,16]

The anterior part of the articular fossa gradually continues anteriorly to the articular eminence, the preglenoid plane, and the infratemporal fossa (see Fig 1-3). Both the articular fossa and eminence contribute to the articulating surface of the TMJ. When viewed in a sagittal plane, they form an S-shaped profile. The steepness of the articular eminence increases during development. At birth, the eminence is flat[21]; as development progresses, the eminence becomes increasingly more prominent. Similarly, with loss of the teeth, the eminence flattens.[22,23] The eminence often flattens with increased function.

The bony roof of the glenoid fossa is thin compared to the surrounding bones. The thinness of this roof precludes heavy condylar loading, indicating that most condylar loads are directed toward the posterior slope of the articular eminence. The nonarticulating surfaces of the glenoid fossa (roof and posterior part) are covered by a thin, vascularized layer of fibrous connective tissue, very similar to periosteum.

Articular Disc

The articular disc, a structure of dense fibrous connective tissue, is interposed between the condylar head and the articular fossa, articular eminence, and preglenoid plane (see Fig 1-2). The disc divides the joint cavity into the two completely separated compartments, the upper discotemporal space and the lower discomandibular space.[24,25] Both compartments are filled with a plasmalike (synovial) fluid, secreted by cells of the synovial lining.

The morphology of the TMJ disc is assumed to compensate for the incongruities between the temporal and mandibular components of the joint during function. In the frontal view, the inferior, concave surface of the disc matches the articular surface of the condylar head. The superior surface of the disc is slightly convex, fitting the concave surface of the articular fossa. The articular disc is firmly attached to the medial and lateral poles of the condyle. These attachments prevent excessive mediolateral mobility of the disc during condylar movements.

In the parasagittal view (anteroposterior section through the joint), the articular disc is divided morphologically into three parts: an anterior band (AB), a thinner intermediate zone (IZ), and a (broader) posterior band (PB). The PB is the thickest. Both the PB and IZ thin laterally; the thinnest portion is located on the most lateral aspect of the IZ (0.4 mm). The AB does not differ in its thickness mediolaterally. The most common explanation for the differential thickness of the disc in the mediolateral direction is the differential loading pattern during mandibular movements (discussed later in the chapter).[15]

Similar to the articular surfaces of the condyle and the articular fossa, the mature articular surface of the disc is not innervated by sensory (nociceptive) nerves. However, during early human postnatal growth, the disc is vascularized throughout its extent and has an abundant supply of fibroblasts.[26,27] During growth, the central part of the articular disc becomes avascular, lacking innervation.[28,29] The fibrous connective tissue of the articular disc is similar in structure to that found lining the condylar head and articular fossa.

As in the superficial fibrous layers of the condylar head and articular fossa, the disc has a relatively random arrangement of predominately type I collagen fibrils, elastic fibers, and glycosaminoglycans comprised of chondroitin sulfate, dermatan sulfate, hyaluronic acid, and keratin sulfate.[30–32] The detailed structure of the individual regions of the disc varies. The IZ of the disc is remarkable for the predominantly wavy anteroposterior orientation of its collagen fibrils.[33–35] The most superficial layers of the IZ (ie, surfaces facing the condylar head and articular fossa) are composed of collagen fibrils that, although primarily arranged in the anteroposterior direction, can also form a randomized pattern in the horizontal plane. These two layers surround the deeper, more loosely arranged connective tissue layer. The latter part of the IZ has thicker and anteroposteriorly oriented collagen fibrils.[36] This specific arrangement of the fibers becomes pronounced as the TMJ matures.[37]

These fibrils in the IZ continue anteriorly and posteriorly, where they become interwoven with the three-dimensional framework of the collagen fibrils, which is the primary structural feature of the AB and PB of the articular disc. The dominant orientation of the fibers in both of these regions of the disc is in the lateromedial and superoinferior directions. Fibers from the PB continue medially and laterally and attach the disc to the subcondylar bone immediately below the medial and lateral poles of the condyles.

The elastic fibers are predominantly located within the superficial layers of the margins of the IZ and follow the general direction of the collagen fibrils. They are of smaller diameter than those found in the AB and PB, as well as in all of the disc attachment tissues.[38]

The mature articular disc contains only a small amount of fibrocartilage cells, predominantly located around its periphery. Whereas the presence of cartilage cells in the central part of the articular disc is likely related to load bearing of the TMJ, this is not true for the periphery of the disc.[39]

As part of the intercellular matrix, the proteoglycan components are primarily chondroitin-6-sulfate and/or dermatan sulfate.[40,41] Concentrations of the individual components are reported to vary with the area of the disc. The highest concentrations are along the surface layer in the IZ. It has been suggested that even in this zone the concentration of proteoglycans is not uniform.[41]

Proteoglycans, along with adjacent collagen fibrils, play a very important role in the resistance and distribution of the compressive forces that are applied to the TMJ during joint loading. Fluid within the body of the disc redistributes itself as the load is applied. It is still not clear whether the difference in the local concentrations of proteoglycans in the IZ has a direct effect on the pattern of redistribution of the fluid in this zone during loading. However, it has been hypothesized that excessive and repetitive loading of the same part of the disc (eg, during clenching) prevents a uniform exchange of fluid throughout the disc and articular areas. It has also been hypothesized that this phenomenon represents the initial stage of mechanical failure of the TMJ, leading ultimately to the development of arthropathy.[42]

The PB of the articular disc continues posteriorly into the richly innervated and vascularized posterior attachment tissue, the bilaminar zone. The posterior attachment is histologically defined as fibroelastic, and its surface is covered by a synovial layer. The posterior attachment can be divided into the temporal, intermediate, and condylar layers or laminae.[35,43,44] The temporal layer or lamina attaches to the most superoposterior areas of the glenoid fossa: the postglenoid process posteriorly, the posterior articular lip, and medially into the petrosquamosal and tympanosquamosal fissures unless the fissures are missing.[18] The inferior lamina is attached to the posterior region of the condylar neck (see Fig 1-2).

Between these two laminae is a loose connective tissue (intermediate portion) that is innervated by sensory fibers, most likely within the vicinity of the local arteries.[20] These blood vessels supply most of the articular disc except for the avascular IZ.[21] The volume of the posterior attachment increases significantly when the disc-condyle complex moves anteriorly, primarily because of the influx of venous blood into the venous plexus that is situated within the intermediate layer of the posterior attachment. Change in volume of the attachment is accompanied by change in its shape and rearrangement of its components.[43,44]

The AB is continuous anteriorly as the anterior (discal) attachment, and it inserts along the anterior margin of the preglenoid plane, well anterior to the articular eminence. The anterior attachment is thicker laterally and thinner medially, where some of the fibers from the AB often appear to be continuous with the superior head of the lateral pterygoid muscle (anteromedially) and probably with the fibers of the masseter and temporal muscles (laterally).[45,46]

The articular disc is firmly attached below the medial and lateral sides (poles) of the condylar head by the collateral (polar) ligaments. Laterally the disc is separated from the articular capsule, while anteriorly the disc continues into this capsule and, in many cases, through the anterior attachment into the tendon of the superior belly of the lateral pterygoid muscle.[47,48]

Articular Capsule

The articular capsule is laterally reinforced by the temporomandibular ligament. This ligament, which has often been described as having both lateral (superficial) and medial (deep) components or layers, is assumed to provide limitations to condylar movements. The major difference between these two layers is in their orientation, caused by their differential attachment to the mandible (see Fig 1-5). The lateral portion originates from the lateral part of the articular tubercle and inserts into the posterior aspect of the lateral side of the condylar neck.[16] The more delicate medial portion has a horizontal orientation and attaches more superiorly on the lateral pole of the condylar head. Because of the superficial position of the temporomandibular ligament relative to the articular capsule, both layers of the ligament attach to the condylar neck inferior to the lateral attachment of the articular capsule.

Historical Review of Studies of Mandibular Movement

The current understanding of condylar function is not complete without a brief review of the development of approaches and methods used to study mandibular movement. The difficulty in developing a system that meets all the requirements necessary to record jaw movement may well explain why so many approaches were taken and different jaw-tracking devices developed. Ideally, such a device should be simple to use but should not be invasive, interfere with hard and soft tissue function, or restrict head movements. In addition, this system should also record mandibular movements in all three dimensions simultaneously with six degrees of freedom.

Only since the development of three-dimensional tracking systems supplemented with sophisticated mathematical transformation of obtained data has it been possible to estimate condylar movements relatively accurately. It is important to stress, however, that all of these systems assume that the mandible is a rigid body, free from bony deformations during mandibular loading.

Two-Dimensional Analysis

Jaw tracking approach

The first analyses of mandibular movement were two-dimensional observations and were mainly studied in the sagittal plane. Because the mandibular condyles are not directly accessible, two approaches were used. The first was purely mechanical, by recording the path of a point lateral to the condyle during mandibular border movements. These movements were traced by a pointer that was rigidly connected to a face-bow and firmly attached to the mandibular teeth (eg, kinematic facebow).

The second, or electro-optical, approach was more sophisticated and involved the use of small markers (in most cases light-emitting diodes), commonly attached to the maxillary and mandibular incisors. Their motion was recorded by sets of cameras. The condylar movement was then calculated by using the geometric relationship between the tracked points and the condyle. Both methods provided information about the condylar movement during superoinferior and anteroposterior translations. However, the electro-optical method had the advantage of the acquisition of a third degree of freedom, ie, rotation, in the parasagittal plane.

As with all anaylses of moving objects, the results of the electro-optical approach to analyze condylar motion during unassisted mandibular opening and closing are described as a combination of rotation and translation. The contribution of each component during the movement changes and is directly related to the amount of mandibular opening. The initial part of opening consists of predominantly condylar rotation that occurs around a stationary transverse axis. If the clinician making the analysis is skilled and the patient is cooperative, this axis is readily localized and used to relate the mandible to the cranium with its condyles in CR position. This position is further recognized as the most repeatable reference position of a mandible as well as a starting point from which all border and functional mandibular movements can be made. As the mandible continues to open, the contribution of anterior translation to the condylar movement increases. These methods, and the results of the studies that used them, have influenced the development of initial concepts of occlusion and articulation that, in some cases, still maintain a very important role in reconstructive dentistry.

Imaging approach

Radiographic tracking of the condylar movement is usually performed by fluoroscopy with the x-ray source positioned in such a way that only one condyle is visible on the fluorescent screen.[49–51] A major drawback of using fluoroscopy for studying condylar movements in normal individuals is its potential for significant overexposure of the subject to x-rays.

Another method, although limited to studies on cadavers, is high-speed cinematography.[50,51] Obviously, studying condylar movements in cadavers is not the same as studying normal in vivo movements. To obtain a dynamic description of condylar motion, a series of tomographic images are taken with the mandible held at different degrees of mouth opening.[52–54] The images are stored on a videotape and then played back sequentially like a cartoon. Despite the excellent animations of the movement of the TMJ complex, this method is still only two dimensional and thus does not allow the analysis of the movement of the entire condylar head in the articular fossa. Furthermore, this method is not suitable for studying functional movements associated with transient events, such as those occurring during sudden articular disc displacements.

More recently, magnetic resonance imaging (MRI) methods, such as echo planar imaging, have been used to image the condyle in vivo during its movement. However, two shortcomings of this method are its low image acquisition rate[1,2,55] and that the observation of the condylar movement is still limited to only one plane.

Three-Dimensional Analysis

Tracking the incisal point

The motion of a mandibular point, most commonly the incisal point, is usually recorded by tracking small magnets or light-emitting diodes placed close to the mandibular incisors. These systems allow tracking of the incisal or any other mandibular point during mandibular movement with six degrees of freedom without the need for any mathematical data transformation. Unlike more complicated systems, the analyzed point in this case is identical to the recorded landmark.

This technique has been widely used because of its theoretical and technical simplicity. Examples of this technology are the Kinesiograph (Myotronics),[56–60] the Sirognathograph (Siemens),[60–64] and the Selspot systems (Innovation Systems).[65–67] These systems are very user friendly to clinicians who have applied them in clinical settings. Deviations of the observed mandibular movement from what is considered to be the ideal are used as an outcome measure for screening and diagnostic purposes in symptomatic and asymptomatic subjects.

Although these tracking systems use a three-dimensional approach to study mandibular movement, they still have no ability to analyze the true contribution of the rotational and translational components to the mandibular movements. Extrapolation of the obtained data beyond the results for the point that has been tracked is invalid.[68] It is thus impossible, using these systems, to determine the precise condylar path.

Tracking the entire mandible

Electro-optical approach with mathematical data transformations
To overcome the limitations of the methods previously described, and to provide a more comprehensive description of mandibular and condylar motion, a new method has been developed. It is based on the principle of acquiring mandibular movement with all six degrees of freedom.[69–76] A kinematic analysis uses mathematical transformation of the obtained data; this allows the three-dimensional reconstruction of the trajectory of any point along the mandible, including those located within the condyles, under the assumption that the mandible is a rigid body. This approach represents a significant step forward with respect to the systems that analyze the two-dimensional movement of a single point on the mandible and then extrapolate the results to include the condyles.[77–79] One of the systems developed was the noninvasive, optoelectronic system Jaws-3D (Metropoly), which minimized restriction of head movement and disturbance of the lip.[80–86]

A novel analysis of the motion data acquired with six degrees of freedom has led to a modification of the theory of mandibular movement during simple unassisted jaw opening and closing. The modified model proposes that the motion of a rigid body (in this case the mandible) occurs around and along an axis of rotation that is moving in space. In other words, the infinitesimal spatial motion of the mandible is expressed as a combination of rotation and simultaneous translation along its rotational axis. Because the rotational axis is continuously moving in space, at any point in time the observed position of the axis is true for that moment only. The term *instantaneous helical axis* is therefore used to describe this moving axis in space. During mandibular motion, the instantaneous helical axis follows a continuous pathway, as previously described by Gibbs et al.[87] If the sampling frequency of the tracking system is sufficiently high, then the result represents a continuous spatial motion of the axis.

This new approach for analyzing mandibular and condylar movements represents a significant improvement over previous methods. It allows extrapolation of the simultaneous rotation and translation of the condyle and provides detailed information of their individual contributions to the overall movement. It therefore yields a more comprehensive description of jaw movements than is obtained by tracking a single mandibular point (eg, the incisal point), located away from the condyle itself. This is important because a symmetric movement of the incisal point does not necessarily indicate symmetric condylar movements and thus a symmetric movement of the mandible as a whole. For example, a difference between the two condylar translations can be compensated for by different amounts of condylar rotation. The result can still be a symmetric movement of the incisal point. However, the spatial location and orientation of the helical axis indicate whether the mandibular movement is indeed symmetric from a bilateral condylar perspective.

Electro-optical approach with mathematical data transformations combined with an imaging technique

The greatest limitation of all previously described methods is their inability to relate the real-time kinematics of all TMJ components to each other and to any other stationary point in the cranium. For example, although the jaw-tracking devices allow reconstruction of the movement of preselected condylar points, the method itself is not capable of relating recorded paths of the condyle to the articular disc and/or articular fossa. This deficiency has clinical importance in certain situations; for example, in the case of a significantly irregular condylar path, it is very difficult to determine whether the specific condylar movement occurred as a result of morphologic irregularities of the articular fossa and/or other abnormalities of the articular disc. In addition, because of its complex nature, motion analysis of a single point selected within the condylar head does not allow reconstruction of the whole condylar movement.

To overcome these deficiencies, a novel methodology was introduced. It involves tracking mandibular movement relative to the cranium and combining the data with the anatomy revealed by means of an imaging technique. Because the movement of the unloaded mandible is complex, consisting of rotational and translatory components, it is necessary to record jaw movement with a system that has the capability of acquiring data with six degrees of freedom (ie, three rotations and three translations), such as Jaws-3D. The combination of motion data with a set of MRI sections of the TMJ allows modeling of the three-dimensional dynamics of the condyle relative to the other components of the TMJ.[2,88] This state-of-the-art method, also termed *dynamic stereometry*, provides an understanding of the time-dependent relationships among the articular surfaces during mandibular movements, such as the distance between each point of the reconstructed condyle and the articular fossa for every moment of mandibular motion.

All of the methods of studying condylar movements that have been previously described reveal interindividual variability, not only in TMJ morphology but also in mandibular movements. Nevertheless, the repeatability of intraindividual observations, although different in their detail and dependent on the sophistication of the method used, tends to support certain conclusions about condylar function. The remainder of this chapter integrates the findings obtained with the latest data acquisition methodology with the current knowledge of TMJ morphology to describe condylar kinematics during various mandibular movements.

Function

With the evolution of the understanding of mandibular function, the concept outlining the optimal position of the terminal mandibular transverse rotational axis during assisted initial symmetric opening and closing (CR) has changed several times. Any change in concept would also have clinical applicability, resulting in a change in definition of CR and thus of the ideal anatomic relationship among the TMJ components. It is no surprise that throughout various studies of TMJ function, one of the most intriguing questions has been the specific relationships among the condylar head, articular disc, and articular fossa while the mandible is in its CR position and thus ideally in maximal intercuspation.

Despite the absense of a verifiable clinical methodology, the relationship among the TMJ components in this mandibular position has been consistently defined in anatomic terms. The first definition described CR as "the most retruded relation of the mandible to the maxilla with its condyles in the most posterior unrestrained position in the glenoid fossae from which lateral mandibular movements can be made."[89] The definition currently in use defines CR as "the maxillo-mandibular relationship in which each condyle articulates with the thinnest avascular portion of the disc (the IZ) in an antero-superior position against the posterior slope of the articular eminence."[90]

Newer technology capable of combining motion and morphology of the TMJ components during condylar movements, however, provides more detailed information about the spatial relationship of these components

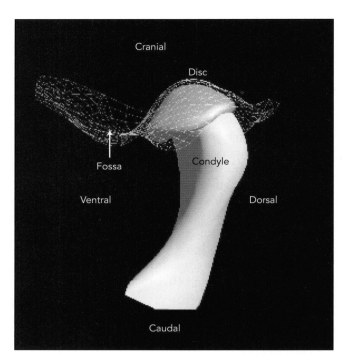

Fig 2-1 TMJ during maximum intercuspation reconstructed from real MRI data (oblique frontal view with the subject looking to the left of the figure). The fossa is represented by a grid, and the disc and the condyle are represented by rendered surfaces. The disc is located between the condyle and the posterior slope of the articular eminence.

when the jaws are closed in maximal intercuspation. For example, it is now well established that in this mandibular position the condylar head is positioned under the PB of the articular disc, so that the disc is located between the condyle and the posterior slope of the articular eminence (Fig 2-1). The collagen fibrils of the temporal and intermediate parts of the posterior discal attachment are generally loosely packed, while the condylar posterior discal attachment wraps the posterior aspect of the condylar head and stabilizes the disc in the anteroposterior direction. Furthermore, stretched anteroposterior-oriented collagen fibers in the articular disc that connect AB to the temporal bone and IZ and PB to the condyle would suggest that the internal morphology of the disc determines the posterior limit of condylar movement.[91]

Mandibular Opening and Closing

As soon as condylar rotation begins during initial mandibular opening, the position of the condylar head immediately

changes relative to the articular disc and articular fossa.[92] Some of the most recent studies using the electro-optical approach have found that the location of the transverse axis of condylar rotation (helical axis) during opening and closing is, on average, 49 mm from the center of the condyle.[93] As expected, the axis of rotation during the opening and closing movement is not stationary relative to the condylar head. Instead, it moves in space with boundaries that are, on average, 5 mm anterior, 28 mm posterior, and 44 mm inferior to the condylar head[93] (Fig 2-2). In general, it is now agreed that during both the initial and final stages of jaw opening, the condyle and the disc move forward simultaneously. In asymptomatic subjects, the axis of rotation moves anteriorly and parallel to itself with little change in its orientation relative to the sagittal plane (4.0 ± 1.5 degrees). This motion has a main posteroanterior direction during opening and in the anteroposterior direction during closing.

This high degree of parallelism between consecutive positions of the rotational axis in space demonstrates the well-known fact that both joints move simultaneously in an anterior direction with corresponding amounts of rotation and translation. This coordinated movement includes rotation and translation of the condylar head along the intermediate zone of the articular disc. These findings are in contrast to the traditional view that the initial part of the opening movement consists of pure condylar rotation, as the disc remains relatively stationary with respect to the articular fossa.

The most recent studies have also demonstrated a negligible mediolateral shift of the mandible during its initial phase of opening, confirmed by relatively small translation of the helical axis (0.9 ± 0.7 mm) in the lateral direction during the entire opening movement.[93] This lateral translation of the mandible has minimal effect on the deviation of the incisal point from the midsagittal plane.[94] Because the articular disc is attached to the condyle at its medial and lateral poles, the differential mobility of the disc-condyle complex around and along the helical axis is thus possible. This may indicate that the discal attachments are sufficiently flexible and that an independent mediolateral movement of the condylar head relative to the disc during mandibular movement is possible. It is therefore reasonable to conclude that part of this lateral mandibular shift can be attributed to the movement of the condylar heads alone. If so, this differential mediolateral component of the anteriorly moving condyles must be of a significantly lesser magnitude than their anterior component.[95] The kinematic observations, described with the helical axis model of condylar rotation during the mandibular opening movement, are therefore supported by the observed morphology of the TMJ complex.

Several hypotheses have been proposed to explain the mechanism that coordinates the disc-condyle complex during the initial phase of jaw opening.[96] For example, one proposes that the activity of the superior head of the lateral pterygoid muscle, through its minor attachment to the AB, pulls the disc forward as soon as mandibular opening begins. Although the muscle is apparently not active at this time, it is possible that it passively pulls the disc forward when the condyle translates forward. Another hypothesis proposes an important role of the elastic fibers within the temporal zone of the AB as the equilibrium of the elastic network system is disrupted during mandibular rotation and translation. A third hypothesis suggests that the disc moves forward as a result of a wedging action of the condylar head against the AB.[97] Finally, it was proposed that the disc follows the movement of the condylar head with help of the polar ligaments.[98] Not all of these hypotheses are mutually exclusive.[97]

As mandibular opening progresses, the condylar head rotates around the helical axis on average 2 degrees for each millimeter of anterior translation along the articular eminence.[85] However, there is great variability in the relationship between condylar rotation and translation during a single opening phase. For example, note in Fig 2-2 that the condylar movement begins mainly with rotation and ends mainly with translation. This results, on average, in 24 degrees of condylar rotation and 13 to 15 mm of condylar translation for maximal mouth opening.[93] The disc follows the general direction of the condylar translation but only half of the distance (5 to 9 mm).[99] One of the theories explaining this discrepancy between the extents of the two translations proposes the presence of a retractive passive force exerted on the disc by the elastic fibers within the PB.[96]

Once maximal jaw opening is achieved, the condyles are usually positioned beyond the apex of the articular eminence on the preglenoid plane. In this most anterior position, the anterior part of the condylar articular surface establishes an intimate contact with the AB and the adjacent part of the IZ of the articular disc. At the same time, the temporal and the intermediate zones of the PB are stretched up to five times.[100] When this occurs, the posterior temporal attachment of the retrodiscal tissue is pressed against the fossa, while the posterior condylar attachment becomes loose beneath the PB of the articular disc. As was mentioned, the intermediate posterior attachment contains an abundant elastic-fiber network that is attached to the walls of the venous plexus, located posterior to the condyle. During this anterior movement of the disc-condyle complex, the elastic fibers facilitate the inflow of blood into the expanded venous network located between the two posterior attachments. The hydrostatic pressure within the posterior attachment thus increases.[101]

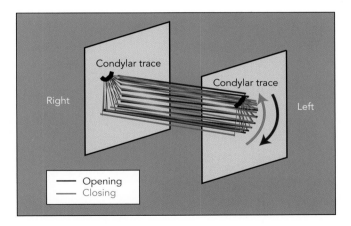

Fig 2-2 Oblique frontal view of the helical axis pathway of a normal subject during (thick blue lines) jaw opening and (thick red lines) jaw closing (subject facing to the left of the figure). (black) Condylar traces. (vertical thin blue and red lines) Distances between the center of the condyle and the helical axis at each instant. (blue boxes) Sagittal planes passing through the condyles. (arrows) Progression of movement. The helical axis remains parallel to itself throughout the whole movement.

Closing movements of the condylar heads are similar to the opening ones but in reverse. As is the case with an opening movement, there are several theories regarding the mechanism of discal control during mandibular closure.[95] The posterior attachment contraction theory, which may be valid for lightly loaded condyles only, proposes that the PB of the articular disc is being pulled back by stretched elastic fibers connecting IZ with the temporal part of the posterior discal attachment.[102,103]

The alternative, the condyle-traction hypothesis,[95] proposes that the condylar head braces the PB and moves the disc posteriorly. One of the most often cited arguments in support of this theory is the observed inferior closing condylar path.[104,105] This discrepancy in condylar paths during opening and closing movements has been explained in part with the inferiorly displaced condylar head resting on thickened PB of the disc during mandibular closure. It is expected that during this phase the PB receives heavy loads and thus a thicker PB is ideal to resist them. Indeed, with its three-dimensional network of collagen fibers and with an increased concentration of glycosaminoglycans, the PB is well suited to receive heavy loads.[106,107]

The observation of the inferior condylar path during mandibular closure has been recently challenged using the latest kinematic methodology.[108] Although there is an agreement between the two theories that the two paths, as well as the ratio of condylar rotation and translation

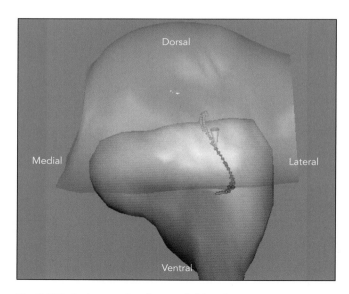

Fig 2-3 Typical example of stress-field paths in an asymptomatic TMJ during jaw opening and closing (superior view). The fossa is translucent. The stress-field paths are almost perfectly coincident during the opening and closing phases, and, in this case, move in the lateral part of the joint.

during mandibular opening and closing movements, are not necessarily identical, Palla et al[108] described the closing condylar path as being superior to the path traced during mandibular opening. This difference in relationship among TMJ components during the two mandibular movements has been explained by the fact that different muscles are used to open and close the mandible, producing different force vectors acting on the mandible and thus the condyles and articular discs. The intra-articular loading is hypothesized to be greater during mandibular closure than during mandibular opening, therefore resulting in a more superior condylar path of closure.

This theory is supported by the observed differences in the amount of separation of the articular components during the two movements.[108] The area of the minimum distance and its variation through time are two important parameters that, after making certain assumptions about the material properties of the articular tissues, reflect the strain (and by inference the stress) of the articular components in the TMJ. Tracking of the geometry of the intra-articular space indicates that it continuously changes with respect to its peak and location. This supports the theory that the zones with the greatest compression and shear (stress fields) shift through the articular tissue during condylar motion. In asymptomatic joints, these shifts of the stress fields occur predominantly within the lateral aspect of the

articular disc in a direction that is independent of the rate of condylar movement. Their locations within the disc are nearly superimposable during the opening and closing mandibular movements (Fig 2-3). In the majority (65%) of the cases that were observed, the stress field translated mediolaterally during opening; in 20% of the cases it translated lateromedially, while the remaining 15% showed an unclear pattern.[109] Unlike the direction of translation, the peak velocity of the stress-field shift does appear to be dependent on the rate of jaw opening and closing.

Mediolateral stress-field translations through the disc also occur during jaw-opening and jaw-closing movements in clicking TMJs. A typical example of stress-field paths in a clicking TMJ during jaw opening and closing is shown in Fig 2-4. One of the significant differences from the asymptomatic TMJs is that the locations of the disc where these stress-field shifts occur during opening and closing are not superimposable.[110] In addition, the average length of the translation of the stress-field shifts is significantly greater than that found in asymptomatic joints. Longer stress-field paths and lack of superimposition of the stress-field traces during opening and closing movements in clicking joints suggest that the areas of the soft tissue of the TMJ that are subject to stress are greater in clicking joints than in asymptomatic joints. The cause may be found in either the reciprocal movement of a displaced disc or in altered muscular activity directly affecting the opening and closing condylar paths.

Another interesting difference between asymptomatic and clicking joints is an overall decrease of the intra-articular distance in the latter. This may indicate thinning of the disc, supported by the results of MRI studies showing that anteriorly displaced discs often appear deformed and mediolaterally stretched.[111] Alternatively, this decrease in intra-articular space may also be explained by the flattening of the condylar heads, a result of the discal and condylar modeling-remodeling process observed in static MRIs.[112]

Mandibular Lateral Border Movements

The lateral border movements of the mandible described in this section occur very seldom during chewing. Most often they may be detected during parafunction (eg, tooth grinding). As is the case during the initial opening of the mandible, the condylar lateral border movements depend on the anatomy of the TMJ and are individually specific. The shape of the medial wall and the roof of the articular fossa, the medial pole of the condyle, the congruency of the articulating disc with the mandibular and temporal articulating surfaces, the tightness of the capsule and the

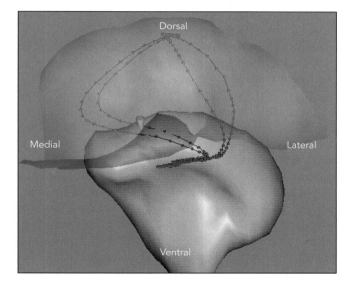

Fig 2-4 Typical example of stress-field paths in a clicking TMJ during jaw opening and closing (superior view). The fossa is translucent. During the opening phase, the stress field moves to the medial part of the joint; during the closing phase, the stress field moves to the lateral part of the joint. The stress-field paths of the opening and closing phases do not coincide because of disc reduction.

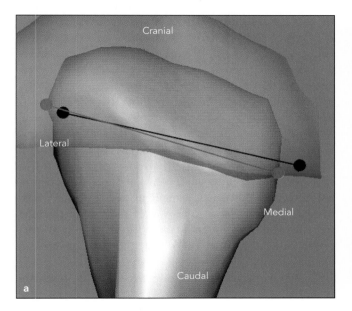

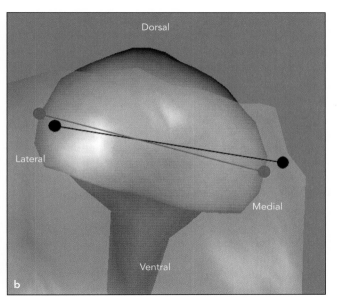

Fig 2-5 Difference in the movement of the medial and lateral condylar poles on the working side during a laterotrusive movement in an asymptomatic subject. (a) Frontal view of a right condyle at the beginning of movement. (b) Cranial view of a right condyle at the beginning of movement. The fossa is translucent. The black line connects the medial and lateral poles at the beginning of the movement and the red line connects them at the end of laterotrusion.

ligaments, and to a lesser extent the result of muscle recruitment, all determine the exact path of the condyles.

In addition to rotation around a vertical axis, the mandible exhibits lateral translation toward the working (chewing) side. During lateral border movement, the balancing-side (b-s) condyle-disc complex translates inferiorly, anteriorly, and medially. Simultaneously, the working-side (w-s) condyle moves superiorly or inferiorly, anteriorly, and slightly laterally.[113] As this mandibular movement to the working side progresses, a significant difference in the movement of the lateral poles of the individual condylar heads is observed. Whereas the lateral pole of the w-s condyle moves in the posterior, superior, and lateral direction, its medial pole moves in the anterior, inferior, and lateral direction. The difference in the movements of the medial and lateral condylar poles of the w-s condyle during a lateral border movement is shown in Fig 2-5.

This differential movement of the individual w-s condylar poles in two of the three directions is not observed on the b-s condylar head. The b-s condylar poles always move in the same mediolateral direction. The result is a lateral translatory movement of the mandible to the chewing side (see Fig 1-5). The amount of this lateral displacement of the condyles varies individually and depends on the same anatomic constraints mentioned previously. There is still a debate concerning which one of these constraints (ie, ligaments and capsule of the w-s TMJ, and the shape and congruency of the b-s condyle with the medial wall of the articulating fossa) is most important in determining the exact direction of the lateral displacement of the mandible.

As is the case during the opening and closing mandibular movements, a mediolateral stress-field shift within the disc does occur during the lateral border movement as well. However, there are significant differences between the working- and balancing-side articular disc tissues with respect to the length of the shift and its peak velocity. For example, the working side exhibits consistently shorter shifts (2.4 ± 2.2 mm) and lower mean velocity than does the balancing side (4.5 ± 2.6 mm).[109]

Mandibular Protrusion

Mandibular protrusion occurs as the mandibular teeth move past their maxillary counterparts in an anterior direction. The condylar movement has been described as primarily translatory. The reverse mandibular movement, retrusion, is similar.

When viewed in the sagittal plane, the paths of the b-s condyle during lateral border movements differ from those during protrusion. The protrusive path is superior to the projected path of the anteromedially moving b-s condyle during the lateral border movement.[114–116] The explanation for this discrepancy is that the b-s condyle closely approaches the medial part of the articular eminence. Because the medial part of the eminence slants inferiorly when viewed in the frontal plane, the path of the medially moving condyle is inferior to the path of the same condyle during mandibular protrusion. It has been also observed that during protrusion the length and the mean peak velocity of stress-field shifts are similar to those recorded during the b-s lateral border movement.[109]

Mandibular Functional (Chewing) Movements

The incisal path of the mandible during masticatory movements has been analyzed with respect to its outline and rate,[87,113,117,118] age[119,120] and gender of the subject,[121] food

characteristics,[113,118,122–125] and occlusal scheme.[113,124] There is great interindividual variability of the chewing path in asymptomatic subjects.[118,124] The movement of the incisal point has also been analyzed in patients with temporomandibular disorders (TMDs).[126–130]

The chewing cycle is divided into an opening stroke, a closing stroke, and a power stroke (see chapter 4), in which the power stroke brings the mandible to maximal intercuspation. After opening, the mandible moves laterally, away from the midline. It is from this position that the fast closing stroke begins in the mediosuperior direction, with a significant posterior component. During the power stroke, the w-s mandibular teeth approach their maxillary counterparts in an anteromedial direction to reach the occlusal phase of the power stroke.[113] Because the bolus is interposed between the teeth, maximal intercuspation is seldom achieved during the first few initial power strokes.

Condylar movements during chewing differ from those recorded during border movements. When traced in all three planes, the condylar paths during unilateral chewing are always observed to be within the areas determined by the tracings produced during mandibular border movements (see Fig 1-14). In addition, chewing movements are not as readily reproducible as the paths of border movements. It is for this reason that, as previously mentioned, tracings of the condylar border movements are used to set the articular components of an articulator.

One of the movements in which the two condylar paths do approximate each other is during an opening mandibular movement. Namely, as the jaws open symmetrically prior to moving toward the working or chewing side, the movements of both condyles appear symmetric and thus similar to those described for the opening stroke of an empty movement.

Similar to empty opening and closing movements, the mandibular instantaneous axis of rotation during chewing is predominantly transversely (mediolaterally) oriented (Fig 2-6a). Mediolateral displacement of the condyles is a result of their translation along the helical axis, whereas their anterior movement results from the anterior displacement of the helical axis. There are significant differences in the amount of total condylar rotation and transverse shift of the condylar heads between the two movements. As expected, the maximal jaw rotation around the helical axis is smaller during chewing (16.2 ± 5.4 degrees) than for deliberate maximum jaw opening and closing (24.3 ± 4.2 degrees).[131] This is obviously due to the fact that jaw opening is less during chewing than during maximum opening.[113] Similarly, the maximal mediolateral translation of the mandible along the helical axis is greater during this phase of the chewing cycle (2.4 ± 0.9 mm) than it is during maximum symmetric opening (0.9 ± 0.7 mm).[131]

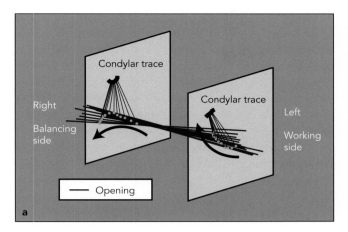

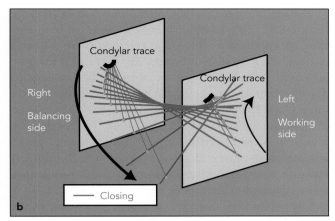

Fig 2-6 Oblique frontal views of typical pathways of the mandibular helical axis in an asymptomatic subject. *(a)* Helical pathway during the opening phase of a masticatory cycle. *(b)* Helical pathway during the closing phase of a masticatory cycle. *(black)* Condylar traces. *(thin lines)* Distances between the center of the condyle and the helical axis at each instant. *(blue boxes)* Sagittal planes passing through the condyles. *(green dots)* Intersections of the helical axes through the sagittal planes, revealing the differences between the movements of the working and the balancing condyles. *(arrows)* Progression of movement.

Fig 2-7 Oblique-frontal view of asymmetric movement of both condyles during the closing phase of a right chewing cycle in an asymptomatic subject. The fossa is translucent. Six positions (in the sequence gray, blue, red, purple, green, and yellow) of the working-side and balancing-side condyle are shown. Note the difference in timing between the working and balancing condyles and how the working condyle reaches its most cranial position before the balancing condyle.

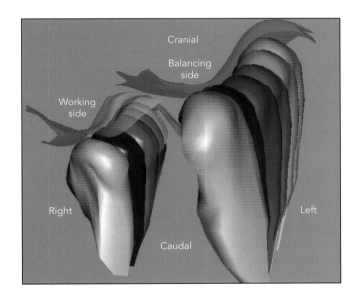

The extent of condylar translation forward corresponds to the amount of mandibular opening during mastication. The latter varies with the type and size of the food being chewed. For example, foods that are associated mainly with vertical mandibular movements (ie, meats) require wider jaw opening.

As the mandible begins closing, it continues to deviate laterally to the working side. It has been observed that, during this part of the chewing cycle, the orientation of the helical axis and its positional relationship relative to both condylar heads differ significantly from any other described movement. The instantaneous axis of rotation of the mandible is no longer perpendicular to the sagittal plane (Fig 2-6b). On the working side, the axis is located posteroinferiorly to the condyle at the beginning of closing and near or sometimes above it at the end of closing. On the balancing side, however, the helical axis is located near or superior to the condyle at the beginning of closing and posteroinferiorly to the condyle at the end of the jaw closing. When this phase of mandibular closing comes to its end, the helical axis is found closer to the w-s condyle than it is to the b-s condyle. As a result, the w-s condyle reaches its most superoposterior position before the b-s condyle, which continues moving in the superior and posterior direction (Fig 2-7).

The exact location of the helical axis and its distance from both condylar heads largely depend on food texture. For example, as the size of the food bolus increases or tougher foods, such as bread with crust and dried beef, are chewed, the helical axis tends to oscillate more in its distance from the w-s condylar head, in both the superoinferior and the anteroposterior directions.[132] At the maximal lateral position of the mandible, just before the power stroke commences, the b-s condyle rests on its anteromedial surface along the posterior incline of the articular eminence. At the same time, the w-s condyle essentially rotates about a vertical axis.[87,108,113]

Just before the power stroke begins, the center of the w-s condyle is dispaced laterally and posteriorly before eventualy regaining its final position in the maximal intercuspation. There has been considerable controversy regarding the loading pattern of the w-s condyle during this phase of the chewing cycle (see chapter 1). Recent studies have shown that the interarticular distance (ie, the distance between the condyle and fossa) in both the w-s and b-s joints is significantly smaller during the power stroke than it is during other phases of the chewing cycle.[133] This suggests that both joints are loaded during the power stroke, and, contrary to earlier interpretations,[87,113] it also indicates that the w-s condyle does not distract at this time. Furthermore, the decrease in the condyle fossa distance during closing is generally more pronounced on the balancing side than on the working side. This likely reflects the fact that overall compression of the b-s disc is greater than that of the w-s disc during chewing. This is in agreement with those models that describe greater reaction force along the b-s condyle during the power stroke of chewing.[134] Nevertheless, this does not indicate that the largest stresses (force/area) necessarily occur along the b-s condyle, because during the power stroke the w-s mandibular corpus is twisted about its long axis. This twisting causes the lower border of the corpus to be everted and the alveolar process (and teeth) to be inverted. This pattern of twisting also causes the lateral aspect of the w-s condyle to be pressed harder against the articular eminence and intervening disc. Thus, although the overall largest reaction force may indeed occur along the b-s condyle, the condylar reaction force may be more concentrated along the w-s condyle (see chapter 1).

This differential loading pattern along the mediolateral direction of the PB and IZ corresponds to the changes in thickness of their respective morphologies.[107] However, the exact magnitude and direction of the loading pattern within the articular disc are related to the resultant muscle force, changing continuously with differential recruitment of the closing muscles.[135,136]

When the teeth are in maximal intercuspation and both condylar heads are braced against the posterior slopes of the articular eminences, the IZ of the articular disc separates the two compartments of the TMJ. During clenching, the condyle tends to move slightly more superoposteriorly, narrowing the joint space between the anterior and superior aspects of the glenoid fossa and the condylar head.[137] The heaviest loads are expected to be located at the PB region, adjacent to the condylar zone of the posterior discal attachment.

Conclusion

Recent advancements in science and technology have significantly improved the understanding of TMJ morphology and mandibular function. The new methods of combining three-dimensional kinematic analysis of any particular point on the mandible (including the condylar head) with MRI have allowed reconstruction of the dynamic relationships among the intra-articular components during various mandibular movements. The most important information from the new data about TMJ morphology and function is that the variability of the former is determined largely by the variability of the latter; ie, it is the demands of mandibular function that induce morphologic adaptations. This is a significant change from many past theories, which generally assumed that form determines function and therefore underestimated the system's capacity to adapt in response to ever-changing functional demands.

This perspective of the stomatognathic system enables dental scientists and clinicians to reassess some of the concepts of maxillomandibular relationships that are based on assumptions of stability of both TMJ morphology and mandibular function. The outcome has important clinical relevance to the diagnosis and treatment of occlusal disharmonies as well as for the management of TMDs. For example, strict adherence to the very narrow definitions of ideal intraindividual and interindividual TMJ morphology and mandibular function has often led clinicians to regard otherwise normal variability in asymptomatic populations as a pathologic condition needing treatment.

Similarly, in patients with a TMD, a narrow focus on variations from the predefined ideal TMJ morphology, position, and function has led clinicians to address these disorders according to certain arbitrary occlusal concepts, instead of relating them to their actual pathophysiology. Frequently, the outcome of this treatment approach was worsening of the signs and symptoms of the TMD as a result of the irreversible procedures used to "correct" morphologic imperfections, as advocated by various mechanistic concepts. TMD patients were therefore at risk for negative outcomes that went beyond the simple failure to respond positively.

On the other hand, success with the clinical procedures that are based on the concepts of stability of TMJ morphology and repeatability of mandibular function can be explained by other confounding variables that are capable of contributing to clinical success (see chapters 14 and 25).

By recognizing the capacity of the stomatognathic system to function in a wide variety of patterns, and appreciating its ability to adapt to functional demands, clinicians should be able to deal more effectively with their patients' problems when they do arise.

References

1. Chen J, Buckwalter K. Displacement analysis of the temporomandibular condyle from magnetic resonance images. J Biomech 1993;26:1455–1462.
2. Price C, Connell DG, MacKay A, Tobias DL. Three-dimensional reconstruction of magnetic resonance images of the temporomandibular joint by I-DEAS. Dentomaxillofac Radiol 1992;21:148–153.
3. Dubrul EL. Sicher's Oral Anatomy. St Louis: Mosby, 1980:91.
4. Costa RL Jr. Asymmetry of the mandibular condyle in Haida Indians. Am J Phys Anthropol 1986;70:119–123.
5. Koppe T, Autrum B, Krczal P. Physiologische Formvarianten am Kiefergelenk des Menschen und der Pongiden. In: Benner KU, Fanghänel J, Kowalewski R, Kubein-Meesenburg D, Randzio J (eds). Morphologie, Funktion und Klinik des Kiefergelenks. Berlin: Quintessenz, 1993:101–109.
6. Meyer H. Das Kiefergelenk. Arch Anat Physiol Wiss Med 1865;719–731.
7. Oberg T, Carlsson GE, Fajers CM. The temporomandibular joint. A morphologic study on a human autopsy material. Acta Odontol Scand 1971;29:349–384.
8. Türp JC, Alt KW, Vach W, Harbich K. On asymmetries of mandibular condyles and rami. In Radlanski R, Renz H (eds). Proceedings of the 10th International Symposium on Dental Morphology, 6–10 Sept 1995. Berlin: Brünne, 1995:444–448.
9. Wendler D, Bergmann M, Schumacher GH, Kunz G. The temporomandibular joint—Structure and function during the course of development [in German]. Anat Anz 1989;169:1–5.
10. Dibbets JM, van der Weele LT. Prevalence of structural bony change in the mandibular condyle. J Craniomandib Disord 1992;6:254–259.
11. Lubsen CC, Hansson TL, Nordstrom BB, Solberg WK. Histomorphometric analysis of cartilage and subchondral bone in mandibular condyles of young human adults at autopsy. Arch Oral Biol 1985;30:129–136.
12. Yale SH, Allison BD, Hauptfuehrer JD. An epidemiological assessment of mandibular condyle morphology. Oral Surg Oral Med Oral Pathol 1966;21:169–177.
13. Pullinger AG, Bibb CA, Ding X, Baldioceda F. Relationship of articular soft tissue contour and shape to the underlying eminence and slope profile in young adult temporomandibular joints. Oral Surg Oral Med Oral Pathol 1993;76:647–654.
14. Pullinger AG, Bibb CA, Ding X, Baldioceda F. Contour mapping of the TMJ temporal component and the relationship to articular soft tissue thickness and disk displacement. Oral Surg Oral Med Oral Pathol 1993;76:636–646.
15. Hansson T, Oberg T, Carlsson GE, Kopp S. Thickness of the soft tissue layers and the articular disk in the temporomandibular joint. Acta Odontol Scand 1977;35:77–83.
16. Hylander WL. Functional anatomy. In: Sarnat BG, Laskin DM (eds). The Temporomandibular Joint: A Biological Basis for Clinical Practice. Philadelphia: Saunders, 1992:60–92.
17. Solberg WK, Hansson TL, Nordstrom B. The temporomandibular joint in young adults at autopsy: A morphologic classification and evaluation. J Oral Rehabil 1985;12:303–321.
18. Dauber W. The adjacent structural relationships of the articular disk of the temporomandibular joint and its functional importance [in German]. Schweiz Monatsschr Zahnmed 1987;97:427–437.
19. Luder HU, Bobst P. Wall architecture and disc attachment of the human temporomandibular joint. Schweiz Monatsschr Zahnmed 1991;101:557–570.
20. Zenker W. Retroarticular plastic pad of the temporomandibular joint and its mechanic significance [in German]. Z Anat Entwicklungsgesch 1956;119:375–388.
21. Wright DM, Moffett BC Jr. The postnatal development of the human temporomandibular joint. Am J Anat 1974;141:235–249.
22. Granados JI. The influence of the loss of teeth and attrition on the articular eminence. J Prosthet Dent 1979;42:78–85.
23. Ogston A. Articular cartilage. J Anat 1876;10:49–74.
24. Fick R. Handbuch der Anatomie und Mechanik der Gelenke. 1. Anatomie der Gelenke. Jena, Germany: Fischer, 1904.
25. Tandler J. Lehrbuch der systematischen Anatomie, vol 1. Leipzig: Vogel, 1919.
26. Moffett BC. The prenatal development of the human temporomandibular joint. Carnegie Contr Embryol 1957;36:19–28.
27. Thilander B, Carlsson GE, Ingervall B. Postnatal development of the human temporomandibular joint. 1. A histological study. Acta Odontol Scand 1976;34:117–126.
28. Boyer CC, Williams TW, Stevens FH. Blood supply of the temporomandibular joint. J Dent Res 1964;43:224–228.
29. Keith DA. Development of the human temporomandibular joint. Br J Oral Surg 1982;20:217–224.
30. Axelsson S, Holmlund A, Hjerpe A. Glycosaminoglycans in normal and osteoarthrotic human temporomandibular joint disks. Acta Odontol Scand 1992;50:113–119.

31. Kobayashi J. Studies on matrix components relevant to structure and function of the temporomandibular joint [in Japanese]. Kokubyo Gakkai Zasshi 1992;59:105–123.

32. Rees LA. The structure and function of the mandibular joint. Br Dent J 1954;96:125–133.

33. Mills DK, Daniel JC, Scapino R. Histological features and in-vitro proteoglycan synthesis in the rabbit craniomandibular joint disc. Arch Oral Biol 1988;33:195–202.

34. Minarelli AM, Del Santo JM, Liberti EA. The structure of the human temporomandibular joint disc: A scanning electron microscopy study. J Orofac Pain 1997;11:95–100.

35. Scapino RP. Histopathology associated with malposition of the human temporomandibular joint disc. Oral Surg Oral Med Oral Pathol 1983;55:382–397.

36. Isacsson G, Isberg AM. Tissue identification of the TMJ disk and disk attachments and related vascularization. Cranio 1985;3:374–379.

37. Goose DH, Appleton J. Human Dentofacial Growth. Oxford: Pergamon Press, 1982.

38. Helmy E, Larke V, Bays R, Sharaway M. Identification of elastic and oxytalin fibers in human cadaver TMJ. J Dent Res 1984;63:228.

39. Carlsson GE, Hassler O, Oberg T. Microradiographic study of human temporomandibular disks obtained at autopsy. J Oral Pathol 1973;2:265–271.

40. Granstrom G, Linde A. Glycosaminoglycans of temporomandibular articular discs. Scand J Dent Res 1973;81:462–466.

41. Kopp S. Topographical distribution of sulfated glycosaminoglycans in the surface layers of the human temporomandibular joint. A histochemical study of an autopsy material. J Oral Pathol 1978;7:283–294.

42. Mohl ND. Functional anatomy of the temporomandibular joint. In: Laskin DM (ed). The President's Conference on the Examination, Diagnosis and Management of Temporomandibular Disorders. Chicago: American Dental Association, 1983:3–12.

43. Scapino RP. The posterior attachment: Its structure, function, and appearance in TMJ imaging studies. 2. J Craniomandib Disord 1991;5:155–166.

44. Scapino RP. The posterior attachment: Its structure, function, and appearance in TMJ imaging studies. 1. J Craniomandib Disord 1991;5:83–95.

45. Meyer LJ. Newly described muscle attachments to the anterior band of the disk of the temporomandibular joint. J Am Dent Assoc 1988;117:437–439.

46. Wilkinson TM. The relationship between the disk and the lateral pterygoid muscle in the human temporomandibular joint. J Prosthet Dent 1988;60:715–724.

47. Heylings DJ, Nielsen IL, McNeill C. Lateral pterygoid muscle and the temporomandibular disc. J Orofac Pain 1995;9:9–16.

48. Meyenberg K, Kubik S, Palla S. Relationships of the muscles of mastication to the articular disc of the temporomandibular joint. Schweiz Monatsschr Zahnmed 1986;96:815–834.

49. Heller U, Palla S. Fluoroscopic analysis of condylar movements in clicking of the temporomandibular joint [in German]. Schweiz Monatsschr Zahnmed 1988;98:465–471.

50. Isberg Holm AM, Westesson PL. Movement of disc and condyle in temporomandibular joints with and without clicking. A high-speed cinematographic and dissection study on autopsy specimens. Acta Odontol Scand 1982;40:165–177.

51. Isberg Holm AM, Westesson PL. Movement of disc and condyle in temporomandibular joints with clicking. An arthrographic and cineradiographic study on autopsy specimens. Acta Odontol Scand 1982;40:151–164.

52. Bell KA, Miller KD, Jones JP. Cine magnetic resonance imaging of the temporomandibular joint. Cranio 1992;10:313–317.

53. Conway WF, Hayes CW, Campbell RL. Dynamic magnetic resonance imaging of the temporomandibular joint using FLASH sequences. J Oral Maxillofac Surg 1988;46:930–938.

54. Sadowsky PL, McCutcheon MJ, Fletcher SG, Lowman JC, Sutton DI. Electronically mediated mandibular positioning for MR images of the TMJ [abstract 1160]. J Dent Res 1990;69(special issue):253.

55. Mansfield P, Maudsley AA. Planar spin imaging by NMR. J Magn Reson 1977;27:101–119.

56. Jankelson B, Swain CW, Crane PF, Radke JC. Kinesiometric instrumentation: A new technology. J Am Dent Assoc 1975;90:834–840.

57. Jankelson B. Measurement accuracy of the mandibular kinesiograph—A computerized study. J Prosthet Dent 1980;44:656–666.

58. Hannam AG, De Cou RE, Scott JD, Wood WW. The relationship between dental occlusion, muscle activity and associated jaw movement in man. Arch Oral Biol 1977;22:25–32.

59. Hannam AG, DeCou RE, Scott JD, Wood WW. The kinesiographic measurement of jaw displacement. J Prosthet Dent 1980;44:88–93.

60. Michler L, Bakke M, Moller E. Graphic assessment of natural mandibular movements. J Craniomandib Disord 1987;1:97–114.

61. Lewin A, van Rensburg LB, Lemmer J. A method of recording the movement of a point on the jaws. J Dent Assoc S Afr 1974;29:395–397.

62. Lemmer J, Lewin A, van Rensburg LB. The measurement of jaw movement. 1. J Prosthet Dent 1976;36:211–218.

63. Lewin A, Lemmer J, van Rensburg LB. The measurement of jaw movement. 2. J Prosthet Dent 1976;36:312–318.

64. Lewin A, Nickel B. The full description of jaw movement. J Dent Assoc S Afr 1978;33:261–267.

65. Karlsson S. Recording of mandibular movements by intra-orally placed light emitting diodes. Acta Odontol Scand 1977;35:111–117.

66. Jemt T, Karlsson S. Computer-analysed movements in three dimensions recorded by light-emitting diodes. A study of methodological errors and of evaluation of chewing behaviour in a group of young adults. J Oral Rehabil 1982;9:317–326.

67. Jemt T, Olsson K. Computer-based analysis of the single chewing cycle during mastication in repeated registrations. J Prosthet Dent 1984;52:437–443.

68. Hobo S. A kinematic investigation of mandibular border movement by means of an electronic measuring system. 2: A study of the Bennett movement. J Prosthet Dent 1984; 51:642–646.

69. Chen J, Siegler S, Schneck CD. The three-dimensional kinematics and flexibility characteristics of the human ankle and subtalar joint. 2. Flexibility characteristics. J Biomech Eng 1988;110:374–385.

70. de Lange A, Huiskes R, Kauer JM. Effects of data smoothing on the reconstruction of helical axis parameters in human joint kinematics. J Biomech Eng 1990;112:107–113.

71. Fioretti S, Jetto L, Leo T. Reliable in vivo estimation of the instantaneous helical axis in human segmental movements. IEEE Trans Biomed Eng 1990;37:398–409.

72. Hart RA, Mote CD Jr, Skinner HB. A finite helical axis as a landmark for kinematic reference of the knee. J Biomech Eng 1991;113:215–222.

73. Ramakrishnan HK, Kadaba MP. On the estimation of joint kinematics during gait. J Biomech 1991;24:969–977.

74. Siegler S, Chen J, Schneck CD. The three-dimensional kinematics and flexibility characteristics of the human ankle and subtalar joints. 1. Kinematics. J Biomech Eng 1988;110: 364–373.

75. Spoor CW, Veldpaus FE. Rigid body motion calculated from spatial co-ordinates of markers. J Biomech 1980;13: 391–393.

76. Spoor CW. Explanation, verification and application of helical-axis error propagation formulas. Hum Mov Sci 1984;3:95–117.

77. Baragar FA, Osborn JW. A model relating patterns of human jaw movement to biomechanical constraints. J Biomech 1984;17:757–767.

78. McMillan AS, McMillan DR, Darvell BW. Centers of rotation during jaw movements. Acta Odontol Scand 1989;47: 323–328.

79. Nattestad A, Vedtofte P. Mandibular autorotation in orthognathic surgery: A new method of locating the centre of mandibular rotation and determining its consequence in orthognathic surgery. J Craniomaxillofac Surg 1992;20: 163–170.

80. Airoldi RL, Gallo LM, Palla S. Precision of the jaw tracking system JAWS-3D. J Orofac Pain 1994;8:155–164.

81. Ernst, BM. Condylar Path and Translatory Velocity Changes in Clicking Temporomandibular Joints [thesis]. Zurich: University of Zurich, 1988.

82. Merlini L, Palla S. The relationship between condylar rotation and anterior translation in healthy and clicking temporomandibular joints: Action of the muscles of mastication. Schweiz Monatsschr Zahnmed 1988;98:1191–1199.

83. Mesqui F, Kaeser F, Fischer P. Real-time noninvasive recording and three-dimensional display of the functional movements of an arbitrary mandible point. Proc SPIE 1985;602: 77–84.

84. Mesqui F, Kaeser F, Fischer P. On-line three-dimensional light spottracker and its application to clinical dentistry. Int Arch Photogrammetry Remote Sensing 1986;26:310–317.

85. Salaorni C, Palla S. Condylar rotation and anterior translation in healthy human temporomandibular joints. Schweiz Monatsschr Zahnmed 1994;104:415–422.

86. Witt E. Variations in Condylar Velocity During Opening and Closing in Healthy Human Temporomandibular Joints [thesis]. Zurich: University of Zurich, 1991.

87. Gibbs CH, Messerman T, Reswick JB, Derda HJ. Functional movements of the mandible. J Prosthet Dent 1971;26: 604–620.

88. Price C. Method of quantifying disc movement on magnetic resonance images of the temporomandibular joint. 1. The method. Dentomaxillofac Radiol 1990;2:59–62.

89. The Glossary of Prosthodontic Terms, ed 1. St Louis: Academy of Denture Prosthetics, 1956.

90. The Glossary of Prosthodontic Terms. J Prosthet Dent 1999; 81:39–110.

91. Eriksson L, Westesson PL, Macher D, Hicks D, Tallents RH. Creation of disc displacement in human temporomandibular joint autopsy specimens. J Oral Maxillofac Surg 1992;50: 869–873.

92. Maeda M, Itou S, Ishii Y, et al. Temporomandibular joint movement. Evaluation of protrusive splint therapy with GRASS MR imaging. Acta Radiol 1992;33:410–413.

93. Gallo LM, Airoldi GB, Airoldi RL, Palla S. Description of mandibular finite helical axis pathways in asymptomatic subjects. J Dent Res 1997;76:704–713.

94. Helkimo M. Studies on function and dysfunction of the masticatory system. 2. Index for anamnestic and clinical dysfunction and occlusal state. Sven Tandlak Tidskr 1974; 67:101–121.

95. Schmolke C. The relationship between the temporomandibular joint capsule, articular disc and jaw muscles. J Anat 1994;184:335–345.

96. Scapino R. Morphology and mechanism of the jaw joint. In: McNeill C (ed). Science and Practice of Occlusion. Chicago: Quintessence, 1997:23–40.

97. Osborn JW. The disc of the human temporomandibular joint: Design, function and failure. J Oral Rehabil 1985;12: 279–293.

98. Sicher H. Functional anatomy of the temporomandibular joint. In: Sarnat BG (ed). The Temporomandibular Joint. Springfield: Thomas, 1964:28–58.

99. Schmolke C, Hugger A. The human temporomandibular joint region in different positions of the mandible. Anat Anz 1999;181:61–64.

100. Wilkinson TM, Crowley CM. A histologic study of retrodiscal tissues of the human temporomandibular joint in the open and closed position. J Orofac Pain 1994;8:7–17.

101. Wish-Baratz S, Ring GD, Hiss J, Shatz A, Arensburg B. The microscopic structure and function of the vascular retrodiscal pad of the human temporomandibular joint. Arch Oral Biol 1993;38:265–268.

102. Mongini F. The Stomatognathic System: Function, Dysfunction and Rehabilitation. Chicago: Quintessence, 1984.

103. Mahan PE. The temporomandibular joint in function and pathofunction. In: Solberg WK, Clark GT (ed). Temporomandibular Joint Problems. Chicago: Quintessence, 1980: 33–42.

104. Wilkinson TM, Gibbs CH. Variations between opening and closing condylar movement paths during chewing [abstract 1150]. J Dent Res 1985;64(special issue):302.

105. Huddleston Slater JJ, Visscher CM, Lobbezoo F, Naeije M. The intra-articular distance within the TMJ during free and loaded closing movements. J Dent Res 1999;78:1815–1820.

106. Scapino RP, Obrez A, Greising D. Organization and function of the collagen fibre system in the human temporomandibular joint disc. Cells Tissues Organs (in press).

107. Nickel JC, McLachlan KR. In vitro measurement of the stress-distribution properties of the pig temporomandibular joint disc. Arch Oral Biol 1994;39:439–448.

108. Palla S, Krebs M, Gallo LM. Jaw tracking and temporomandibular joint animation. In: McNeill C (ed). Science and Practice of Occlusion. Chicago: Quintessence, 1997:365–378.

109. Palla S, Gallo LM, Gossi D. Dynamic Stereometry of the temporomandibular joint. Orthod Craniofac Res 2003;6 (suppl 1):37–47.

110. Gossi DB, Gallo LM, Bahr E, Palla S. Dynamic intra-articular space variation in clicking TMJs. J Dent Res 2004;83: 480–484.

111. Chen YJ, Gallo LM, Palla S. The mediolateral temporomandibular joint disc position: An in vivo quantitative study. J Orofac Pain 2002;16:29–38.

112. Rao VM, Babaria A, Manoharan A, et al. Altered condylar morphology associated with disc displacement in TMJ dysfunction: Observations by MRI. Magn Reson Imaging 1990; 8:231–235.

113. Gibbs CH, Lundeen HC. Jaw movements and forces during chewing and swallowing and their clinical significance. In: Lundeen HC, Gibbs CH (eds). Advances in Occlusion. Boston: Wright, 1982:2–32.

114. Fischer R. The opening movements of the mandible and their reproduction in the articulator [in German]. Schweiz Mschr Zahnmed 1935;45:867–899.

115. Dupas PH, Picart B, Graux F, Lefevre C. Effect of clutch surface changes on the computerized pantographic reproducibility index and the Fischer angle. J Prosthet Dent 1987; 57:625–630.

116. Starcke EN. The history of articulators: Pursuing the evolution of the incisal-pin and guide. 2. J Prosthodont 2001; 10:113–121.

117. Proschel P, Hofmann M, Ott R. Ortho-function of the masticatory system [in German]. Dtsch Zahnarztl Z 1985;40: 186–191.

118. Proschel P, Hofmann M. Problems in interpreting functional mandibular movements. 1. The effects of multifactorial influences on the interpretability of recordings of masticatory movements [in German]. Dtsch Zahnarztl Z 1987;42:696–700.

119. Karlsson S, Carlsson GE. Characteristics of mandibular masticatory movement in young and elderly dentate subjects. J Dent Res 1990;69:473–476.

120. Kiliaridis S, Karlsson S, Kjellberg H. Characteristics of masticatory mandibular movements and velocity in growing individuals and young adults. J Dent Res 1991;70:1367–1370.

121. Wilding RJ, Lewin A. The determination of optimal human jaw movements based on their association with chewing performance. Arch Oral Biol 1994;39:333–343.

122. Plesh O, Bishop B, McCall W. Effect of gum hardness on chewing pattern. Exp Neurol 1986;92:502–512.

123. Proschel P, Hofmann M. Frontal chewing patterns of the incisor point and their dependence on resistance of food and type of occlusion. J Prosthet Dent 1988;59:617–624.

124. Chew CL, Lucas PW, Tay DK, Keng SB, Ow RK. The effect of food texture on the replication of jaw movements in mastication. J Dent 1988;16:210–214.

125. Horio T, Kawamura Y. Effects of texture of food on chewing patterns in the human subject. J Oral Rehabil 1989;16: 177–183.

126. Mongini F, Tempia-Valenta G, Conserva E. Habitual mastication in dysfunction: A computer-based analysis. J Prosthet Dent 1989;61:484–494.

127. Ozaki Y, Shigematsu T, Takahashi S. Analysis of the chewing movement in temporomandibular disorders. Bull Tokyo Dent Coll 1990;31:91–103.

128. Kuwahara T, Bessette RW, Maruyama T. Chewing pattern analysis in TMD patients with unilateral and bilateral internal derangement. Cranio 1995;13:167–172.

129. Kuwahara T, Bessette RW, Maruyama T. Chewing pattern analysis in TMD patients with and without internal derangement. 2. Cranio 1995;13:93–98.

130. Kuwahara T, Bessette RW, Maruyama T. Chewing pattern analysis in TMD patients with and without internal derangement. 1. Cranio 1995;13:8–14.

131. Gallo LM, Fushima K, Palla S. Mandibular helical axis pathways during mastication. J Dent Res 2000;79:1566–1572.

132. Gallo LM, Brasi M, Ernst B, Palla S. Relevance of mandibular helical axis analysis in functional and dysfunctional TMJs. J Biomech (in press).

133. Fushima K, Gallo LM, Krebs M, Palla S. Analysis of the TMJ intraarticular space variation: A non-invasive insight during mastication. Med Eng Phys 2003;25:181–190.

134. Hylander WL. Experimental analysis of temporomandibular joint reaction force in macaques. Am J Phys Anthropol 1979;51:433–456.

135. Throckmorton GS, Groshan GJ, Boyd SB. Muscle activity patterns and control of temporomandibular joint loads. J Prosthet Dent 1990;63:685–695.

136. Trainor PG, McLachlan KR, McCall WD. Modelling of forces in the human masticatory system with optimization of the angulations of the joint loads. J Biomech 1995;28:829–843.

137. Kuboki T, Azuma Y, Orsini MG, Takenami Y, Yamashita A. Effects of sustained unilateral molar clenching on the temporomandibular joint space. Oral Surg Oral Med Oral Pathol Oral Radiol Endod 1996;82:616–624.

CHAPTER 3

TMJ Growth, Adaptive Modeling and Remodeling, and Compensatory Mechanisms

Boudewijn Stegenga and Lambert G. M. de Bont

The temporomandibular joint (TMJ) is part of the locomotor system, consisting of interdependent connective tissues. It serves the essential purposes of maintaining the stability of the mandibular position and efficient movement during mandibular function.[1] In addition, the joint is an important regional field, contributing to the growth of the mandible.[2]

In his monumental study of 400 patients with TMJ osteoarthrosis, Boering[3] noted that 55% had a shortening of the mandibular ramus (Figs 3-1a and 3-1b). He also noted that at least 25% of these patients reported manifestation of their first symptoms before puberty. Such patients had flattened and shortened condyles caused by condylar deformity and disturbance of normal growth.[4] In a subsequent prospective study, a characteristic compensatory growth pattern, resulting in a backward growth rotation, was observed (see Figs 3-1a and 3-1b).[5] Thus, knowledge of the growth and adaptive mechanisms of the joint's tissues provides a biologic basis for understanding the maladaptive responses underlying temporomandibular disorders.

This chapter describes the tissues making up the TMJ, focusing on their development and capacity to adapt to environmental influences.

Definition of Terms

This chapter uses several terms that must be defined. The basic terms are *modeling* and *remodeling*. The process of modeling is required for reshaping and resizing to maintain the shape, proportions, and relationships of a bone during

its growth[2] and for adaptation after growth has ceased. The process of remodeling (often called *internal* or *haversian remodeling*) is associated with the resorption and deposition of bone internally, but it does not reshape or resize bone along its surfaces. Enlargement and simultaneous displacement of bone occur through a combination of bone deposition and resorption, which takes place at multiple sites at the same time in a complex three-dimensional variety of directions.[2] It is the composite of all these processes that produces growth. Bone may form either in cartilage by the process of endochondral bone formation or in membranous connective tissue by the process of intramembranous bone formation, which occurs by calcification of osteoid matrix derived from undifferentiated mesenchymal cells.

The tissues of the human body respond to changes in functional demand by tissue *adaptation*, resulting in changes in shape by a process that continues throughout life. This involves a balance between synthesis and breakdown (ie, between anabolic and catabolic activity) within the tissues, aimed at maintaining structural and functional integrity. When this process occurs at a molecular level and does not involve any change in the histologic or ultrastructural appearance of the tissue, the process is referred to as tissue *turnover*.[6]

Johnson[7] classified "remodeling" of a joint into three categories, although here we will use "modeling," the correct terminology by today's standards:

1. Progressive modeling, resulting from excessive proliferation and formation of new cartilage, with subsequent mineralization and conversion to bone
2. Regressive modeling, ie, resorption of the subchondral bone by osteoclasts, resulting in cavities that become

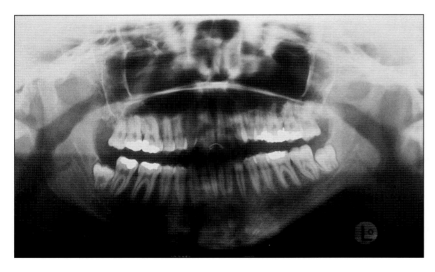

Fig 3-1a Shortening of the left mandibular ramus in a young patient. (From Stegenga et al.[4] Reprinted with permission.)

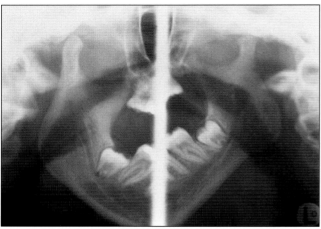

Fig 3-1b Transpharyngeal radiographs of the patient in Fig 3-1a, revealing the small condylar head, which has grown backward. Note the antegonial notching on the left side. (From Stegenga et al.[4] Reprinted with permission.)

filled with connective tissue, while the tissue of the articular zone remains intact

3. Circumferential (peripheral) modeling, which can lead to formation of osteophytes

An imbalance between synthesis and breakdown can jeopardize the system's integrity; this is referred to as *maladaptation*.

Another response to altered loading is *deformation*, ie, a change in shape in response to compression, tension, or shear; the change may be temporary or permanent. A temporary response is usually *compensatory*. An example is the viscoelastic deformation of the disc to compensate for the incongruity of the bony surfaces during joint movements. Another example of compensation is a (usually temporary) muscular response to altered circumstances. When a compensatory response is out of control, it can jeopardize the system's continued undisturbed functioning; this situation is termed *decompensation*.

Developmental Changes

Unlike most of the synovial joints of the body, the TMJ does not form in a primary cartilaginous matrix. Meckel's cartilage is the primary cartilage of the first branchial arch, and it forms the malleus and incus bones, the anterior malleolar ligament, and the sphenomandibular ligament, but it does not contribute to the formation of the TMJ. The TMJ is formed from a secondary cartilage that arises ectopically rather than from the primary cartilage, and it is transformed into bone except at its proximal end, where it forms an articulation with the temporal bone. Unlike in the long bones, where the epiphyseal and articular cartilages are separated by bone tissue, in the mandibular condyle the growth cartilage is near the surface of the bone just beneath the fibrous articular layer. It quickly undergoes atrophic change in the absence of function but regains its endochondral capability when

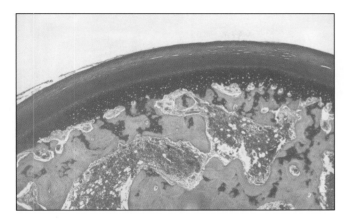

Fig 3-2 Section through the condylar head of a 14-year-old boy, revealing endochondral ossification. (Alcian blue PAS, 22× magnification.)

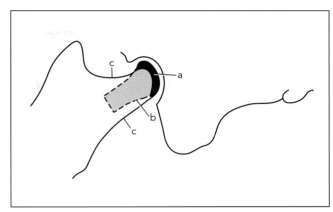

Fig 3-3 As (a) the condylar cartilage proliferates in an upward and backward direction, it is progressively replaced by (b) a medullary core of endochondral bone, while (c) the cortical bone of the mandibular neck and other parts of the ramus undergoes growth along the periosteal and endosteal surfaces. (Redrawn from Enlow[2] with permission.)

functional demands are reestablished.[8,9] Thus, the cartilage of the mandibular condyle provides endochondral bone growth, regional adaptive growth, and a moveable articulation.

The mandibular condyle plays an important role in mandibular and craniofacial development. The condylar process continues to grow by endochondral ossification of the secondary cartilage (Fig 3-2) in response to functional requirements. This process of endochondral bone growth produces a core of fine cancellous bone located specifically in the medullary part of the condyle and its neck (Fig 3-3).

However, the process of mandibular growth involves more than condylar growth. Each part of the mandible actively participates, and a widespread distribution of modeling fields covers the entire bone, both inside (endosteal surfaces) and outside (periosteal surfaces) (Fig 3-4).[2] At each site, growth represents adaptations to the localized developmental, biomechanical, and physiologic circumstances that are present.[2] The growing bone undergoes modeling to relocate its parts. For example, the growing ramus is displaced in a posterior direction, and the area that was part of the ramus becomes modeled into an addition to the mandibular body, which in this way gains in length. Also, when the ramus grows posteriorly, the mandibular condyle simultaneously grows upward and backward by the process of endochondral bone formation to maintain its relationship with the temporal bone. By contrast, an intramembranous type of growth takes place in the other parts of the ramus because of the tensile relationships of the periosteum with the muscles of mastication.[2] The glenoid fossa

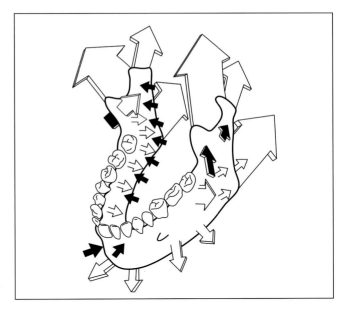

Fig 3-4 Three-dimensional directions of mandibular growth. (*white arrows*) Surfaces that are depository in nature. (*black arrows*) Resorptive periosteal surfaces. (Redrawn from Enlow[2] with permission.)

and articular eminence in the temporal bone also form by intramembranous ossification.

The postnatal development of the TMJ has been described in a study of 61 humans with ages ranging from 2 days to 27 years.[10] In neonates, the cartilage layer con-

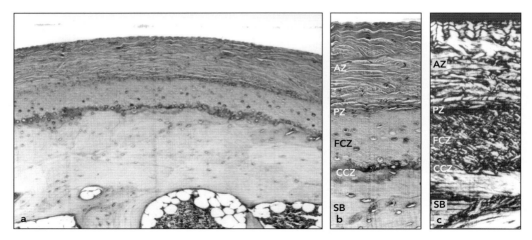

Fig 3-5 *(a)* Section through a healthy condylar head, viewed under transmitted light microscopy. (Hematoxylin-eosin stain; original magnification ×27.) *(b)* Enlarged view of the section in Fig 3-5a, showing the different zones: (AZ) Articular zone; (PZ) proliferative zone; (FCZ) fibrocartilaginous zone; (CCZ) calcified cartilage zone; (SB) subchondral bone. (Original magnification ×56.) *(c)* Same area shown in Fig 3-5b, viewed under polarized light. (AZ) Articular zone; (PZ) proliferative zone; (FCZ) fibrocartilaginous zone; (CCZ) calcified cartilage zone; (SB) subchondral bone. (Original magnification ×56.)

stitutes a large part of the condyle, and the outermost layer is richly vascularized. However, the condylar cartilage gradually decreases in thickness, and by 5 to 6 years of age it constitutes only a thin zone on the top of the condyle. In neonates, the temporal component is flat and lined by vascularized connective tissue, but, by the age of 3 years, the articular layer becomes avascular and contains few cells. A fibrocartilage layer is lacking in the fossa but is present on the articular eminence.

At birth, the TMJ lies almost in line with the occlusal plane.[11] Continued postnatal growth is largely dependent on the normal relationship of bone, muscles, and teeth. The condyle contributes to the continuing growth of the ramus in a posterosuperior direction until growth ceases and the joint is then positioned superior to the occlusal plane.

Condylar Fibrocartilage

The fibrocartilage of the growing mandibular condyle consists of several distinct zones, each with a characteristic organization and alignment of collagen fibrils (Fig 3-5). The fibrils in the articular zone are arranged in densely packed sheets running parallel to the articular surface.[12,13] This layer passively adapts to the underlying tissue layers. The next layer, the fibrocartilaginous zone, contains dense, fibrous connective tissue in which the fibrils are organized in bundles with random orientation.[12] The bundles in the

calcified cartilaginous zone are also randomly oriented, although those just adjacent to the subchondral bone have a radial orientation.[12]

Although many authors have described the presence of a distinct proliferative zone containing undifferentiated mesenchyme,[12,14–18] Luder[13] has noted the presence of chondrocyte clusters in the superficial and deep zones as well, indicating that proliferation does not seem to be confined only to this proliferative zone. Luder[13] also observed hyaline-like fibrocartilage to be present in more than 40% of young adults, especially in areas with an irregular cartilage-bone interface, suggesting active bone modeling.[13]

The architecture of adult articular tissue differs from that observed in growing individuals.[10,19] In the latter, the fibrocartilaginous layer forms a growth zone, which plays an important role in normal development of the joint. In areas with rapid growth, the undifferentiated cells transform into prechondrocytes and hypertrophying chondrocytes. The rapidity of growth is to a large extent related to the hypertrophying cartilage cells. Growth is rapid up to the age of 15 years, after which it progressively decreases until adulthood is reached. Hypertrophic cartilage has been reported to be present only in individuals younger than 30 years,[15,17,19] after which it is replaced by fibrocartilage.[20] These latter changes are largely confined to the load-bearing superior and anterior areas of the condyle, while its posterior slope maintains the same appearance seen during growth. These findings are in agreement with earlier reports.[10,13,17,18,21]

Maintenance of cells in non–load-bearing areas and reduction in cellularity in load-bearing areas point to the utilization of fibrocartilage as a substitute for hypertrophic cartilage.[17,19] Studies suggest that the tissue's cellularity is reduced or even disappears from this zone soon after cessation of condylar growth.[15,18] Following endochondral ossification during growth, a compact subchondral bone plate is formed.[20]

Articular Disc

A concentration of mesenchymal cells between the developing temporal bone and mandibular condyle produces the articular disc, the capsule of the TMJ, and the lateral pterygoid muscle.[22] The embryonic disc is vascularized until it becomes loaded by jaw movements in utero.[23] At birth, the disc is flat on its superior surface because the articular eminence has not yet developed. By the time the primary teeth occlude, the temporal component develops its curvature,[24] and the disc becomes biconcave. After approximately 20 years of jaw function, the compressed central part of the disc changes into fibrocartilage.

Whenever the disc is loaded, its inclined planes will seat it in a stable relationship with the condyle.[25] The opening rotation of the condyle causes the disc to lie against the more posterior region of the condyle, where it is more stable. During translation, the disc is passively carried along in an anterior direction.[25,26]

Light microscopy of the articular disc reveals a tight, fibrous connective tissue composed of collagen fiber bundles[27] and elastic fibers,[28] especially in the anterior and medial parts.[29] Scanning electron microscopy reveals that the collagen fiber bundles are running in all directions, although the main alignment is anteroposterior.[30] The disc is designed to withstand compressive and shearing loads and has viscoelastic properties, and its resistance is strengthened by the arrangement of the collagen fibers.[31,32] It also has a self-centering capability; when compressed, the joint space is narrowed and the thinnest portion of the disc is brought between the bones.[25,33] On release of pressure, the elastic fibers restore the shape of the disc, which then allows a thicker portion to fill the joint space.[23,25] Thus, the disc is pliable and easily deformed. However, the disc is not capable of cellular modeling,[23] and loading produces only elastic or plastic deformation.

The morphology of the posterior part of the disc is especially important for the stability of the disc-condyle complex. This part has the highest resistance of all the parts of the disc.[27] However, flattening of the posterior band of the disc can occur with sustained loads in a posterosuperior direction.[25] As the disc becomes increasingly

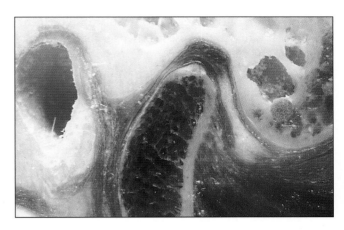

Fig 3-6 Sagittal section through a TMJ showing flattening of the posterior band of a deranged disc. (From Stegenga et al.[4] Reprinted with permission.)

deformed by such compression, it gradually loses its thickened peripheral bands, and hence its self-seating capacity, and becomes (more) deranged (Fig 3-6).[23]

Temporal Component

The articular eminence of the TMJ, as a mechanical constraint, dictates the movement of the condyle-disc complex. It shows a symmetric growth pattern and grows rapidly, attaining almost half of its adult form by the age of 2 years.[34] Bone deposition along the articular eminence leads to a steeper slope. This process occurs parallel to eruption of the primary incisors, the permanent first molars, and the permanent second molars.[24] The eminence increases in height rapidly until the age of 7 years; growth almost ceases during the period of the mixed dentition, and the eminence acquires its final height by the age of 20 years.[35] Growth of the articular eminence creates incongruities between the loading surfaces that predispose to stress concentration in the anterior region of the condyle, making this area prone to degenerative alterations.[36]

It has been suggested that a steep articular eminence can predispose to temporomandibular dysfunction. However, an arthrotomographic study revealed that the articular eminence is steeper in asymptomatic volunteers with normal disc position than in patients with TMJ disc derangement.[37] These authors found that osseous changes in the form of modeling or osteoarthrosis are the important factors that influence the steepness of the eminence. Therefore, they concluded that a gradual flattening of the eminence is not causally related to the disc displacement, but rather it is due to the osseous changes that develop as sequelae to the derangement.[37]

Adaptive Modeling

After growth has stopped, structural changes continue to occur in both the soft and the mineralized tissues of the joint. Such modeling changes reflect the functional demands on the joint structures.[38] Modeling is characterized by slow morphologic changes under physiologic circumstances that permit adaptation of the shape of the joint components and, in this way, maintain joint function. In experimental studies, condylar cartilage hyperplasia has been observed in response to mandibular protrusion,[39] mandibular retrusion,[40] surgical induction of disc displacement,[41] disc perforation,[42] and removal of the disc.[43]

More extensive modeling can lead to morphologic changes that may interfere with joint function. Such morphologic variations have been documented and demonstrate that modeling changes are common in the TMJs of young adults.[15,44] With nonphysiologic loads, structural changes associated with tissue breakdown are dominant (regressive modeling).

The characteristic mechanisms of modeling are observed in maladaptive (ie, osteoarthritic) joints as well. This makes it difficult to distinguish between what can be regarded as a normally adapted joint and one that has become maladapted and pathologically involved. A useful criterion is related to the integrity of the articular tissue.[21] Thus, osteoarthrosis represents changes associated with breakdown of the articular surface layer, resulting in fibrillation, fissuring, and erosion.

Blackwood[45] described three types of modeling in different age groups. He concluded that the proliferative cell zone is mainly responsible for the dimensional changes in the articular surface and that the fibrous surface layer does not participate in this process. Subsequent studies confirmed that increased loading stimulates cellular proliferation and cartilage formation from the undifferentiated mesenchyme.[14] The amount of undifferentiated mesenchyme appears to vary inversely with the thickness of the soft tissue covering of the condyle and the amount of loading. These studies also showed that the condyle has a higher modeling capacity than the temporal component. However, Rabie et al[46] have shown that forward mandibular positioning elicited a cellular response in both the condyle and the glenoid fossa and that the number of replicating mesenchymal cells is proportional to the bone-forming potential at that site.

The pathways of mesenchymal cells differ in the condyle and the temporal bone component because of the different mechanisms of bone formation at these sites. In the temporal bone component, mesenchymal cells directly differentiate into osteoblasts before ultimately forming bone. In the condyle, mesenchymal cells first undergo a transitory stage of cartilage formation before being replaced by bone after vascular invasion.[47,48] In the condyle, these cells are located mainly in the proliferative layer,[49,50] and in the glenoid fossa they can be seen as a row of cells beneath the articular layer.[51]

The ability of the articular disc to remodel is very limited (if present at all),[23] and loading produces only viscoelastic or plastic deformation. Deformation in the area of the posterior band takes place principally on the lower side of the disc.[52] It has been suggested that this type of deformation is related to an increased risk of progression from a reducing disc derangement to a nonreducing disc derangement.[53]

The disc attachments merge with the articular capsule around the periphery of the disc, thus dividing the joint cavity into separate superior and inferior compartments.[23] The capsule and capsular ligaments consist of a well-vascularized, loose collagenous tissue containing elastic fibers and sensory nerve endings. Therefore, when this tissue is overloaded (eg, stretched beyond the habitual range), it commonly responds with an inflammatory reaction (Fig 3-7a) that is a common source of joint pain. The pain elicits a protective muscular response that permits the tissue to heal. The capsular attachment of the articular disc is reinforced at the lateral and medial condylar poles, thereby restraining its movement relative to the condyle to mainly a rotational component.[54] However, it is more flexible at other sites owing to the presence of elastic fibers.

Adaptive changes occurring within these tissues can have mechanical implications. For example, when the reinforced attachments of the disc to the condyle are overextended (ie, elongated because of plastic deformation) as a response to gradual or repetitive stretching, the sliding component of the movements in the lower joint compartment may increase, allowing the disc to become hypermobile relative to the condyle.

Another well-documented response to repetitive compression and/or shear involves decreased vascularity and fibrosis. The nature of this response is determined by the magnitude and direction of the forces acting on the joint. For example, repetitive loading of the retrodiscal tissues may induce adaptive changes aimed at making the tissue more resistant to compression, ie, fibrosis and cartilaginous changes compatible with the formation of a nonvascularized and noninnervated "pseudodisc."[55–57] However, chronic excessive compression can also result in decompen-

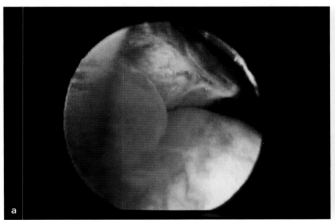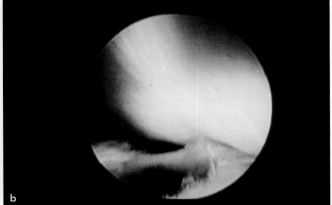

Fig 3-7 Arthroscopic views of tissue responses to overloading. *(a)* Inflammatory response to soft tissue impingement. *(b)* Perforation of the retrodiscal tissue.

sation in the form of thinning, overextension, inflammation, and perforation (Fig 3-7b).

Disc derangement also appears to be associated with adaptive changes of the soft tissues that cover the articular eminence.[58] Increased thickness of the articular surface layer has been observed in TMJs with a completely displaced disc with a normal, biconcave shape and in joints with a chronic, nonreducing, deformed biconvex disc. This increase in articular soft tissue thickness has been interpreted as an adaptive mechanism to maintain the condylar path and to withstand excessive loading.[58]

The capacity for adaptation of the bony structures in children and adolescents allows modeling to occur in the TMJ during orthodontic treatment[59,60] and after surgical repositioning of the condyles.[61] Magnetic resonance images have shown that progressive remodeling of the condyle and temporal part of the joint occurs within 3 months after insertion of a Herbst appliance.[62] Furthermore, adaptive changes of the condyle and fossa have been found in more than half of joints after mandibular midline osteodistraction.[63]

Control of Growth and Adaptation

The control of growth of an organism, organ, or tissue depends on the interaction between genetic and environmental factors. The extent of the environmental influences depends on the tissue under consideration and the severity of these external effects. All tissues require an adequate level of nutrition and an appropriate hormonal balance for growth to be within normal limits.

Although the overall shape of the mandible is, at least in part, genetically determined, there are many variations in the size and shape of the components of the TMJ and their relationship to each other (Fig 3-8). These developmental variations likely reflect variations in function, both of the mandible itself and of its surrounding structures. This also applies to the period after growth has ceased and skeletal maturation has been achieved. The process of modeling continues so that adaptation in structure can meet changing functional demands. Loss of the teeth, for example, results not only in resorption of the alveolar process but also in changes in the shape of other sites of the mandible, presumably in response to changes in the surrounding "functional matrix."[64]

However, the original functional matrix concept should not be overextended. In his revision of the functional matrix hypothesis, Moss[65] suggested that genomic and epigenetic factors interact and that neither alone is a sufficient cause of morphologic change. Although it has been demonstrated that the condylar cartilage is endowed with an adaptive modeling potential, it also possesses an intrinsic growth potential.[66]

The clinical importance of the mandibular condyle has generated investigations focusing on its natural growth and its adaptive potential in response to changes in mandibular position.[67–69] This research has identified cellular influences on condylar growth, which result in questions that can only be answered on a molecular level. Rabie and Hägg[70] reported on the influence of various growth factors and other regulatory factors that are endogenously

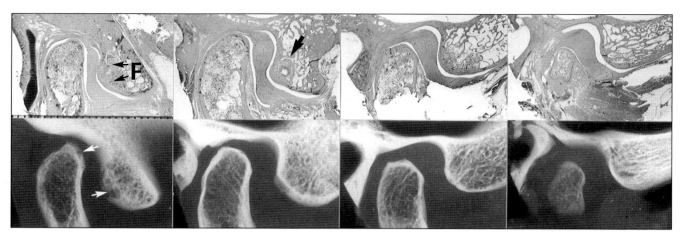

Fig 3-8 *(top row)* Light microscopic sections and *(bottom row)* corresponding radiographs of a right TMJ with an anteriorly displaced disc. *(top and bottom, right to left)* Medial to lateral cuts. The first (medial) cut shows the disc in a normal position. The disc position and shape alter as the cuts move from medial to lateral. *(white arrows)* Erosions of the condyle and eminence. *(black arrows)* The marrow spaces in the eminence show fibrosis (F). (Hematoxylin-eosin, original magnification ×1.6.)

expressed by cells in the mandibular condyle. The process of condylar growth appears to follow a sequence of events that can be outlined as follows[70]:

Cells in the proliferative layer express Sox 9 transcription factor required for the differentiation of mesenchymal cells to chondroblasts.[71] Chondroblasts engage in cartilage formation marked by the synthesis of type II collagen, the main type of collagen that forms the framework of the cartilage matrix in the growing condyle. Chondrocytes express Sox 9 transcription factor that regulates the synthesis of type II collagen and subsequently affects condylar cartilage formation. These cells continue to mature and progress towards hypertrophy. Hypertrophic chondrocytes secrete type X collagen, the matrix for the hypertrophic cartilage destined for endochondral ossification. Cells in the upper zone of the hypertrophic cartilage secrete vascular endothelial growth factor, which regulates the neovascularization of the hypertrophic cartilage and influences the removal of the cartilage matrix. Erosion of the hypertrophic cartilage continues as neovascularization, and the formation of marrow tissue and resorptive tissue progresses. The invading blood vessels bring osteogenic progenitor mesenchymal cells into the mineralization front and later differentiate into osteoblasts and engage in osteogenesis.

Based on this work, cellular and molecular changes in the condyle during mandibular advancement have been compared. Forward mandibular positioning appears to lead to an increase in the number of replicating mesenchymal cells,[46] an increase in the factors regulating chondrocyte differentiation and maturation,[72] and an increase in the level of expression of vascular endothelial growth factor, the central regulator of vascularization,[73] thus leading to new bone formation in the condyle.

Threats to the TMJ As a Biologic System

Growth Disturbances

The two basic varieties of abnormal growth are excessive and impaired growth. Mandibular dysfunction in growing individuals can be associated with reduced mandibular growth as well as with reactive hyperplastic growth of the condylar and coronoid processes and in the gonial region. A common example of excessive growth is unilateral condylar hyperplasia, which is a good illustration of the impressive adaptive capacity and compensatory mechanisms of the human body. Ongoing unilateral growth of the condyle causes facial asymmetry, chin deviation to the contralateral side, and a tilted occlusal plane that is caused by the compensatory eruption of the maxillary teeth (Fig 3-9a).[74] After condylectomy, the adaptive and compensatory changes appear to be reversible within about a year (Figs 3-9b and 3-10).

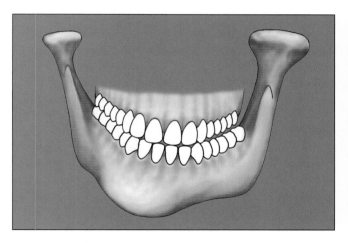

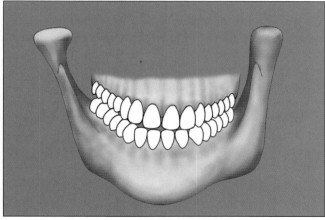

Fig 3-9a Condylar hyperplasia. Ongoing growth of the condyle results in changes in the position of the chin, alveolar process, and teeth. (From Stegenga et al.[4] Reprinted with permission.)

Fig 3-9b Result of condylectomy: adaptive modeling that resolves the asymmetry. (From Stegenga et al.[4] Reprinted with permission.)

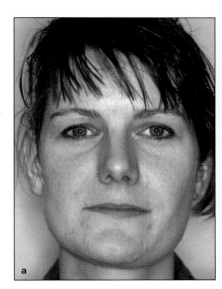

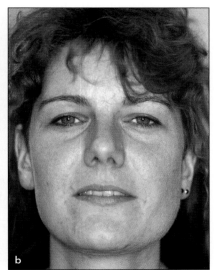

Fig 3-10 (a) Asymmetry of the face, resulting from condylar hyperplasia in a 27-year-old woman. (b) 1 year after condylectomy. (From Stegenga et al.[4] Reprinted with permission.)

Another example of excessive growth is reactive coronoid hyperplasia. It has been suggested that the temporal muscle plays an etiologic role in this process.[75] Permanent disc displacement, with associated restriction in condylar translatory capacity, has been shown to induce temporal muscle hyperactivity,[76] which can impair local circulation in its tendon, favoring degenerative changes and subsequent reactive bone hyperplasia.

Impaired growth may be developmental (eg, craniofacial microsomia) or may occur secondary to trauma, ionizing radiation, infection, systemic arthropathy, and neoplasia. *Postcondylar fracture syndrome* refers to several adaptive alterations that can occur following condylar fracture.[77] These include a shortened ramus and restricted translation on the injured side, slow compensatory eruption of the teeth on the contralateral side, and secondary changes in the remainder of the facial skeleton.[78] A common sequela of juvenile idiopathic arthritis affecting the TMJ in children is facial deformity caused by destruction of the condylar growth site.

Diagnostically, it is important to distinguish whether a specific TMJ disorder is caused by or results from a disturbance of mandibular growth. A follow-up study of Boering's patients showed that differences in the heights of the mandibular rami were observed significantly more often in patients with unilateral permanent disc displacement than in control individuals.[79] In addition, an association between facial asymmetry and TMJ disc displacement has been reported in children and adults.[80,81] However, a cause-effect relationship has not been established.

A series of studies in growing rabbits have addressed the influence of experimentally induced disc displacement on mandibular growth. When the retrodiscal tissue was kept intact, mandibular growth slowed on the disc displacement side, resulting in a shorter ramus, reactive hyperplastic growth in the gonial region associated with antegonial notching,[82] a midline shift toward the ipsilateral side, and an inferiorly directed forward-growth tendency.[83] It has been suggested that the excessive bone growth in the gonial region compensates for the shortening of the mandibular ramus.[84] When the disc was experimentally displaced and the retrodiscal tissue was transsected, shortening of the mandible resulted from reduction of condylar height secondary to degenerative changes.[85] These experimental results were confirmed in patients with an onset of permanent disc derangement before the end of the growth spurt, in whom craniofacial height was consistently shorter on the affected side, resulting in deviation of the chin to that side.[75]

Maladaptive Changes

Like any biologic system, the mandibular locomotor apparatus is subjected to potentially harmful influences. The connective tissues making up the TMJ display a dynamic balance between form and function. All have the capacity to adapt to changing functional demands, each within tissue-specific limits.[1,86] As long as the system remains in this state, normally the patient will not report symptoms or functional disturbances.

Altered loading induces an adaptive response aimed at achieving a tissue structure that is able to withstand the load imposed on the tissue. This adaptive mechanism, indicated by the addition of bone in response to mechanical stimuli, has been referred to as *progressive remodeling*. When the tissue-specific physiologic limits are exceeded, protective and compensatory mechanisms that are aimed at preventing, limiting, or repairing damage are recruited.[86] This frequently involves temporary adjustments within or outside the involved tissues that may result in repair or regeneration or to a more permanently changed state of equilibrium. An example of the former is the compensatory muscular response to joint pain from an injury (splinting), providing sufficient rest to the joint to permit healing. An example of the latter is the compensatory changes occur-

ring within the retrodiscal tissue, involving decreased vascularity and innervation, fibrosis, and the presence of cartilage cells that have been reported to be related to an anteriorly positioned disc[87–89] or to aging.[90] These changes produce transient (or sometimes permanent) signs and symptoms that usually are compatible with continued function and do not justify active treatment. Thus, adaptation and compensation are the primary mechanisms to overcome the many adverse influences imposed on the joint.

However, the adaptive and compensatory mechanisms are limited in each of the tissues of the TMJ. This limitation is highly variable among individuals and probably declines gradually with age. Persistent damaging influences can exceed the tissue's adaptive capacity and exhaust the compensatory mechanisms. In these cases, regressive remodeling (ie, maladaptation) and decompensation, accompanied by destructive morphologic changes as well as by pain and other clinically evident signs and symptoms, become manifest. However, the majority of signs and symptoms have a tendency to subside with time, indicating that the body is able to continue functioning even under less-than-desirable circumstances.[3,91] Although osteoarthritis is frequently characterized by crepitation and accompanied by deformation of the condyle, there is rarely any pain originating from the joint surfaces.[91] Therefore, the end stage of the disease has been referred to as *residual osteoarthrosis*.[92]

Although the etiologic factors that play the major role in disturbing the balance between damaging influences and the adaptive capacity of the joint tissues remain obscure, overloading (either absolute or relative) seems to be a common denominator. Over the years, trauma has been implicated as a major cause of TMJ disorders, either primarily or secondarily. Macrotrauma can result in soft tissue injuries such as tearing, laceration, or rupture of a disc attachment or of the lateral ligament and capsule. Traumatic arthritis is the immediate response, characterized by joint effusion resulting from increased vascular permeability or from intra-articular bleeding following tissue rupture. The patient reports pain and an acute malocclusion (ie, a sudden change in tooth contact). There is usually a remission of the acute symptoms within a few days. However, intra-articular bleeding can give rise to the formation of adhesions and fibrosis, both of the capsule and in the joint cavity. Isberg et al[93] described the formation of vascularized and innervated intra-articular hyperplastic tissue related to trauma and disc displacement that can cause a sharp, shooting pain with jaw motion.

Microtraumatic events, repetitive small injuries that cause soft and hard tissue responses, are also often mentioned as a significant etiologic factor in producing TMJ disorders. The roles of bruxism, condylar hypermobility, recurrent condylar dislocation, retrusive guidance by the dental occlusion directing the condyle posteriorly in the fossa, and partial or complete tooth loss and loss of molar support in particular[94,95] have been stressed repeatedly. However, a causal relationship between bruxism and temporomandibular disorders has not been established.[96] Moreover, neither hypermobility[97] nor lack of molar support[98] necessarily leads to osteoarthritis (see chapter 25).

Luder[99] observed that degenerative changes in the human TMJ depend on (in order of significance) age, loss of molar support, disc position, and load bearing. In comparison with all other factors examined, age seemed to play by far the most important role. This association could reflect an intrinsic accumulation of tissue damage caused by a gradual decline in cellular capacity for adaptation, as typically occurs with aging.[99] Mechanical factors, such as loss of molar support, also appear to be involved, particularly in the initiation of lesions on the load-bearing articular surfaces of the condyle and articular eminence of younger individuals.[99] Disc displacement only seems to play a role in association with loss of molar support. Load bearing of the condyle and temporal components seem to play a significant role only in association with aging. It has been suggested that, because the initial articular tissue disintegration at a young age is observed mainly on load-bearing surfaces, this most likely arises under the influence of mechanical factors.[99] In contrast, lesions on non–load-bearing surfaces, which must depend on factors other than mechanical ones, become significant only at an advanced age and therefore develop secondarily.[99–101]

Summary

The maintenance of the TMJ in a functional state involves the interdependence of the tissues making up the joint. The fibrocartilage is supported by the subchondral bone and is dependent on the synovial fluid for its nutrients, metabolic exchange, protection, and lubrication. The synovial membrane is supported by the joint capsule. The major part of the load during functional movements is absorbed by involuntary contraction of the muscles supporting the joint in response to proprioceptive information from the muscles and capsular ligaments. Compression of the joint surfaces and stretching of the ligaments contribute to load absorption. The shearing stress is reduced by a very effective lubrication mechanism (see chapter 7). This supporting system is essential for normal joint function.

Absolute (eg, traumatic) overloading can exceed the intact adaptive capacity of the tissues making up this system. Under these circumstances, compensatory responses from the adjacent structures and therapeutic support usually are sufficient to permit healing, unless the influences contributing to overloading are not eliminated. This is frequently the case when the capacity of the tissues involved in the supporting system is intrinsically reduced. This makes the joint vulnerable even to normal loading (relative overloading), which may be sufficient to exceed the tissue's capacity to adapt.

The joint organ is the outcome of the development of a functioning system. In young people, adaptation is based on a combination of growth, modeling, and remodeling.[102] In adults, since growth is no longer occurring, adaptation depends primarily on modeling and remodeling processes.[103] As a result, there are wide variations in the morphology, adaptive capacity, and functional demands of the human TMJ. There are also variations in the relationship of the condyle to the fossa and in the position of the articular disc. In addition, a joint that has adapted to an abnormal situation by recovery or repair may be clinically healthy despite the presence of signs and symptoms (such as clicking). Unfortunately, such phenomena often are erroneously regarded as an indication of an abnormality requiring treatment.[86] Instead, clinicians should realize that the body may have introduced compensatory mechanisms, resulting in nonpathologic clinical characteristics that have been present for many years.

Influences imposing loads on the masticatory apparatus, mechanisms of adaptation and compensation, and the emergence of symptoms are interrelated and provide the biologic basis for clinical practice. Whether or not symptoms will arise in the masticatory system depends primarily on the equilibrium between harmful influences and the patient's capacity for adaptation. It appears that this balance is difficult to maintain in the age group between 20 and 45 years.[104]

With persistent nonphysiologic loading, the masticatory system's structures can lose their ability to adapt and compensate, thus resulting in a state of maladaptation and decompensation. Provocation of reproducible symptoms during the clinical examination indicates the presence of a disturbance that may be either compensated or decompensated. The former require no treatment or, at most, therapeutic efforts aimed at supporting the adaptive and compensatory mechanisms to prevent a transition toward maladaptation and decompensation. The amount of structural change depends on the intensity, frequency, duration, and direction of the loads.[105] Therefore, to provide a rational basis for treatment, it is important to determine the nature and relative contribution of the harmful influences as comprehensively as possible. In addition, the clinician should determine the direction of loading that provokes the symptoms, which may be specific (symptoms are provoked only in one main direction) or nonspecific (symptoms are provoked in various directions).

In a thorough history, information about the patient's complaints and harmful influences is collected. The clinical examination serves to determine whether or not specific structures are adapted by determining the extent to which passive mouth opening and the range of movement is limited[106,107] and whether loading of the joint surfaces and ligamentous and muscular structures reproduces the patient's complaints.[108,109]

One might expect that diagnostic imaging would reveal which TMJs are compromised and in need of treatment. However, it has been shown that the appearance of the TMJ structures on diagnostic images is of minor importance both diagnostically and therapeutically. In spite of radiographically visible osseous changes and/or soft tissue displacements or deformities, adaptation of the fibrocartilaginous articular surfaces may permit normal function. Moreover, epidemiologic and clinical studies have shown that TMJs with obvious radiographic changes often display insignificant or no clinical symptoms (see chapter 10).[79,110]

References

1. Stegenga B. Osteoarthritis of the temporomandibular joint organ and its relationship to disc displacement. J Orofac Pain 2001;15:193–205.

2. Enlow DH. The condyle and facial growth. In: Sarnat BG, Laskin DM (eds). The Temporomandibular Joint: A Biological Basis for Clinical Practice, ed 4. Philadelphia: Saunders, 1992:48–59.

3. Boering G. Temporomandibular Joint Osteoarthrosis [thesis]. Groningen, The Netherlands: University of Groningen, 1966 (reprinted in English, 1994).

4. Stegenga B, Vissink A, de Bont LGM. Mondziekten en kaakchirurgie. Assen, The Netherlands: Van Gorcum, 2000.

5. Dibbets JM. Juvenile temporomandibular joint dysfunction and craniofacial growth [thesis]. Groningen, The Netherlands: University of Groningen, 1977.

6. Meikle MC. Remodeling. In: Sarnat BG, Laskin DM (eds). The Temporomandibular Joint: A Biological Basis for Clinical Practice, ed 4. Philadelphia: Saunders, 1992:93–107.

7. Johnson LC. Kinetics of osteoarthritis. Lab Invest 1959;8: 1223–1238.

8. Glineburg RW, Laskin DW, Blaustein DI. The effects of immobilization of the primate temporomandibular joint. J Oral Maxillofac Surg 1982;40:3–8.

9. Lydiatt DD, Davis LF. The effects of immobilization on the rabbit temporomandibular joint. J Oral Maxillofac Surg 1985;43:188–193.

10. Thilander B, Carlsson GE, Ingervall B. Postnatal development of the human temporomandibular joint. 1. A histological study. Acta Odontol Scand 1976;34:117–126.

11. Bell WE. Temporomandibular Disorders. Classification, Diagnosis, Management, ed 3. Chicago: Year Book Medical, 1990.

12. de Bont LGM, Boering G, Havinga P, Liem RSB. Spatial arrangement of collagen fibrils in the articular cartilage of the mandibular condyle: A light microscopic and scanning electron microscopic study. J Oral Maxillofac Surg 1984;42: 306–313.

13. Luder HU. Frequency and distribution of articular tissue features in adult human mandibular condyles: A semiquantitative light microscopic study. Anat Rec 1997;248:18–28.

14. Hansson TL, Öberg T, Carlsson GE, Kopp S. Thickness of the soft tissue layers and the articular disk in the temporomandibular joint. Acta Odontol Scand 1977;35:77–83.

15. Lubsen CC, Hansson TL, Nordström BB, Solberg WK. Histomorphometric analysis of cartilage and subchondral bone in mandibular condyles of young human adults at autopsy. Arch Oral Biol 1985;30:129–136.

16. Slootweg PJ, de Wilde PCM. Condylar pathology in jaw dysfunction: A semi-quantitative study. J Oral Pathol 1985;14: 690–697.

17. Lubsen CC, Hansson TL, Nordström BB, Solberg WK. Histomorphometry of age and sex changes in mandibular condyles of young human adults. Arch Oral Biol 1987;32: 729–733.

18. Bibb CA, Pullinger AG, Baldioceda F. The relationship of undifferentiated mesenchymal cells to TMJ articular tissue thickness. J Dent Res 1992;71:1816–1821.

19. Öberg T, Carlsson GE. Macroscopic and microscopic anatomy of the temporomandibular joint. In Zarb GA, Carlsson GE (eds). Temporomandibular Joint Function and Dysfunction. Copenhagen: Munksgaard, 1979:101–118.

20. Luder HU. Age changes in the articular tissue of human mandibular condyles from adolescence to old age: A semiquantitative light microscopic study. Anat Rec 1998;251: 439–447.

21. Moffett BC, Johnson LC, McCabe JB, Askew HC. Articular remodeling in the adult human temporomandibular joint. Am J Anat 1964;115:119–141.

22. Van der Linden EJ, Burdi AR, de Jongh HJ. Critical periods in the prenatal morphogenesis of the human lateral pterygoid muscle, the mandibular condyle, the articular capsule and medial articular capsule. Am J Orthod 1987;91:22–28.

23. Moffett BC. Histologic aspects of temporomandibular joint derangements. In: Moffett BC (ed). Diagnosis of Internal Derangements of the Temporomandibular Joint. Seattle: University of Washington, 1984:47–49.

24. Dibbets JM, Dijkman GE. The postnatal development of the temporal part of the human temporomandibular joint. A quantitative study on skulls. Anat Anz 1997;179:569–572.

25. Osborn JW. The disc of the human temporomandibular joint: Design, function and failure. J Oral Rehabil 1985;12:279–293.

26. Roth TE, Goldberg JS, Behrents RG. Synovial fluid pressure determination in the temporomandibular joint. Oral Surg Oral Med Oral Pathol Oral Radiol Endod 1984;57:583–588.

27. Mills DK, Fiandaca DJ, Scapino RP. Morphologic, microscopic, and immunohistochemical investigations into the function of the primate TMJ disc. J Orofac Pain 1994;8:136–154.

28. Nagy NB, Daniel JC. Distribution of elastic fibers in the developing rabbit craniomandibular joint. Arch Oral Biol 1991;36:15–23.

29. Luder HD, Bobst P. Wall architecture and disc attachment of the human temporomandibular joint. Schweiz Monatsschr Zahnmed 1991;101:557–570.

30. de Bont LGM, Liem RSB, Havinga P, Boering G. Fibrous component of the temporomandibular joint disk. Cranio 1985;3:368–373.

31. Shengyi T, Xu Y. Biomechanical properties and collagen fiber orientation of TMJ discs in dogs. 1. Gross anatomy and collagen fiber orientation of the discs. J Orofac Pain 1991;5:28–34.

32. Chin LP, Aker FD, Zarrinnia K. The viscoelastic properties of the human temporomandibular joint disc. J Oral Maxillofac Surg 1996;54:315–318.

33. van Blarcom CW. Glossary of Prosthodontics, ed 6. J Prosthet Dent 1994;71:43–104.

34. Katsavrias EG. Changes in articular eminence inclination during the craniofacial growth period. Angle Orthod 2002;72:258–264.

35. Katsavrias EG, Dibbets JM. The growth of articular eminence height during craniofacial growth period. Cranio 2001;19:13–20.

36. Nickel JC, McLachlan KR. An analysis of surface congruity in the growing human temporomandibular joint. Arch Oral Biol 1994;39:315–332.

37. Ren YF, Isberg A, Westesson PL. Steepness of the articular eminence in the temporomandibular joint: Tomographic comparison between asymptomatic volunteers with normal disk position and patients with disk displacement. Oral Surg Oral Med Oral Pathol Oral Radiol Endod 1995;80:258–266.

38. Carlsson GE, Öberg T. Remodeling of the temporomandibular joint. In: Zarb GE, Carlsson GE (eds). Temporomandibular Joint Function and Dysfunction. Copenhagen: Munksgaard, 1979:155–174.

39. McNamara JA, Hinton RJ, Hoffman DL. Histologic analysis of temporomandibular adaptation to protrusive function in young adult rhesus monkeys. Am J Orthod 1982;82:288–298.

40. Isberg AM, Isacsson G. Tissue reaction of the temporomandibular joint following retrusive guidance of the mandible. Cranio 1986;4:413–418.

41. Ali A, Sharawy M. Enlargement of the rabbit mandibular condyle after experimental induction of anterior disc displacement: A histomorphometric study. J Oral Maxillofac Surg 1995;53:544–560.

42. Axelsson S, Holmlund A, Hjerpe A. An experimental model of osteoarthritis in the temporomandibular joint of the rabbit. Acta Odontol Scand 1992;50:273–280.

43. Hinton RJ. Alteration in rat condylar cartilage following discectomy. J Dent Res 1992;71:1292–1297.

44. Solberg WK, Hansson TL, Nordström B. The temporomandibular joint in young adults at autopsy: A morphologic classification and evaluation. J Oral Rehabil 1985;12:303–321.

45. Blackwood HJJ. Adaptive changes in the mandibular joints with function. Dent Clin North Am 1966;10:559–566.

46. Rabie AB, Wong L, Tsai M. Replicating mesenchymal cells in the condyle and glenoid fossa during mandibular forward positioning. Am J Orthod Dentofac Orthop 2003;123:49–57.

47. Caplan AI. Mesenchymal stem cells. J Orthop Res 1991;9:641–650.

48. Bruder SP, Fink DJ, Caplan AI. Mesenchymal stem cells in bone development, repair and skeletal regeneration therapy. J Cell Biochem 1994;56:283–294.

49. Luder HU. Postnatal Development, Aging, and Degeneration of the Temporomandibular Joint in Humans, Monkeys, and Rats. Monograph No. 29, Craniofacial Growth Series. Ann Arbor, MI: Center for Human Growth and Development, University of Michigan, 1993.

50. Kantomaa T. New aspects of the histology of the mandibular condyle in the rat. Acta Anat 1986;126:218–222.

51. Hinton RJ, Carlson DS. Histological changes in the articular eminence and mandibular fossa during growth in the rhesus monkey (Macaca mulatta). Am J Anat 1983;166:99–116.

52. Kondoh T, Westesson PL, Takahashi T, Seto K. Prevalence of morphological changes in the surfaces of the temporomandibular joint disc associated with internal derangement. J Oral Maxillofac Surg 1998;56:339–343.

53. Westesson P-L, Lundh H. Arthrographic and clinical characteristics of patients with disk displacement who progressed to closed lock during a 6-month period. Oral Surg Oral Med Oral Pathol Oral Radiol Endod 1989;67:654–657.

54. DuBrul EL. The biomechanics of the oral apparatus. In: DuBrul EL, Menekrats A (eds). The Physiology of Oral Reconstruction. Chicago: Quintessence, 1981:13–53.

55. Hall MB, Brown RW, Baughman RA. Histological appearance of the bilaminar zone in internal derangement of the temporomandibular joint. Oral Surg Oral Med Oral Pathol 1984;58:375–381.

56. Kurita K, Westesson P-L, Sternby NH, et al. Histologic features of the temporomandibular joint and posterior disk attachment: Comparison of symptom-free persons with normally positioned disks and patients with internal derangement. Oral Surg Oral Med Oral Pathol Oral Radiol Endod 1989;67:635–643.

57. Björnland T, Refsum SB. Histopathologic changes of the temporomandibular joint disk in patients with chronic arthritic disease. A comparison with internal derangement. Oral Surg Oral Med Oral Pathol 1994;77:572–578.

58. Jonsson G, Eckerdal O, Isberg A. Thickness of the articular soft tissue of the temporal component in temporomandibular joints with and without disk displacement. Oral Surg Oral Med Oral Pathol Oral Radiol Endod 1999;87:20–26.

59. Stöckli PW, Willert HG. Tissue reactions in the temporomandibular joint resulting from anterior displacement of the mandible in the monkey. Am J Orthod 1971;60: 142–155.

60. Woodside DG, Metaxas A, Altuna G. The influence of functional appliance therapy on glenoid fossa remodeling. Am J Orthod Dentofac Orthop 1987;92:181–198.

61. Hoppenreijs TJ, Freihofer HP, Stoelinga PJ, Tuinzing DB, van't Hof MA. Condylar remodeling and resorption after Le Fort I and bimaxillary osteotomies in patients with anterior open bite. A clinical and radiological study. Int J Oral Maxillofac Surg 1998;27:81–91.

62. Ruf S, Pancherz H. Temporomandibular growth adaptation in Herbst treatment: A prospective magnetic resonance imaging and cephalometric roentgenographic study. Eur J Orthod 1998;20:375–388.

63. Harper RP, Bell WH, Hinton RJ, Browne R, Cherkashin AM, Samshukov ML. Reactive changes in the temporomandibular joint after mandibular midline osteodistraction. Br J Oral Maxillofac Surg 1997;35:20–25.

64. Moss ML, Salentijn L. The primary role of functional matrices in facial growth. Am J Orthod 1969;55:566–577.

65. Moss ML. The functional matrix hypothesis revisited. 4. The epigenetic antithesis and resolving synthesis. Am J Orthod Dentofac Orthop 1997;112:410–417.

66. Copray JCVM. Growth Regulation of Mandibular Condylar Cartilage In Vitro [thesis]. Groningen, The Netherlands: University of Groningen, 1984.

67. Petrovic AG, Stutzmann JJ, Oudet CL. Control processes in the postnatal growth of the condylar cartilage of the mandible. In: McNamara JA (ed). Determinants of Mandibular Form and Growth. Monograph No. 4, Craniofacial Growth Series. Ann Arbor, MI: Center for Human Growth and Development, University of Michigan, 1975:101–153.

68. McNamara JA Jr, Carlson DS. Quantitative analysis of temporomandibular joint adaptations to protrusive function. Am J Orthod 1979;76:593–611.

69. Kantomaa T, Pirttiniemi P. Differences in biologic response of the mandibular condyle to forward traction or opening of the mandible. An experimental study in the rat. Acta Odontol Scand 1996;54:138–144.

70. Rabie ABM, Hägg U. Factors regulating mandibular condylar growth. Am J Orthod Dentofacial Orthop 2002;122: 401–409.

71. Bi W, Deng J, Zhang Z, Behringer RR, De Crombrugghe B. Sox 9 is required for cartilage formation. Nat Genet 1999; 22:85–89.

72. Rabie AB, She TT, Hägg U. Functional appliance therapy accelerates and enhances condylar growth. Am J Orthod Dentofacial Orthop 2003;123:40–48.

73. Rabie AB, Leung FY, Chayanupatkul A, Hägg U. The correlation between neovascularization and bone formation in the condyle during forward mandibular positioning. Angle Orthod 2002;72:431–438.

74. de Bont LGM, Blankestijn J, Panders AK, Vermeij A. Unilateral condylar hyperplasia combined with synovial chondromatosis of the temporomandibular joint. J Oral Maxillofac Surg 1985;13:32–36.

75. Isberg A. Temporomandibular Joint Dysfunction. A Practitioner's Guide. London: Martin Dunitz, 2001.

76. Isberg A, Widmalm SE, Ivarsson R. Clinical, radiographic and electromyographic study of patients with internal derangement of the temporomandibular joint. Am J Orthod 1985;88:453–460.

77. Assael LA. Surgical management of condylar fractures. In: Manson P (ed). Management of Facial Injuries. Philadelphia: Lippincott, 1990.

78. Assael LA. Hard tissue trauma. In: Kaplan S, Assael LA (eds). Temporomandibular Disorders: Diagnosis and Treatment. Philadelphia: Saunders, 1991:224–237.

79. de Leeuw R. A 30-Year Follow-Up of Non-Surgically Treated Temporomandibular Joint Osteoarthrosis and Internal Derangement [thesis]. Groningen, The Netherlands: University of Groningen, 1994.

80. Schellhas KP, Piper MA, Omlie MR. Facial skeleton remodeling due to temporomandibular joint degeneration: An imaging study of 100 patients. Am J Neuroradiol 1990;11; 541–551; Am J Roentgenol 1990;155:373–383.

81. Westesson P-L, Tallents RH, Katzberg RW. Radiographic assessment of asymmetry of the mandible. Am J Neuroradiol 1994;15:991–999.

82. Legrell PE., Isberg A. Mandibular height asymmetry following experimentally induced temporomandibular joint disk displacement in rabbits. Oral Surg Oral Med Oral Pathol Oral Radiol Endod 1998;86:280–285.

83. Legrell PE, Isberg A. Mandibular length and midline asymmetry after experimentally induced temporomandibular joint disk displacement in rabbits. Am J Orthod Dentofac Orthop 1999;115:247–253.

84. Dibbets JM, van der Weele LTh, Boering G. Craniofacial morphology and temporomandibular joint dysfunction in children. In: Carlson DS, McNamara JA, Ribbens KA (eds). Developmental Aspects of Temporomandibular Joint Disorders. Monograph No. 16, Craniofacial Growth Series. Ann Arbor, MI: Center for Human Development, University of Michigan, 1985:151–182.

85. Hatala MP, Macher DJ, Tallents RH, Spoon M, Subtelny JD, Kyrkanides S. Effect of a surgically created disk displacement on mandibular symmetry in the growing rabbit. Oral Surg Oral Med Oral Pathol Oral Radiol Endod 1996;82: 625–633.

86. Stegenga B, de Bont LGM, Boering G, van Willigen JD. Tissue responses to degenerative changes in the temporomandibular joint. A review. J Oral Maxillofac Surg 1991; 49:1079–1088.

87. Scapino RP. Histopathology associated with malposition of the human temporomandibular joint disc. Oral Surg Oral Med Oral Pathol Oral Radiol Endod 1983;55:382–397.

88. Isberg A, Isacsson G. Tissue reactions associated with internal derangement of the temporomandibular joint. A radiographic, cryomorphologic, and histologic study. Acta Odontol Scand 1986;44:159–164.

89. McCoy JM, Gotcher JE, Chase DC. Histologic grading of TMJ tissues in internal derangement. Cranio 1986;4:213–128.

90. Pereira FJ Jr, Lundh H, Westesson P-L. Age-related changes of the retrodiscal tissues in the temporomandibular joint. J Oral Maxillofac Surg 1996;54:55–61.

91. de Leeuw R, Boering G, Stegenga B, de Bont LGM. Clinical signs of TMJ osteoarthrosis and internal derangement 30 years after nonsurgical treatment. J Orofac Pain 1994;8:18–24.

92. Stegenga B, de Bont LGM, Boering G. Classification of osteoarthrosis and internal derangement of the temporomandibular joint. 2. Specific diagnostic criteria. Cranio 1992;10:107–116.

93. Isberg A, Isacsson G, Johansson AS, Larson O. Hyperplastic soft tissue formation in the temporomandibular joint associated with internal derangement. Oral Surg Oral Med Oral Pathol Oral Radiol Endod 1986;61:32–38.

94. Kopp S. Clinical findings in temporomandibular joint osteoarthrosis. Scand J Dent Res 1977;85:434–443.

95. Holmlund A, Hellsing G, Axelsson S. The temporomandibular joint: A comparison of clinical and arthroscopic findings. J Prosthet Dent 1989;62:61–65.

96. Lobbezoo F, Lavigne GJ. Do bruxism and temporomandibular disorders have a cause-and-effect relationship? J Orofac Pain 1997;11:15–23.

97. Dijkstra PU, de Bont LGM, Stegenga B, Boering G. Temporomandibular joint osteoarthrosis and generalized joint hypermobility. Cranio 1992;10:221–227.

98. Holmlund A, Axelsson S. Temporomandibular joint osteoarthrosis. Correlation of clinical and arthroscopic findings with degree of molar support. Acta Odontol Scand 1994;52:214–218.

99. Luder HU. Factors affecting degeneration in human temporomandibular joints as assessed histologically. Eur J Oral Sci 2002;110:106–113.

100. Toller PA. Osteoarthrosis of the mandibular condyle. Br Dent J 1973;134:223–231.

101. Pereira FJ Jr, Lundh H, Westesson P-L. Morphologic changes in the temporomandibular joint in different age groups. An autopsy investigation. Oral Surg Oral Med Oral Pathol Oral Radiol Endod 1994;78:279–287.

102. Hinton RJ, Carlsson DS. Effect of function on growth and remodeling of the temporomandibular joint. In: McNeill C (ed). Science and Practice of Occlusion. Chicago: Quintessence, 1997:95–110.

103. de Bont LGM, Stegenga B, Boering G. Hard tissue pathology. A. Osteoarthritis. In: Thomas M, Bronstein SL (eds). Arthroscopy of the Temporomandibular Joint. Philadelphia: Saunders, 1992:258–275.

104. LeResche L. Epidemiology of temporomandibular disorders: Implications for the investigation of etiologic factors. Crit Rev Oral Biol Med 1997;8:291–305.

105. Karaharju-Suvanto T, Peltonen J, Laitinen O, Kahri A. The effect of gradual distraction of the mandible on the sheep temporomandibular joint. Int J Oral Maxillofac Surg 1996;25:152–156.

106. Hesse JR, Naeije M, Hansson TL. Craniomandibular stiffness toward maximum mouth opening in healthy subjects: A clinical and experimental investigation. J Craniomandib Disord Fac Oral Pain 1990;4:257–266.

107. Stegenga B, de Bont LGM, de Leeuw R, Boering G. Assessment of mandibular function impairment associated with temporomandibular joint osteoarthrosis and internal derangement. J Orofac Pain 1993;7:183–195.

108. Bates RE, Gremillion HA, Stewart CM. Degenerative joint disease. 1. Diagnosis and management considerations. Cranio 1994;11:284–290.

109. Pereira FJ Jr, Lundh H, Westesson P-L, Carlsson LE. Clinical findings related to morphologic changes in TMJ autopsy specimens. Oral Surg Oral Med Oral Pathol Oral Radiol Endod 1994;78:288–295.

110. Mejersjö C, Hollender L. TMJ pain and dysfunction: Relation between clinical and radiographic findings in the short and long-term. Scand J Dent Res 1984;92:241–248.

Sensory and Motor Neurophysiology of the TMJ

Barry J. Sessle

This chapter provides an overview of the neural mechanisms related to the sensory and neuromuscular functions of the temporomandibular joint (TMJ) and the associated musculature and discusses their clinical correlates. Particular emphasis is given to TMJ and muscle pain. Review references are provided for readers who are interested in the details of the studies noted in the text.

Peripheral Sensory Mechanisms

Receptors and Primary Afferents

Musculoskeletal tissues such as the TMJ and adjacent musculature are supplied by primary afferent nerve fibers that terminate in sense organs (receptors) that respond to peripheral stimulation of the tissues.[1–3] Most of the small-diameter, slowly conducting primary afferents terminate as free nerve endings that are activated by noxious stimuli; these are termed *nociceptors*. The larger-diameter, faster-conducting primary afferents end as low-threshold receptors (eg, Ruffini-like and Pacinian-like receptors) that respond to non-noxious mechanical stimuli or movements. These so-called specialized receptors typically have epithelial or connective tissue cell specializations embracing the afferent ending. In most muscles, some of these large-diameter afferents are associated with muscle spindles and Golgi tendon organs that respond, respectively, to muscle stretch and contractile tension.

Activation of nociceptors leads to the generation of action potentials in their associated afferent fibers. These signals are conducted to the central nervous system (CNS) and can lead to the perceptual, reflex, and other behavioral responses characterizing pain. In contrast, the various low-threshold receptors and their afferent input to the CNS are thought to play a role in perceptual as well as reflex responses related to non-noxious joint position and movement as well as to muscle stretch and tension. The contribution of joint receptors to joint position sense, relative to muscular and cutaneous receptors, has been the subject of considerable debate. It is currently thought that their role is quite limited and only becomes significant at extreme joint positions.[4,5] Nonetheless, it is important to keep in mind that the human mandible is a single bone with right and left articulations, which differ from most other joints in the body because the condyles not only rotate but also translate. Therefore, nociceptive as well as non-nociceptive afferent input from the TMJ and associated masticatory muscles into the CNS is conceivably associated with central integrative processes that are somewhat different from those in other joints.

The TMJ is supplied by afferent fibers that are carried principally in the auriculotemporal branch of the trigeminal nerve; the richest innervation is in the posterolateral aspect of the TMJ capsule in most species. Some of the innervating fibers may not be afferents but rather are efferents of the sympathetic nervous system.[1–3,6,7] Although several studies suggest that the articular surfaces and disc of the TMJ are not innervated, other studies contradict this conclusion.[8,9] The TMJ contains numerous free nerve endings, but more specialized receptors are sparse and indeed may be nonexistent in some species. Nearly all the afferents that supply these specialized and nonspecialized receptors are less than 10 μm in diameter (ie, belonging to fiber groups II, III, and IV, known in another classification scheme as Aβ, Aδ, and C fibers), particularly in the case of those species lacking specialized receptors.

The few electrophysiologic investigations that have recorded the response properties of TMJ afferents [1,5,10,11] have documented low-threshold non-nociceptive afferents with either rapidly adapting or slowly adapting responses to joint movement or change in position. These responses have been implicated in both mandibular movement and position sense (kinesthesia). Nonetheless, other nonarticular primary afferents may show activity during jaw movements.[5,12] These include afferents supplying the muscle spindles that are present in some masticatory muscles, as well as some skin and intraoral afferents. By their movement-related activity, these nonarticular afferents may thereby contribute to kinesthetic sense and motor control, although these movement-related orofacial afferent inputs to the CNS can be modulated (eg, inhibited) by central mechanisms involved in sensorimotor control.

Several pieces of evidence indicate that afferent inputs to the CNS also occur from nociceptors in the TMJ and associated muscles[1–3,13–15]:

1. Pain can be evoked from the TMJ as well as from the craniofacial musculature.
2. Reflex muscle responses can be elicited by high-threshold stimulation of afferents supplying the TMJ and masticatory muscles.
3. These tissues contain several chemical mediators (eg, leukotrienes) involved in peripheral mechanisms of inflammation and pain.
4. Free nerve endings are common in these tissues, which are innervated by small-diameter, slowly conducting (group III and IV [Aδ and C fibers]) afferents, the afferent groups that are associated with nociceptive fibers elsewhere in the body.
5. Slowly conducting afferents supplying the TMJ or muscles respond to noxious mechanical and chemical stimuli.
6. Some afferents supplying the TMJ and associated muscles, especially the small-diameter fibers, contain substance P and other neuropeptides (such as calcitonin gene–related peptide [CGRP]), which are neurochemicals implicated in nociception and neurogenic inflammation.

Nociceptive afferent endings in general are activated by chemical products that are released from cells or vessels damaged by a peripheral noxious stimulus (eg, prostaglandins, K^+, and bradykinins). The activation of the nociceptive endings causes action potentials to be generated and conducted into the CNS along the nociceptive afferents. A large number of factors and chemical mediators have been identified that can influence the excitability of nociceptive endings.[7,13–17] These influences are outlined in chapter 6. They include damage of peripheral tissues (including nerves), which can result in inflammation and involve products released from blood vessels or from cells of the immune system. In addition, substances that are synthesized in the primary afferent cell body and released peripherally from the afferent fibers themselves, ie, neurochemicals, may influence the excitability of the nociceptive afferents; examples include neuropeptides such as substance P and CGRP and neurotrophins such as nerve growth factor.

Under certain conditions, substances such as norepinephrine may be released from the sympathetic efferents that innervate many peripheral tissues, and they can modulate the excitability of the nociceptive afferents and thereby contribute to the pain in conditions such as complex regional pain syndromes. Tissue trauma, for example, may lead to upregulation of α-adrenergic receptors on nociceptive afferents so that the afferents now become sensitive to norepinephrine. Sometimes the peripheral damage can lead to nerve sprouting or abnormal nerve changes that are associated with so-called ectopic or aberrant neural discharges, and these phenomena are of pathophysiologic significance in neuropathic pain conditions.

Peripheral Sensitization

These effects of tissue damage and inflammation are relevant in many painful conditions that dentists or related specialists typically treat, such as pulpitis, mucositis, and myositis, as well as arthritic conditions affecting the TMJ. Thus, it is important to know that tissue damage or inflammation can produce an increased excitability of the nociceptors at the site of injury.[7,14,16,18] This is termed *nociceptor* or *peripheral sensitization*.

An important process in producing peripheral sensitization is the release of the neurochemicals noted above (eg, substance P and CGRP), which are synthesized in the primary afferent cell bodies of nociceptive afferents and are released from their afferent endings (Fig 4-1). These

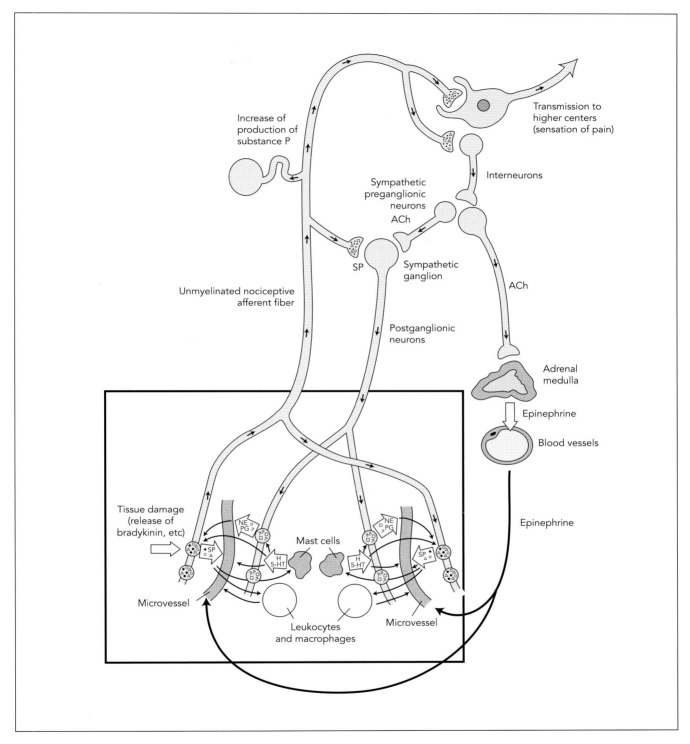

Fig 4-1 Summary of events occurring in peripheral tissues, in primary afferent and sympathetic neurons, and in nociceptive neurons of the V brainstem (orofacial dorsal horn) during pain and inflammation. The boxed area encompasses the peripheral events. (•) Substance P (SP); (□) norepinephrine (NE); (O, △) other mediators; (?) prostaglandins (PG) and other mediators that may be present in sympathetic (postganglionic) efferents; (H) histamine; (5-HT) 5-hydroxytryptamine (serotonin); (ACh) acetylcholine. (From Lund and Sessle.[7] Reprinted with permission.)

Table 4-1	Pain features that may be explained by peripheral sensitization of nociceptive afferents of central sensitization of central nociceptive neurons	
Pain feature	**Nociceptive afferent**	**Central nociceptive neuron**
Allodynia	Decreased activation threshold	Decreased activation threshold
Hyperalgesia	Increased suprathreshold responsiveness	Increased suprathreshold responsiveness
Pain spread	Involvement of adjacent afferent endings	Receptive field expansion
Spontaneous pain	Spontaneous activity	Spontaneous activity

neuropeptides may act on platelets, macrophages, mast cells, and other cells of the immune system to release inflammatory mediators such as histamine, serotonin (5-HT), bradykinin, and cytokines. This results in what has been termed *neurogenic inflammation*, because it is initially generated by substances released from the afferent nerve fiber endings and is characterized by redness, edema, and local temperature increases, which, together with pain, represent the cardinal signs of inflammation.

The inflammatory mediators, in addition to producing inflammation, can act on the nociceptive afferent endings and increase their excitability, ie, peripheral sensitization. The increased excitability of the nociceptors can be reflected in their spontaneous activity, lowered activation thresholds, and increased responsiveness to subsequent noxious stimuli that appear to contribute, respectively, to the spontaneous pain, allodynia (pain produced by a stimulus that is normally non-noxious), and hyperalgesia (increased sensitivity to noxious stimuli) that are features of many chronic or persistent pain conditions (Table 4-1). The inflammatory mediators may also diffuse through the peripheral tissues and influence the excitability of endings of adjacent nociceptive afferents and thereby initiate peripheral processes that also contribute to the spread of pain.

This increased nociceptor activity may also lead to an increased afferent barrage into the CNS, where functional changes can occur in central nociceptive processing that contribute to persistent pain. This is described in more detail later in the chapter, but these central processes, termed *central sensitization*, are especially involved in so-called secondary hyperalgesia, in which increased pain sensitivity occurs well beyond the site of tissue injury. The peripheral processes involving peripheral sensitization of nociceptive afferent endings at the site of injury, in contrast, appear to represent the principal mechanism accounting for the increased pain sensitivity at the site of injury (primary hyperalgesia).

Clinical Implications

An understanding of the chemical mechanisms involved in the activation or sensitization of the nociceptive afferents has led to the development of therapeutic agents targeting specific peripheral mechanisms. Examples include the commonly used nonsteroidal anti-inflammatory drugs and salicylates such as aspirin as well as many newly developed analgesics such as cyclooxygenase-2 (COX-2) inhibitors. These drugs achieve their principal anti-inflammatory and analgesic effects in peripheral orofacial tissues by reducing inflammation associated with tissue injury, by modulating nociceptive afferent excitability, or by altering the hyperalgesia associated with transient orofacial pain conditions.

Also important are the clinical implications of recent discoveries of additional mechanisms in peripheral nerve endings that are involved in pain. They include the discovery of transient receptor potential (TRP) mechanisms, such as vanilloid receptor 1 (VR1 or TRPV1), that account for the sensitivity to heat, cold, and chemicals such as capsaicin (the pungent ingredient in hot peppers). In addition, chemical mediators long associated with nociceptive transmission or modulation within the CNS (eg, the excitatory amino acid, glutamate; γ-aminobutyric acid [GABA]; and opioid-related substances) have recently been shown to act peripherally to influence the excitability of the nociceptive afferents.[3,19–21] For example, glutamate is also synthesized by primary afferent cell bodies and may be released from peripheral afferent nerve endings. When applied to the TMJ or jaw muscles, it can excite nociceptive afferents supplying these structures and produce transient pain by activating excitatory amino acid receptors (N-methyl-D-aspartate [NMDA] and non-NMDA receptors) located on the afferent endings.

In contrast, the peripheral application of GABA can depress the activity of these afferent inputs into the CNS, as can the opiate drug morphine. These two chemical substances appear to depress the activity of the nociceptive afferents by interacting with GABA and opioid receptors, respectively, on the nociceptive afferent endings. It is also of interest that sex differences have been found in some of these peripheral actions of glutamate and morphine (but not GABA),[3,21] which raises the possibility that peripherally based physiologic mechanisms may contribute to the sex differences in the prevalence of many chronic pain conditions, such as some of the temporomandibular disorders (TMDs).

Moreover, the existence of numerous chemical mediators means that a number of potential targets exist; this fact holds promise for the development of new and more effective therapeutic approaches that act peripherally to modify pain without the undesirable side effects that characterize most of the centrally acting analgesic drugs currently in use. However, the multiplicity of chemical mediators involved in peripheral nociceptive afferent activation and sensitization and related events (eg, inflammation) also implies that the clinical use of a drug that targets only one of the many mechanisms underlying pain may have limited clinical efficacy unless the particular pain is shown to operate by a chemical process in which the targeted mechanism is crucial.

Afferent Projections to the Central Nervous System

Most primary afferents supplying the orofacial region have their cell bodies in the trigeminal (V) ganglion. The cell bodies of TMJ afferents are found in the posterolateral aspect of the ganglion, where the cell bodies of some jaw muscle afferents are also located.[22,23] The sizes of the TMJ cell bodies span the range representing both nociceptive and non-nociceptive (eg, mechanosensitive) afferents; the smaller size range of the masticatory muscle primary afferent cell bodies in the ganglion suggests that they may be mainly related to high-threshold muscle afferents. The primary afferent cell bodies of muscle spindle afferents supplying most jaw muscles are located within the CNS, in the V mesencephalic nucleus.[1,5,12,23]

When applied to TMJ or jaw muscle tissues, certain histochemicals can be taken up by the afferent fiber endings and transported centrally, resulting in labeling in the rostral and caudal components of the trigeminal (V) brainstem sensory nuclear complex.[22,23] The rostral projection of some of these afferents is consistent with findings of neurons in the rostral subnuclei responsive to innocuous TMJ stimuli or jaw movements.[1,23] The caudal projection of some of the afferents is supported by studies using antidromic stimulation techniques that have shown that single, slowly conducting nociceptive afferents supplying the TMJ or jaw-closing muscles project to subnucleus caudalis of the V brainstem complex.[3]

Brainstem and Thalamocortical Sensory Mechanisms

Brainstem

As previously noted, the small-diameter primary afferents innervating the TMJ and jaw muscles and most other orofacial tissues project into the brainstem and terminate centrally in the V brainstem sensory nuclear complex. At their central terminals they have been shown to release excitatory neurochemicals such as excitatory amino acids and neuropeptides that are involved in the activation of second-order neurons in the V brainstem complex.[24,25] The V brainstem complex can be subdivided into the main, or principal sensory, nucleus and the spinal tract nucleus, which comprises three subnuclei: oralis, interpolaris, and caudalis (Fig 4-2).

Low-threshold mechanoreceptive neurons

The rostral components of the V brainstem complex (main sensory nucleus, subnucleus oralis, and subnucleus interpolaris) are considered to be the essential brainstem regions relaying sensory information related to so-called fine touch. However, over the past 30 years, it has become increasingly clear that many neurons that receive and faithfully transmit detailed somatosensory information about light tactile stimuli delivered to localized regions of the face and mouth are abundant not only in the rostral components of the V brainstem complex but also in the subnucleus caudalis.[1,15,18] These neurons are referred to as *low-threshold mechanoreceptive (LTM) neurons* because they receive low-threshold A-fiber afferent inputs and thereby are activated by light tactile stimuli. The LTM neurons provide the higher levels of the brain with detailed information about the modality and spatiotemporal features (eg, location and intensity) of orofacial tactile stimuli.

Although there has only been limited study of neurons in the V brainstem complex that are responsive to low-threshold input from the TMJ or other musculoskeletal tissues, some low-threshold neurons can be excited by jaw movements, especially jaw opening, and their activation apparently reflects input from low-threshold TMJ mechanoreceptors or stretch-sensitive receptors in the jaw muscles.[1,23] These brainstem neurons are thought to

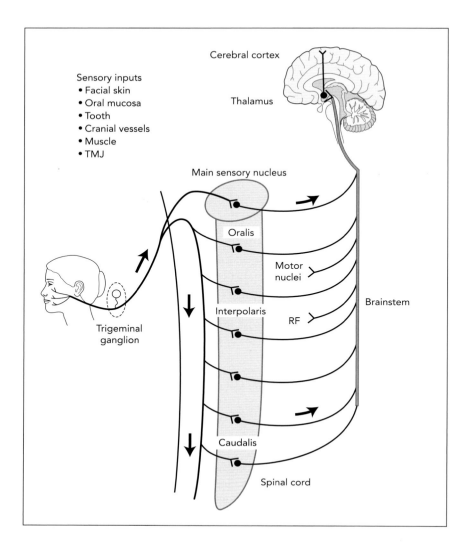

Fig 4-2 Major somatosensory pathway from the face and mouth. Trigeminal (V) primary afferents have their cell bodies in the trigeminal ganglion and project to second-order neurons in the V brainstem sensory nuclear complex. These neurons may project to neurons in higher levels of the brain (eg, in the thalamus) or in brainstem regions such as the cranial nerve motor nuclei or the reticular formation (RF). The sensory inputs also include orofacial afferents supplying the cornea and sinuses (eg, maxillary). Also, not shown are the projections of some cervical nerve afferents and cranial nerve VII, IX, X, and XII afferents to the V brainstem complex and the projection of many V, VII, IX, and X afferents to the solitary tract nucleus. (From Sessle.[15] Reprinted with permission.)

contribute to reflex brainstem circuits regulating masticatory muscle activity (see the section on neuromuscular mechanisms) or to ascending sensory pathways (eg, to thalamus and cortex) involved in jaw position sense (see the section on mandibular kinesthesia).

Nociceptive-specific and wide dynamic range neurons

There is considerable evidence that the subnucleus caudalis is the principal brainstem relay site of V nociceptive information from neurons responsive to nociceptive afferent input[1,2,7,14,15,18,26–29]:

1. The subnucleus caudalis has a laminated structure and cell types that morphologically resemble those of the spinal dorsal horn, which is the essential region of the spinal cord involved in pain. Its laminae include the superficial laminae I and II, the so-called substantia gelatinosa (SG).

2. The great majority of the small-diameter (Aδ- and C-fiber) primary afferents carrying nociceptive information from the orofacial tissues terminate in the subnucleus caudalis. These small-diameter afferents terminate in laminae I, II, V, and VI of the subnucleus caudalis, whereas the larger A-fiber primary afferents conducting low-threshold mechanosensitive (tactile) information terminate primarily in laminae III through VI of the subnucleus caudalis as well as in the more rostral components of the V brainstem complex. The termination sites of TMJ and muscle afferents include especially the superficial laminae of the subnucleus caudalis as well as its deeper lamina, ie, sites where trigeminal nociceptive neurons responsive to stimulation of craniofacial deep tissues are located.

3. Transection of the V spinal tract at the rostral pole of the subnucleus caudalis, a neurosurgical procedure in humans termed *V tractotomy*, produces relief of the excruciating pain of V neuralgia and a marked reduction in the patient's ability to perceive noxious stimuli (especially those applied to the face); analogous lesions in experimental animals reduce behavioral, autonomic, and muscle reflex responses to noxious facial stimuli. These findings suggest that the caudalis lesion is interfering with the relay of nociceptive signals from the brainstem terminals of the small-diameter nociceptive primary afferents to second-order neurons in the subnucleus caudalis.

4. Increases in immunocytochemical markers of neuronal activity, such as Fos protein, occur in caudalis neurons following noxious stimulation of craniofacial tissues, including the TMJ or jaw muscles.

5. Electrophysiologic recordings of the activity of brainstem neurons have revealed that many neurons in the subnucleus caudalis, as in the spinal dorsal horn, can be activated by noxious stimulation of cutaneous or deep tissues.

6. The output of caudalis neurons includes regions of the brain involved in pain processing. Many of these features of the subnucleus caudalis are similar to those of the spinal dorsal horn; consequently, the subnucleus caudalis is now often termed the *medullary dorsal horn*. However, there are some important differences that call into question whether a complete structural and functional homology between subnucleus caudalis and spinal dorsal horn exists; for example, the rostral and caudal parts of the subnucleus caudalis have different functions (described later).

The recordings showing that many subnucleus caudalis neurons can be activated by cutaneous noxious stimuli have documented that they are concentrated in the superficial (I and II) and deep laminae (V and VI). In contrast, the LTM neurons predominate in laminae III and IV. The nociceptive neurons have been classified on the basis of their functional properties as either nociceptive-specific (NS) neurons or wide dynamic range (WDR) neurons. The NS neurons receive small-diameter nociceptive afferent inputs from Aδ and/or C fibers and respond only to noxious stimuli (eg, pinch or heat) applied to a localized region of the face or mouth, the so-called neuronal receptive field (RF). The WDR neurons, in contrast, receive large-diameter as well as small-diameter A-fiber and C-fiber input and can be excited by both non-noxious (eg, tactile) stimuli and noxious stimuli applied to their RF.

The RF of the WDR neurons is generally larger than that of the NS neurons. Many subnucleus caudalis NS and WDR neurons can be excited only by natural stimulation of cutaneous or mucosal tissues, and they respond with a progressively increasing discharge as the intensity of the peripheral noxious stimulus is gradually increased or as more of the RF is stimulated. These various RFs and response properties are consistent with a role for both NS and WDR neurons in the detection, localization, intensity coding, and discrimination of superficial noxious stimuli.[15,26]

These properties of subnucleus caudalis neurons clearly point to a crucial role played by both NS and WDR neurons in superficial pain, yet very few caudalis NS and WDR neurons appear to be activated exclusively by cutaneous (or mucosal) stimuli. Indeed, while the vast majority of caudalis NS and WDR neurons have a superficial RF, most of these also can be excited by one or more other afferent inputs as well as by cutaneous or mucosal afferent inputs (Fig 4-3). Furthermore, some have a deep tissue RF (eg, in TMJ and muscle) as well as an RF in the superficial craniofacial tissues. For example, in the rat and cat, electrical or noxious mechanical stimuli that activate small-diameter primary afferents supplying jaw or tongue muscles or the TMJ may activate as many as 60% of the NS and WDR neurons.[7,14,15]

Furthermore, an algesic chemical (eg, mustard oil, capsaicin, or glutamate) that produces pain in humans can also activate a substantial proportion of NS and WDR neurons when the chemical is applied to the TMJ or jaw muscle[14,21,31] (Fig 4-4). In contrast, very few LTM neurons receive these convergent excitatory inputs from deep as well as superficial tissues. In addition, very few subnucleus caudalis NS and WDR neurons are activated exclusively by deep noxious stimuli, so the vast majority of the caudalis neurons transmitting deep nociceptive information receive additional inputs from afferents supplying other tissues, including skin. These features are thought to contribute to pain spread and referral (discussed later in the chapter).

There may also be sex differences in subnucleus caudalis nociceptive neuronal responses to deep noxious stimuli[31] which, along with the sex differences in responsivity of TMJ and jaw muscle primary afferents to some noxious or pain-modulatory chemicals applied to TMJ or jaw muscles, might be factors contributing to sex differences in the reports of TMJ and myofascial pain in humans.

Different parts of the subnucleus caudalis may have different functional roles. The rostral and caudal portions of the subnucleus have different neuronal RF and response properties and appear to be differentially involved in the autonomic and muscle reflex responses to noxious craniofacial stimulation[27,32] (see the section on neuromuscular mechanisms). Moreover, the subnucleus caudalis is not the only component of the V brainstem complex with a nociceptive role, because more rostral

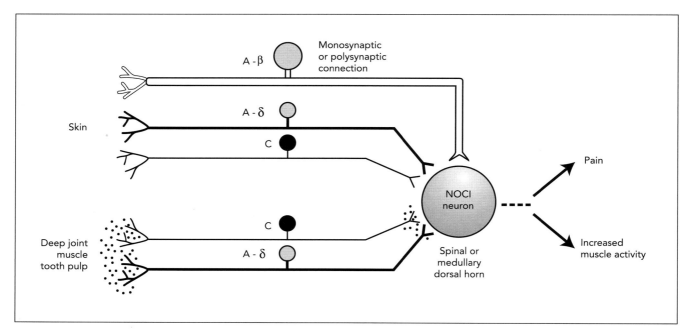

Fig 4-3 Convergence of afferent inputs onto nociceptive neurons in the trigeminal subnucleus caudalis (medullary dorsal horn) or its analogous structure in the spinal cord. Some afferents are excited only by superficial afferent inputs from the skin (or mucosa); others are excited by superficial and one or more of the deep afferent inputs (eg, from the TMJ, muscle, or tooth pulp). (A-β) Aβ afferent; (A-δ) Aδ afferent; (C) C afferent; (NOCl) nitrosyl chloride. (Modified from Hu[30] with permission.)

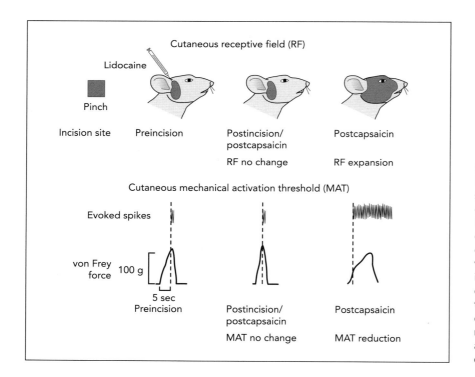

Fig 4-4 Central sensitization induced by noxious stimulation of the TMJ in a nociceptive-specific neuron, recorded in rat subnucleus caudalis. If the skin overlying the TMJ was locally anesthetized, then a surgical incision of the skin did not induce any evidence of central sensitization. However, it did not prevent the occurrence of central sensitization induced by application of the algesic chemical capsaicin to the TMJ itself. Central sensitization was reflected by an increase in the cutaneous pinch receptive field size of the neuron and a decrease in the mechanical activation threshold (Lam et al, unpublished data, 2005).

Fig 4-5 Neurochemical processes related to nociceptive transmission in the trigeminal subnucleus caudalis. In the example, activation of nociceptive fibers leads to the release of glutamate (Glu) and substance P (SP), which are conveyed across a synapse to a wide dynamic range (WDR) neuron that projects to the thalamus. Glutamate binds and activates either N-methyl-D-aspartate (NMDA) or alpha-amino-3-hydroxy-5-methyl-4-isoxazole propionate (AMPA) receptors, while substance P binds and activates the neurokinin 1 (NK-1) receptors. The afferent fibers can activate the WDR neuron directly or indirectly via contacts onto excitatory interneurons. Several intracellular signal transduction pathways have been implicated in modulating the responsiveness of the nociceptive neurons, including the protein kinase A and protein kinase C pathways. The neurons can themselves modulate nearby cells by synthesis and release of prostaglandins (PGs) via cyclooxygenase (COX), and nitric oxide (NO) via nitric oxide synthase (NOS). Glia can modulate nociceptive processing by release of cytokines and prostaglandins. Descending terminals of fibers originating in regions such as the nucleus raphe magnus (NRM) or locus coeruleus (LC) can release serotonin (5HT) or norepinephrine (NE). The major proposed receptors for these neurotransmitters are also depicted. Drugs that alter these receptors or neurotransmitters have potential as analgesics. (TGG) Trigeminal ganglion; (M-ENK) met-enkephalin; (δ/μ) delta/mu opiod receptors; (5HT1$_{A/D}$) 5HT receptors; (α2) noradreneurgic receptors; (GABA) γ-aminobutyric acid (GABA$_B$) GABA$_B$ receptor. (From Hargreaves.[33] Reprinted with permission.)

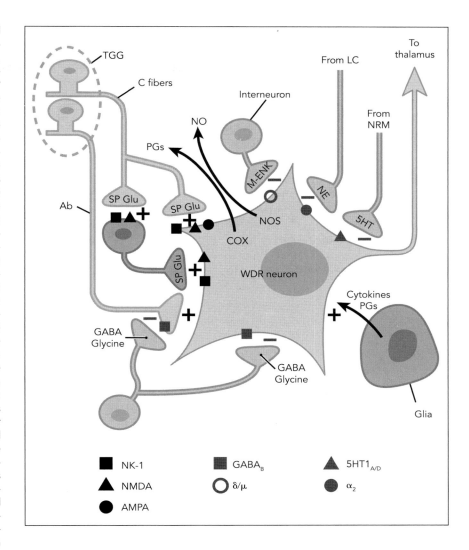

components of the V brainstem complex (eg, the subnuclei interpolaris and oralis) have NS and WDR neurons, and lesions of rostral components can disrupt some craniofacial pain behaviors. In addition, the rostral nociceptive neurons have cutaneous RFs that are usually localized to intraoral or perioral areas, and many of them can be activated by tooth pulp stimulation.[1,15,28,32] These findings suggest that the more rostral components may play a role in intraoral and perioral nociceptive processing, in contrast to the role of subnucleus caudalis in pain, which may be primarily involved in processing of nociceptive information from facial skin and deep tissues.

Neurochemicals and nociceptive transmission

It was briefly noted previously that excitatory amino acids, including glutamate and aspartate, and neuropeptides, including substance P, CGRP, and neurokinin A, are released in the central endings of V nociceptive primary afferents in the V brainstem complex. Figure 4-5 shows examples of this process. For example, the release of glutamate from the afferent endings in the subnucleus caudalis leads to the activation of caudalis nociceptive neurons by a process involving ionotropic receptors for glutamate, NMDA and non-NMDA (eg, alpha-amino-3-hydroxy-5-methyl-4-isoxazole-propionate [AMPA]) receptors, as well as metabotropic glutamate receptors (see Fig 4-5).

These different types of glutamate receptor in the caudalis neurons have different physiologic characteristics and actions. Activation of the AMPA receptor, for example, is rapid and short lived, whereas the NMDA receptor has a longer period of activation. Both receptor types appear to be important in the process of central sensitization (see the section on modulation of somatosensory transmission). Their activation can be counteracted by AMPA receptor antagonists, such as CNQX, and NMDA receptor antagonists, such as MK-801 and APV. These features appear to apply to nociceptive transmission in subnucleus caudalis from the TMJ and jaw muscle afferents because glutamate receptor antagonists can block such transmission.[15,21]

The neuropeptide substance P also contributes to nociceptive mechanisms. Like glutamate, it is synthesized by the primary afferent cell body and is transported to the peripheral endings of small-diameter primary afferents (as already discussed) as well as to the central endings of these primary afferents, such as those in the subnucleus caudalis (see Fig 4-5). Noxious craniofacial stimulation can cause the release of substance P, which then acts on so-called neurokinin receptors in the caudalis nociceptive neurons to produce a long-latency, sustained excitation of the nociceptive neurons that can be blocked by substance P antagonists.[15,25] Recent findings have revealed that CGRP, which is also released from both the peripheral and central endings of small afferents, may also play a role in nociceptive transmission.[34,35]

It has recently become clear that there are complex cellular mechanisms underlying the release and actions of glutamate and the neuropeptides. For example, the release of glutamate may be influenced by the action of adenosine triphosphate (ATP) on purinergic receptors on the central endings of V nociceptive afferents within subnucleus caudalis; the source of the ATP is unclear but may include non-neural cells in the subnucleus caudalis. Non-neural cells such as glia also appear to be a source of other modulatory influences on these neurochemical mechanisms underlying nociceptive transmission[35,36] (see Fig 4-5).

This neurochemical substrate has limited expression in the more rostral components of the V brainstem complex, and there is evidence that the nociceptive processing within them (eg, in the subnucleus oralis) is largely dependent on the functional integrity of the subnucleus caudalis. The subnucleus caudalis, via ascending projections, some of which are derived from its SG, exerts a modulatory influence on oralis nociceptive processing through NMDA and purinergic receptor mechanisms based within the subnucleus caudalis itself.[15,28,37]

Projections from the Trigeminal Brainstem Sensory Nuclear Complex

Many neurons in all components of the V brainstem complex are relay neurons that project to the thalamus either directly or indirectly via polysynaptic pathways that may involve the reticular formation.[1,2,14,38] These projections carry signals that reach the higher brain centers involved in somatosensory perception (eg, touch and pain) and other functions (eg, emotion and motivation). Some of the projections to the reticular formation, as well as projections to the cranial nerve motor nuclei, contribute to the brainstem neural circuitry underlying autonomic and muscle reflex responses to craniofacial stimuli (see the section on neuromuscular mechanisms).

Other neurons may have only intrinsic projections; that is, their axons do not leave the V brainstem complex but instead terminate within it. One example is the intrinsic projections from the subnucleus caudalis that influence the activity of nociceptive neurons in subnucleus oralis. Of particular note are the neurons in the SG of the subnucleus caudalis. The axons of most SG neurons terminate locally within the V brainstem complex and release neurochemicals such as enkephalin or GABA. The SG receives input from fibers originating in other areas in the brain in addition to craniofacial afferent input, and it represents one of the main sites by which these peripheral afferents and brain centers modulate somatosensory transmission through the action of these neurochemicals (see the section on modulation of somatosensory transmission).

Thalamus and Cortex

The projections from the V brainstem complex to the thalamus can result in the activation of neurons in parts of the lateral thalamus (eg, the ventrobasal complex), the posterior nuclear group, and the medial thalamus.[1,2,38] These thalamic regions contain LTM and nociceptive (NS and WDR) neurons that receive craniofacial somatosensory information relayed through the V brainstem complex. The LTM and nociceptive neurons are somatotopically organized in the ventrobasal thalamus; most of the ventrobasal LTM and nociceptive neurons are relay neurons that project directly to neurons in the overlying somatosensory cerebral cortex, and they have functional properties that indicate that their principal role is in the sensory-discriminative aspects of touch and pain, respectively. For example, like nociceptive neurons in the subnucleus caudalis, ventrobasal thalamic NS and WDR neurons have an RF that is localized within the craniofacial region. These neurons show graded responses to noxious craniofacial stimuli.

Nociceptive neurons in the medial thalamus (eg, intralaminar nuclei and parafascicular nucleus) on the other hand, generally have an extensive RF (eg, face and limbs). In addition, they exhibit other properties and connections (eg, with the anterior cingulate cortex, discussed later) that are more in keeping with a role in the affective or motivational dimensions of pain.

In the face, primary somatosensory cortex (SI) LTM neurons are abundant and have localized cutaneous or mucosal RFs and graded responses to orofacial tactile stimuli; they are implicated in the cortical processing underlying localization and intensity discrimination of tactile stimuli. The SI area also contains NS and WDR neurons.[2,39,40] In general, their properties are similar to those of subnucleus caudalis or ventrobasal nociceptive neurons, indicating a role for them in pain localization and intensity coding, ie, the sensory-discriminative dimension of pain.

Nociceptive neurons also occur in other cortical regions, such as the insula and anterior cingulate cortex, which have been implicated in the affective dimension of pain. The relevance of these cortical features to human pain processes is underscored by recent brain imaging findings that noxious stimulation in humans can activate several cortical regions, including the somatosensory cortex, insula, and anterior cingulate cortex.[41,42]

There is, however, limited information available about the way in which nociceptive information from the TMJ or the masticatory muscles is processed in the thalamus or cerebral cortex. Low-threshold stimulation of jaw, tongue, or facial muscle afferent inputs has been shown to activate neurons in the ventrobasal thalamus, face SI, or primary motor cortex (MI) of cats or monkeys.[1,2,43,44] Some of these MI neurons respond to external loads applied to jaw muscles or to small-amplitude sinusoidal jaw movements, which suggests that they may be receiving input from jaw muscle spindles.[44] The deep input to the face MI in the monkey, nonetheless, is much less prominent than that from superficial craniofacial mechanoreceptors (eg, in facial skin, mucosa, and periodontal tissues around the teeth); this contrasts with the prominent representation of deep inputs to the limb motor cortex. The sensory inputs to the face SI and MI from deep and superficial receptors are important in sensing mandibular jaw position (kinesthesia) and in providing sensory feedback from craniofacial receptors that may be used in the motor control of craniofacial movements (see the sections on neuromuscular mechanisms and mandibular kinesthesia).

Modulation of Somatosensory Transmission

Craniofacial somatosensory transmission in the brainstem, thalamus, and somatosensory cortex can be modulated at each of these levels. The modulation in the thalamus and cortex in large part reflects modifications of the sensory signals occurring first in the V brainstem complex. The intricate organization of each subdivision of the V brainstem complex and the variety of inputs to each from peripheral craniofacial tissues or from different parts of the brain provide important substrates for numerous interactions between the various inputs. For example, the responses of V brainstem neurons to craniofacial tactile stimuli can be suppressed by influences derived from structures within the V brainstem complex itself as well as from other parts of the brainstem and higher centers (eg, periaqueductal gray matter and somatosensory cortex).[1,18,45]

Nociceptive transmission can also be modulated by a variety of influences. Several brain areas in the thalamus, reticular formation, limbic system, and cerebral cortex provide so-called descending inputs to the V brainstem complex and influence the activity of NS and WDR neurons in this site.[1,18,45,46] Through these influences, perceptual, emotional, autonomic, and neuroendocrine responses to noxious stimuli can be totally or partly inhibited or facilitated. There can be differences in these modulatory effects from one person to another, which helps explain why pain is a highly personal experience that is susceptible to a variety of biologic, pharmacologic, psychological, genetic, and environmental influences.

Inhibitory Influences

The descending modulatory inputs to the V brainstem complex release one or more endogenous neurochemical substances, some of which underlie facilitatory influences on nociceptive transmission (discussed in the next section); other substances primarily exert inhibitory influences on the activity of NS and WDR neurons by presynaptic or postsynaptic regulatory mechanisms. These neurochemicals include serotonin (5-HT), GABA, norepinephrine, and opioids such as the enkephalins.

The so-called descending inhibitory influences have particularly powerful modulatory effects on nociceptive transmission that use these neurochemical substrates. These emanate from several CNS structures, including the periaqueductal gray matter, the rostroventral medulla/nucleus raphe magnus, the locus coeruleus and parabrachial area of the pons, the anterior pretectal nucleus, and the somatosensory and motor areas of the cerebral cortex.[18,45,46] Electrical or chemical stimulation of these sites activates descending pathways projecting to the V brainstem complex and can inhibit V brainstem neuronal and associated reflex and behavioral responses to noxious craniofacial stimuli in experimental animals, including responses to deep musculoskeletal stimuli.[47] This suggests that pain in deep craniofacial tissues can be influenced by these descending modulatory influences, and such processes may be operative in TMJ and myofascial pain. Furthermore, stimulation of some of these structures can relieve pain in human patients.[48]

Some of these descending pathways influence nociceptive transmission by the release from their endings of certain of the chemicals previously mentioned (eg, 5-HT). Other pathways may cause the release of chemicals such as the enkephalins and GABA from the endings of interneurons intrinsic to the V brainstem complex (eg, in the SG of the subnucleus caudalis), and these particular chemicals act respectively on opiate or GABA receptors within the subnucleus caudalis. The enkephalins, for example, can suppress the activity of caudalis NS and WDR neurons, and these inhibitory influences are thought to contribute to the analgesic efficacy of the narcotic opiate-related analgesic drugs (eg, morphine). However, the action of these opiate-related drugs is more complex. In addition to their actions in peripheral tissues (as described earlier), they can also act on opiate receptors at other levels of the brain (eg, amygdala, cortex, and periaqueductal gray matter). This can influence nociceptive processing per se at these levels, or it can lead to the activation of descending influences at these sites that act on nociceptive transmission at lower levels, such as the V brainstem complex.[15,45,49]

A variety of behavioral and environmental events can also involve the descending influences and thereby modify pain.[18,45] For example, if a patient's expectations that a drug will produce a powerful analgesic effect are increased, this can result in a considerable increase in the drug's analgesic properties. This is related to the so-called placebo effect, which involves changes in the descending modulatory influences in pain and, in part, endogenous opioid processes. The descending influences can also come into play in the cognitive processes associated with the context or environment in which a noxious stimulus is experienced, and even a person's personality, emotional state, and previous life experiences can modify the descending influences. Changes in the CNS processes underlying neuroendocrine function (eg, hormone levels) and sleep, and even nutritional and genetic factors, also can influence pain expression, in part by affecting the function of some descending influences.

Nociceptive transmission can also be modulated by so-called segmental or afferent influences, in addition to the various descending influences previously noted.[1,18,45] These segmental influences can be initiated by stimulation of peripheral afferents and involve the interneuronal circuitry existing within the subnucleus caudalis (and the spinal dorsal horn). Some of these modulatory effects have clinical relevance because acupuncture and transcutaneous electrical nerve stimulation activate afferent inputs that may, for example, inhibit the responses of V brainstem nociceptive neurons evoked by noxious orofacial stimuli. These clinical procedures are thought to act mainly by activating small-diameter afferent input into the CNS, although there is evidence that nociceptive transmission can also be suppressed by non-noxious (eg, vibratory or tactile) stimuli that excite large-diameter afferent nerve fibers.

It is also noteworthy that small-fiber afferent inputs from spatially dispersed regions of the body may inhibit neuronal nociceptive responses to other small-fiber afferent inputs, so-called diffuse noxious inhibitory controls; in other words, pain evoked from one part of the body can inhibit pain in another part of the body. This is thought to be an important factor in the pain relief that can occur in so-called counterirritation and has been shown to be effective in diminishing craniofacial pain.[18,45]

Facilitatory Influences

Some of the descending influences on somatosensory transmission can produce facilitatory instead of inhibitory influences and thereby contribute to the augmentation of pain that can occur in certain situations, such as when an individual is experiencing anxiety or some forms of stress.[41,45] Peripheral afferent inputs into the CNS may also induce facilitation of nociceptive transmission under some conditions, and the extensive convergence of afferent input onto nociceptive neurons plays a role. Inflammation or injury of peripheral tissues or nerve fibers may produce a barrage of nociceptive primary afferent inputs into the CNS, which can lead to prolonged augmentation of nociceptive neuronal properties in the subnucleus caudalis (and spinal dorsal horn), or central sensitization.

Inputs from deep tissues are especially effective in inducing central sensitization in the subnucleus caudalis.[7,14,15,18,37,46] For example, the injection of the small-fiber irritant mustard oil or capsaicin into the TMJ or masticatory muscles produces a barrage of action potentials that are conducted into the brainstem along the afferent nerve fibers supplying the injected tissues. On reaching the subnucleus caudalis, this deep afferent input produces the release of neurochemicals from the afferent endings onto NS and WDR neurons, leading to a cascade of intracellular events, manifesting as an increased neuronal excitability. The net result of these changes is an increased central excitatory state that is dependent on peripheral nociceptive afferent input for its initiation, although it may not be fully dependent on peripheral afferent drive for its maintenance. Chapters 5 and 6 outline these processes in more detail.

Neuronal Changes

The increased excitability, or central sensitization, may be reflected as an increase in spontaneous activity, expansion of the neuronal cutaneous and/or deep RF, lowering of the activation threshold, and augmentation of the responses of both NS and WDR caudalis neurons to craniofacial stimuli (see Fig 4-4). The nociceptive neuronal changes reflecting central sensitization are thought to result in part from a disinhibition, an unmasking, and an increased efficacy of the extensive convergent afferent inputs that are a feature of the NS and WDR neurons[15,17,46] (see chapter 5). This disinhibition may involve counteraction of some of the descending modulatory influences previously described. In addition to the neuronal changes, central sensitization induced by the afferent input barrage is also associated with increased electromyographic (EMG) activity in both jaw-opening and jaw-closing muscles in experimental animals.[15,18] This increased muscle activity involves a reflex pathway that relays in the subnucleus caudalis (also see the following section on neuromuscular mechanisms).

Central sensitization is usually reversible after a transient, uncomplicated trauma or inflammation, but, depending on the type of injury or inflammation, the resulting central sensitization also can be associated with pain behavior that can last for hours, days, or even weeks. The factors accounting for why central sensitization can resolve after most injuries, but is maintained with others, is a topic of considerable current research. Clinically, maintenance of central sensitization is thought to contribute to the spontaneous pain, allodynia, hyperalgesia, and pain spread or referral that characterize many cases of persistent pain following injury or inflammation. Inflammation is not, however, a necessary condition for the induction of central sensitization. For example, the injection of glutamate into deep craniofacial tissues, which does not appear to produce any substantive inflammatory

reaction, is very effective in inducing central sensitization in subnucleus caudalis NS and WDR neurons.[21]

Injury to afferent nerves can also trigger other mechanisms that can result in central sensitization.[17,18] These include the initiation of abnormal impulses in the injured afferents, sprouting of the afferents into peripheral tissues, formation of neuromas, phenotypic changes in the afferents, development of functional contacts between sympathetic efferents and nociceptive afferents, structural reorganization of the central endings of primary afferents in the CNS as a result of central sprouting, and activation of microglia in the CNS. These changes associated with the afferent fibers and their central consequences, such as central sensitization and changes (eg, disinhibition) in segmental or descending influences, can persist for long periods and lead to the development of neuropathic pain conditions. Chapters 5 and 6 provide a more extensive review of these mechanisms.

The central sensitization induced by afferent inputs underscores the fact that the afferents and the brainstem nociceptive circuitry are not "hard wired" but are plastic. In other words, neuroplastic changes can occur in the RF and response properties of the nociceptive neurons as a result of peripheral tissue damage or inflammation, including trauma induced during dental surgical procedures. In some cases, structural as well as functional changes can occur. These neuroplastic changes underlying central sensitization appear important in the development of chronic pain conditions, thereby providing justification for the emerging view that chronic pain is a disease or disorder in itself.

Central sensitization in V nociceptive pathways is not restricted to the subnucleus caudalis but also occurs in nociceptive neurons in the subnucleus oralis of the V brainstem complex as well as in higher brain regions such as the ventrobasal thalamus. Nonetheless, the importance of the subnucleus caudalis in V nociceptive mechanisms is emphasized by recent findings that it is responsible for the expression of central sensitization in these structures by way of its projections to both the subnucleus oralis and the ventrobasal thalamus.[47] Furthermore, the increases in jaw muscle activity that can be reflexly induced by deep craniofacial noxious stimuli and that accompany the central sensitization process are also dependent on the functional integrity of the subnucleus caudalis, because it is a vital interneuronal relay site in these reflex effects.[18,21]

Several neuropeptides (eg, substance P and CGRP) and excitatory amino acids (eg, glutamate) appear to be crucial for the production of central sensitization (see Fig 4-5). For example, both NMDA and non-NMDA (eg, AMPA) glutamate receptor subtypes underlie the involvement of excitatory amino acids in nociceptive processing, but NMDA receptor mechanisms are especially important in the production of central sensitization. This explains why centrally acting NMDA receptor antagonists are particularly effective in preventing, for example, the increased jaw muscle activity and the RF expansion and related hyperexcitability of V brainstem nociceptive neurons induced by afferent inputs from TMJ or masticatory muscle tissues.[14,15,46] As noted in chapter 5 several other neurochemicals that are released from central neurons (eg, in the SG of the caudalis) of the glia may modulate these central effects; these include opioids, ATP, 5-HT, and GABA.

Clinical Implications

There are several clinical implications of these various features of central sensitization. Because NMDA receptor antagonists are particularly effective in blocking central sensitization within the V brainstem complex, they might be useful clinically as analgesics. However, glutamate release and NMDA receptor activation are common in many regions of the CNS involved in functions other than nociceptive transmission; therefore, NMDA antagonists may have limited application for pain relief because of their potential side effects associated with interfering with other functions. The challenge in developing clinically useful NMDA receptor antagonists is to produce a drug that is very effective in suppressing central sensitization but does not produce undesirable side effects (eg, nausea and drowsiness).

Also of clinical relevance is the importance of afferent inputs in the initiation of central sensitization and their possible role in its maintenance. This role is underscored by recent unpublished data (Lam et al, 2005) showing that surgical incision of the facial skin and subcutaneous tissues can induce central sensitization in subnucleus caudalis nociceptive neurons that can be prevented by prior local anesthesia of the incised tissues. These findings support the incorporation of clinical approaches (eg, preemptive analgesia and long-acting local anesthetics) that reduce nociceptive afferent input into the CNS and thus reduce the risk that central sensitization will develop or be maintained.

The properties of the subnucleus caudalis nociceptive neurons and their susceptibility to central sensitization also are relevant to the spread and referral of pain. Most caudalis NS and WDR neurons have a cutaneous RF as well as a deep RF, and nociceptive afferent input from deep tissues such as the TMJ and jaw muscles is especially effective in inducing an expansion of both cutaneous and deep RFs in these neurons. These features may explain

the poor localization, spread, and referral of pain that is typical of deep pain conditions involving the TMJ and associated jaw musculature.

In addition, the RF changes that are a feature of central sensitization may be accompanied by an increased responsiveness of the nociceptive neurons and a lowering of their threshold for activation by peripheral stimuli. As previously noted, these additional features of central sensitization and neuroplasticity are thought to contribute to the tenderness, hyperalgesia, and allodynia of superficial as well as deep tissues that characterize many cases involving injury to the TMJ and other deep tissues in the craniofacial region (see Table 4-1). It was also pointed out earlier that the central sensitization process induced in the V brainstem complex by deep nociceptive afferent inputs is associated with increased EMG activity in jaw-opening and jaw-closing muscles in animals. It has been suggested that these neuromuscular changes may represent a "splinting" effect that counteracts excessive movement and so protects the articular or muscular tissues from further damage. This neuromuscular effect is in keeping with the general concept of the pain-adaptation model (see chapter 6).

In addition, it is important to recall that peripheral sensitization can also contribute to pain spread, hyperalgesia, and allodynia by increasing the excitability and decreasing the activation threshold of primary afferents. Thus, many pain conditions may, in fact, involve a mixture of peripheral sensitization and central sensitization phenomena.

Neuromuscular Mechanisms and Sensorimotor Control

Recent reviews[50,51] have discussed the structural and functional features of the craniofacial musculature and its motor units and muscle fibers. This section focuses on the brainstem and higher brain center mechanisms involved in the reflex regulation and sensorimotor coordination of the craniofacial musculature associated with TMJ function.

The TMJ, muscle, and other craniofacial afferent inputs that access the brainstem, thalamus, and cerebral cortex not only are involved in perceptual processes but also may be involved at each of these levels in sensorimotor integration and control. The craniofacial neuromuscular system can be influenced reflexly by the receptors in TMJ and muscle tissues; these include the free nerve endings in these tissues as well as the specialized receptors in the TMJ and craniofacial muscles (eg, muscle spindles and Golgi tendon organs) that were outlined in the section on peripheral sensory mechanisms. Thus, the neuromuscular system can be reflexly influenced by the afferent inputs into the brainstem from those receptors that signal joint position, muscle stretch or tension, pain, and so on. The central mechanisms responsible for motor control of the craniofacial muscles include the brainstem sensory and motor nuclei, adjacent brainstem interneuronal sites, and higher brain centers that project to and modulate these sensory and motor substrates.[1,5,12,50,52]

Brainstem Mechanisms

Several reflex responses involving brainstem circuits and their modulation by afferent and descending influences can be elicited by mechanical stimulation of the jaw-closing muscles. For example, stretch of these muscles evokes myotatic reflexes through activation of jaw muscle spindle afferents. The primary cell bodies of these spindle afferents are in the V mesencephalic nucleus, from which impulses in the central axon can monosynaptically activate jaw-closing motoneurons in the V motor nucleus. Non-noxious stimulation of TMJ tissues also evokes reflex responses in the tongue and other craniofacial muscles. In addition to the brainstem-based reflex responses evoked by these non-noxious stimuli, afferent signals are also sent to higher brain centers involved in sensorimotor control of the muscles.

Brainstem circuits underlie the reflex changes in heart rate, blood pressure, breathing, and salivation as well as the more complex pain-avoidance behaviors that can be evoked by noxious stimulation of craniofacial tissues. On the basis of these various types of response, several behavioral paradigms have been developed to study the effects of noxious craniofacial stimuli in humans; these include changes in autonomic function (eg, heart rate), muscle reflexes, and facial expression as well as more subjective indicators of pain (eg, intensity and unpleasantness) measured psychometrically by visual analog scales, the McGill Pain Questionnaire, and other scales.[18,53] Behavioral animal models of orofacial pain have also recently been used to replicate trigeminal neuropathic or inflammatory pain, for example, by inducing chronic constriction injury of the infraorbital or inferior alveolar nerve or the application of inflammatory irritants such as formalin, Freund's adjuvant, or mustard oil to the TMJ, jaw muscles, or other craniofacial tissues.[17,18,29,46,54]

In the case of the reflex effects of noxious stimulation of TMJ or muscle tissues, high-intensity stimulation can elicit the jaw-opening reflex, and some stimuli can evoke transient inhibitory effects.[1,2] Application of algesic chemicals such as hypertonic saline, capsaicin, glutamate, or mustard oil to the TMJ, jaw muscles, or other craniofacial tissues of anesthetized animals[7,14,15,18,21] can activate neurons in the subnucleus caudalis. The activation and connection of these neurons with the brainstem reflex centers, such as the V motor nucleus, can result in prolonged increases in EMG activity of both the jaw-opening and jaw-closing muscles, as previously noted (Fig 4-6). Furthermore, the evoked EMG activity may be blocked by application of NMDA receptor antagonists to the subnucleus caudalis, indicating that these central receptors and related secondary messenger systems are involved in the EMG changes reflexly evoked in the jaw muscles by the application of mustard oil or glutamate to the TMJ or masticatory muscles, just as they are in the neuroplastic changes in the subnucleus caudalis (as mentioned previously).

It is also noteworthy that a central opioid-based depression of the EMG changes may be "triggered" by noxious stimulation of the TMJ. This finding suggests that deep nociceptive afferent inputs to the brainstem evoke central NMDA-dependent neuronal activity in the subnucleus caudalis and associated neuromuscular changes but that these neural changes are limited by the recruitment of central opioid mechanisms also evoked by the noxious stimulation. Further evidence for changes in central inhibitory as well as excitatory mechanisms in response to deep craniofacial stimuli is outlined in chapter 5.

These findings in animals underscore the close interplay between sensory and motor pathways. In addition, the reflex effects of noxious stimuli on jaw muscle activity in animals are of clinical relevance because they bear on the underlying pathophysiologic mechanisms involved in many musculoskeletal disorders manifesting pain in humans, such as certain TMDs and tension-type headache. The animal data indicate that excitatory reflex pathways do exist from the peripheral orofacial nociceptors (via caudalis nociceptive neurons) to the α motoneurons in the V motor nucleus supplying the jaw-opening and jaw-closing muscles. While it has been suggested that the co-contraction of these muscles may provide a splinting effect that limits jaw movements in pathophysiologic conditions affecting deep tissues such as the TMJ and masticatory muscles, there is no consensus as to whether the EMG activity of these muscles decreases, increases, or remains unchanged during experimentally induced or clinical orofacial pain in humans, and a number of factors have been invoked as accounting for the disparity in experimental and clinical pain data.[14,15,56]

Moreover, even when increased EMG jaw muscle activity in humans has been reported, its relatively small magnitude contrasts with the robust and prolonged EMG jaw muscle increases reflexly induced in animals by algesic stimuli to TMJ and other craniofacial tissues. Nonethe-

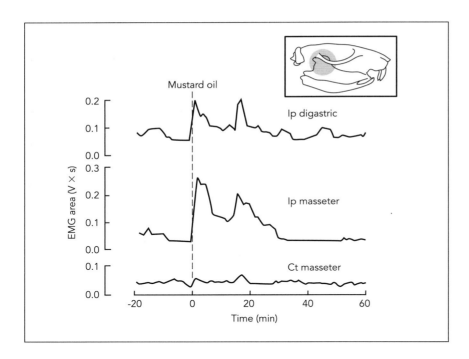

Mustard oil

Ip digastric

Ip masseter

Ct masseter

EMG area (V × s)

Time (min)

Fig 4-6 Increases over time in jaw muscle electromyographic (EMG) activity reflexly induced by injection of the algesic chemical mustard oil into the rat TMJ region. The EMG activity has been rectified and integrated. Note the biphasic character of the increase. (Ip) Ipsilateral; (Ct) contralateral. *(inset)* Site of mustard oil injection. (From Yu et al.[55] Reprinted with permission.)

less, although the exact same postural EMG pattern may not occur in awake humans as it does in anesthetized animals when an algesic chemical is infused into the TMJ or jaw muscles, alterations can occur in humans as well as animals in the normal alternating activity of the jaw-opening and jaw-closing muscles during mastication in the presence of noxious orofacial stimulation (see chapter 6). These alterations include an enhancement of EMG jaw-closing activity during jaw opening and vice versa.

Such findings appear inconsistent with many current and long-held concepts related to the etiology of TMD pain, in particular the so-called vicious cycle that is conceptualized in terms of muscle hyperactivity leading to pain, which in turn leads to more muscle hyperactivity, and so on. Although strenuous exercise reflecting increased muscle activity can lead to microtrauma in muscles and connective tissue that is usually followed by pain that peaks in about 24 hours (postexercise muscle soreness), it is unclear whether these processes characterize TMD myofascial pain. Also, most elements of the vicious cycle have not been experimentally tested or proven, although the animal data previously noted do clearly show that noxious stimulation can reflexly induce an increase in jaw muscle activity.

A concept of pain adaptation has recently been proposed (see chapter 6). According to this model, pain can cause agonist muscles to become less active during a move-ment (eg, the anterior digastric muscle during the jaw-opening phases of mastication) and antagonist muscles (eg, masseter) to become more active in this movement, thereby limiting jaw mobility and possibly aiding healing.

Higher Center Mechanisms

It was noted earlier that many V brainstem neurons relaying to the thalamus or other brain regions are subject to segmental (afferent) modulation and to descending modulation from various cortical and subcortical structures. Because many of these neurons also contribute to reflex and other behavioral responses to stimulation of TMJ and other orofacial tissues, these reflex responses can also be regulated by such modulatory influences. These descending modulatory influences include those from the amygdala and other parts of the limbic system, the lateral hypothalamus, the lateral habenular nucleus, the basal ganglia, the anterior pretectal nucleus, the red nucleus, the cerebellum, the sensorimotor cerebral cortex, and the cortical masticatory areas.

One particularly important cortical area exerting descending influences on brainstem and other subcortical regions is the face MI. Recent studies using intracortical microstimulation in monkeys have revealed that each muscle or movement is represented multiple times within the MI, leading to the current view that each output zone of the MI controls one of the many contextual functions in which a muscle participates.[44,57] This concept of multiple representation includes not only elemental movements, such as jaw opening and tongue protrusion, but also complex activities, such as mastication and swallowing. In the monkey, mastication and swallowing can be evoked not only by intracortical microstimulation of the classic masticatory area lateral to the face MI, but also from within the face MI and even within the face primary sensory cortex (SI). Furthermore, selective cold block or ablation of each of these regions disrupts chewing and swallowing to varying degrees, indicating that each may be involved differentially in the production and patterning of chewing and swallowing.[44,57,58]

Further evidence for the role of these three cortical regions in semiautomatic (eg, chewing and swallowing) as well as elemental movements comes from studies using single neuron recordings in monkeys and other mammals. In monkeys, for example, many face MI and SI neurons discharge in relation to chewing or swallowing. Many also discharge in association with more elemental movements; some are active in relation to jaw movements and many others are active in relation to tongue movements.[43,44,58] These findings are supported by evidence that ablation or cold block of the monkey's face MI or SI disrupts the animal's ability to perform a learned tongue task but causes much less disruption of a biting task.[44,58]

The neuronal and ablation findings previously noted also underscore the importance of the somatosensory cortex as well as the motor cortex in the fine motor control of orofacial movements. The face SI can influence orofacial movements by its projections to the face MI and other cortical areas and to subcortical regions such as the V brainstem complex and the cranial nerve motor nuclei. The face SI has a somatotopically arranged array of sensory inputs that are predominantly from facial skin and intraoral structures but may also include some inputs from deep tissues (eg, muscle). The face MI also receives input from afferents supplying deep and especially superficial tissues (eg, skin, mucosa, and periodontal tissues) of the face, mouth, and jaws. The studies of deep afferent input to the face MI and SI have not yet provided a clear delineation of what proportion of these derive from TMJ tissues. Nonetheless, the convergence of these various inputs may be related to mandibular kinesthesia. The substantial number of face MI neurons that receive bilateral input from the orofacial tissues is probably related to the need for bilateral sensorimotor coordination in orofacial muscle function. The face MI may use its orofacial afferent inputs for generating and regulating orofacial movements in order to refine ongoing cortical motor activity and shape the appropriate motor response. For example, it can participate in the control of voluntary orofacial movements such as the manipulation of the food bolus after it is placed in the mouth.

Thus, both the face MI and SI may use orofacial afferent inputs to guide, correct, and control movement by the use of sensory cues prior to movement and by using sensory information generated during movement. These processes may involve intracortical processing, cortical gating, transfer of somatosensory information, and, by cortical projections descending to subcortical sites, modulation and selection of somatosensory information ascending through subcortical relay neurons in the V brainstem complex and thalamus.[44,58]

A role for the face MI in orofacial motor skill acquisition is also suggested by recent findings in monkeys and humans of face MI neuroplasticity associated with the learning of a novel tongue-protrusion task.[57,59] These studies underscore the crucial role played by the face MI in sensorimotor integration and control and its remarkable capacity for neuroplasticity that may reflect dynamic, adaptive cortical mechanisms mediating complex motor and cognitive phenomena related to motor learning and memory. They also suggest that there may be cortical templates for a variety of familiar, learned orofacial motor activities. Such findings are fundamental to understanding how all animals (including humans) learn and acquire a new skill, how they adapt or fail to adapt to an altered oral environment, and how clinical approaches aimed at restoring orofacial function (eg, fixed partial dentures, dentures, and implants) may produce their rehabilitative effect.

Mandibular Kinesthesia and Bite Force Regulation

There are other integrative sensory and motor functions that may involve TMJ and muscle receptors. For example, a subject's estimation of the position, speed, and direction of jaw movements and the thickness and hardness of objects between the teeth relies heavily on a fully integrated nervous system.[1,60] For these purposes, the subject usually generates voluntary jaw muscle effort and uses this "sense of effort" together with the continuous afferent input from multiple intraoral and extraoral sites.

One such sensorimotor function is jaw position sense, called *mandibular kinesthesia*. When subjects open and close their mouth repeatedly to conceptualized target positions, they do so more accurately near dental intercuspation and near complete jaw opening than at half-open positions.[2,61] This function could conceivably depend on afferent inputs to the cerebral cortex (eg, the face SI and MI) from the TMJ or jaw muscles or even cutaneous sites.[1,2,5] The use of local anesthesia and capsular pressure changes to alter TMJ afferent input has revealed that the kinesthetic sense used when efforts are made to self-position the jaw at specified gapes is partly the result of mechanoreceptors in the TMJ capsule and ligament.[1,2] However, input from jaw muscle afferents may also contribute, and there is evidence supporting the involvement of muscle spindles in kinesthesia in other parts of the body.

Subjects with some forms of TMD have an impaired mandibular kinesthetic sense, lateral jaw position sense, and reduced control over the direction of movement.[1,2] As noted earlier, pain can influence muscle activity, and there are reports that myalgic pain reduces the precision in reaching a preset vertical jaw position.[62] However, other studies[62] have not demonstrated significant differences in jaw position sense between normal subjects and those with fatigued muscles, arthrogenic disorders, or myogenic pain, suggesting that only strongly fatigued muscles may lead to an impaired sense of jaw position.

Another integrative function is the regulation of bite force. The control of bite force is needed for the regulation of interocclusal and articular forces as well as for compression and tension in muscle and bone. Bite forces are subject to ongoing modification in many orofacial motor behaviors, eg, the slow, closing phase of the chewing cycle, tooth clenching, and biting. Afferent inputs into the CNS from orofacial tissues is crucial in this control and exerts their effects both reflexly at the brainstem level and consciously at higher brain levels (eg, the cerebral cortex).

The potential mechanoreceptors for signaling regional distortions of the craniofacial tissues include the TMJ, muscle, periodontal, and mucosal mechanoreceptors; periosteal and sutural receptors; and Golgi tendon organs. Afferent input from periodontal mechanoreceptors, along with tonically active muscle spindle input, appears to be particularly important in bite force regulation and can enhance the activity of the jaw-closing muscles by positive feedback. Further details of the factors influencing bite force are provided in chapter 6 and in other reviews.[2,5,60]

Acknowledgments

The research studies by the author noted in this chapter were supported by grant MT-4918 from the Canadian Institutes of Health Research and by grants DE04786 and DE15420 from the US National Institute of Dental and Craniofacial Research.

References

1. Dubner R, Sessle BJ, Storey AT. The Neural Basis of Oral and Facial Function. New York: Plenum Press, 1978.
2. Hannam AG, Sessle BJ. Temporomandibular neurosensory and neuromuscular physiology. In: Zarb G, Carlsson G, Sessle BJ, Mohl N (eds). Temporomandibular Joint and Masticatory Muscle Disorders. Copenhagen: Munksgaard, 1994: 67–100.
3. Cairns BE. Nociceptors in the orofacial region—TMJ and muscle. In: Schmidt RF, Willis WD (eds). Pain Encyclopedia. Heidelberg: Springer (in press).
4. Gandevia SC, Refshauge KM, Collins DF. Proprioception: Peripheral inputs and perceptual interactions. Adv Exp Med Biol 2002;508:61–68.
5. Miles TS. Mastication. In: Miles TS, Nauntofte B, Svensson P (eds). Clinical Oral Physiology. Copenhagen: Quintessence, 2004:219–243.
6. Widenfalk B, Wiberg M. Origin of sympathetic and sensory innervation of the temporomandibular joint. A retrograde axonal tracing study in the rat. Neurosci Lett 1990;109: 30–35.
7. Lund JP, Sessle BJ. Neurophysiological mechanisms related to chronic pain disorders of the temporomandibular joint and masticatory muscles. In: Zarb G, Carlsson G, Sessle B, Mohl N (eds). Temporomandibular Joint and Masticatory Muscle Disorders. Copenhagen: Munksgaard, 1994:188–207.
8. Dreesen D, Halata Z, Strasmann T. Sensory innervation of the temporomandibular joint in the mouse. Acta Anat 1990; 139:154–160.
9. Kido MA, Kiyoshima T, Kondo T, et al. Distribution of substance P and calcitonin gene-related peptide-like immunoreactive nerve fibers in the rat temporomandibular joint. J Dent Res 1993;72:592–598.
10. Klineberg IJ. Structure and function of temporomandibular joint innervation. Ann R Coll Surg Engl 1971;49:268–288.
11. Lund JP, Matthews B. Response of temporomandibular joint afferents recorded in the gasserian ganglion of the rabbit to passive movements of the mandible. In: Kawamura Y, Dubner R (eds). Oral-Facial Sensory and Motor Functions. Tokyo: Quintessence, 1981:153–160.
12. Lund JP, Scott G, Kolta A, Westberg KG. Role of cortical inputs and brainstem interneuron populations in patterning mastication. In: Nakamura Y, Sessle BJ (eds). Neurobiology of Mastication. From Molecular to Systems Approach. Amsterdam: Elsevier, 1999:504–514.
13. Kopp S. Neuroendocrine, immune, and local responses related to temporomandibular disorders. J Orofac Pain 2001; 15:9–28.
14. Sessle BJ. The neural basis of temporomandibular joint and masticatory muscle pain. J Orofac Pain 1999;13:238–245.
15. Sessle BJ. Acute and chronic craniofacial pain: Brainstem mechanisms of nociceptive transmission and neuroplasticity, and their clinical correlates. Crit Rev Oral Biol Med 2000;11:57–91.

16. Hargreaves KM. Neurochemical factors in injury and inflammation of orofacial tissues. In: Lund JP, Lavigne GJ, Dubner R, Sessle BJ (eds). Orofacial Pain. From Basic Science to Clinical Management. Chicago: Quintessence, 2001:59–66.

17. Woda A. Mechanisms of neuropathic pain. In: Lund JP, Lavigne GJ, Dubner R, Sessle BJ (eds). Orofacial Pain. From Basic Science to Clinical Management. Chicago: Quintessence, 2001:67–78.

18. Svensson P, Sessle BJ. Orofacial pain. In: Miles TS, Nauntofte B, Svensson P (eds). Clinical Oral Physiology. Copenhagen: Quintessence, 2004:93–139.

19. Julius D. The molecular biology of thermosensation. In: Dostrovsky JO, Carr DB, Koltzenburg M (eds). Proceedings of the 10th World Congress on Pain, Progress in Pain Research and Management, vol 24. Seattle: IASP Press, 2003:63–70.

20. Dray A. Future pharmacologic management of neuropathic pain. J Orofac Pain 2004;18:381–385.

21. Lam DK, Sessle BJ, Cairns BE, Hu JW. Neural mechanism of temporomandibular joint and masticatory muscle pain: A possible role for peripheral glutamate receptor mechanisms. Pain Res Manage (in press).

22. Shigenaga Y, Sera M, Nishimori T, et al. The central projection of masticatory afferent fibers to the trigeminal sensory nuclear complex and upper cervical spinal cord. J Comp Neurol 1988;268:489–507.

23. Capra NF, Dessem D. Central connections of trigeminal primary afferent neurons: Topographical and functional considerations. Crit Rev Oral Biol Med 1992;4:1–52.

24. Bereiter DA, Benetti AP. Excitatory amino release within spinal trigeminal nucleus after mustard oil injection into the temporomandibular joint region of the rat. Pain 1996; 67:451–459.

25. Messlinger KB, Ellrich J. Processing of nociceptive inputs from different tissues to the spinal trigeminal nucleus and release of immunoreactive substance P. In: Nakamura Y, Sessle BJ (eds). Neurobiology of Mastication. From Molecular to Systems Approach. Amsterdam: Elsevier, 1999:177–188.

26. Dubner R. Recent advances in our understanding of pain. In: Klineberg I, Sessle BJ (eds). Oro-Facial Pain and Neuromuscular Dysfunction: Mechanisms and Clinical Correlates. Oxford, England: Pergamon Press, 1985:3–19.

27. Bereiter DA, Hiraba H, Hu JW. Trigeminal subnucleus caudalis: Beyond homologies with the spinal dorsal horn. Pain 2000;88:221–224.

28. Woda A. Pain in the trigeminal system: From orofacial nociception to neural network modeling. J Dent Res 2003;82: 764–768.

29. Ro JY, Capra NF, Masri R. Contribution of peripheral N-methyl-D-aspartate receptors to c-fos expression in the trigeminal spinal nucleus following acute masseteric inflammation. Neuroscience 2004;123:213–219.

30. Hu JW. Cephalic myofascial pain pathways. In: Olesen J, Schoenen J (eds). Tension-type Headache: Classification, Mechanisms, and Treatment. New York: Raven Press, 1993: 69–77.

31. Okamoto K, Hirata H, Takeshita S, Bereiter DA. Response properties of TMJ neurons in superficial laminae at the spinomedullary junction of female rats vary over the estrous cycle. J Neurophysiol 2003;89:1467–1477.

32. Sessle BJ. Orofacial pain. In: Merskey H, Besson JD, Loeser I, Dubner R (eds). The Paths of Pain. 1975–2005. Seattle: IASP Press, (in press).

33. Hargreaves KM. Pain mechanisms of the pulpodentin complex. In: Hargreaves KM, Goodis HE (eds). Seltzer and Bender's Dental Pulp. Chicago: Quintessence, 2002:184.

34. Hill RG. New targets for analgesic drugs. In: Dostrovsky JO, Carr DB, Koltzenburg M (eds). Proceedings of the 10th World Congress on Pain, Progress in Pain Research and Management, vol 24. Seattle: IASP Press, 2003:419–436.

35. Watkins LR, Milligan ED, Maier SF. Immune and glial involvement in physiological and pathological exaggerated pain states. In: Dostrovsky JO, Carr DB, Koltzenburg M (eds). Proceedings of the 10th World Congress on Pain, Progress in Pain Research and Management, vol 24. Seattle: IASP Press, 2003:369–385.

36. Tsuda M, Shigemoto-Mogami Y, Koizumi S, et al. P2X4 receptors induced in spinal microglia gate tactile allodynia after nerve injury. Nature 2003;424:778–783.

37. Chiang CY, Hu B, Park SJ, et al. Purinergic and NMDA-receptor mechanisms underlying tooth pulp stimulation-induced central sensitization in trigeminal nociceptive neurons. In: Dostrovsky JO, Carr DB, Koltzenburg M (eds). Proceedings of the 10th World Congress on Pain, Progress in Pain Research and Management, vol 24. Seattle: IASP Press, 2003:345–354.

38. Craig AD, Dostrovsky JO. Processing of nociceptive information at supraspinal levels. In: Yaksh TL, Lynch C III, Zapol WM, et al (eds). Anesthesia: Biologic Foundations. Philadelphia: Lippincott-Raven, 1997:625–642.

39. Chudler EH, Anton F, Dubner R, Kenshalo DR Jr. Responses of nociceptive neurons in monkeys and pain sensation in humans elicited by noxious thermal stimulation: Effect of interstimulus interval. J Neurophysiol 1990;63:559–569.

40. Iwata K, Tsuboi Y, Tashiro A, Sakamoto M, Sumino R. Integration of tooth-pulp pain at the level of cerebral cortex. In: Nakamura Y, Sessle BJ (eds). Neurobiology of Mastication. From Molecular to Systems Approach. Amsterdam: Elsevier, 1999:471–481.

41. Bushnell MC. Perception and behavioral modulation of pain. In: Lund JP, Lavigne GJ, Dubner R, Sessle BJ (eds). Orofacial Pain. From Basic Science to Clinical Management. Chicago: Quintessence, 2001:107–114.

42. Davis KD. The neural circuitry of pain as explored with functional MRI. Neurological Res 2000;22:313–317.

43. Luschei ES, Goldberg LJ. Neural mechanisms of mandibular control: Mastication and voluntary biting. In: Brooks VB (ed). Handbook of Physiology. Motor Control, vol 2. Washington: American Physiological Society, 1981:1237–1274.

44. Sessle B, Yao D, Yamamura K. Face primary motor cortex and somatosensory cortex: Input and output properties and functional interrelationships in the awake monkey. In: Nakamura Y, Sessle BJ (eds). Neurobiology of Mastication. From Molecular to Systems Approach. Amsterdam: Elsevier, 1999:482–493.

45. Maixner W. Pain modulatory systems. In: Lund JP, Lavigne GJ, Dubner R, Sessle BJ (eds). Orofacial Pain. From Basic Science to Clinical Management. Chicago: Quintessence, 2001:79–91.

46. Ren K, Dubner R. Central nervous system plasticity and persistent pain. J Orofac Pain 1999;13:155–163.

47. Chiang CY, Sessle BJ, Hu JW. Parabrachial area and nucleus raphe magnus–induced modulation of electrically evoked trigeminal subnucleus caudalis neuronal responses to cutaneous or deep A-fiber and C-fiber inputs in rats. Pain 1995;62:61–68.

48. Linderoth B, Meyerson BA. Central nervous system stimulation for neuropathic pain. In: Hannson PT, Fields HL, Hill RG, Marchettini P (eds). Neuropathic Pain: Pathophysiology and Treatment. Seattle: IASP Press, 2001:223–249.

49. Kalso E. Opioids for chronic noncancer pain. In: Dostrovsky JO, Carr DB, Koltzenburg M (eds). Proceedings of the 10th World Congress on Pain, Progress in Pain Research and Management, vol 24. Seattle: IASP Press, 2003:751–765.

50. Miller A. The Neuroscientific Principles of Swallowing and Dysphagia. San Diego: Singular, 1999:284.

51. Miles TS. Masticatory muscles. In: Miles TS, Nauntofte B, Svensson P (eds). Clinical Oral Physiology. Copenhagen: Quintessence, 2004:199–217.

52. Lund JP, Kolta A, Westberg KG, Scott G. Brainstem mechanisms underlying feeding behaviours. Curr Opin Neurobiol 1998;8:718–724.

53. Raineville P. Measurement of pain. In: Lund JP, Lavigne GJ, Dubner R, Sessle BJ (eds). Orofacial Pain. From Basic Science to Clinical Management. Chicago: Quintessence, 2001:95–105.

54. Iwata K, Tsuboi Y, Shima A, et al. Central neuronal changes after nerve injury: Neuroplastic influences of injury and aging. J Orofac Pain 2004;18:293–298.

55. Yu XM, Sessle BJ, Vernon H, Hu JW. Effects of inflammatory irritant application to the rat temporomandibular joint on jaw and neck muscle activity. Pain 1995;60:143-149.

56. Svensson P, Graven-Nielsen T. Craniofacial muscle pain: Review of mechanisms and clinical manifestations. J Orofac Pain 2001;15:117–145.

57. Sessle BJ, Yao D. Contribution of plasticity of sensorimotor cerebral cortex to development of communication skills. Behav Brain Sci 2002;25:638–639.

58. Murray GM, Lin LD, Yao D, Sessle BJ. Sensory and motor functions of face primary somatosensory cortex in the primate. In: Rowe MJ, Iwamura Y (eds). Somatosensory Processing: From Single Neuron to Brain Imaging. Amsterdam: Harwood Academic, 2001:113–130.

59. Svensson P, Romaniello A, Arendt-Nielsen L, Sessle BJ. Plasticity in corticomotor control of the human tongue musculature induced by tongue-task training. Exp Brain Res 2003;152:42–51.

60. Trulsson M, Essick GK. Mechanosensation. In: Miles TS, Nauntofte B, Svensson P (eds). Clinical Oral Physiology. Copenhagen: Quintessence, 2004:165–197.

61. Nielsen IL, Ogro J, McNeill C, Danzig WN, Goldman SM, Miller AJ. Alteration in proprioceptive reflex control in subjects with craniomandibular disorders. J Craniomandib Disord Facial Oral Pain 1987;1:170–178.

62. Dahlstrom L, Haraldson T, Carlsson GE. Perception of jaw position during different conditions. J Craniomandib Disord 1989;3:147–151.

Persistent Orofacial Pain

Ronald Dubner and Ke Ren

Pain produced by transient stimuli, such as touching a hot stove, is protective. Such stimuli warn of impending tissue damage and injury to most of the tissues and organs of our body. Pain that occurs after an athletic injury or due to surgery is also protective and forces us to rest the injured part. This type of pain usually subsides in a few days or weeks. However, in some cases the pain is chronic; it persists long after the injury has apparently healed, possibly for months or years. This type of pain is nonprotective. Chronic persistent pain is often difficult to treat and leads to a reduction in quality of life, increased medical costs, and loss of personal income.

Studies conducted in the past two decades have helped to unravel the mysteries of chronic pain. We know that there are changes at the site of injury as well as long-term changes in the central nervous system (CNS) that contribute to an increase in intensity and persistence of pain.

Activity-Induced Plasticity in the CNS

Both tissue and nerve injury can produce prolonged changes in the nervous system.[1] Tissue damage results in an increased sensitivity of receptors that respond specifically to tissue damage, called *nociceptors*, at the site of injury. This is called *peripheral sensitization*. The nociceptors exhibit spontaneous activity, lowered thresholds, and increased responsiveness to subsequent painful stimuli. Peripheral sensitization is also dependent on the environment of the receptor, which changes with injury. There is a release of multiple chemical mediators, eg, bradykinin, prostaglandins, neuropeptides such as substance P (SP), and a lowered pH. The increased nociceptor activity ultimately leads to an increased neuronal barrage

into the CNS and functional changes in the spinal cord and brain that contribute to an increase in pain. These changes in the CNS are referred to as *central sensitization*. The increase in pain at a site of injury is called *hyperalgesia*. Often injury leads to pain in response to nonpainful stimuli, which is referred to as *allodynia*. In addition to spontaneous pain, the most common signs and symptoms of chronic pain are allodynia and hyperalgesia in response to mechanical stimuli.

Similarly, nerve damage also can lead to increased activity at the site of injury. Cut or damaged nerves emit new axon sprouts and form *neuromas*, or bundles of axon sprouts. The neuromas emit spontaneous nerve activity that travels to the spinal cord or brain.[2] Neuromas are also sensitive to mechanical, thermal, and chemical stimulation. Spontaneous nerve activity also originates from the cell bodies of damaged nerves located in the dorsal root or trigeminal ganglia. The increase in nerve activity arising from neuromas and the dorsal root/trigeminal ganglia results in hyperexcitability or hypersensitivity in the CNS, contributing to the hyperalgesia, allodynia, and spontaneous pain. As with tissue damage, we refer to these changes as *central sensitization*. Thus, both tissue and nerve injury can lead to prolonged changes in the nervous system.

Nociceptive systems (ie, those that signal approaching or actual tissue damage) contain specialized neurons, transmitters, and receptors in the periphery, the spinal and medullary dorsal horns, and at supraspinal sites. We now know that information about tissue damage is transmitted to the forebrain via multiple pathways whose temporal and spatial distribution of activity ultimately results in the experience of pain. It is important to recognize that activity in these specialized pathways is not immutable and can be modified by a number of the mechanisms discussed below.

Mechanisms of Central Sensitization

Signals from peripheral nociceptors in the face and mouth travel along the smallest nerve fibers and terminate in the spinal cord and the trigeminal equivalent of the spinal cord in the brain. The terminals of these nerve fibers release a number of chemical mediators, including glutamate, the major excitatory neurotransmitter in the dorsal horn, and neuropeptides such as SP and calcitonin gene–related peptide (CGRP). These chemical mediators contribute to an increase in the excitability of neurons in the dorsal horn of the spinal cord and medulla via actions at ionotropic receptors and G protein–coupled receptors, leading to central sensitization.[3,4] The increase in the excitability of dorsal horn neurons is brought about by a cascade of events, including neuronal depolarization, removal of the voltage-dependent magnesium block of the N-methyl-D-aspartate (NMDA) receptor, calcium entry into the cells, phosphorylation of the NMDA receptor, a change in the cell's kinetics, and resulting hyperexcitability or an increase in synaptic strength. The critical role of NMDA receptors in central sensitization has been shown by a number of researchers.[3–5] NMDA receptor antagonists can, dose-dependently, either act at the agonist recognition site or block ion channel permeability and completely reverse inflammatory thermal or mechanical hyperalgesia after intrathecal injection.[5] The presence of ionotropic, calcium permeable, alpha-amino-3-hydroxy-5-methyl-4-isoxazole propionate (AMPA) glutamate receptors in the spinal cord suggests that they may also play a role in central sensitization via calcium entry as well as interaction with the NMDA receptor.

The metabotropic glutamate receptors (mGluRs) are a family of large monomeric receptors that are coupled to effector systems via activation of G proteins. There are eight mGluRs that are further classified into three groups (I to III) according to their amino acid homology. Most studies indicate that the group I mGluR1/5 receptors are involved in nociceptive responses.[6] The role of mGluRs appears to be more prominent after prolonged noxious stimuli, and spinal mGluRs are required for the generation of inflammation-evoked spinal hyperexcitability.[6] Peripheral inflammation results in up-regulation of mGluR mRNA in the spinal cord.[7] Recent studies indicate that mGluR activation at the level of the spinal cord is involved in the initiation of behavioral hyperalgesia by leading to the mobilization of calcium from intracellular stores and activating kinases that phosphorylate and prime the NMDA receptor for subsequent channel activa-

tion and calcium permeability.[8] Thus, both metabotropic and ionotropic glutamate receptors play important roles in the development of central sensitization and persistent pain.

SP plays a role in dorsal horn hyperexcitability, presumably by increasing neuronal depolarization, releasing the magnesium block of NMDA receptors, and contributing to phosphorylation of the NMDA receptor via activation of second messenger pathways. Antagonists of the neurokinin 1 (NK-1) or SP receptor, injected intrathecally, reverse inflammatory hyperalgesia in a dose-dependent fashion.[9]

Neurotrophins such as nerve growth factor (NGF) and brain-derived neurotrophic factor (BDNF) not only contribute to establishing the development and connectivity of the nervous system, but they also play a role in sensitization after peripheral tissue injury.[10] A number of chemical mediators in the inflammatory medium such as cytokines (interleukin 1β and tumor necrosis factor α [TNF-α]) are inducers of NGF production from keratinocytes and fibroblasts. NGF in turn activates mast cells, which then release substances such as histamine and serotonin, and this indirectly results in peripheral sensitization of nociceptors. NGF has another important target: primary afferent neurons that express the receptor tyrosine kinase A (trkA) at their peripheral terminals. Binding to trkA can have two effects: (1) local changes may occur at the site of the peripheral terminal, where the intracellular domain of trkA leads to phosphorylation of ion channels or receptors, thus altering nociceptor sensitivity and peptide release; (2) retrograde transport of the NGF-trkA complex back to the dorsal root/trigeminal ganglion alters the transcription of neuropeptides involved in the sensitization process. NGF is up-regulated in the sciatic nerve after inflammation.[11] The increased levels of NGF after inflammation appear to contribute to an increase in the synthesis of neuropeptides such as SP, CGRP, and BDNF, which ultimately participate in the development of hyperalgesia.[12,13] Importantly, the application of NGF antibody prevents inflammatory hypersensitivity and hyperalgesia.[12,14]

Model of Neuronal Plasticity

A number of years ago, the authors proposed a model[1] in which increased nociceptor activity at the site of tissue or nerve injury leads to spinal cord dorsal horn hyperexcitability and behavioral hyperalgesia. Increased neural activity from the periphery leads to increased depolarization at excitatory amino acid receptor sites. This depolarization is facilitated by neuropeptide (SP, CGRP) release. The cascade of events leading to synaptic strengthening at the NMDA receptor site is initiated, leading to central sensitization. The result is an expansion of receptive fields, hyperexcitability, and an increase in pain. This hyperexcitability, or increased depolarization, if excessive, can lead to a pathologic state by promoting excitotoxicity, cell dysfunction, and a loss of inhibitory mechanisms. The combined effects of excessive excitation and loss of inhibition further contribute to the expansion of receptive fields, hyperexcitability, and amplification and prolongation of pain.

Hyperexcitability and Central Sensitization in the Trigeminal System

Most of our knowledge about mechanisms of persistent pain is based on studies at spinal cord levels; therefore, it is important to determine whether trigeminal mechanisms of pain are different from pain mechanisms originating from other body sites. In recent years, investigators have concentrated on developing animal models of deep pain in the craniomandibular region and pursuing studies of the function of the trigeminal brain stem nuclei and surrounding structures in persistent deep tissue inflammatory hyperalgesia and nerve injury pain conditions. Recent studies have reported the presence of central sensitization in trigeminal nociceptive pathways following orofacial noxious stimulation. The neuronal hyperexcitability, manifested in part as increases in peripheral receptive field size, suggests a functional plasticity of sensory neurons. In the medullary dorsal horn (trigeminal subnucleus caudalis), stimulation of craniofacial muscle afferents results in prolonged facilitatory effects on nociceptive neurons, including the expansion of receptive fields.[15] Cutaneous formalin injection can evoke a nociceptive neuronal response that lasts for more than 30 minutes.[16] Strassman et al[17] have shown that chemical stimulation of the dura receptive fields with inflammatory mediators sensitizes trigeminal primary afferent neurons innervating the intracranial meninges. Further studies indicate that the sensitization of meningeal sensory neurons leads to activation and sensitization of central trigeminal neurons that receive convergent input from the dura and skin.[18] Local anesthesia of the dura abolishes the response to dural stimulation but has minimal effect on the increased responses to

cutaneous stimulation, suggesting the involvement of a central mechanism in maintaining the hyperexcitability.

Injection of inflammatory agents such as complete Freund's adjuvant (CFA) or carrageenan into the hind paw of the rat produces edema, redness, and hyperalgesia that is limited to the injected paw and can begin as early as 5 to 10 minutes after injection, lasting up to 2 weeks.[8,19] This model has been adapted to the orofacial region, and mechanical stimulation has been used to measure hyperalgesia and allodynia.[20] The mechanical threshold is assessed with von Frey filaments. The response to suprathreshold stimuli can be evaluated using a range of filament forces.[21] A nonlinear regression analysis of the stimulus-response function can be used to calculate an EF50, the filament force that produces a response 50% of the time. The development of mechanical allodynia and hyperalgesia follows a pattern similar to that found after hind-paw stimulation, peaking at 4 to 24 hours and persisting for at least 2 weeks.

The authors have analyzed the effects of CFA-induced orofacial inflammation on the response properties of neurons in trigeminal subnucleus caudalis, the rostral extension of the upper cervical dorsal horn, also referred to as the *medullary dorsal horn (MDH)*.[22] MDH neurons were recorded extracellularly and classified as low threshold mechanoreceptive, wide dynamic range (WDR), or nociceptive specific (NS), similar to their categorization in the spinal dorsal horn. After producing inflammation of the temporomandibular joint (TMJ) with CFA, it was found that the receptive fields (RFs) of MDH nociceptive neurons were significantly enlarged. This finding confirmed previous results.[15] The enlarged RFs were found both in neurons whose RFs included the facial skin over the TMJ as well as in neurons whose RFs were entirely outside the zone of injury. Medullary dorsal horn neuronal hyperexcitability produced by central sensitization is manifested as an enlargement of RFs, and its presence outside the zone of injury suggests central sensitization. Responses to thermal stimuli were significantly greater in inflamed animals than in control animals, also suggesting hyperexcitability. These findings indicate that MDH hyperexcitability and central sensitization contribute to mechanisms of persistent pain associated with orofacial deep tissue injury.

Deep Versus Cutaneous Orofacial Tissue Injury

At both the trigeminal and spinal levels, C-fiber inputs produce more robust and longer-lasting neuronal hyperexcitability following stimulation of nerves within muscle than they do following cutaneous nerve stimulation.[23] There is a selective expansion of the deep mechanoreceptive fields of the trigeminal nociceptive neurons after mustard oil application into the tongue muscle versus application into the facial skin.[24] The stimulus-induced expression of Fos, the protein product of the immediate early gene, c-Fos, has been widely used as a measure of nociceptive neuronal activation.[25] Fos protein–like immunoreactivity is induced in the trigeminal pathways after noxious stimulation.[26] The authors systematically examined the effects of persistent orofacial deep versus cutaneous tissue injury on neuronal activation in the trigeminal brain stem nuclei.[27] The results demonstrate that TMJ tissue injury produces more robust central hyperexcitability than does perioral cutaneous tissue injury and resembles that seen in the hind-paw inflammation model.[19,28] TMJ inflammation induced significantly stronger neuronal activation than did perioral cutaneous inflammation, as indicated by trigeminal nociceptive neuronal hyperexcitability, increases in Fos protein expression, and an increase in opioid gene expression.[20,22,27,29]

Interestingly, Fos expression induced by TMJ and perioral inflammation parallels the intensity and course of the inflammation.[27] This observation suggests that the increase in intensity and persistence of Fos protein expression may be associated with a maintained increase in peripheral neural input from the site of injury.

NMDA receptor activation also plays an important role in trigeminal central hyperexcitability after injury. Trigeminal Fos activation after noxious stimulation is selectively attenuated by administration of NMDA receptor antagonists,[30,31] suggesting an NMDA receptor–related central sensitization at the trigeminal level. These findings have clinical relevance. An increase in deep tissue (ie, TMJ, muscle) C-fiber input after inflammation and strong central neuronal activation may initiate and maintain central hyperexcitability and contribute to persistent pain associated with temporomandibular disorders (see below).

Subnucleus Interpolaris/ Caudalis Transition Zone

Using Fos protein expression as a marker of neuronal activation, it has been found that orofacial noxious input activates two distinct regions in the spinal trigeminal nucleus, the trigeminal subnucleus interpolaris/caudalis transition zone (Vi/Vc) and the caudal subnucleus caudalis contiguous with the upper cervical dorsal horn

(Vc/C1,2; also previously referred to as the MDH).[26,32] The Vi/Vc is at the convergence of the caudal Vi and rostral Vc at the obex level. The ventral portion of the Vc is pushed dorsomedially by Vi. The Fos protein labeling in Vc/C1,2 is quite homologous to the spinal dorsal horn, with detailed somatotopic representation. This region is involved in sensory discriminative aspects of pain originating in the trigeminal dermatomes.[10] In contrast to Vc/C1,2 Fos labeling, the Vi/Vc Fos activation is more diverse. Some somatotopy exists in the Vi/Vc, eg, mandibular structures such as the TMJ and the masseter muscle send afferent terminals to the dorsomedial Vi/Vc, and corneal and frontal nerve afferents are found in the ventral Vi/Vc.[27] Fos protein immunoreactivity is predominantly ipsilateral only in the dorsal portion of Vi/Vc. The most prominent features of Vi/Vc include converging input from all trigeminal dermatomes as well as deep and cutaneous tissues and equivalent bilateral representations in the ventral portion of Vi/Vc.

The finding that inflammation-induced Fos protein activation in the Vi/Vc is mostly not somatotopically represented has led to the idea that it has a role other than discriminative sensory function. One hypothesis is that it has a function in autonomic and visceral processing.[30] Trigeminal neurons send input to the submedius nucleus of the thalamus, the hypothalamus, and the parabrachial nucleus, structures that are involved in somatovisceral and somatoautonomic processing.[33] The authors directly tested this hypothesis by investigating the contribution of the adrenals and vagal afferent input to the expression of Fos protein in Vi/Vc following inflammation of the masseter muscle. In addition, there was intense Fos activation bilaterally in nucleus tractus solitarius (NTS). Vagotomy and adrenalectomy, each combined with masseter inflammation, resulted in a significant decrease in the Fos expression in Vi/Vc and NTS produced by the masseter inflammation. In contrast to the effect of these lesions at the Vi/Vc level, there were no significant changes in Fos expression at the Vc/C1,2 level. Two important findings have emerged from these studies. First, they support the hypothesis that stress and vagal input contribute predominantly and bilaterally to masseteric-induced Fos expression in the Vi/Vc. Second, stress and vagal input have minimal effect in the Vc/C1,2 laminated region of the trigeminal nucleus.[30] This finding suggests that somatovisceral and somatoautonomic inputs are integrated at bilateral sites to enhance coordinated responses to deep tissue injury of mandibular musculature and the TMJ.[10]

The previous studies also led to the hypothesis that identification of the rostral projections of neurons activated in the Vi/Vc after inflammation would lead to a better understanding of their functional implications.

Trigeminal brain stem neurons are known to project to somatosensory as well as somatovisceral and somatoautonomic regulatory centers in the brain stem, hypothalamus, and thalamus. The authors studied the projection of neurons to four sites: nucleus submedius of the thalamus (Sm), ventroposterior medial thalamic nucleus (VPM), lateral hypothalamus (LH), and parabrachial nucleus of the midbrain (PB).[33] FluoroGold (Fluorochrome) retrograde tracing and Fos protein immunochemistry were used to identify neurons that projected to any of these sites and were activated by masseter CFA-induced inflammation. The rostral projections of trigeminal neurons exhibited a bilateral projection pattern with a unilateral predominance. The major population of trigeminal Fos-activated neurons that projected to the Sm was found at the ventral pole of the bilateral Vi/Vc. These findings confirm other studies reporting Sm projections from more rostral trigeminal nuclei in single retrograde labeling experiments.[33] Very few double-labeled neurons were found in the laminated Vc/C1,2. Another region of dense double labeling near this site was the bilateral caudal ventrolateral medulla. A small population of Fos-activated neurons in the Vi/Vc was labeled from PB injections, but the largest population was located in the ipsilateral dorsal pole of Vi/Vc. In caudal Vc/C1,2, there were double-labeled neurons following PB injections, with most found ipsilateral to the site of inflammation and located in the superficial laminae. Compared to the Sm and PB groups, the major population of activated neurons labeled from LH was in the caudal ventrolateral medulla. Surprisingly, very few Fos-positive cells in the Vi/Vc and in the laminated Vc/C1,2 were labeled following injection of FluoroGold into the VPM. In summary, there were dramatic differences in labeling dependent upon the rostral site of FluoroGold injection. In the bilateral Vi/Vc, the percentage of neurons projecting to the Sm was significantly greater than that projecting to LH and VPM, particularly in the ventral zone. In the ipsilateral laminated Vc/C1,2, the PB was the major site of rostral projection of activated neurons, with a secondary site in the ipsilateral dorsal Vi/Vc region. In the bilateral caudal ventrolateral medulla and NTS, there were significant projections to the Sm, PB, and LH, but not to VPM.

The previous findings confirm that there are heterogeneous populations of neurons in the ventral portion of the Vi/Vc. There are neurons that are activated bilaterally by anesthesia.[26] Others are activated by corneal stimulation, and corneal afferents provide ipsilateral afferent input to the region.[34] These findings also strengthen the view that the Vi/Vc plays an important role in the response to deep tissue injury.[10] The neurons in the dorsal pole receive primary afferent input from the TMJ and masseter muscle unilaterally and project mainly to PB and not to VPM or Sm. The neurons in the ventral pole respond to deep tissue input bilaterally and likely receive this input polysynaptically because masseter and TMJ afferents do not terminate in this region. The major projections from Vi/Vc are to Sm and PB, supporting the conclusion that this region plays a role in autonomic and hormonal functions and in emotionality.[30,33] The bilateral neuronal activation in this transition zone may also facilitate integration of sensorimotor functions associated with recuperation from injury.

Descending Modulation

The studies previously described have focused almost entirely on the role of primary afferent neurons and intrinsic spinal cord and trigeminal brain stem neurons in dorsal horn plasticity and hyperexcitability. The role of the third major component in the spinal and medullary dorsal horns, the axon terminals of extrinsic neurons originating mainly from descending brainstem pathways, until recently has been neglected in the mechanisms of central sensitization. Descending mechanisms are important because they provide the neural networks by which cognitive, attentional, and motivational aspects of the pain experience modulate nociceptive transmission.[35]

We have shown at the spinal cord level that descending modulation increases after inflammation to modulate central sensitization and that the effects can be both facilitatory and inhibitory. In our more recent studies,[36–38] Fos protein immunoreactivity as a measure of neuronal activity in the spinal cord and behavioral models of hyperalgesia have been combined to evaluate the contribution of specific brain stem nuclei to the modulation of neuronal activity in the spinal dorsal horn. Lesions were made in nucleus raphe magnus (NRM) of the medulla using the neurotoxin 5,7-DHT, which destroys serotonin-containing axons descending to the spinal dorsal horn. Five to seven days after injection of the neurotoxin into the NRM, the inflammatory agent CFA was injected into the hind paw of the rats. There was a significant enhancement of the behavioral hyperalgesia after the injection of the neurotoxin as compared with a vehicle injection. There also was an increase in Fos protein labeling in all laminae of the spinal dorsal horn. These findings suggest that destruction of the 5-HT-containing neurons in the NRM results in a reduction in the net descending inhibitory effects from the NRM on dorsal horn neurons, leading to a further increase in spinal cord central sensitization. Focal lesions of the locus caeruleus are also followed by an increase in spinal Fos expression and hyperalgesia after inflammation.[39]

In contrast, lesions of nucleus reticularis gigantocellularis (NGC) in the medulla led to opposite effects. The NGC lesions were made bilaterally with ibotenic acid, which produces excitotoxic destruction of the neurons. Two to three days later, CFA was injected into the ipsilateral hind paw, and after 24 hours there was a reduction in the hyperalgesia and in Fos protein immunoreactivity in the spinal cord. It appears that NGC lesions have the net effect of reducing hyperalgesia, suggesting that the net descending effects from NGC are facilitatory.[37,40]

Trigeminal nociceptive transmission is also subject to descending modulation from rostral brain stem structures, including the rostral ventromedial medulla (RVM). The authors examined the hypothesis that the Vi/Vc plays a prominent role in the activation of RVM modulatory circuitry since it has major projections to rostral brain sites involved in autonomic function, stress, and emotionality.[34,41] The same double-labeling method previously described was used and FluoroGold was injected into the RVM. Fos activation was produced by injection of CFA into the masseter muscle. Consistent with previous studies described, Fos protein was expressed in the Vi/Vc and the laminated Vc/C1,2. Double-labeled neurons were found bilaterally in the ventral portion of the Vi/Vc but not in the dorsal portion. In the Vc/C1,2, Fos was expressed mainly in the superficial laminae, but double-labeled neurons were mainly found in the deep laminae. The hypothesis that Vi/Vc neurons had reciprocal connections with RVM was then tested using an anterograde tracer, Phaseolus vulgaris leucoagglutinin (PHA-L), or the retrograde tracer, FluoroGold. Similar to the earlier studies, it was found that Fos-labeled Vi/Vc neurons send axons to RVM. Clusters of axon terminals labeled with PHA-L injected into the RVM were observed at the level of the Vi/Vc, including a dense labeling in the ventral pole of Vi/Vc, suggesting RVM terminals at this site in Vi/Vc.

To directly test the role of these connections in behavioral hyperalgesia and allodynia, excitotoxic lesions of RVM neurons were produced with ibotenic acid in a first set of experiments, and lesions of the ventral pole of Vi/Vc were produced in a second set.[41] Unilateral CFA-induced inflammation of the masseter muscle produced mechanical allodynia and hyperalgesia in the orofacial region overlapping the masseter muscle. The allodynia/hyperalgesia was significantly attenuated in rats receiving the ibotenic injection into the RVM 5 days prior to the induced inflammation. These findings indicate that modulatory inputs from the RVM enhance the hyperalgesia/allodynia found after masseter inflammation. It appears that descending facilitation contributes significantly to the hyperexcitability in this model of inflammatory hyperalgesia. Ibotenic acid lesions of the ventral Vi/Vc resulted in similar attenuation of the hyperalgesia/allodynia, suggesting that the Vi/Vc is a component of an upstream sensory pathway leading to RVM activation and resulting in descending facilitation. Although other studies suggest that descending facilitation and inhibition originate from the same sites and that the net effect is stimulus-intensity dependent,[42] descending facilitatory effects also appear to originate from different brain stem sites than those involved in descending inhibition.[37] The net descending effect is dependent on the total activity originating from these multiple sites after inflammation. The findings support the authors' overall hypothesis that the ventral pole of Vi/Vc is involved in the coordination of bilateral sensorimotor functions of the trigeminal system associated with the response to deep tissue injury. This response includes roles in nociceptive sensory processing, somatovisceral and somatoautonomic function, and descending modulation. These results indicate that tissue injury, and likely nerve injury, lead to activation of Vi/Vc and alter diverse neural functions in the craniofacial and oral regions.

It is clear that different behavioral or physiological conditions can shift the balance of descending modulation from inhibition to facilitation and vice versa. This shift in the balance may be one mechanism underlying patient susceptibility to deep tissue chronic pain conditions. In patients suffering from deep pain conditions, where central sensitization appears to be a prominent component (see above), such as temporomandibular disorders, fibromyalgia, and low back pain, the diffuse nature and amplification of pain may be due in part to changes in descending modulation with an enhancement of descending facilitation.[43]

Clinical Implications

These findings of activity-induced neuronal plasticity at peripheral and CNS sites have important clinical implications. The problem of persistent pain can now be attacked in the periphery at the site of injury and at CNS sites. This knowledge can be used in the development of new approaches to the management of persistent or chronic pain. It also teaches us about mechanisms of pain that can also be applied in the diagnosis of clinical conditions. Two illustrations of the clinical implications of this new knowledge are discussed below.

The knowledge that increases in nociceptor activity can lead to long-term hyperexcitability in the nervous system and amplification of pain led to the use of preoperative administration of drugs, such as local anesthetics or nonsteroidal anti-inflammatory agents, that act to reduce or block activity in peripheral nociceptors. Support for this idea has been provided by clinical studies demonstrating that presurgical administration of local anesthetics reduced postoperative pain in comparison to surgery performed without local anesthesia[44] or postoperative infiltration of local anesthetic.[45] A major concern about these studies was that the agents had effects beyond the surgical period and therefore were interfering not only with the neural barrage as a result of the surgical procedure, but also with neural activity produced by the inflammatory process initiated by the surgery. A recent study has separated intraoperative from postoperative effects of the peripheral neuronal barrage on the development of pain after oral surgery.[46] Patients were given a short-acting local anesthetic (lidocaine) preoperatively, and then general anesthesia was induced and third molar teeth extracted. A second intraoral injection consisting of a long-acting local anesthetic (bupivacaine) or saline was administered at the end of the surgery. Pain during the first 4 hours was significantly less in the group receiving bupivacaine postoperatively compared with the other group. At 48 hours, pain was also significantly lower in this same group, and no effect was demonstrated for the preoperative lidocaine. These findings indicate that the blockade of postoperative nociceptive input reduces pain long after the anesthetic effects have terminated. In contrast, blockade of the intraoperative nociceptive input on postoperative pain showed no effect in this model, suggesting that the nociceptive input during the brief period of the oral surgery produced minimal central sensitization as compared with the prolonged postoperative nociceptive input. Most importantly, these results indicate that blockade of nociceptive input emanating from the site of injury during the postoperative period is a critical component of the analgesic process of attenuating pain following surgery. However, surgical procedures that have a much longer intraoperative period than that associated with oral surgery may produce more significant central sensitization that would be blocked by a local anesthetic. The use of local anesthetics to block central sensitization can also be used as an aid in the diagnosis of temporomandibular disorders and other chronic orofacial pain conditions.

Another perspective on how knowledge of mechanisms can improve our ability to manage persistent pain comes from a study of a 52-year-old woman who developed severe shooting pains in the elbow following ulnar nerve transposition surgery.[47] After 18 months of various treatments that resulted in partial relief, she experienced severe pain in the forearm and hand. Clinical examination revealed spontaneous pain in the forearm and pain evoked by light touch from a cotton wisp on the elbow, forearm, and hand, indicating mechanical allodynia, which was shown to be mediated by activation of large myelinated or A beta afferent fibers normally activated by touch. As discussed earlier, this type of allodynia has been shown to be related to the development of central sensitization.[48,49] Two minutes after the injection of 1.5% lidocaine into the hyperpigmented region at the elbow, the injected site was completely anesthetized and the allodynia had disappeared from all areas. It was proposed that the A beta–mediated allodynia was due to input from a nociceptive focus at the original site of injury, which dynamically maintained altered central processing, resulting in touch being perceived as pain.[47] The peripheral input was proposed to potentially originate from several sources: neuromas, sympathetic stimulation, or soft tissue injury. Blocking this input caused the central processing to revert to normal, eliminating the allodynia. This example points out that peripheral nerve injury can lead to activation of peripheral nerve fibers by multiple mechanisms. Although the role of nerve injury pain in temporomandibular disorders is poorly understood, it might be useful in some cases to exploit the concept that foci of peripheral nerve activity involving C-fiber input may contribute to these disorders. The methods described above certainly can be used in such an effort.

These clinical studies illustrate the importance of peripheral sensitization and central sensitization in mechanisms of ongoing pain. We should not think of peripheral or central sensitization, nor descending modulation, as being a pathologic change in the nervous system. Rather, these phenomena should be regarded as part of the normal function of nociceptive systems in response to persistent injury. This normal function is protective after an injury occurs, as we guard the injured site while we recuperate and heal the injury. However, under some circumstances, the changes in the CNS may persist, even after the peripheral tissue injury has completely healed. Future research is needed to better understand why some people develop such nonprotective disturbances of the CNS that lead to the abnormal persistence of pain.

Summary

Nerve signals arising from sites of tissue or nerve injury lead to long-term changes in the CNS and contribute to hyperalgesia and the amplification and persistence of pain. These nociceptor activity–dependent changes are referred to as *central sensitization*. Central sensitization involves an increase in the excitability of medullary and spinal dorsal horn neurons brought about by a cascade of events, including neuronal depolarization; removal of the voltage-dependent magnesium block of the NMDA receptor; release of calcium from intracellular stores; phosphorylation of the NMDA, AMPA, and NK-1 receptors via activation of protein kinases; a change in the cell's excitability; and an increase in synaptic strength. Central sensitization occurs in trigeminal nociceptive pathways, and more robust neuronal hyperexcitability occurs following deep tissue versus cutaneous stimulation. Using Fos protein immunocytochemistry, it has been found that two distinct regions are activated in the trigeminal brain stem nuclei, namely the Vi/Vc and the caudal subnucleus caudalis. The latter is very similar to the spinal dorsal horn and is involved in the sensory discriminative aspects of pain. In contrast, the ventral pole of Vi/Vc is unique; in addition to its role in nociceptive sensory processing of mainly deep tissues, it is involved bilaterally in somatovisceral and somatoautonomic processing, activation of the pituitary-adrenal axis, and descending modulatory control. These findings support the overall hypothesis that the ventral pole of Vi/Vc is involved in the coordination of bilateral sensorimotor functions of the trigeminal system associated with the response to deep tissue injury.

Acknowledgments

The authors' studies presented in this chapter were supported by NIH grants DE11964 and DA10275.

References

1. Dubner R. Neuronal plasticity and pain following peripheral tissue inflammation or nerve injury. In: Bond MR, Charlton JE, Woolf CJ (eds). Proceedings of the VIth World Congress on Pain. Amsterdam: Elsevier, 1991:264–276.
2. Devor M. The pathophysiology of damaged peripheral nerves. In: Wall PD, Melzack R (eds). Textbook of Pain, ed 3. Edinburgh: Churchill Livingstone, 1994:79–100.
3. Dubner R, Ruda MA. Activity-dependent neuronal plasticity following tissue injury and inflammation. Trends Neurosci 1992;15:96–103.
4. Woolf CJ, Thompson SWM. The induction and maintenance of central sensitization is dependent on N-methyl-D-aspartic acid receptor activation: Implications for the treatment of postinjury pain hypersensitivity states. Pain 1991;44:293–299.
5. Ren K, Hylden JLK, Williams GM, Ruda MA, Dubner R. The effects of a non-competitive NMDA receptor antagonist, MK-801, on behavioral hyperalgesia and dorsal horn neuronal activity in rats with unilateral inflammation. Pain 1992;50:331–334.
6. Neugebauer V, Lucke T, Schaible HG. Requirement of metabotropic glutamate receptors for the generation of inflammation-evoked hyperexcitability in rat spinal cord neurons. Eur J Neurosci 1994;6:1179–1186.
7. Boxall SJ, Berthele A, Laurie DJ, et al. Enhanced expression of metabotropic glutamate receptor 3 messenger RNA in the rat spinal cord during ultraviolet irradiation induced peripheral inflammation. Neuroscience 1998;82:591–602.
8. Guo W, Zou S, Guan Y, et al. Tyrosine phosphorylation of the NR2B subunit of the NMDA receptor in the spinal cord during the development and maintenance of inflammatory hyperalgesia. J Neurosci 2002;22:6208–6217.
9. Ren K, Iadarola MJ, Dubner R. An isobolographic analysis of the effects of N-methyl-D-aspartate and NK-1 tachykinin receptor antagonists on inflammatory hyperalgesia in the rat. Br J Pharmacol 1996;117:196–202.
10. Ren K, Dubner R. Central nervous system plasticity and persistent pain. J Orofac Pain 1999;13:155–163.
11. Donnerer J, Schuligoi R, Stein C. Increased content and transport of substance P and calcitonin gene-related peptide in sensory nerves innervating inflamed tissue: Evidence for a regulatory function of nerve growth factor in vivo. Neuroscience 1992;49:693–698.
12. Lewin GR, Rueff A, Mendell LM. Peripheral and central mechanisms of NGF-induced hyperalgesia. Eur J Neurosci 1994;6:1903–1994.
13. Leslie TA, Emson PC, Dowd PM, Woolf CJ. Nerve growth factor contributes to the up-regulation of growth-associated protein 43 and preprotachykinin A messenger RNAs in primary sensory neurons following peripheral inflammation. Neuroscience 1995;67:753–761.
14. Woolf CJ, Safieh-Garabedian B, Ma QP, Crilly P, Winter J. Nerve growth factor contributes to the generation of inflammatory sensory hypersensitivity. Neuroscience 1994;62:327–331.
15. Hu JW, Sessle BJ, Raboisson P, Dallel R, Woda A. Stimulation of craniofacial muscle afferents induces prolonged facilitatory effects in trigeminal nociceptive brainstem neurones. Pain 1992;48:53–60.
16. Raboisson P, Dallel R, Clavelou P, Sessle BJ, Woda A. Effects of subcutaneous formalin on the activity of trigeminal brain stem nociceptive neurones in the rat. J Neurophysiol 1995;73:496–505.
17. Strassman AM, Raymond SA, Burstein R. Sensitization of meningeal sensory neurons and the origin of headaches. Nature 1996;384:560–564.
18. Burstein R, Yamamura H, Malick A, Strassman AM. Chemical stimulation of the intracranial dura induces enhanced responses to facial stimulation in brain stem trigeminal neurons. J Neurophysiol 1998;79:964–982.
19. Hargreaves K, Dubner R, Brown F, Flores C, Joris J. A new and sensitive method for measuring thermal nociception in cutaneous hyperalgesia. Pain 1988;32:77–88.

20. Ren K. An improved method for assessing mechanical allodynia in the rat. Physiol Behav 1999;67;711–716.

21. Anseloni VCZ, Weng H–R, Terayama R, et al. Age-dependency of analgesia elicited by intraoral sucrose in acute and persistent pain models. Pain 2002;97:93–103.

22. Iwata K, Tashiro A, Tsuboi Y, et al. Medullary dorsal horn neuronal activity in rats with persistent temporomandibular joint and perioral inflammation. J Neurophysiol 1999;82:1244–1253.

23. Wall PD, Woolf CJ. Muscle but not cutaneous C-afferent input produces prolonged increases in the excitability of the flexion reflex in the rat. J Physiol 1984;356:443–458.

24. Yu X-M, Sessle BJ, Hu JW. Differential effects of cutaneous and deep application of inflammatory irritant on mechanoreceptive field properties of trigeminal brain stem nociceptive neurons. J Neurophysiol 1993;70:1704–1707.

25. Munglani R, Hunt SP. Molecular biology of pain. Br J Anaesth 1995;75:186–192.

26. Strassman AM, Vos BP. Somatotopic and laminar organization of Fos-like immunoreactivity in the medullary and upper cervical dorsal horn induced by noxious facial stimulation in the rat. J Comp Neurol 1993;331:495–516.

27. Zhou QQ, Imbe H, Dubner R, Ren K. Persistent Fos protein expression after orofacial deep or cutaneous inflammation in rats: Implications for persistent orofacial pain. J Comp Neurol 1999;412:276–291.

28. Iadarola MJ, Brady LS, Draisci G, Dubner R. Enhancement of dynorphin gene expression in spinal cord following experimental inflammation: Stimulus specificity, behavioral parameters and opioid receptor binding. Pain 1988;35:313–326.

29. Imbe H, Ren K. Orofacial deep and cutaneous tissue inflammation differentially upregulates preprodynorphin mRNA in the trigeminal and paratrigeminal nuclei of the rat. Mol Brain Res 1999;67:87–97.

30. Bereiter DA, Bereiter DF, Hathaway CB. The NMDA receptor antagonist MK-801 reduces Fos-like immunoreactivity in central trigeminal neurons and blocks select endocrine and autonomic responses to corneal stimulation in the rat. Pain 1996;64:179–189.

31. Mitsikostas DD, Sanchez del Rio M, Waeber C, Moskowitz MA, Cutrer FM. The NMDA receptor antagonist MK-801 reduces capsaicin-induced c-fos expression within rat trigeminal nucleus caudalis. Pain 1998;76:239–248.

32. Hathaway CB, Hu JW, Bereiter DA. Distribution of Fos-like immunoreactivity in the caudal brainstem of the rat following noxious chemical stimulation of the temporomandibular joint. J Comp Neurol 1995;356:444–456.

33. Ikeda T, Terayama R, Jue S-K, Sugiyo S, Dubner R, Ren K. Differential rostral projections of caudal brainstem neurons receiving trigeminal input after masseter inflammation. J Comp Neurol 2003;465:220–233.

34. Bereiter DA, Hathaway CB, Benetti AP. Caudal portions of the spinal trigeminal complex are necessary for autonomic responses and display Fos-like immunoreactivity after corneal stimulation in the cat. Brain Res 1994;657:73–82.

35. Casey KL. Forebrain mechanisms of nociception and pain: Analysis through imaging. Proc Natl Acad Sci U S A 1999; 96:7668–7674.

36. Wei F, Ren K, Dubner R. Inflammation-induced Fos protein expression in the rat spinal cord is enhanced following dorsolateral or ventrolateral lesions. Brain Res 1998;782: 136–141.

37. Wei F, Dubner R, Ren K. Nucleus reticularis gigantocellularis and nucleus raphe magnus in the brain stem exert opposite effects on behavioral hyperalgesia and spinal Fos expression after peripheral inflammation. Pain 1999;80:127–141.

38. Ren K, Dubner R. Enhanced descending modulation of nociception in rats with persistent hindpaw inflammation. J Neurophysiol 1996;76:3025–3037.

39. Tsuruoka M, Willis WD. Bilateral lesions in the area of the nucleus locus caeruleus affect the development of hyperalgesia during carrageenan-induced inflammation. Brain Res 1996;726:233–236.

40. Urban MO, Gebhart GF. Supraspinal contributions to hyperalgesia. Proc Natl Acad Sci U S A 1999;96:7687–7692.

41. Sugiyo S, Dubner R, Ren K. Trigeminal transition zone-RVM reciprocal connection and orofacial hyperalgesia. Presented at the 82nd IADR/AADR/CADR Meeting, Honolulu, 10–13 Mar 2004.

42. Gebhart GF. Descending modulation of pain. Neurosci Biobehav Rev 2004;729–737.

43. Maixner W, Fijllingim R, Sigurdsson A, Kincaid S, Silva S. Sensitivity of patients with painful temporomandibular disorders to experimentally evoked pain: Evidence for altered temporal summation of pain. Pain 1998;76:71–81.

44. Tverskoy M, Cozacov C, Ayache M, Bradley EL, Kissin I. Postoperative pain after inguinal herniorrhaphy with different types of anesthesia. Anesth Analg 1990;70:29–35.

45. Ejlersen E, Andersen HB, Eliasen K, Mogensen T. A comparison between preincisional and postincisional lidocaine infiltration and postoperative pain. Anesth Analg 1992;74: 495–498.

46. Gordon SM, Brahim JS, Dubner R, McCullagh LM, Sang CN, Dionne RA. Attenuation of pain in a randomized trial by suppression of peripheral nociceptive activity in the immediate postoperative period. Anesth Analg 2002;95:1351–1357.

47. Gracely RH, Lynch SA, Bennett GJ. Painful neuropathy: Altered central processing maintained dynamically by peripheral input. Pain 1992;51:175–194.

48. Ren K, Dubner R. NMDA receptor antagonists attenuate mechanical hyperalgesia in rats with unilateral inflammation of the hindpaw. Neurosci Lett 1993;163:22–26.

49. Ma QP, Woolf CJ. Progressive tactile hypersensitivity: An inflammation-induced incremental increase in the excitability of the spinal cord. Pain 1996;67:97–106.

Muscular Pain and Dysfunction

James P. Lund

Anyone who has experienced persistent or chronic pain knows that it affects movements. When the jaw, neck, or back muscles are sore, we say that they are "stiff" because it takes an effort to get them to contract, and our range of motion is limited. Pain in the legs can cause us to limp and can make running impossible, while pain in the arms can make it impossible to lift even moderately heavy weights. In this chapter, the effects of nociceptor inputs on our motor systems and the impact of this information on the proposed etiologies of chronic musculoskeletal pain states are discussed. (For further discussion of muscular pain mechanisms, see chapter 33.)

Nociceptive Reflexes

Sudden stimulation of nociceptors triggers short-latency reflex responses in the affected body part that tend to remove it from the source of pain. When nociceptors in the hand or foot are activated, this triggers a flexion-withdrawal reflex in which the flexor muscles of the limb are activated while their antagonists, the extensor muscles, are inhibited concurrently. If the reflex occurs in a leg, the extensors of the other leg are activated (crossed-extension reflex), which helps to maintain balance. Thus, even simple spinal reflexes like these are coordinated in a purposeful way.

The trigeminal nerve (cranial nerve V) equivalent of the flexion-withdrawal reflex is the jaw-opening (JO) reflex. It can be triggered by the stimulation of intraoral and facial nociceptors and by non-noxious inputs from

mechanoreceptors. For instance, sharp taps on the teeth, which stimulate rapidly adapting periodontal pressoreceptors, can trigger the reflex. The jaw-closing muscles are the extensors of the mandible, and they are strongly inhibited by inputs that cause the JO reflex in all animals tested as well as in humans. In animals, the flexor muscles (the digastrics and mylohyoids) are excited at disynaptic latency. We do not know why these muscles are not excited during the JO reflex in humans, even when the stimulus is highly noxious.[1]

The response of human masseter and temporal muscles evoked by mechanical stimuli or electrical shocks is shown by electromyography (EMG) to consist of early and late periods of suppression, often called *silent period 1 (SP1)* and *silent period 2 (SP2)*, respectively. Miles et al[2] concluded that the two responses in humans were produced by early and late inhibitory postsynaptic potentials in the trigeminal motoneurons at latencies of about 10 and 40 milliseconds, respectively. Cruccu and Romaniello[1] used a CO_2 laser to selectively stimulate heat nociceptors and showed that only SP2 was present in healthy humans, at a latency of about 70 milliseconds. They concluded that SP1 is a response to low-threshold afferents, while SP2 is the reaction to the stimulation of nociceptors.

The reflexes evoked by the stimulation of nociceptors do not increase in amplitude if the stimulus is rapidly repeated. Instead, the response quickly fades away (habituates), even when the interval between stimuli is relatively long. Furthermore, the JO reflex in humans is also easily suppressed by prior activation of other sensory inputs, a phenomenon described as *conditioning*.[1]

Protection During Biting and Chewing

Acute stimulation of orofacial nociceptors usually occurs when either the head or mandible is in movement. If an animal runs into an object, the resulting stimulation of mechanoreceptors and nociceptors can have several reflex effects. It can stop locomotion or change the pattern to avoid the obstruction, and it can trigger the flexion reflex of the neck muscles.

Many pieces of evidence gained from animal and human experiments show that reflex responses change markedly during movement. If the movements are rhythmic, such as those in mastication or locomotion, the reflex responses almost always vary with the phase of movement.[3] For instance, if nociceptors are stimulated during walking, the flexion reflex only occurs during the swing phase, when the foot is off the ground. When the foot is carrying the weight of the body (stance phase), flexion does not occur, and instead the extensor muscle activity is reflexly facilitated to thrust the limb away while also maintaining balance. Although other mechanisms are involved, the main reason that reflex responses vary in phase with the cycle of rhythmic movements is that the reflex circuits are under the control of the systems that generate the movements.

The fundamental pattern of mastication, ie, the alternating opening and closing of the mandible with accompanying protrusion and retrusion of the tongue and contraction-relaxation of facial muscles, is produced by two collections of neurons, one on each side of the hindbrain, that are reciprocally connected.[4] Neural circuits like these are called *central pattern generators (CPGs)*.

During mastication, oral nociceptors are almost always stimulated during the jaw-closing phase of the movement by various events: biting something hard or sharp, biting the tongue, or applying pressure to a sore tooth. Therefore, the JO reflex is most important when there is a need to protect against tissue damage during the phase in which the jaw-closing motoneurons are most active and thus very difficult to inhibit. In animals, but not humans, the suprahyoid motoneurons are activated to counteract the closing forces, but during this phase these motoneurons are relatively inexcitable.

However, when a trigeminal sensory nerve is stimulated during the jaw-closing phase at an intensity high enough to activate nociceptors, the jaw-closing muscle bursts are strongly inhibited, and in animals there is a large digastric response. The net result is prevention of full closure and a shortening of the jaw closing phase.[3] To enable this to happen, the CPG appears to facilitate nociceptor interneurons in the JO reflex circuits during the jaw-closing phase. Some of these interneurons inhibit the jaw-closing motoneurons; in animals, but not humans, a second group facilitates JO motoneurons. This increase in the efficacy of the JO reflex during mastication is an excellent example of the general rule that CPGs modify reflex responses to increase protection and improve the performance of movement.

Relationship Between Persistent Pain and Movement

Although the simple reflex responses to repetitive stimulation of nociceptors rapidly habituate, people who live with chronic musculoskeletal pain often have difficulty moving easily, and their patterns of movement are often abnormal, from both their point of view and that of an observer.

Vicious Cycle Theory

For the whole of the 20th century and into the 21st, it has been generally accepted by the health professions, the public, and the pharmaceutical industry that abnormal patterns of muscle contraction are, in large part, responsible for maintaining pain.[5–7] It was suggested that muscle pain became chronic because stimulation of nociceptors by an initial injury led to tonic excitation of motoneurons (hyperactivity). Researchers believed that muscular hyperactivity led to spasm, fatigue, and overwork and that this process led to further stimulation of nociceptors, resulting in a pain-spasm-pain cycle that came to be called the *vicious cycle*.[8] This vicious cycle theory was used to explain the etiology of temporomandibular disorders[9,10] (TMDs) and of a number of similar conditions elsewhere in the body.

The model was attractive because it supported beliefs that almost anything that caused pain in a jaw muscle or the temporomandibular joint (TMJ), or that altered such muscle activity, could initiate or maintain a TMD. It was compatible with the idea that such conditions had a multifactorial etiology, and it provided a theoretical framework for treatments that were aimed at changing muscle activity. Such treatments included direct approaches, such as biofeedback or physical therapy, as well as mechanical therapies that were presumed to improve muscle function by correcting "abnormal" dentofacial anatomy with occlusal appliances, repositioning appliances, occlusal adjustments, prosthetic reconstruction, orthodontics, TMJ surgery, and orthognathic surgery.

In the late 1980s, the clinical and experimental evidence in favor of the vicious cycle model was analyzed. This model predicts that EMG activity in painful muscles at rest and during contraction should be higher than normal. The analysis included studies in which EMG activity in groups of patients with a variety of chronic musculoskeletal pain conditions was compared with EMG activity in appropriate control groups at rest and during movements. In general, no significant difference in resting EMG activity was found between the groups; furthermore, when the muscles were contracting and shortening (also called *concentric contraction*), EMG activity or force output was actually lower in the patient groups.[11–13] For instance, Molin[14] showed that maximum biting force was about 40% lower in a group of female patients with myofascial pain than in a group of age-matched control subjects.

Although disuse of muscles undoubtedly occurs in the presence of chronic pain, the results of several studies have suggested that pain, whatever its origin, inhibits motoneuronal output to contracting muscles. For instance, maximum biting force is reduced during the pain that follows third molar extraction,[15] while blocking pain restores a subject's ability to contract muscles forcefully.

One of the principal signs of a TMD is an inability to open the mouth widely,[17] and a reduction in range of motion is a characteristic of several other chronic musculoskeletal pain conditions. Although reduced activity in agonist muscles (eg, the digastric and mylohyoid muscles during jaw opening) probably contributes to this limitation of movement, several studies have shown that EMG activity in the antagonist muscles (eg, the masseters) of the patient groups appears to be higher than normal during their attempts to function.[11–13,18]

Pain-Adaptation Model

Based on the previous findings, it was concluded that the vicious cycle model was not consistent with the available data. Another model, called the *pain-adaptation model*, was proposed to explain the relationship between persistent pain and the associated motor signs and symptoms that were described in the previous section.[11] The new model was based on three testable hypotheses: *(1)* that persistent pain has general effects on the body that include changes in facial expression and body posture; *(2)* that persistent activation of nociceptors in a body part inhibits local motoneurons of muscles that are acting as agonists and facilitates antagonist motoneurons through segmental reflexes and by modifying the output of CPGs; and *(3)* that nociceptors in skin, teeth, connective tissue, muscle, and joints have similar effects on the motor system.

The reduction in range of motion and the inability to lift heavy loads, bite hard, or move quickly in the presence of pain are usually characterized as dysfunctions. From a bioengineering standpoint, this is reasonable because people are mechanically less efficient when in pain. However, these pain-related changes should be viewed as adaptive because they help to prevent further damage and promote healing. It is also suggested that pain-induced changes in facial expression and body posture are adaptive because they tend to elicit sympathy and help for the sufferer.

Effects of Persistent Experimental Pain on Motor and Sensory Systems

Several experiments have been carried out with normal subjects to see if experimental pain can induce the signs and symptoms that characterize chronic pain conditions.

Muscle tonus

As noted in a previous section, the jaw muscles of TMD patients are not hyperactive at rest. Stohler et al[19] carried out a crossover study of normal human subjects to directly test the hypothesis that tonic muscle pain does not increase resting EMG activity. They recorded resting EMG activity with surface electrodes over the masseter and temporal muscles on both sides, first under baseline conditions, then after a continuous infusion of 5% saline into one masseter muscle that caused a moderate level of pain, and finally while the subjects imagined pain of similar intensity (sham pain). They found that mean resting activity was increased in all muscles relative to baseline during both pain and sham pain, but there were no significant differences between the pain and sham pain states. Activity in the muscles of facial expression changed in both pain and sham pain, and this appeared to be responsible for the increase in EMG activity during these two states. The authors concluded that muscular pain does not cause an increase in tonus in the damaged muscle or in its synergists. This was confirmed by Svensson et al,[20] who injected hypertonic saline into the masseter and anterior tibial muscles and found no evidence of increases in resting activity.

Stretch reflex

A number of studies have been carried out in the last few years to assess the effects of experimental pain on the stretch reflex in humans and animals. The motivation for many of these studies was the suggestion that nociceptors could cause resting muscle hyperactivity in patients with chronic pain through the excitation of fusimotor neurons, which reduces the clinical relevance of the studies (see previous section). Nevertheless, the results of some animal studies suggested that injections of pain-producing substances can activate the fusimotor system,[21] although other animal studies showed inhibition[22] or mixed effects.[23]

The equivocal nature of the animal evidence is also reflected in the results of the human studies. Several studies carried out by the Aalborg University group and their collaborators have shown increases in stretch reflex amplitude in masseter and temporal muscles after injections of algesic substances,[24] suggesting that nociceptor input increases fusimotor drive. However, the same group showed that responsiveness of single motor units in the masseter fell after hypertonic saline injections and had to conclude that fusimotor drive also had decreased.[25]

Mastication, locomotion, and other types of movement

Recently, it has been shown that the major motor signs and symptoms that accompany chronic pain states can be induced experimentally by painful infusions of hypertonic saline into the muscles of normal volunteers. As Stohler[18] has shown, the results of the great majority of studies are highly consistent with the predictions of the pain-adaptation model. For instance, Arendt-Nielsen et al[26] found that normal subjects adopted the gait and EMG pattern of patients with chronic lower back pain when 5% saline was injected into the dorsal paraspinal muscles, because the activity of these muscles increased when they were acting as antagonists. Experimentally induced masticatory muscle pain also brings on signs and symptoms of a TMD.[18] Svensson et al[27] showed that injections of hypertonic saline into both masseter muscles reduce the activity of the muscles during the jaw-closing phase (suppression of agonists) and increase it during the jaw-opening phase (activation of antagonists) of mastication.

Obrez and Stohler[28] found that the amplitude of mandibular border movements recorded on a Gothic arch plate (protrusion and left and right lateral excursions) was significantly reduced during saline-induced masseter pain. They also found that the apex of the Gothic arch moved forward and laterally during pain, which would be interpreted clinically as a shift in centric relation. Obrez and Stohler concluded that the occlusal changes that some TMD patients report could be a consequence of pain rather than its cause, which is one more piece of evidence that occlusal discrepancies are not an important etiologic factor in TMDs.

Consistent with the fact that maximum occlusal force is significantly reduced in some patients with a TMD,[14] Svensson et al[20] showed that injections of hypertonic saline into the masseter muscle caused a significant decrease in maximum occlusal force in normal human subjects. Similarly, Graven-Nielsen et al[29] showed that intramuscular injections of hypertonic saline into leg muscles reduced maximal voluntary contraction during knee extension. However, they also showed that the mechanical properties of the muscle fibers were not significantly changed.

During voluntary contractions much of the input to the motoneurons originates in the motor cortex, and Svensson et al[30] showed that tonic muscle pain suppresses responses in muscles of the hand to magnetic stimulation of the cortex. Although it is possible that some of this suppression is occurring within the cortex, the response to direct stimulation of corticobulbar fibers was also reduced, suggesting that most of the nociceptor-induced depression of the pathway is taking place at the segmental level. Although there are monosynaptic connections between motor cortex neurons and motoneurons supplying the hand and jaw muscles, most of the connections are made through segmental interneurons, and it is probable that these are subject to the same modulation by nociceptor inputs as other interneuron groups.

Conclusion

The rationale underlying most commonly used therapies for myogenous TMDs and similar conditions elsewhere in the body is that they reduce tonic muscle hyperactivity that has been perpetuated by a vicious cycle of pain-spasm-pain. In addition, some of these therapies are presumed to modify abnormal patterns of movement or posture that are causing fatigue, spasm, and trauma to muscles and joints. It is now clear that muscular hyperactivity is not the basis for these disorders and that the other signs of motor dysfunction are a consequence of nociceptor activity or perhaps a response to pain of central origin.

This lack of fundamental validity of the traditional conceptions of chronic muscular pain helps to explain why it is difficult to show that most nonpharmacologic therapies are more effective than placebo for treating these disorders (see chapter 24 and 25). It also helps to clarify why there are large populations of patients with chronic muscular pain who have failed to respond to multiple therapies. Hopefully, new therapeutic avenues will be forthcoming from innovative studies and discoveries in the laboratory and in the clinic; in the meantime, conservative and reversible therapies should be used to manage these complex disorders.

References

1. Cruccu G, Romaniello A. Jaw-opening reflex after CO_2 laser stimulation of the perioral region in man. Exp Brain Res 1998;118:564–568.

2. Miles TS, Türker KS, Nordstrom MA. Reflex responses of motor units in human masseter muscle to electrical stimulation of the lip. Exp Brain Res 1987;65:331–336.

3. Rossignol S, Lund JP, Drew T. The role of sensory inputs in regulating patterns of rhythmical movements in higher vertebrates. A comparison between locomotion, respiration, and mastication. In: Cohen AH, Rossignol S, Grillner S (eds). Neural Control of Rhythmic Movements in Vertebrates. New York: John Wiley and Sons, 1988:201–283.

4. Lund JP, Kolta A, Westberg K-G, Scott G. Brainstem mechanisms underlying feeding behaviors. Curr Opin Neurobiol 1998;8:718–724.

5. Hough T. Ergographic studies in muscle soreness. Am J Physiol 1902;7:76–92.

6. De Vries HA. Quantitative electromyographic investigation of the spasm theory of muscle pain. Am J Phys Med 1966;45:119–134.

7. Kamyszek G, Ketcham R, Garcia R Jr, Radke J. Electromyographic evidence of reduced muscle activity when ULF-TENS is applied to the Vth and VIIth cranial nerves. Cranio 2001;19:162–168.

8. Travell J, Rinzler S, Herman M. Pain and disability of the shoulder and arm. Treatment by intramuscular infiltration with procaine hydrochloride. JAMA 1942;120:417–422.

9. Schwartz LL. A temporomandibular joint pain-dysfunction syndrome. J Chronic Dis 1956;3:284.

10. Okeson JP. Fundamentals of Occlusion and Temporomandibular Disorders. St Louis: Mosby, 1985.

11. Lund JP, Donga R, Widmer CG, Stohler CS. The pain-adaptation model: A discussion of the relationship between chronic musculoskeletal pain and motor activity. Can J Physiol Pharmacol 1991;69:683–694.

12. Lund JP, Stohler CS, Widmer CG. The relationship between pain and muscle activity in fibromyalgia and similar conditions. In: Vaeroy H, Merskey H (eds). Progress in Fibromyalgia and Myofascial Pain. Amsterdam: Elsevier, 1993:311–327.

13. Lund JP. Pain and movement. In: Lund JP, Lavigne GJ, Dubner R, Sessle BJ (eds). Orofacial Pain: From Basic Science to Clinical Management. Chicago: Quintessence, 2001:151–163.

14. Molin C. Vertical isometric muscle forces of the mandible. A comparative study of subjects with and without manifest mandibular pain dysfunction syndrome. Acta Odontol Scand 1972;30:485–499.

15. High AS, Macgregor AJ, Tomlinson GE, Salkouskis PM. A gnathodynamometer as an objective means of pain assessment following wisdom tooth removal. Br J Oral Maxillofac Surg 1988;26:284–291.

16. Arvidsson I, Eriksson E, Knutsson E, Arner S. Reduction of pain inhibition on voluntary muscle activation by epidural analgesia. Orthopedics 1986;9:1415–1419.

17. Dworkin SF, LeResche L. Research diagnostic criteria for temporomandibular disorders: Review, criteria, examinations and specifications, critique. J Craniomandib Disord 1992;6:301–355.

18. Stohler CS. Craniofacial pain and motor function: Pathogenesis, clinical correlates, and implications. Crit Rev Oral Biol Med 1999;10:504–508.

19. Stohler CS, Zhang X, Lund JP. The effect of experimental jaw muscle pain on postural muscle activity. Pain 1996;66: 215–221.

20. Svensson P, Graven-Nielsen T, Matre D, Arendt-Nielsen L. Experimental muscle pain does not cause long-lasting increases in resting electromyographic activity. Muscle Nerve 1998;21:1382–1389.

21. Matre DA, Sinkjaer T, Knardahl S, Andersen JB, Arendt-Nielsen L. The influence of experimental muscle pain on the human soleus stretch reflex during sitting and walking. Clin Neurophysiol 1999;110:2033–2043.

22. Mense S, Skeppar P. Discharge behaviour of feline gamma-motoneurones following induction of an artificial myositis. Pain 1991;46:201–210.

23. Ro JY, Capra NF. Modulation of jaw muscle spindle afferent activity following intramuscular injections with hypertonic saline. Pain 2001;92:117–127.

24. Wang K, Svensson P, Arendt-Nielsen L. Effect of tonic muscle pain on short-latency jaw-stretch reflexes in humans. Pain 2000;88:189–197.

25. Svensson P, Miles TS, Graven-Nielsen T, Arendt-Nielsen L. Modulation of stretch-evoked reflexes in single motor units in human masseter muscle by experimental pain. Exp Brain Res 2000;132:65–71.

26. Arendt-Nielsen L, Graven-Nielsen T, Svarrer H, Svensson P. The influence of low back pain on muscle activity and coordination during gait: A clinical and experimental study. Pain 1995;64:231–240.

27. Svensson P, Houe L, Arendt-Nielsen L. Bilateral experimental muscle pain changes electromyographic activity of human jaw-closing muscles during mastication. Exp Brain Res 1997;116:182–185.

28. Obrez A, Stohler CS. Jaw muscle pain and its effect on gothic arch tracings. J Prosthet Dent 1996;74:393–398.

29. Graven-Nielsen T, Lund H, Arendt-Nielsen L, Danneskiold-Samsoe B, Bliddal H. Inhibition of maximal voluntary contraction force by experimental muscle pain: A centrally mediated mechanism. Muscle Nerve 2002;26:708–712.

30. Svensson P, Miles TS, McKay D, Ridding MC. Suppression of motor evoked potentials in a hand muscle following prolonged painful stimulation. Eur J Pain 2003;7:55–62.

TMJ Osteoarthritis

Stephen B. Milam

The temporomandibular joint (TMJ) is a load-bearing synovial joint that, like other load-bearing joints, is subject to breakdown by damaging molecular events triggered by overloading or systemic disease. TMJ overloading, consisting of either repetitive or extreme mechanical loads, results in a pathologic state if the intrinsic healing or adaptive capacity of the joint is exceeded. Systemic factors (eg, immune dysfunction) may also contribute to TMJ osteoarthritis or a variety of other distinct forms of arthritis of the TMJ (eg, rheumatoid arthritis) that share common pathogenic mechanisms (eg, molecular events mediated by interleukin 1β [IL-1β] or tumor necrosis factor α [TNF-α]). The impact of these systemic factors is presumably either the amplification of molecular events generated by mechanical loading or the enhancement of susceptibility to injury. The factors contributing to individual variations in adaptive capacity of the TMJ have not been examined thoroughly to date. However, it is likely that variables such as genetic background, age, sex, and diet determine an individual's susceptibility to degenerative TMJ disease.

Osteoarthritis Versus Osteoarthrosis

The term *osteoarthritis* refers to an inflammatory condition affecting an articulation that results in erosion and fibrillation of articular cartilage and degeneration of adjacent subchondral bone. Over recent years, the term *osteoarthrosis* has evolved to distinguish a noninflammatory condition producing similar degenerative changes. However, there is little scientific evidence to support the notion that distinct pathophysiologic processes are involved in these conditions. Rather, it is likely that the condition referred to as *osteoarthrosis* represents a subacute or chronic process that

has an inflammatory component. This is suggested by studies that have identified inflammatory biochemicals in fluid and tissue samples obtained from symptomatic, but not clinically inflamed, TMJs.[1–6] For this reason, *osteoarthritis* will be used in this chapter to refer to a degenerative disease of joints, believed to be initiated by excessive or protracted mechanical loads, that involves inflammatory biochemicals in the pathophysiologic process.

Despite distinctions in the pathophysiologic mechanisms of other inflammatory joint diseases, some biochemicals believed to be involved in the genesis of osteoarthritis are also involved in the genesis of other joint diseases (eg, rheumatoid arthritis). Given the similarities in some of the mechanisms involved in these diseases, it is not surprising to find common approaches to therapy (eg, nonsteroidal anti-inflammatory drugs [NSAIDs]). However, given the dissimilarities in these diseases, therapies that are effective for one condition may be relatively ineffective for other conditions.

Osteoarthritis Versus Aging

Clinical signs of TMJ osteoarthritis are more common in older populations.[7,8] For example, the prevalence of TMJ crepitation increases with age (Fig 7-1). This is true for both males and females.[9] However, Haskin and colleagues[10] noted that contemporary studies of the TMJ have not adequately distinguished age-related changes in joint structure and function from pathologic changes associated with degenerative arthritides, including osteoarthritis. With the anticipation that new diagnostic techniques will someday permit clinical researchers to probe the human TMJ at the molecular level, it will be important to distinguish pathologic states from normal aging processes.

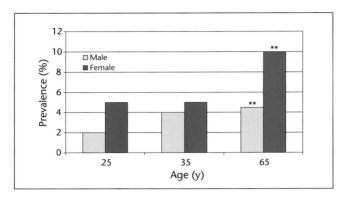

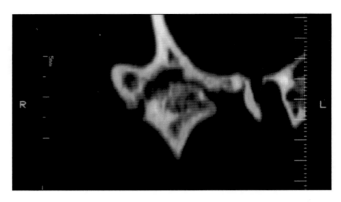

Fig 7-1 Prevalence of TMJ crepitation. The prevalence increases with age. **Statistically significant difference (*P* < .05) at age 65 years versus age 25 years. (Data from Agerberg and Bergenholtz.[3])

Fig 7-2 Computed tomogram (coronal view) of an osteoarthritic TMJ. Note the irregular contours of the articular surfaces of the mandibular condyle and glenoid fossa. This patient exhibited a restricted mandibular range of motion, marked crepitation, and pain isolated to the preauricular region.

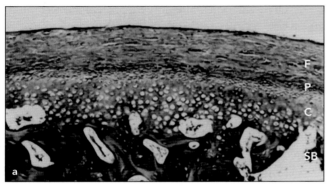

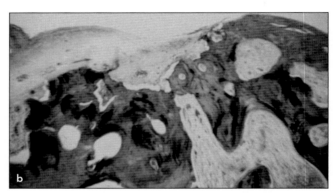

Fig 7-3 *(a)* Normal mandibular condyle. The normal mandibular condyle is covered by a fibrocartilage with distinct cellular layers: (F) fibrous layer; (P) prechondroblastic layer; (C) cartilaginous layer; (SB) subchondral bone. *(b)* Osteoarthritic mandibular condyle. Fibrocartilage is lost in the osteoarthritic mandibular condyle, and the contour of the subchondral bone is irregular.

Characteristics of TMJ Osteoarthritis

TMJ osteoarthritis is typically a slowly progressive, asymmetric disease resulting in the destruction of articular tissues. Some degenerative conditions, such as idiopathic condylar resorption, progress very rapidly in relatively young individuals and may represent either a distinct pathologic entity or osteoarthritis in a highly susceptible individual.

Clinically, individuals suffering from TMJ osteoarthritis experience pain of variable intensity, restricted jaw movement, and joint sounds (eg, crepitation). Contemporary serologic studies, including erythrocyte sedimentation rate or C-reactive protein level, rheumatoid factor, uric acid, and antinuclear antibody panels, are usually within normal range. Common radiographic changes associated with TMJ osteoarthritis include flattening or irregularities of the surface of the mandibular condyle and glenoid fossa (Fig 7-2). Other radiologic findings have been described, including reduction of joint space, condylar lipping (ie, osteophytes), and subchondral bone sclerosis.[11–13]

The molecular events involved in the pathogenesis of TMJ osteoarthritis have only been partially characterized.[14,15] However, it is apparent that, in susceptible individuals, excessive or protracted mechanical loads are capable of triggering a cascade of molecular events that lead to the degradation of the fibrocartilage and bone in the TMJ. Histologic and biochemical studies have provided evidence of a breakdown or loss of fibrocartilage covering the articular surfaces of the mandibular condyle and temporal bone[1,10,11,16] (Fig 7-3).

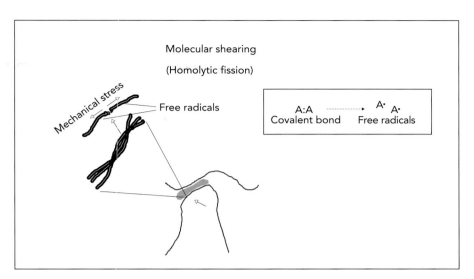

Fig 7-4 Free radical production by molecular shearing. Under extreme mechanical loading conditions, molecules in a tissue can be torn apart (covalent bonds holding the molecule together can be broken). If covalent bonds break symmetrically (one electron composing the covalent bond goes with one piece of the molecule and the other electron goes with the other piece of the molecule [insert]), then two free radicals (A• [insert]) are formed. Each piece of the fragmented molecule contains an unpaired electron derived from the broken covalent bond. This process is known as *homolytic fission*.

Among the earliest molecular events involved in the pathogenesis of osteoarthritis are the disruption of the collagenous components of the fibrocartilage and the subsequent loss of proteoglycans and glycosaminoglycans.[1,14,16–18] The loss of these molecules eventually leads to articular tissues that lack resiliency to the compressive and shearing loads generated during jaw movement. As a result, the affected joint becomes increasingly susceptible to structural damage with repetitive mechanical loading. In addition, molecules or fragments of molecules liberated from these damaged articular tissues may contribute to the progression of disease by evoking inflammatory responses from resident cell populations.

Mechanical Loads and Biologic Signals

There are at least two mechanisms through which mechanical loads can trigger molecular events that may culminate in degenerative joint disease in susceptible individuals. First, mechanical loads can result in the production of highly reactive molecules, termed *free radicals*.[15] Free radicals can damage important molecules of the articular tissues and synovial fluid as well as trigger cellular responses (eg, gene transcription) that can lead to degenerative joint disease. Second, mechanical loads can stimulate sensory neurons supplying the nerve-rich regions of the TMJ (eg, retrodiscal tissues and capsular ligament) resulting in release of neu-

ropeptides and perhaps other molecules, such as nitric oxide, that may also contribute to disease by initiation of neurogenic inflammation.[2,3,14,19,20]

Free Radicals and TMJ Osteoarthritis

Free radicals are molecular species, capable of independent existence, that contain one or more unpaired electrons (an electron that occupies an atomic orbit by itself). Free radicals may be produced in the TMJ by molecular shearing resulting from excessive mechanical loads[15] (Fig 7-4). Under extreme conditions, the covalent bonds holding the molecule together can be broken, and the molecules in a tissue can be torn apart. When covalent bonds break symmetrically—one electron composing the covalent bond goes with one piece of the molecule and the other electron goes with the other piece of the molecule—two free radicals are formed. Each piece of the fragmented molecule contains an unpaired electron derived from the broken covalent bond. This process is known as *homolytic fission*.

Free radicals can also be produced in hypoxic tissues on restoration of oxygenation by a mechanism referred to as *hypoxia-reperfusion injury* (Fig 7-5). In the TMJ, focal regions may become hypoxic if intra-articular pressures exceed the end-capillary perfusion pressures of the blood vessels supplying affected articular tissues.[15] This condition could arise during sustained or forceful elevation of the mandible (eg, clenching). Under these hypoxic conditions, resident cell populations may rapidly undergo

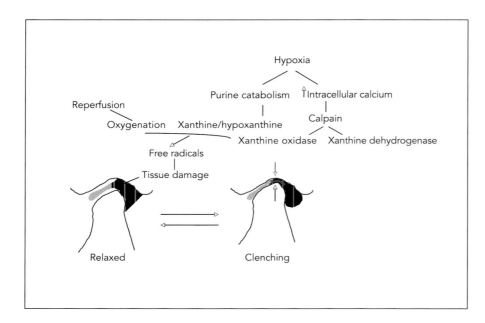

Fig 7-5 Hypoxia-reperfusion injury. Articular tissues may become hypoxic if intra-articular pressures exceed the end-capillary perfusion pressures of blood vessels supplying regions of the TMJ. This condition could arise during sustained or forceful elevation of the mandible (eg, clenching). Under these hypoxic conditions, resident cell populations may rapidly undergo metabolic changes that involve (1) elevations of intracellular calcium with activation of calpain, an enzyme that drives the conversion of xanthine dehydrogenase to xanthine oxidase, and (2) increased purine catabolism, resulting in the production of xanthine and hypoxanthine. Injury may result when perfusion of the previously hypoxic tissue is reestablished (eg, during jaw-opening movement that results in a reduction in intra-articular pressure). Under this condition, oxygen-derived free radicals that may damage affected tissues are generated. It is believed that this mechanism may contribute to progressive loss of the structural integrity of articular tissues subjected to excessive cyclic loads.

metabolic changes. Injury may result when perfusion of the previously hypoxic tissue is reestablished—for example, when jaw-opening movement results in a reduction in intra-articular pressure. Under this condition, oxygen-derived free radicals that may damage affected tissues are generated.

Finally, resident cell populations may generate free radicals as a direct or indirect result of their stimulation. For example, some synoviocytes (macrophage-type) may generate free radicals on stimulation by cytokines, tissue debris, microbes, or foreign material such as wear debris from a TMJ implant.

Free radicals are generally unstable and highly reactive. They initiate molecular reactions (ie, oxidation reduction) that can activate or inactivate molecules. The vulnerability of specific molecules to modification by free radicals is dependent on their structure. Some molecules, such as fibronectin and hyaluronic acid, appear to be extremely vulnerable, while others, including type I collagen, albumin, and matrix metalloproteinases, appear to be relative resistant.[4] Under some conditions, free radicals can destroy vulnerable molecules in TMJ tissues or synovial fluid.

It has been proposed that articular disc displacements result from a failure of the lubrication system that is initiated by free radicals.[21,22] Hyaluronic acid, a key element of this system, is susceptible to degradation by free radicals.[23] Therefore, it has been speculated that the degradation of hyaluronic acid by free radicals generated in susceptible TMJs unmasks enzymes (ie, phospholipases) that are normally inhibited by hyaluronic acid.[21,22] These active phospholipases, which apparently are relatively resistant to degradation by free radicals, in turn degrade surface phospholipids that cover the articular surfaces of the joint and function as critical elements of the lubrication system of the joint. As the lubrication system fails because of degradation of these critical phospholipids, friction between the articular surfaces of the joint increases. This increasing friction contributes to articular disc displacement, as the disc is "pushed" from its normal position.[21,22] In this model, free radicals contribute to articular disc displacement by initiation of events that culminate in a disruption of the lubrication system of the joint. The model is also consistent with the view that a disease state precedes articular disc displacement (see chapter 8).

Fig 7-6 Regulation of gene transcription by free radicals. Free radicals can evoke a transient rise in intracellular calcium, leading to the activation of specific kinases capable of phosphorylating inhibitory κβ (IκΒ). In an unphosphorylated state, IκΒ binds to the nuclear factor κβ (NFκΒ) transcription factor complex in the cytoplasm of the cell, preventing its translocation to the cell nucleus. Phosphorylated IκΒ dissociates from the NFκΒ complex, allowing this complex to move to the nucleus, where it associates with specific DNA sequences located upstream of specific genes. On binding to these DNA sequences, the NFκΒ complex facilitates transcription of targeted genes production of mRNAs used as templates for protein synthesis. Among the proteins synthesized by this action are specific cytokines (eg, interleukin 1β [IL-1β], tumor necrosis factor α [TNF-α], interleukin 6 [IL-6]) that have been implicated in the pathogenesis of some TMJ arthritides, including osteoarthritis. By this mechanism, free radicals may initiate molecular cascades triggered by the actions of these potent cytokines.

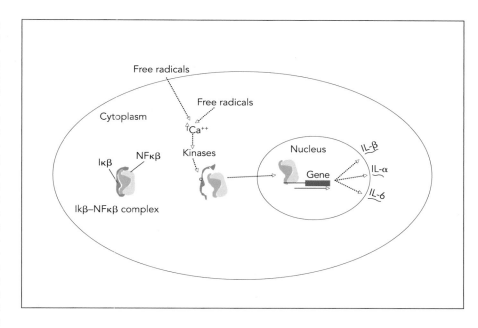

In some instances, free radicals can also initiate reactions that lead to molecular crosslinking.[24] This may occur when two free radicals react with one another, resulting in the sharing of their unpaired electrons and the subsequent formation of a covalent bond linking the two molecular species together. This process has been implicated in the genesis of TMJ adhesions that can contribute to joint disease by restriction of movement.[24]

Free radicals also can affect the production of other molecules involved in the pathogenesis of TMJ osteoarthritis by activation of gene transcription.[15] For example, free radicals can initiate gene transcription in some cells by activation and translocation of a transcription factor complex known as *nuclear factor κβ (NFκΒ)* (Fig 7-6). It appears that free radicals can evoke a transient rise in intracellular calcium in some cells, leading to the activation of specific kinases, which are enzymes capable of phosphorylating targeted proteins.[25,26,27] Some of the affected kinases phosphorylate a protein termed *inhibitory κβ (IκΒ)* In an unphosphorylated state, IκΒ binds to the NFκΒ complex in the cytoplasm of the cell, preventing the translocation of this complex to the nucleus. Phosphorylated IκΒ dissociates from the NFκΒ complex, allowing this complex to move to the nucleus, where it associates with specific DNA sequences located upstream of specific genes. On binding to the DNA sequences, the NFκΒ complex facilitates transcription of these genes. Among the genes affected by this action are specific cytokines (eg, TNF-α and IL-1β) that have been implicated in the pathogenesis of some TMJ arthritides, including osteoarthritis.

Neuropeptides and TMJ Osteoarthritis

Neuropeptides are released from peripheral terminals of stimulated sensory nerves supplying the TMJ[2,3,19,28] (Fig 7-7). Some neuropeptides released in this fashion, such as substance P (SP) and calcitonin gene–related peptide (CGRP), are proinflammatory and can initiate molecular cascades implicated in the pathogenesis of osteoarthritis.[10,14] In the TMJ, sensory nerve endings containing these proinflammatory neuropeptides are derived from the trigeminal (V) ganglion and dorsal root ganglion (C2–C5) neurons. Terminals from these neurons are found predominantly in retrodiscal tissues as well as in the capsular ligament supporting the

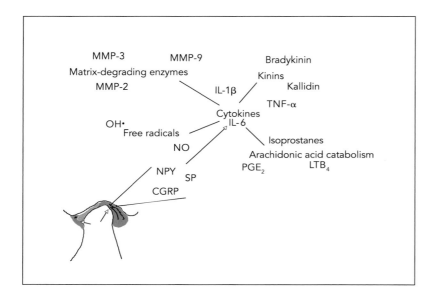

Fig 7-7 Neurogenic inflammation. Sensory nerve terminals from neurons located in the trigeminal ganglia and C2–C5 dorsal root ganglia contain proinflammatory neuropeptides, such as substance P (SP), calcitonin gene–related peptide (CGRP), and neuropeptide Y (NPY). These sensory nerve terminals are found predominantly in retrodiscal tissues, as well as in the capsular ligament supporting the TMJ. Mechanical stimulation of these nerve endings with joint movement leads to the release of neuropeptides that evoke inflammatory responses in adjacent articular tissues. These responses involve the release of potent cytokines (interleukin 1β [IL-1β], tumor necrosis factor α [TNF-α], interleukin 6 [IL-6]), the production of active matrix-degrading enzymes (matrix metalloproteinases [MMP-2, MMP-3, and MMP-9]), the generation of free radicals (OH• and NO), increased production of prostanoids and leukotrienes by arachidonic acid catabolism (prostaglandin E_2 [PGE_2] and leukotriene B_4 [LTB_4]), and the genesis of bradykinin.

TMJ.[19,29–32] It is believed that mechanical stimulation of these nerve endings with joint movement leads to the release of neuropeptides that evoke inflammatory responses in adjacent articular tissues. Under normal circumstances, this mechanism may be important for normal adaptive or healing responses. However, under pathologic conditions, release of these proinflammatory neuropeptides may contribute to excessive tissue degradation and inflammatory pain.

Opioids (eg, morphine) can prevent the release of these proinflammatory peptides when administered to affected joints by intra-articular injection. Clinical trials of intra-articular morphine have demonstrated efficacy in the reduction of postsurgical pain after knee surgery.[33–40] However, recent studies of the efficacy of intra-articular morphine administered to diseased human TMJs have yielded equivocal results.[41–44]

Cytokines and TMJ Osteoarthritis

Cytokines are extremely potent peptides that are produced by some cells in articular tissues of the TMJ.[10,45–47] Cytokines released from stimulated cells diffuse through tissues or fluids in the joint and stimulate local cell populations that express receptors for these molecules. By this mechanism, cells communicate over relatively long distances.

IL-1β, TNF-α, and interleukin 6 (IL-6) have been identified in fluids and tissues obtained from diseased human TMJs.[5,10,45–49] IL-1β, TNF-α, and IL-6 may contribute to TMJ osteoarthritis via several mechanisms:

1. Stimulation of the synthesis and activation of matrix-degrading enzymes
2. Alteration of extracellular matrix synthesis
3. Stimulation of arachidonic acid catabolism, resulting in the production of prostanoids (eg, prostaglandin E_2 [PGE_2]) and leukotrienes (eg, leukotriene B_4 [LTB_4])
4. Generation of free radicals by stimulated resident cells (eg, synoviocytes and macrophages)
5. Up-regulation of proinflammatory neuropeptide synthesis by sensory neurons
6. Stimulation of sensory nerve terminals

As previously mentioned, these cytokines are extremely potent. For example, primary cultures of primate TMJ chondrocytes respond to femtomolar (10^{-15} M) concentrations of IL-1β.[50] This concentration is below the detection limits of contemporary assays used to quantitate

Fig 7-8 Activation of latent matrix metalloproteinases (MMPs) by both enzymatic and nonenzymatic processes. MMPs are endopeptidases (ie, enzymes) capable of degrading the articular tissues of the TMJ. These enzymes require zinc (Zn^{++}) as a cofactor for activity. To date, four MMPs (MMP-1, MMP-2, MMP-3, and MMP-9) have been implicated in TMJ osteoarthritis. MMPs are produced in a latent, inactive form that contains a leader sequence at the amino terminus. These enzymes are subsequently activated either by cleavage of this leader sequence by other enzymes (enzymatic processing) or by oxidative degradation of the leader sequence by free radicals (nonenzymatic processing). (insert) Nonenzymatic activation of MMP-2 by free radicals in vitro. In lanes 1 and 2, basal MMP-2 activity is demonstrated by a standard zymographic technique (dotted arrow). In lane 2, additional MMP-2 activity (solid arrow) is generated by free radicals induced by the addition of hydrogen peroxide. This additional enzymatic activity is the result of the nonenzymatic activation of MMP-2.

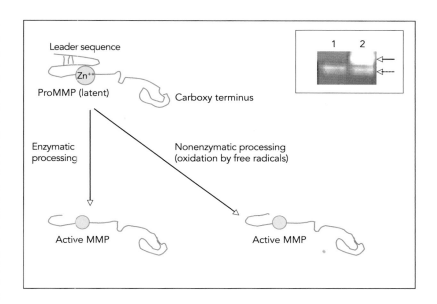

these molecules in fluids and tissues obtained from diseased TMJs. Therefore, despite the fact that clinical investigators typically do not detect elevated cytokine levels in all symptomatic TMJ subjects, it is possible that higher levels are present in biologically relevant concentrations.

Proteases and TMJ Osteoarthritis

Enzymes (proteases) that degrade cartilage and bone have been implicated in the pathogenesis of TMJ osteoarthritis.[6,48,51–59] Among those enzymes capable of degrading articular tissues of the TMJ, the endopeptidases, known as *matrix metalloproteinases (MMPs)*, appear to be the most abundant. These enzymes require zinc as a cofactor and can be inactivated by tetracyclines that chelate zinc.

Of the 15 known MMPs, four (MMP-1, MMP-2, MMP-3, and MMP-9) have been implicated in TMJ osteoarthritis. Collectively, these enzymes are capable of degrading collagens (I, II, III, IV, V, VII, VIII, IX, X, XI, and XIV), proteoglycans (aggrecan, versican, link protein, entactin, and decorin),

and other extracellular matrix molecules (fibronectins, tenascin, laminins, osteonectin, elastin, and fibrin) that are found in various articular tissues of the TMJ.

Some MMPs are produced in a latent, inactive form and are subsequently activated by the actions of other enzymes. Some MMPs can cleave latent MMPs, resulting in their activation. Latent MMPs may also be activated by free radicals via a nonenzymatic mechanism. Latent MMP-2 and MMP-9 can be activated in vitro by this mechanism (Fig 7-8).

Active MMPs are regulated in the TMJ by molecules termed *tissue inhibitors of metalloproteinases (TIMPs)*.[53] As the name implies, these proteins bind to activated MMPs and inhibit their action. Two TIMPs (TIMP-1 and TIMP-2) have been isolated from TMJ tissues or fluids.[55,59–61] Both TIMPs have been recovered from diseased human TMJs in oxidized forms, suggesting modification by free radicals. In vitro studies (Zardeneta and Milam, unpublished data, 2000) have provided evidence that oxidized TIMPs do not effectively inhibit active MMPs (Figs 7-9 and 7-10). This suggests that excessive free radical production in the TMJ creates an imbalance between MMP activation and inhibition (ie, by TIMPs), resulting in increased tissue degradation.

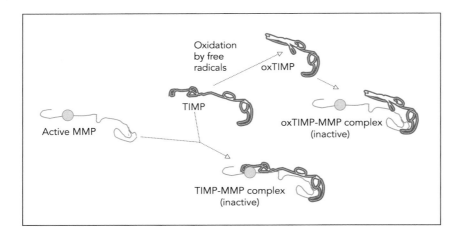

Fig 7-9 Tissue inhibitors of metalloproteinases (TIMPs) inhibit active matrix metalloproteinases (MMPs) under normal conditions. TIMPs are proteins that bind to and inhibit active MMPs. At least two TIMPs (TIMP-1 and TIMP-2) have been recovered from diseased human TMJs by lavage or arthrocentesis procedures. Some of the TIMPs recovered from these diseased TMJs were found to be oxidized (oxTIMP), presumably because of the actions of free radicals. In vitro evidence (see Fig 7-10) suggests that oxTIMPs do not effectively inhibit active MMPs.

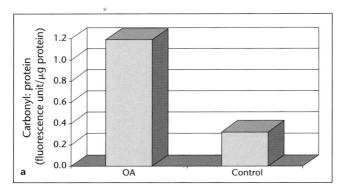

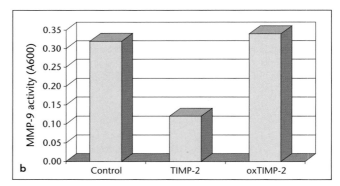

Fig 7-10 Oxidized tissue inhibitor of metalloproteinases (oxTIMP) recovered from osteoarthritic human TMJs. (Zardeneta and Milam, unpublished data, 2000.) (a) The relative amounts of oxidized TIMP-2 recovered from osteoarthritic (OA) human TMJs were compared to the amounts recovered from a control sample of TIMP-2 (control) by measurement of the carbonyl content of the protein. Carbonyl groups are formed in proteins by oxidation reactions typically driven by free radicals. The carbonyl content of TIMP-2 recovered from osteoarthritic human TMJs by lavage of the superior joint space was significantly higher than that recovered from the control sample ($P < .01$). (b) In vitro studies demonstrate that oxidized TIMP-2 (oxTIMP-2) does not effectively inhibit matrix metalloproteinases (MMPs), in this instance MMP-9. For these experiments, intact TIMP-2 or oxTIMP-2 (oxidized by a 5-minute exposure to 1 mM of H_2O_2) was added to a reaction mixture containing active MMP-9 and enzyme substrate (cowhide azure). Degradation of the substrate was assessed by colorimetric assay (A600). The control sample consisted of substrate and active enzyme without TIMP-2. The data indicated that intact TIMP-2 significantly inhibited MMP-9 activity ($P < .001$). However, oxTIMP-2 did not inhibit degradation of the substrate by MMP-9.

Fatty Acid Catabolites and TMJ Osteoarthritis

Cell membranes serve as rich reservoirs of structurally diverse fatty acid derivatives that are precursors of biologically active molecular species generated by the actions of specific phospholipases (eg, phospholipase A_2). The activation of phospholipases is a key element in the regulation of the production of these biologically active molecules from cell membrane fatty acids. Some cytokines, neuropeptides, and free radicals are capable of generating signals that culminate in the activation of these important enzymes.[62–71] Products of membrane fatty acid catabolism by activated phospholipases include prostaglandins and leukotrienes that have been implicated in inflammation and the genesis of hyperalgesia (Fig 7-11).

Fig 7-11 Phospholipid catabolism. Arachidonic acid is generated by the enzymatic action of phospholipases on cell membrane phospholipids. Prostaglandins (eg, PGF2α, PGI$_2$, PGE$_2$, and PGD$_2$), implicated in the pathogenesis of TMJ osteoarthritis and pain, are generated by actions of cyclooxygenases (COX-1, COX-2, and COX-3) are currently known to exist. COX-1 is constitutively expressed in most tissues, providing a continuous supply of prostanoids required for various tissue functions. COX-2 is synthesized in response to injury in most tissues, resulting in an increase production of prostanoids above normal baseline. Cytokines such as interleukin 1β (IL-1β) and tumor necrosis factor a (TNF-α) are capable of stimulating the synthesis of COX-2 by sensitive cell populations. COX-3 was recently discovered in central nervous tissues and is believed to influence nociception by production of centrally active prostanoids. Acetaminophen is an effective inhibitor of COX-3. Leukotrienes (eg, LTA$_4$, LTB$_4$, LTC$_4$, and LTD$_4$) and hydroxy fatty acids are derived from arachidonic acid by action of lipoxygenases, some of which may be activated by cytokines, such as IL-1β and TNF-α. Leukotriene B$_4$ (LTB$_4$) can promote bone resorption, and the hydroxyeicosatetraenoic acids (eg, 5-HETE and 12-HETE) and hydroperoxyeicosatetraenoic acids (eg 5-HPETE and 12-HPETE) may function as algesic substances, activating nociceptive responses to joint injury. Finally, isoprostanes (eg, 8-iso-PGE$_2$ and 8-iso-PGF$_{2α}$) may be generated by nonenzymatic oxidation (ie, by free radicals) of arachidonic acid, resulting in the production of extremely potent prostanoids that have been implicated in a variety of physiologic responses, including nociception.

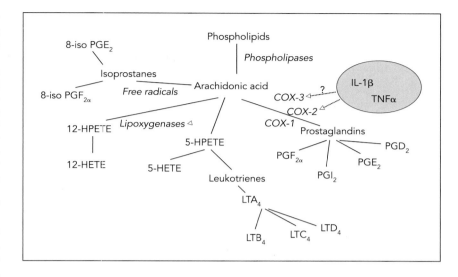

Prostaglandins

Biologically active prostanoids are produced by catabolism of arachidonic acid by the action of cyclooxygenases (COXs). Arachidonic acid is generated by the enzymatic action of phospholipases on cell membrane phospholipids. At least three COXs (COX-1, COX-2, and COX-3) are currently known to exist.[62,66,72–74] COX-1 is constitutively expressed in most tissues, providing a continuous supply of prostanoids required for various tissue functions. COX-2 is not typically expressed in most tissues under normal conditions. However, COX-2 is synthesized after injury or induction of inflammation, resulting in an increased production of prostanoids above the normal baseline level. Cytokines, such as IL-1β and TNF-α, are capable of stimulating the synthesis of COX-2 by sensitive cell populations (see Fig 7-11). COX-3 was recently discovered in central nervous tissues and is believed to influence nociception by production of centrally active prostanoids.[75,76] Acetaminophen, which has little inhibitory effect on COX-1 and COX-2, is an effective inhibitor of COX-3.[77,78]

Prostaglandins have been implicated in the genesis of joint pain by both peripheral and central mechanisms.[79] For example, PGE$_2$ and prostaglandin I$_2$ (PGI$_2$) produce hyperalgesic responses in rats after intradermal administration.[80] Recent evidence suggests that some prostaglandins (ie, PGE$_2$) may be important regulators of chondrogenesis.[81–83] PGE$_2$ stimulates the synthesis of cartilage-specific type II collagen by cultured chondrocytes. However, this effect appears to be indirect and may be mediated, at least in part, by insulin-like growth factor 1 (IGF-1). IGF-1 is a hormone released from chondrocytes on stimulation by PGE$_2$.[83] In vitro studies have provided evidence that some (eg, indomethacin and ketoprofen), but not all (eg, etodolac), NSAIDs inhibit chondrogenesis, as assessed by cartilage-specific collagen synthesis.[84] Although controversial, this observation suggests that chronic administration of some NSAIDs to manage TMJ osteoarthritis may have detrimental effects on cartilage. However, this suggestion should be tempered by the realization that the fibrocartilages of the TMJ are distinct from the hyaline cartilages of other load-bearing joints and may not be subjected to similar regulatory mechanisms. Clearly, further study is warranted on this subject, particularly in light of the popular use of NSAIDs by patients with TMJ osteo-arthritis.

Isoprostanes

Isoprostanes are prostanoids produced by nonenzymatic oxidation of arachidonic acid and may be more potent than their COX-derived prostanoid counterparts.[85] Oxidation reactions producing isoprostanes are generated by free radicals. Some isoprostanes (ie, 8-iso prostaglandin E_2 and 8-iso prostaglandin $F_{2\alpha}$) reduce mechanical and thermal withdrawal thresholds in rats and stimulate sensory neural impulses in vitro, indicating that some isoprostanes may be important mediators of nociception.[85] Other studies have implicated isoprostanes in the pathogenesis of some degenerative arthritides.[86] However, to date there have been no reported studies of isoprostane production in the TMJ. Therefore, the role of isoprostanes in the genesis of TMJ osteoarthritis, other degenerative joint diseases, and TMJ arthralgia is unknown.

Leukotrienes and Hydroxy Fatty Acids

Leukotrienes and hydroxy fatty acids are derived from arachidonic acid by the action of lipoxygenases[87,88] (see Fig 7-11). Some leukotrienes (LTB_4) have been detected in lavage fluid samples obtained from diseased TMJs and have been implicated in degradation of bone.[88–91] For example, LTB_4 applied adjacent to the cranial periosteum evokes the formation of osteoclasts and subsequent bone resorption at the injection site.[89,90]

The substances 5-(S)-hydroxyeicosatetraenoic acid (5-HETE), 15-(S)-hydroxyeicosatetraenoic acid (15-HETE), 12-(S)-hydroperoxyeicosatetraenoic acid (12-HPETE), and 15-(S)-hydroperoxyeicosatetraenoic acid (15-HPETE),which are hydroxy fatty acid products of arachidonic acid generated by the action of lipoxygenases, have been implicated as mediators of nociception.[92,93] These HETEs and HPETEs are capsaicin-like endogenous substances that can stimulate primary afferent nociceptors.[93] Capsaicin is the substance in chili peppers that produces a burning sensation when applied to tissues. This noxious sensation results from stimulation of specific receptors expressed by nociceptive neurons, termed *transient receptor potential vanilloid 1 (TRPV1)*. Stimulation of nociceptive neurons via TRPV1 activation also results in the release of neuropeptides (eg, SP and CGRP) from their terminals. As previously mentioned, these neuropeptides can promote inflammation by stimula-

tion of adjacent cell populations, such as endothelial cells and synoviocytes.

Possible Factors in Susceptibility to TMJ Osteoarthritis

The TMJ is unique compared to other load-bearing synovial joints. It is capable of both hinge and sliding movements, which produce both compressive and shearing loads. The articular surfaces of the TMJ are composed of fibrocartilages that are distinct, in both molecular composition and material properties, from the hyaline cartilages of load-bearing joints of the appendicular skeleton.[94] There is also evidence that the molecular events that control the development, and perhaps the healing responses, of the TMJ are distinct from those involved in the development and healing of other load-bearing synovial joints.[95,96]

One of the most dramatic attributes of the TMJ, compared to other load-bearing synovial joints, is its remarkable adaptive capacity. For example, most oral and maxillofacial surgeons have witnessed almost complete modeling and remodeling of the TMJ following subcondylar fractures in some individuals (Fig 7-12).

Because of this remarkable regenerative capacity, it is difficult to comprehend that degenerative TMJ diseases, such as osteoarthritis, are common and can affect young individuals. It is becoming increasingly apparent that an individual's susceptibility to degenerative TMJ disease is likely governed by a number of factors, including sex-based determinants (eg, estrogen), diet, genetic background, and psychological stress.

Estrogens

Epidemiologic studies indicate a female predisposition for some TMJ diseases, including osteoarthritis.[94,97] For this reason, several investigators have focused studies on the potential roles of sex hormones in the pathogenesis of degenerative TMJ diseases.

Clinical investigations have implicated estrogens in certain temporomandibular disorders.[97,98] Pain felt in the preauricular region is more common in females of childbearing age. Furthermore, postmenopausal women who receive estrogen replacement therapy totaling 185 mg or more per year are more than 1.8 times more likely to be referred for treatment of a temporomandibular disorder than are postmenopausal women who do not take estrogens.[97]

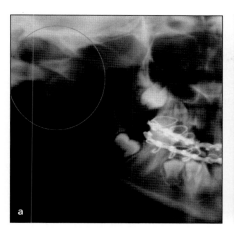
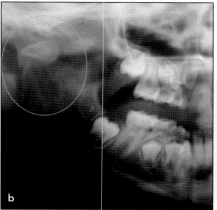
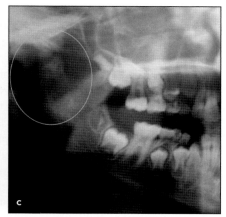
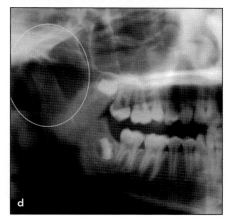

Fig 7-12 Adaptive modeling and remodeling of the TMJ. *(a)* Day 0. An 11-year-old boy sustained a subcondylar fracture treated with closed reduction. *(b)* Six weeks after injury. Position of fractured condyle after maxillomandibular fixation (48 hours) and guiding elastics were stopped. *(c)* Sixteen weeks after injury. Marked adaptive modeling and remodeling is visible. *(d)* Forty-seven months after injury. A normal joint architecture is observed.

Estrogens are synthesized from cholesterol. Estrogen mimetics can also be introduced from environmental sources. However, the extent to which these latter molecules contribute to the pathophysiology of TMJ osteoarthritis is unknown. Estrogens exert their action via estrogen receptors (ERs) that are expressed by a variety of cells in different tissues. Estrogen receptors have been identified in articular tissues of the TMJ.[99–101]

At least two distinct ERs are known (ERα and ERβ). However, polymorphisms of both ERs have also been described. ER polymorphisms are created by mutations of the ER genes. These mutations result in the synthesis of ERs that may differ in either affinity for estrogens or in signaling efficiency. Therefore, ER polymorphisms appear to govern an individual's response to estrogens, likely accounting for the variability in responses to estrogens and estrogen-related disease susceptibility observed in the general population. For example, abnormal ossification of spinal ligaments has recently been associated with specific ER polymorphisms.[102] Other diseases, including osteoporosis, rheumatoid arthritis, and breast cancer, may occur with a higher prevalence in women who express certain ER polymorphisms not expressed by other women of similar age.

Estrogens can evoke both genomic responses (ie, by initiation of gene transcription) and nongenomic responses (ie, responses that are rapid and not dependent on protein synthesis) in various cell populations that constitute the articular tissues of the TMJ. Kapila and Xie[103] have provided evidence that estrogens may contribute to TMJ osteoarthritis by promotion of joint hypermobility. These investigators examined the effects of estrogen priming on TMJ articular disc cell responses to relaxin, a hormone that induces extracellular matrix turnover in fibrocartilaginous tissues. Relaxin, which contributes to the expansion of the pelvic girdle during pregnancy through this turnover mechanism, and has been implicated in generalized joint hypermobility. Priming of TMJ articular disc cells with 17β-estradiol significantly potentiated matrix metalloproteinase synthesis in response to relaxin stimulation.[103] In fact, the maximum expression of these enzymes occurred at relaxin concentrations that were 10- to 100-fold lower in estrogen-primed cells than in unprimed cells. This study suggests that estrogens could increase susceptibility to TMJ osteoarthritis by

(1) altering production of matrix-degrading enzymes (in this instance in response to hormonal stimulation) and *(2)* promoting joint hypermobility that leads to unfavorable biomechanics.

Abubaker et al[104] studied the effects of sex hormones on collagen and total protein content of articular discs of the TMJ in rats. They reported that intact males expressed more collagen and total protein in articular discs than did intact females. They also noted that oophorectomized animals expressed more collagen in articular discs than did intact females, an effect reversed by estrogen supplementation.[104] Collectively, these data indicate that functional ERs are expressed in the TMJ and that estrogen appears to influence the composition and remodeling of the extracellular matrices of the articular tissues of the TMJ. It is speculated that in some females these changes may increase the predisposition to degenerative joint diseases such as articular disc displacements and osteoarthritis.

Epidemiologic studies have suggested that women seek treatment for painful temporomandibular disorders more often than men.[97,98,105,106] A potential explanation for this finding is that women may experience more pain than men for a similar temporomandibular disorder. This notion is supported by animal studies demonstrating that females and males differ with respect to TMJ nociception.[107–109] In these experiments, neural responses in the trigeminal brainstem complex to noxious stimulation of the rat TMJ were assessed by detection of an early response gene product called *c-Fos*. C-Fos is a transcription factor that is synthesized rapidly, typically within 10 to 20 minutes of stimulation. It is detected using standard immunohistochemical staining methods applied to tissue sections obtained from appropriate brainstem regions. Neurons that stain positive for c-Fos represent those neurons that were activated by a recent stimulus, in these instances by noxious stimulation of the rat TMJ. Using this approach, Bereiter[107] has observed significantly more neural activity in female animals after stimulation of the TMJ than in male animals subjected to a similar stimulus.

Therefore, estrogens may influence an individual's susceptibility to TMJ osteoarthritis and pain by a variety of mechanisms. This liability may be dependent on several variables, including local estrogen concentration and the presence of specific ER variants (ie, specific ERα and/or ERβ forms), governed by expression of one or more of the known ER polymorphisms.

Diet

Based on contemporary models of this disease, one can easily speculate that the mechanical properties of foods could contribute to TMJ osteoarthritis; hard mechanical diets may contribute to injury by increasing masticatory demands and subsequent joint loads. However, the pain often experienced by osteoarthritic patients typically exerts a self-limiting effect by forcing patients to softer diets. Perhaps more important are the contributions of certain diets to the genesis of molecules that have clearly been implicated in the pathophysiology of TMJ osteoarthritis. As previously described, molecules such as the prostanoids and leukotrienes are generated from substrates derived from molecules (eg, fatty acids) obtained through dietary intake. The adage "we are what we eat" appears to be correct.

This is best illustrated in recent studies of the effects of 3-omega fatty acids on inflammation.[110–114] Fish oils are rich in 3-omega fatty acids. Ingestion of 3-omega fatty acids leads to the production of eicosapentaenoic acid (EPA) and docosahexaenoic acid (DHA), which are similar in structure to arachidonic acid. Recall that arachidonic acid, derived from a saturated fatty acid diet (6-omega fatty acids), is the precursor of the proinflammatory prostaglandins and leukotrienes. Following ingestion of 3-omega fatty acids, EPA and DHA production can lead to the genesis of novel prostaglandins and leukotrienes that are less inflammatory than their arachidonic acid–derived counterparts. Some EPA and DHA derivatives may actually be anti-inflammatory.[111]

To date, 13 clinical trials have collectively provided evidence that dietary intake of 3-omega fatty acids can significantly reduce signs and symptoms of arthritis at daily doses of 2.6 to 7.1 g, yielding plasma EPA levels exceeding 3% of total fatty acid content.[111] The effects of a 3-omega fatty acid diet on inflammation and disease are typically delayed in onset, requiring intake for 18 to 24 weeks. Furthermore, the benefits of this diet are rapidly lost once 3-omega fatty acid ingestion is terminated.

The effects of 3-omega fatty acid ingestion on the pathogenesis of TMJ osteoarthritis are currently unknown. Likewise, contributions of saturated fatty acid diets to TMJ disease susceptibility are unknown. However, based on existing clinical data obtained from studies of other arthritides, it is reasonable to assume that diet can profoundly influence disease susceptibility by affecting the supply of molecules that are known to be involved in pathogenic mechanisms.

Genetic Background

There is little doubt that genetic background is a significant determinant of an individual's susceptibility to disease. There is evidence suggesting that susceptibility to pain and disease may be governed by subtle variations in the genes expressed by specific individuals. Many, if not all, genes have been subjected to mutations that have functional consequences for proteins that are subsequently expressed; a given protein may be more or less potent as a result of a subtle mutation of its gene. Therefore, gene polymorphisms may account for much of an individual's susceptibility to TMJ disease. In rodents, a mutation affecting the normal production of the α1 chain of type XI collagen appears to greatly increase an animal's susceptibility to the development of TMJ osteoarthritis.[115] Furthermore, recent clinical studies have provided evidence that polymorphisms of the catechol-o-methylytransferase gene (COMT) may be an important determinant of pain experienced by an individual following injury to the masticatory muscles.[116]

Psychological Stress

Psychological stress is believed to be a significant risk factor for certain individuals who are susceptible to TMJ disease. Many investigators have attributed excessive parafunctional joint loading (bruxism and jaw clenching) as the primary mechanism by which psychological stress contributes to such disease. However, recent evidence suggests that psychological stress may evoke significant biologic responses that could be important in the genesis of pain associated with TMJ osteoarthritis.

Nerve growth factor (NGF) has been implicated in the genesis of muscle, neuropathic, and sympathetically maintained pain (ie, complex regional pain syndrome).[117–120] In normal human subjects, recombinant human NGF can evoke moderate to severe pain affecting the jaw musculature following local or systemic administration.[121,122] After sensory nerve injury in rats, sympathetic neurons sprout into the dorsal root ganglia cell bodies for the injured nerve.[117,119,123,124] This mechanism is believed to underlie some types of chronic pain states that appear to involve sympathetic input, such as sympathetically maintained pain, complex regional pain syndromes, and reflex sympathetic dystrophy. This phenomenon can be recreated in the absence of nerve injury by intrathecal administration of NGF.[117] Therefore, it is believed that NGF, produced in response to injury, may stimulate sympathetic neurons to sprout into adjacent sensory ganglia. This unusual physical relationship between sensory neurons and sympathetic neurons could afford a mechanism for sympathetic neurons to regulate activities of affected sensory neurons.

Some patients with degenerative TMJ disease, such as osteoarthritis, complain of marked tactile allodynia affecting the region overlying the diseased joint. Light tactile stimulation of the affected area typically elicits a complaint of moderate to severe burning pain. In some individuals with this clinical presentation, sympathetic blockade by stellate ganglion block provides significant, but temporary, relief of this pain. This phenomenon is more commonly observed in TMJ patients who have undergone multiple TMJ surgical procedures. These observations suggest that some patients with degenerative TMJ disease, particularly those who have undergone TMJ surgery, may experience sympathetically maintained pain, possibly involving the mechanism previously described.

Females appear to be more sensitive to NGF than do males.[121] The primary receptor for NGF is the tyrosine kinase A (trkA) receptor. Interestingly, congenital insensitivity to pain with anhidrosis (inability to sweat), an autosomal-recessive disorder also characterized by recurrent episodic fevers, absence of reaction to noxious or painful stimuli, and self-mutilation, is the result of a mutation of the TRKA gene.[125–127] The TRKA gene is regulated by estrogen; the TRKA gene has an estrogen response element in the 5' untranslated region. Females synthesize more trkA than do their male counterparts, accounting for the increased sensitivity to NGF among women.

Animal and human studies have provided evidence that psychological stress increases plasma NGF concentrations.[128,129] In one study of US soldiers scheduled to parachute for the first time, serum NGF levels increased approximately 70% the night before the jump relative to the levels in controls (soldiers not slated to parachute in the near future), presumably as a result of psychological stress associated with the anticipated jump.[130]

Psychological stress can also have a profound effect on the hypothalamic-pituitary-adrenal axis (HPA axis). Acute psychological stress can evoke the release of corticotropin-releasing factor, a peptide released by the hypothalamus that can act at all levels of the neural axis to produce analgesia.[131] Moreover, chronic stress and activation of the HPA axis may contribute to a variety of human disorders, including obesity, depression, and memory loss.[132] Recent evidence indicates that genetic factors may explain variations in the HPA axis response among individuals responding to stress.[133]

Therefore, chronic psychological stress may contribute to symptoms of TMJ osteoarthritis and other degenerative TMJ diseases by a variety of mechanisms. These may include (1) an increased occurrence of parafunctional habits such as clenching and bruxism that intensify or sustain joint loading, (2) stimulation of the production or release of potent biochemicals (eg, NGF) that may contribute to the genesis of pain, and (3) protracted activation of the HPA axis, leading to complex systemic effects (eg, depression) that may be important in the pathogenesis of TMJ disease and associated sequelae. Future research will be required to determine the mechanisms and extent to which psychological stress contributes to degenerative TMJ diseases as well as to identify factors that may govern an individual's susceptibility to the physiologic effects of psychological stress.

Future Directions

Advancements in imaging and molecular biology promise the rapid expansion of our knowledge of various diseases and great improvements in our diagnostic capabilities. For example, nanotechnologies now permit high-resolution imaging studies designed to localize targeted molecules in humans.[134] This approach employs biodegradable nanoparticles tagged with antibodies or ligands directed to targeted molecules. These nanoparticles can be colabeled with gadolinium. The tagged, gadolinium-labeled nanoparticles, administered systemically or locally, concentrate at sites that contain the targeted molecules, providing a greatly enhanced gadolinium signal that can be detected with a standard 1.5-T magnetic resonance imaging protocol. Conceivably, this minimally invasive technology could facilitate sophisticated human studies of biochemicals (eg, active MMPs) involved in the pathogenesis of degenerative TMJ diseases. It is also possible that such technology could provide a vehicle for the targeted delivery of substances that will modify or ablate molecular events involved in TMJ osteoarthritis.

Pain is the primary motivator for patients who seek treatment for TMJ osteoarthritis. TMJ arthralgia can be severe, resulting in restriction of mandibular range of movement and thereby contributing to sequelae (eg, TMJ adhesions or ankylosis) associated with TMJ osteoarthritis and other degenerative TMJ arthritides. Novel approaches to the management of intractable pain are emerging from basic studies of nociception. For example, selective neuroablative methods employing saporin, a toxin that produces cell death by inhibition of protein synthesis, have the potential to eliminate persistent pain while preserving other neural functions.[135,136]

Saporin is a highly toxic substance that must gain entry into cells to be effective. However, it does not penetrate cell membranes efficiently. Recently, saporin has been conjugated with SP.[135] This hybrid molecule, SP-saporin, binds to SP receptors expressed predominantly by nociceptive neurons. When SP-saporin binds to NK-1 via the SP portion of the molecule, NK-1 and the bound SP-saporin conjugate are internalized in targeted NK-1–expressing neurons. Saporin gains access to sensory neurons by this mechanism, resulting in protein inhibition and neuronal death. Neurons that do not express NK-1 (ie, proprioceptive and motor neurons) are unaffected; that is, they cannot bind and internalize the SP-saporin conjugate. Animal studies have provided evidence that this approach can eliminate responsiveness to painful stimulation while preserving other neural functions.[135]

Advancements in tissue engineering and applications of multipotent cell populations (eg, stem cells) offer promise in the rejuvenation of osteoarthritic TMJs. Resurfacing procedures for the treatment of degenerative arthritides affecting joints of the appendicular skeleton have already reached clinical phases of study. Recent innovations in cell culturing, cell or tissue delivery systems, and guided tissue repair (eg, transforming growth factors and angiogenic growth factors) promise to one day repair diseased TMJs with living tissue constructs that offer substantial advantages over contemporary alloplastic devices.

Summary

The molecular events that underlie the pathogenesis of TMJ osteoarthritis and associated arthralgia are complex (Fig 7-13). Contemporary models suggest that excessive or protracted mechanical loads initiate a cascade of molecular events, including the generation of free radicals, the release of proinflammatory neuropeptides, signaling by potent cytokines, and the production and activation of matrix-degrading enzymes. These events culminate in failure of the lubrication system and destruction of the articular surfaces of joints in susceptible individuals. An individual's susceptibility to the development of TMJ osteoarthritis may be determined by several factors, including sex, age, dietary preferences, and psychological stress, expressed against a genetic background. Future therapies targeting key elements of this cascade, including inhibition of cytokines, inactivation of MMPs, scavenging of free radicals, and inhibition of common signal transduction pathways such as NFκβ, may prove to be extremely effective in the prevention or treatment of TMJ osteoarthritis.

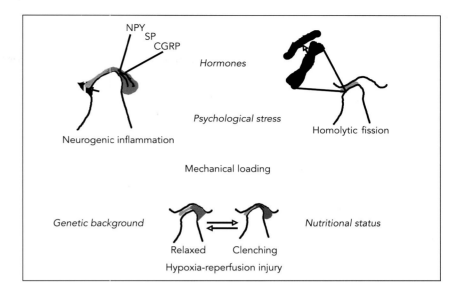

Fig 7-13 Susceptibility to TMJ osteoarthritis. It is likely that several factors contribute to an individual's susceptibility to TMJ osteoarthritis, including the genetic background of the individual, nutrition, hormonal status, and physiologic responses to psychological stress. These factors may modify molecular events initiated by excessive or protracted mechanical loads, triggering a disease state in susceptible individuals. (NPY) Neuropeptide Y; (SP) substance P; (CGRP) calcitonin gene–related peptide.

References

1. Israel HA, Saed-Nejad F, Ratcliffe A. Early diagnosis of osteoarthrosis of the temporomandibular joint: Correlation between arthroscopic diagnosis and keratan sulfate levels in the synovial fluid. J Oral Maxillofac Surg 1991;49:708–711.

2. Holmlund A, Ekblom A, Hansson P, Lind J, Lundeberg T, Theodorsson E. Concentrations of neuropeptides substance P, neurokinin A, calcitonin gene–related peptide, neuropeptide Y and vasoactive intestinal polypeptide in synovial fluid of the human temporomandibular joint. A correlation with symptoms, signs and arthroscopic findings. Int J Oral Maxillofac Surg 1991;20:228–231.

3. Alstergren P, Appelgren A, Appelgren B, Kopp S, Lundeberg T, Theodorsson E. Co-variation of neuropeptide Y, calcitonin gene-related peptide, substance P and neurokinin A in joint fluid from patients with temporomandibular joint arthritis. Arch Oral Biol 1995;40:127–135.

4. Zardeneta G, Milam SB, Schmitz JP. Iron-dependent generation of free radicals: Plausible mechanisms in the progressive deterioration of the temporomandibular joint. J Oral Maxillofac Surg 2000;58:302–308.

5. Sato J, Segami N, Nishimura M. Expression of interleukin 6 in synovial tissues in patients with internal derangement of the temporomandibular joint. Br J Oral Maxillofac Surg 2003;41:95–101.

6. Zardeneta G, Milam SB, Lee T, Schmitz JP. Detection and preliminary characterization of matrix metalloproteinase activity in temporomandibular joint lavage fluid. Int J Oral Maxillofac Surg 1998;27:397–403.

7. Akerman S, Kopp S, Rohlin M. Macroscopic and microscopic appearance of radiologic findings in temporomandibular joints from elderly individuals. An autopsy study. Int J Oral Maxillofac Surg 1988;17:58–63.

8. Nannmark U, Sennerby L, Haraldson T. Macroscopic, microscopic and radiologic assessment of the condylar part of the TMJ in elderly subjects. An autopsy study. Swed Dent J 1990;14:163–169.

9. Agerberg G, Bergenholtz A. Craniomandibular disorders in adult populations of West Bothnia, Sweden. Acta Odontol Scand 1989;47:129–140.

10. Haskin CL, Milam SB, Cameron IL. Pathogenesis of degenerative joint disease in the human temporomandibular joint. Crit Rev Oral Biol Med 1995;6:248–277.

11. Ma XC, Zou ZJ, Zhang ZK, Wu QG. Radiographic, pathological and operative observations of cases with TMJ disturbance syndrome. Int J Oral Surg 1983;12:299–308.

12. Stegenga B, de Bont LG, van der Kuijl B, Boering G. Classification of temporomandibular joint osteoarthrosis and internal derangement. 1. Diagnostic significance of clinical and radiographic symptoms and signs. Cranio 1992;10:96–106.

13. Bates RE Jr, Gremillion HA, Stewart CM. Degenerative joint disease. I. Diagnosis and management considerations. Cranio 1993;11:284–290.

14. Milam SB, Schmitz JP. Molecular biology of temporomandibular joint disorders: Proposed mechanisms of disease. J Oral Maxillofac Surg 1995;53:1448–1454.

15. Fukuoka Y, Hagihara M, Nagatsu T, Kaneda T. The relationship between collagen metabolism and temporomandibular joint osteoarthrosis in mice. J Oral Maxillofac Surg 1993;51:288–291.

16. Ratcliffe A, Israel H. Proteoglycan components of articular cartilage in synovial fluids as potential markers of osteoarthritis of the temporomandibular joint. In: Sessle BJ, Bryant PS, Dionnes RA (eds). Temporomandibular Disorders and Related Pain Conditions. Progress in Pain Research and Management, vol 4. Seattle: IASP Press, 1995:141–150.

17. Hinton RJ. Alterations in rat condylar cartilage following discectomy. J Dent Res 1992;71:1292–1297.

18. Milam SB, Zardeneta G, Schmitz JP. Oxidative stress and degenerative temporomandibular joint disease: A proposed hypothesis. J Oral Maxillofac Surg 1998;56:214–223.

19. Kido MA, Kiyoshima T, Kondo T, et al. Distribution of substance P and calcitonin gene–related peptide-like immunoreactive nerve fibers in the rat temporomandibular joint. J Dent Res 1993;72:592–598.

20. Hutchins B, Patel H, Spears R. Attenuation of pro-inflammatory neuropeptide levels produced by a cyclooxygenase-2 inhibitor in an animal model of chronic temporomandibular joint inflammation. J Orofac Pain 2002;16:312–316.

21. Nitzan DW. The process of lubrication impairment and its involvement in temporomandibular joint disc displacement: A theoretical concept. J Oral Maxillofac Surg 2001;59:36–45.

22. Nitzan DW, Etslon I. Adhesive force: The underlying cause of the disc anchorage to the fossa and/or eminence in the temporomandibular joint—A new concept. Int J Oral Maxillofac Surg 2002;31:94–99.

23. McCord JM. Free radicals and inflammation: Protection of synovial fluid by superoxide dismutase. Science 1974;185:529–531.

24. Dijkgraaf LC, Zardeneta G, Cordewener FW, et al. Crosslinking of fibrinogen and fibronectin by free radicals: A possible initial step in adhesion formation in osteoarthritis of the temporomandibular joint. J Oral Maxillofac Surg 2003;61:101–111.

25. Zamamiri-Davis F, Lu Y, Thompson JT, et al. Nuclear factor-κB mediates over-expression of cyclooxygenase-2 during activation of RAW 264.7 macrophages in selenium deficiency. Free Radic Biol Med 2002;32:890–897.

26. Chen F, Castranova V, Shi X, Demers LM. New insights into the role of nuclear factor-κB, a ubiquitous transcription factor in the initiation of diseases. Clin Chem. 1999;45:7–17.

27. Schreck R, Rieber P, Baeuerle PA. Reactive oxygen intermediates as apparently widely used messengers in the activation of the NF-κB transcription factor and HIV-1. EMBO J. 1991;10:2247–2258.

28. Hutchins B, Spears R, Hinton RJ, Harper RP. Calcitonin gene–related peptide and substance P immunoreactivity in rat trigeminal ganglia and brainstem following adjuvant-induced inflammation of the temporomandibular joint. Arch Oral Biol 2000;45:335–345.

29. Ichikawa H, Matsuo S, Wakisaka S, Akai M. Fine structure of calcitonin gene–related peptide-immunoreactive nerve fibres in the rat temporomandibular joint. Arch Oral Biol 1990;35:727–730.

30. Johansson AS, Isacsson G, Isberg A, Granholm AC. Distribution of substance P–like immunoreactive nerve fibers in temporomandibular joint soft tissues of monkey. Scand J Dent Res 1986;94:225–232.

31. Haeuchi Y, Matsumoto K, Ichikawa H, Maeda S. Immunohistochemical demonstration of neuropeptides in the articular disk of the human temporomandibular joint. Cells Tissues Organs 1999;164:205–211.

32. Shimizu S, Kido MA, Kiyoshima T, Tanaka T. Postnatal development of substance P–, calcitonin gene–related peptide– and neuropeptide Y–like immunoreactive nerve fibres in the synovial membrane of the rat temporomandibular joint. Arch Oral Biol 1996;41:749–759.

33. Drosos GI, Vlachonikolis IG, Papoutsidakis AN, Gavalas NS, Anthopoulos G. Intra-articular morphine and postoperative analgesia after knee arthroscopy. Knee 2002;9:335–340.

34. Ho ST, Wang TJ, Tang JS, Liaw WJ, Ho CM. Pain relief after arthroscopic knee surgery: Intravenous morphine, epidural morphine, and intra-articular morphine. Clin J Pain 2000;16:105–109.

35. Ritter MA, Koehler M, Keating EM, Faris PM, Meding JB. Intra-articular morphine and/or bupivacaine after total knee replacement. J Bone Joint Surg Br 1999;81:301–303.

36. Rosseland LA, Stubhaug A, Skoglund A, Breivik H. Intra-articular morphine for pain relief after knee arthroscopy. Acta Anaesthesiol Scand 1999;43:252–257.

37. Likar R, Kapral S, Steinkellner H, Stein C, Schafer M. Dose-dependency of intra-articular morphine analgesia. Br J Anaesth 1999;83:241–244.

38. De Andres J, Valia JC, Barrera L, Colomina R. Intra-articular analgesia after arthroscopic knee surgery: Comparison of three different regimens. Eur J Anaesthesiol 1998;15:10–15.

39. Kalso E, Tramer MR, Carroll D, et al. Pain relief from intra-articular morphine after knee surgery: A qualitative systematic review. Pain 1997;71:127–134.

40. Liu K, Wang JJ, Ho ST, Liaw WJ, Chia YY. Opioid in peripheral analgesia: Intra-articular morphine for pain control after arthroscopic knee surgery. Acta Anaesthesiol Sin 1995;33:217–221.

41. List T, Tegelberg A, Haraldson T, Isacsson G. Intra-articular morphine as analgesic in temporomandibular joint arthralgia/osteoarthritis. Pain 2001;94:275–282.

42. Kunjur J, Anand R, Brennan PA, Ilankovan V. An audit of 405 temporomandibular joint arthrocenteses with intra-articular morphine infusion. Br J Oral Maxillofac Surg 2003;41:29–31.

43. Bryant CJ, Harrison SD, Hopper C, Harris M. Use of intra-articular morphine for postoperative analgesia following TMJ arthroscopy. Br J Oral Maxillofac Surg 1999;37:391–396.

44. Furst IM, Kryshtalskyj B, Weinberg S. The use of intra-articular opioids and bupivacaine for analgesia following temporomandibular joint arthroscopy: A prospective, randomized trial. J Oral Maxillofac Surg 2001;59:979–983.

45. Habu M, Tominaga K, Sukedai M, et al. Immunohistochemical study of interleukin-1beta and interleukin-1 receptor antagonist in an antigen-induced arthritis of the rabbit temporomandibular joint. J Oral Pathol Med 2002;31:45–54.

46. Ogura N, Tobe M, Sakamaki H, et al. Interleukin-1 beta induces interleukin-6 mRNA expression and protein production in synovial cells from human temporomandibular joint. J Oral Pathol Med 2002;31:353–360.

47. Sandler NA, Buckley MJ, Cillo JE, Braun TW. Correlation of inflammatory cytokines with arthroscopic findings in patients with temporomandibular joint internal derangements. J Oral Maxillofac Surg 1998;56:534–543.

48. Puzas JE, Landeau JM, Tallents R, Albright J, Schwarz EM, Landesberg R. Degradative pathways in tissues of the temporomandibular joint. Use of in vitro and in vivo models to characterize matrix metalloproteinase and cytokine activity. Cells Tissues Organs 2001;169:248–256.

49. Rossomando EF, White LB, Hadjimichael J, Shafer D. Immunomagnetic separation of tumor necrosis factor alpha. 1. Batch procedure for human temporomandibular fluid. J Chromatogr 1992;583:11–18.

50. Milam SB. Cell-Extracellular Matrix Interactions with Special Emphasis on the Primate Temporomandibular Joint [thesis]. San Antonio: University of Texas Health Science Center, 1990.

51. Breckon JJ, Hembry RM, Reynolds JJ, Meikle MC. Identification of matrix metalloproteinases and their inhibitor in the articular disc of the craniomandibular joint of the rabbit. Arch Oral Biol 1996;41:315–322.

52. Ijima Y, Kobayashi M, Kubota E. Role of interleukin-1 in induction of matrix metalloproteinases synthesized by rat temporomandibular joint chondrocytes and disc cells. Eur J Oral Sc 2001;109:50–59.

53. Kapila S, Lee C, Richards DW. Characterization and identification of proteinases and proteinase inhibitors synthesized by temporomandibular joint disc cells. J Dent Res 1995;74:1328–1336.

54. Kiyoshima T, Kido MA, Nishimura Y, et al. Immunocytochemical localization of cathepsin L in the synovial lining cells of the rat temporomandibular joint. Arch Oral Biol 1994;39:1049–1056.

55. Kubota T, Kubota E, Matsumoto A, et al. Identification of matrix metalloproteinases (MMPs) in synovial fluid from patients with temporomandibular disorder. Eur J Oral Sci 1998;106:992–998.

56. Marchetti C, Cornaglia I, Casasco A, Bernasconi G, Baciliero U, Stetler-Stevenson WG. Immunolocalization of gelatinase-A (matrix metalloproteinase-2) in damaged human temporomandibular joint discs. Arch Oral Biol 1999;44:297–304.

57. Tanaka A, Kawashiri S, Kumagai S, et al. Expression of matrix metalloproteinase-2 in osteoarthritic fibrocartilage from human mandibular condyle. J Oral Pathol Med 2000;29:314–320.

58. Bae JW, Takahashi I, Sasano Y, et al. Age-related changes in gene expression patterns of matrix metalloproteinases and their collagenous substrates in mandibular condylar cartilage in rats. J Anat 2003;203:235–241.

59. Srinivas R, Sorsa T, Tjaderhane L, et al. Matrix metalloproteinases in mild and severe temporomandibular joint internal derangement synovial fluid. Oral Surg Oral Med Oral Pathol Oral Radiol Endod 2001;91:517–525.

60. Kanyama M, Kuboki T, Kojima S, et al. Matrix metalloproteinases and tissue inhibitors of metalloproteinases in synovial fluids of patients with temporomandibular joint osteoarthritis. J Orofac Pain 2000;14:20–30.

61. Shinoda C, Takaku S. Interleukin-1 beta, interleukin-6, and tissue inhibitor of metalloproteinase-1 in the synovial fluid of the temporomandibular joint with respect to cartilage destruction. Oral Dis 2000;6:383–390.

62. Hla T, Neilson K. Human cyclooxygenase-2 cDNA. Proc Natl Acad Sci U S A 1992;89:7384–7388.

63. O'Neill GP, Ford-Hutchinson AW. Expression of mRNA for cyclooxygenase-1 and cyclooxygenase-2 in human tissues. FEBS Lett 1993;330:156–160.

64. Ristimaki A, Garfinkel S, Wessendorf J, Maciag T, Hla T. Induction of cyclooxygenase-2 by interleukin-1 alpha. Evidence for post-transcriptional regulation. J Biol Chem 1994;269:11769–11775.

65. Tung JT, Fenton JI, Arnold C, et al. Recombinant equine interleukin-1beta induces putative mediators of articular cartilage degradation in equine chondrocytes. Can J Vet Res 2002;66:19–25.

66. Crofford LJ, Wilder RL, Ristimaki AP, et al. Cyclooxygenase-1 and -2 expression in rheumatoid synovial tissues. Effects of interleukin-1 beta, phorbol ester, and corticosteroids. J Clin Invest 1994;93:1095–1101.

67. Karimi K, Kool M, Nijkamp FP, Redegeld FP. Substance P can stimulate prostaglandin D_2 and leukotriene C_4 generation without granule exocytosis in murine mast cells. Eur J Pharmacol 2004;489:49–54.

68. Pitcher GM, Henry JL. Mediation and modulation by eicosanoids of responses of spinal dorsal horn neurons to glutamate and substance P receptor agonists: Results with indomethacin in the rat in vivo. Neuroscience 1999;93: 1109–1121.

69. Gecse A, Kis B, Mezei Z, Telegdy G. Effects of inflammatory neuropeptides on the arachidonate cascade of platelets. Int Arch Allergy Immunol 1999;118:166–170.

70. Szarek JL, Spurlock B, Gruetter CA, Lemke S. Substance P and capsaicin release prostaglandin E_2 from rat intrapulmonary bronchi. Am J Physiol 1998;275(5 pt 1):L1006—L1012.

71. Tsuji F, Hamada M, Shirasawa E. Tachykinins as enhancers of prostaglandin E_2–induced intraocular inflammation. Ocul Immunol Inflamm 1998;6:19–25.

72. Quinn JH, Kent JH, Moise A, Lukiw WJ. Cyclooxygenase-2 in synovial tissue and fluid of dysfunctional temporomandibular joints with internal derangement. J Oral Maxillofac Surg 2000;58:1229–1232.

73. Yoshida H, Fukumura Y, Fujita S, Nishida M, Iizuka T. The distribution of cyclooxygenase-1 in human temporomandibular joint samples: An immunohistochemical study. J Oral Rehabil 2001;28:511–516.

74. Shaftel SS, Olschowka JA, Hurley SD, Moore RH, O'Banion MK. COX-3: A splice variant of cyclooxygenase-1 in mouse neural tissue and cells. Brain Res Mol Brain Res 2003;119:213–215 [Erratum 2004;123:136].

75. Kis B, Snipes JA, Isse T, Nagy K, Busija DW. Putative cyclooxygenase-3 expression in rat brain cells. J Cereb Blood Flow Metab 2003;23:1287–1292.

76. Schwab JM, Beiter T, Linder JU, et al. COX-3—A virtual pain target in humans? FASEB J 2003;17:2174–2175.

77. Botting RM. Mechanism of action of acetaminophen: Is there a cyclooxygenase 3? Clin Infect Dis 2000;31(suppl 5):S202—S210.

78. Chandrasekharan NV, Dai H, Roos KL, et al. COX-3, a cyclooxygenase-1 variant inhibited by acetaminophen and other analgesic/antipyretic drugs: Cloning, structure, and expression. Proc Natl Acad Sci U S A 2002;99:13926–13931.

79. Schaible HG, Ebersberger A, Von Banchet GS. Mechanisms of pain in arthritis. Ann NY Acad Sci 2002;966:343–354.

80. Taiwo YO, Levine JD. Effects of cyclooxygenase products of arachidonic acid metabolism on cutaneous nociceptive threshold in the rat. Brain Res 1990;537:372–374.

81. Tashjian AH Jr, Voelkel EF, Lazzaro M, et al. Alpha and beta human transforming growth factors stimulate prostaglandin production and bone resorption in cultured mouse calvaria. Proc Natl Acad Sci U S A 1985;82:4535–4538.

82. Gay SW, Kosher RA. Prostaglandin synthesis during the course of limb cartilage differentiation in vitro. J Embryol Exp Morphol 1985;89:367–382.

83. Di Battista JA, Dore S, Martel-Pelletier J, Pelletier JP. Prostaglandin E_2 stimulates incorporation of proline into collagenase digestible proteins in human articular chondrocytes: Identification of an effector autocrine loop involving insulin-like growth factor I. Mol Cell Endocrinol 1996;123:27–35.

84. Goldring MB, Sohbat E, Elwell JM, Chang JY. Etodolac preserves cartilage-specific phenotype in human chondrocytes: Effects on type II collagen synthesis and associated mRNA levels. Eur J Rheumatol Inflamm 1990;10:10–21.

85. Evans AR, Junger H, Southall MD, et al. Isoprostanes, novel eicosanoids that produce nociception and sensitize rat sensory neurons. J Pharmacol Exp Ther 2000;293:912–920.

86. Basu S, Whiteman M, Mattey DL, Halliwell B. Raised levels of F(2)-isoprostanes and prostaglandin F(2alpha) in different rheumatic diseases. Ann Rheum Dis 2001;60:627–631.

87. Goodwin JS. Are prostaglandins proinflammatory, antiinflammatory, both or neither? J Rheumatol (suppl)1991;28:26–29.

88. Quinn JH, Bazan NG. Identification of prostaglandin E_2 and leukotriene B_4 in the synovial fluid of painful, dysfunctional temporomandibular joints. J Oral Maxillofac Surg 1990;48:968–971.

89. Garcia C, Boyce BF, Gilles J, et al. Leukotriene B_4 stimulates osteoclastic bone resorption both in vitro and in vivo. J Bone Miner Res 1996;11:1619–1627.

90. Flynn MA, Qiao M, Garcia C, Dallas M, Bonewald LF. Avian osteoclast cells are stimulated to resorb calcified matrices by and possess receptors for leukotriene B_4. Calcif Tiss Int 1999;64:154–159.

91. Garcia C, Qiao M, Chen D, et al. Effects of synthetic peptido-leukotrienes on bone resorption in vitro. J Bone Miner Re. 1996;11:521–529.

92. Shin J, Cho H, Hwang SW, et al. Bradykinin-12-lipoxygenase-VR1 signaling pathway for inflammatory hyperalgesia. Proc Natl Acad Sci U S A 2002;99:10150–10155.

93. Hwang SW, Cho H, Kwak J, et al. Direct activation of capsaicin receptors by products of lipoxygenases: Endogenous capsaicin-like substances. Proc Natl Acad Sci U S A 2000; 97:6155–6160.

94. Milam SB. Pathophysiology and epidemiology of the TMJ. J Musculoskel Neuron Interact 2003;3:382–390.

95. Luyten F. A scientific basis for the regeneration of synovial joints. Oral Surg Oral Med Oral Pathol Oral Radiol Endod 1997;83:167–169.

96. Thomas JT, Lin K, Nandedkar M, Camargo M, Cervenka J, Luyten FP. A human chondrodysplasia due to a mutation in a TGF-beta superfamily member. Nat Genet 1996;12: 315–317.

97. LeResche L, Saunders K, Von Korff MR, Barlow W, Dworkin SF. Use of exogenous hormones and risk of temporomandibular disorder pain. Pain 1997;69:153–160.

98. LeResche L. Epidemiology of temporomandibular disorders: Implications for the investigation of etiologic factors. Crit Rev Oral Biol Med 1997;8:291–305.

99. Abubaker AO, Raslan WF, Sotereanos GC. Estrogen and progesterone receptors in temporomandibular joint discs of symptomatic and asymptomatic persons: A preliminary study. J Oral Maxillofac Surg 1993;51:1096–1100.

100. Aufdemorte TB, Van Sickels JE, Dolwick MF, et al. Estrogen receptors in the temporomandibular joint of the baboon (Papio cynocephalus): An autoradiographic study. Oral Surg Oral Med Oral Pathol 1986;61:307–314.

101. Campbell JH, Courey MS, Bourne P, Odziemiec C. Estrogen receptor analysis of human temporomandibular disc. J Oral Maxillofac Surg 1993;51:1101–1105.

102. Ogata N, Koshizuka Y, Miura T, et al. Association of bone metabolism regulatory factor gene polymorphisms with susceptibility to ossification of the posterior longitudinal ligament of the spine and its severity. Spine 2002;27:1765–1771.

103. Kapila S, Xie Y. Targeted induction of collagenase and stromelysin by relaxin in unprimed and beta-estradiol-primed diarthrodial joint fibrocartilaginous cells but not in synoviocytes. Lab Invest 1998;78:925–938.

104. Abubaker AO, Hebda PC, Gunsolley JN. Effects of sex hormones on protein and collagen content of the temporomandibular joint disc of the rat. J Oral Maxillofac Surg 1996;54:721–727.

105. Carlsson GE, LeResche L. Epidemiology of temporomandibular disorders. In: Sessle BJ, Bryant PS, Dionnes R (eds). Temporomandibular Disorders and Related Pain Conditions. Progress in Pain Research and Management, vol 4. Seattle: IASP Press, 1995:211–226.

106. Von Korff M, Dworkin SF, LeResche L, Kruger A. An epidemiologic comparison of pain complaints. Pain 1988;32:173–183.

107. Bereiter DA. Sex differences in brainstem neural activation after injury to the TMJ region. Cells Tissues Organs 2001; 169:226–237.

108. Hathaway CB, Hu JW, Bereiter DA. Distribution of Fos-like immunoreactivity in the caudal brainstem of the rat following noxious chemical stimulation of the temporomandibular joint. J Comp Neurol 1995;356:444–456.

109. Bereiter DA, Bereiter DF. Morphine and NMDA receptor antagonism reduce c-fos expression in spinal trigeminal nucleus produced by acute injury to the TMJ region. Pain 2000;85:65–77.

110. Cleland LG, James MJ, Proudman SM. The role of fish oils in the treatment of rheumatoid arthritis. Drugs 2003;63: 845–853.

111. Cleland LG, James MJ, Proudman SM. Omega-6/omega-3 fatty acids and arthritis. World Rev Nutr Diet 2003;92:152–168.

112. Mantzioris E, Cleland LG, Gibson RA, Neumann MA, Demasi M, James MJ. Biochemical effects of a diet containing foods enriched with n-3 fatty acids. Am J Clin Nutr 2000;72:42–48.

113. James MJ, Gibson RA, Cleland LG. Dietary polyunsaturated fatty acids and inflammatory mediator production. Am J Clin Nutr 2000;71:343S–348S.

114. Cleland LG, Neumann MA, Gibson RA, Hamazaki T, Akimoto K, James MJ. Effect of dietary n-9 eicosatrienoic acid on the fatty acid composition of plasma lipid fractions and tissue phospholipids. Lipids 1996;31:829–837.

115. Xu L, Flahiff CM, Waldman BA, et al. Osteoarthritis-like changes and decreased mechanical function of articular cartilage in the joints of mice with the chondrodysplasia gene (cho). Arthr Rheum 2003;48:2509–2518.

116. Zubieta JK, Heitzeg MM, Smith YR, et al. *COMT* val158met genotype affects mu-opioid neurotransmitter responses to a pain stressor. Science 2003;299:1240–1243.

117. Jones MG, Munson JB, Thompson SW. A role for nerve growth factor in sympathetic sprouting in rat dorsal root ganglia. Pain 1999;79:21–29.

118. McLachlan EM, Hu P. Axonal sprouts containing calcitonin gene–related peptide and substance P form pericellular baskets around large diameter neurons after sciatic nerve transection in the rat. Neuroscience 1998;84:961–965.

119. Woolf CJ. Phenotypic modification of primary sensory neurons: The role of nerve growth factor in the production of persistent pain. Philos Trans R Soc Lond B Biol Sci 1996; 351:441–448.

120. Amann R, Schuligoi R, Herzeg G, Donnerer J. Intraplantar injection of nerve growth factor into the rat hind paw: Local edema and effects on thermal nociceptive threshold. Pain 1996;64:323–329.

121. Petty BG, Cornblath DR, Adornato BT, et al. The effect of systemically administered recombinant human nerve growth factor in healthy human subjects. Ann Neurol 1994;36:244–246.

122. Svensson P, Cairns BE, Wang K, Arendt-Nielsen L. Injection of nerve growth factor into human masseter muscle evokes long-lasting mechanical allodynia and hyperalgesia. Pain 2003;104:241–247.

123. Ramer M, Bisby M. Reduced sympathetic sprouting occurs in dorsal root ganglia after axotomy in mice lacking low-affinity neurotrophin receptor. Neurosci Lett 1997;228:9–12.

124. Ramer MS, Thompson SW, McMahon SB. Causes and consequences of sympathetic basket formation in dorsal root ganglia. Pain 1999;(suppl 6):S111–S120.

125. Indo Y. Genetics of congenital insensitivity to pain with anhidrosis (CIPA) or hereditary sensory and autonomic neuropathy type IV. Clinical, biological and molecular aspects of mutations in *TRKA(NTRK1)* gene encoding the receptor tyrosine kinase for nerve growth factor. Clin Auton Res 2002;12(suppl 1):I20–I32.

126. Houlden H, King RH, Hashemi-Nejad A, et al. A novel *TRKA* (*NTRK1*) mutation associated with hereditary sensory and autonomic neuropathy type V. Ann Neurol 2001;49:521–525.

127. Indo Y, Mardy S, Miura Y, et al. Congenital insensitivity to pain with anhidrosis (CIPA): Novel mutations of the *TRKA* (*NTRK1*) gene, a putative uniparental disomy, and a linkage of the mutant *TRKA* and *PKLR* genes in a family with CIPA and pyruvate kinase deficiency. Hum Mutat 2001;18:308–318.

128. Spillantini MG, Aloe L, Alleva E, De Simone R, Goedert M, Levi-Montalcini R. Nerve growth factor mRNA and protein increase in hypothalamus in a mouse model of aggression. Proc Natl Acad Sci U S A 1989;86:8555–8559.

129. Aloe L, Alleva E, Bohm A, Levi-Montalcini R. Aggressive behavior induces release of nerve growth factor from mouse salivary gland into the bloodstream. Proc Natl Acad Sci U S A 1986;83:6184–6187.

130. Aloe L, Bracci-Laudiero L, Alleva E, Lambiase A, Micera A, Tirassa P. Emotional stress induced by parachute jumping enhances blood nerve growth factor levels and the distribution of nerve growth factor receptors in lymphocytes. Proc Natl Acad Sci U S A 1994;91:10440–10444.

131. Lariviere WR, Melzack R. The role of corticotropin-releasing factor in pain and analgesia. Pain 2000;84:1–12.

132. Raber J. Detrimental effects of chronic hypothalamic-pituitary-adrenal axis activation. From obesity to memory deficits. Mol Neurobiol 1998;18:1–22.

133. Veenema AH, Meijer OC, de Kloet ER, Koolhaas JM. Genetic selection for coping style predicts stressor susceptibility. J. Neuroendocrinol 2003;15:256–267.

134. Wickline SA, Lanza GM. Nanotechnology for molecular imaging and targeted therapy. Circulation 2003;107:1092–5.

135. Mantyh PW, Rogers SD, Honore P, et al. Inhibition of hyperalgesia by ablation of lamina I spinal neurons expressing the substance P receptor. Science 1997;278:275–279.

136. Wiley RG, Lappi DA. Destruction of neurokinin-1 receptor expressing cells in vitro and in vivo using substance P-saporin in rats. Neurosci Lett 1997;230:97–100.

TMJ Disc Derangements

Boudewijn Stegenga and Lambert G. M. de Bont

In most classifications of temporomandibular disorders (TMDs), internal derangements are regarded as a separate category of intracapsular conditions.[1] However, although conceptually different, there is much overlap in the clinical course of temporomandibular joint (TMJ) disc derangements and osteoarthritis, and these two disorders are intimately related.[2] There is consensus that degenerative changes and mechanical derangements often occur concomitantly, but it is also recognized that each can occur separately in some patients. Several studies have also shown that degenerative changes in the articular surfaces may be present in a joint with a normal disc position.[3–5] However, overloading of the joint structures because of mechanically unfavorable occurrences can also lead to maladaptive changes in the joint surfaces (see chapters 1 and 7). In this chapter, possible mechanisms underlying disc derangements in the TMJ are discussed against the background of past and current research in this field.

Definition of Terms

The frequently used term *internal derangement* is an orthopedic term, defined as "a localized mechanical fault interfering with smooth joint movement."[6,7] The term *derangement* refers to a disarranged condition, focusing on a disturbance in mechanical operations—a joint that does not function as it should. Thus, *internal derangement* is a classification, not a diagnosis. For a diagnosis to be made, the structures that are deranged must be identified.

Those movement disturbances in which the articular disc plays a central role are referred to as *disc derangements* or *disc-interference disorders*.[8] Because the mechanical derangement is the central issue, this group of joint disorders is basically noninflammatory. Furthermore, derangement is basically a disturbance and, therefore, conceptually different from degeneration, in which normal tissue is converted into or replaced by tissue of an inferior quality. The latter occurs when adaptation is unsuccessful and is classified as *osteoarthrosis*. When inflammation and degeneration occur together, the condition is reclassified as an inflammatory degenerative disorder of the joint, ie, *osteoarthritis*.[8]

Although used widely, the term *disc displacement* is misleading. It implies that the disc previously was in a "normal" position, presumably with the posterior band positioned superior to the condyle in the so-called 12-o'clock position. However, disc positions that deviate from this "normal" position do not always induce clinical symptoms; consequently, strict adherence to the normal 12-o'clock criterion leads to overdiagnosis of disc derangements.[9] The concept that an anterior disc position associated with an otherwise healthy joint should be considered a normal variation is supported by many autopsy, clinical, and imaging studies in asymptomatic subjects and patients without a TMD.[4,10–19]

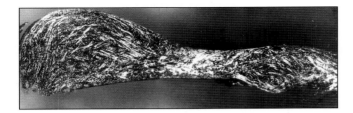

Fig 8-1 Sagittal section of a complete articular disc under polarized light. The posterior band is on the left. Note the different organizations and alignments of the collagen fibers throughout the tissue.

Structure and Function of the Disc and Retrodiscal Tissue

The disc consists of dense fibrous or fibrocartilaginous tissue with collagen fiber bundles running in all directions (Fig 8-1).[20] The inner layer consists mainly of anteroposteriorly oriented collagen fibers and leafletlike proteoglycans, whereas the superior and inferior surface layers consist mainly of anteroposteriorly and mediolaterally running collagen fibers and small proteoglycans.[21,22] Therefore, these layers are considered to have different biomechanical properties, which could lead to shear stress.[23] Another reason that local shear stress likely occurs in the disc during loading is that not all areas of the disc are deformed in the same direction, because the articular surfaces that compress the disc are not parallel to each other.[24,25] Shear stress can result in fatigue, damage, and plastic (irreversible) deformation of dense fibrous tissue or fibrocartilage.[26,27]

The collagen fiber network maintains the tensile strength in cartilage, while proteoglycans, with their hydrophilic glycosaminoglycan side chains, provide the tissue with an osmotic swelling pressure. A reduced glycosaminoglycan content of the cartilage is an early finding in the development of osteoarthritis in other joints.[28] The fibrocartilage of the disc has a relatively high content of collagen and a low content of glycosaminoglycans.[29] However, in osteoarthritic TMJs, the disc has been shown to contain a proportionally reduced content of glycosaminoglycans.[30]

The periphery of the disc is attached by a looser tissue to the capsule that encloses the joint, thereby separating it into upper and lower joint compartments (Fig 8-2).[31] Rees[32] described the retrodiscal tissue as having two laminae, hence the term *bilaminar zone*. It has been assumed for many years that the elastic tissue in the upper lamina serves to retract the disc back into the mandibular fossa when the mouth is closed. However, Osborn[24] pointed out that the elastic tissue helps to prevent the bilaminar

region from being trapped between the disc and eminence (and condyle) as the condyle-disc complex slides back on closing. This view is supported by the observations of Wilkinson and Crowley.[33] They found that, during condylar excursions, the tissue pressure is balanced by the movement of blood in and out of the venous plexus in the retrodiscal tissue (ie, the genu vasculosum or "vascular knee"), which expands to approximately four or five times its original volume on mouth opening so that a negative pressure arises within it.[33–35] This sets up a "pumping" mechanism that is of great importance for the joint's nutrition and lubrication and it remains largely intact even with displacement of the disc.[33]

On mouth opening and closing, the disc and condyle slide along the articular eminence (see Fig 8-2). The surface contours of these bony structures are not congruent, especially over the crest of the eminence.[36] Therefore, the fibrocartilage on the condyle and temporal bone is not well suited for load distribution or lubrication.[37] However, owing to its flexibility, the disc is able to distribute loads over these bony surfaces and to maintain relatively frictionless sliding between them, because its shape varies as it translates forward from the articular fossa to the convexity of the articular eminence.[38] Thus, the structural and mechanical integrity of the disc enable the joint to function smoothly.

The superior and inferior laminae of the retrodiscal tissue, the medial and lateral disc attachments to the condyle, and the shape of the discs provide stability for the disc. The morphology of the posterior band of the disc is especially important for the stability of the disc-condyle complex.[24,39–41] Of all parts of the disc, the posterior band has the greatest mechanical resistance.[42] However, deformation (eg, thickening or flattening, depending on the direction of loading) can occur with sustained loads.

Mandibular movement is characterized by a combination of rotation and translation. Although the rotation of the condyle occurs mainly in the lower joint space, it is

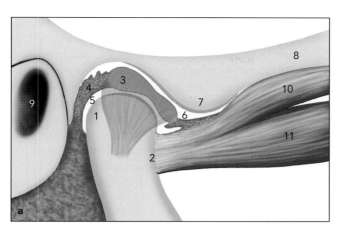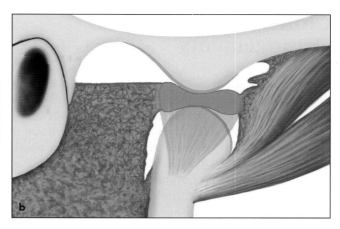

Fig 8-2 *(a)* Sagittal representation of the TMJ in a closed-mouth position. (1) Condylar head; (2) pterygoid fovea; (3) articular disc; (4) retrodiscal tissue; (5) lower joint compartment; (6) upper joint compartment; (7) articular eminence; (8) zygomatic arch; (9) ear canal; (10) lateral pterygoid muscle, upper head; (11) lateral pterygoid muscle, lower head. *(b)* Sagittal representation of the TMJ in an open-mouth position. (From Stegenga et al.[31] Reprinted with permission.)

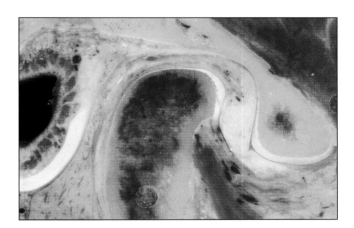

Fig 8-3 TMJ exhibiting disc derangement, evident overstretching of the retrodiscal tissue, and deformation of the disc.

accompanied by a translational component in the upper joint space.[43,44] The disc moves passively with the condyle, unfolding and stretching the predominantly elastic superior lamina of the retrodiscal tissue, which simultaneously rotates the disc in a posterior direction relative to the condyle. During closing, the predominantly ligamentous inferior lamina passively limits forward rotation of the disc on the condyle,[45,46] thus serving as a "check ligament."[8] Anterior disc displacement can only occur in the presence of an overstretched inferior lamina of the retrodiscal tissue, as was shown in an experimental study on fresh human postmortem material.[41] Thus, deformation of the posterior band, together with overstretching of the inferior lamina of the retrodiscal tissue, is necessary for the development of an anterior disc derangement (Fig 8-3). The superior stratum is less important in this respect.[41]

Clinical Course of Disc Derangements

Disc derangement is a commonly observed phenomenon, usually presenting classic clinical signs and symptoms: clicking (characteristic of a reducing disc derangement) and "closed lock" (characteristic of a permanent disc derangement).[7] The disc is usually displaced or dislocated in an anteromedial direction, but it may also occur in a lateral or posterior direction.[47,48] Disc derangements progress in several stages, from "disc displacement with reduction" to "disc displacement without reduction,"[49–51] in which not only the position of the disc but also its configuration is changing (see Figs 16-1 and 16-2 in chapter 16).[52]

The assumption of a progressive course has been based mainly on retrospective and cross-sectional studies. Lundh et al[53] showed that 9% of reducing disc derangements progressed to nonreducing disc derangement within 3 years. However, reducing disc displacements can also remain constant for many years.[54] That a clicking joint does not necessarily (or even usually) progress to locking has been suggested by several controlled studies[55–57] and supported by recent research addressing the natural course of events in TMJs with disc derangements. Sato et al,[58] for example, found that, in patients with reducing disc derangement who do not undergo treatment, the range of movement tends to increase over time, while joint pain fluctuates and clicking tends to persist.

In painful clicking joints, the glycosaminoglycan concentration (reduction of which is thought to be an early sign of osteoarthritis) is retained in both the disc and the retrodiscal tissue without any sign of degeneration of the matrix.[29] Thus, in patients with reducing disc derangement and pain, in spite of the changed load on the retrodiscal tissue, adaptation appears to be sufficient and degenerative changes do not appear to develop. Patients with permanent disc derangement, on the other hand, show reduction in the chondroitin sulfate concentration, which probably is the result of osteoarthritic degeneration.[29] This matrix degeneration is not confined to the discs but simultaneously involves its attachment in a way that may affect tissue function.[29] It can, therefore, be inferred that maladaptive alterations can weaken the posterior disc attachment, resulting in disc derangement.

It has been suggested that reducing disc derangements have a greater tendency to progress to nonreducing disc derangements when the posterior band of the disc shows considerable plastic deformation.[59] This deformation has been shown to occur mainly on the underside of the disc[60] and appears to be due to proliferation of the connective tissue on the disc surface,[61] which is thought to be caused by compressive loading of the displaced disc during condylar movement.[62] Lack of a normal relationship between the disc and the condyle has been suggested to be the most important factor in the initiation of disc deformation,[63] while variations in configuration of the deformed discs may be the result of differing loading conditions. In TMJs with a nonreducing disc, biconcave shapes, thickening of the posterior band, evenly thickened discs, and biconvex and folded shapes are found in almost equal numbers.[64]

A gradual flattening of the eminence has been suggested to reflect the progress of TMJ disc derangement from an early reducing stage to the more advanced nonreducing stage.[65] Contrary to what has been frequently assumed, it is not the steepness of the eminence that predisposes to disc derangement. Rather, osseous adaptive modeling changes occur in response to the derangement, increasing the steepness of the eminence.[65]

Kurita et al[66] followed the natural course of patients with permanent disc derangement over a 2.5-year period. About 75% improved (40% became spontaneously asymptomatic and 33% remained symptomatic but had fewer symptoms) while 25% experienced no alleviation of their symptoms. Those with radiographically visible and clinically detectable degenerative changes had a poorer prognosis. Several other studies have shown that, in the majority of patients with disc derangement without reduction, the signs and symptoms gradually resolve regardless of the type of treatment, or even without treatment.[67–69]

In joints with a permanent derangement, the disc may become immobile and remain in a nonfunctional anterior position. This seems to promote the development of fibrous adhesions in the superior joint compartment.[70,71] Furthermore, lack of movement influences the pumping action that delivers nutrients from the synovial fluid to the articular cartilage, which may induce or aggravate the degeneration.[72]

Proposed Etiologic Events

Some individuals are more prone to develop disc derangement than are others. Over the years, many etiologic factors have been proposed to explain the occurrence of disc derangement. For the disc to displace or dislocate, the functional capability of the ligaments that attach the disc to the condyle must be compromised by deterioration, elongation, or detachment. Usually, plastic deformation of the disc impairs its seating ability.

For many years, it was assumed that the superior head of the lateral pterygoid muscle actively pulls the disc anteriorly. It was therefore suggested that disc derangements are associated with spasm of this muscle.[73,74] The upper head of the lateral pterygoid muscle has its main insertion at the pterygoid fovea (see Fig 8-2),[46,75,76] but medial fibers may attach to the disc-capsule complex.[45,77] However, although the medial part of the disc develops as a condensation in the tendon of the superior head of the lateral pterygoid muscle,[78,79] only a few fibers, if any, have been shown to insert directly into the disc. The main function of this muscle is reflected by its relatively high proportion of low–stimulation threshold and fatigue-resistant fibers, indicating a continuous holding action with low levels of force.[80,81]

Trauma

Trauma is probably the most commonly mentioned cause of disc derangements. Macrotrauma to the joint usually results in soft tissue injury (stretching, tearing, laceration, or rupture) of the disc attachment, lateral ligament, or capsule. The immediate response is a traumatic arthritis and effusion resulting from increased vascular permeability or intra-articular bleeding following tissue rupture. The acute symptoms usually subside within a few days. However, bleeding can result in fibrosis and adhesions or the formation of intra-articular hyperplastic tissue,[82] leading to pain and restricted mobility. Common traumatic events include those that cause overextension of the mandible, such as prolonged maximal opening during a dental procedure, endotracheal intubation, or yawning.[83] Microtrauma (ie, repetitive small injuries) that causes a soft tissue response, such as plastic deformation of the ligaments,[39] may also lead to permanent intra-articular changes that can have long-term consequences. However, several studies have failed to confirm such a relationship.[83,84]

A relationship between indirect whiplash trauma and TMJ injuries has been suggested.[85,86] (see chapter 18). However, these studies illustrate the high prevalence of disc displacement in patients with TMJ symptoms rather than a relationship with whiplash trauma, because the prevalence of anteriorly positioned discs in these reports is similar to the prevalence in patients referred for magnetic resonance imaging who have no specific history of whiplash trauma.[84,87] It is, therefore, not surprising that a prospective study could not confirm such a relationship.[88]

Joint Laxity

It has also been proposed that lax joint ligaments are associated with disc derangements, which is supported by the following findings: Two thirds of TMJs with a reducing disc displacement are hypermobile, and two thirds of hypermobile TMJs have disc displacement with reduction.[89] Systemic joint laxity has been found to be significantly more prevalent in patients with TMJ disc displacement than in those with other types of TMD or in asymptomatic control subjects.[90] Altered collagen metabolism may also play a role in joint laxity,[90] and the collagen composition in TMJs with painful disc displacement and in asymptomatic joints has been found to differ.[91] However, the high prevalence of disc derangement does not parallel the prevalence of joint laxity in the general population. Moreover, Dijkstra et al[92] have shown that there is no significant relationship between TMJ mobility and peripheral joint mobility, nor do TMJ osteoarthrosis and internal derangement seem to be related to generalized joint hypermobility.[93]

Hormonal factors may also play a role in the development of disc displacement, as indicated by the female predominance of this condition.[94,95]

Bruxism

Bruxism has also been implicated as a factor in disc derangements. Such behavior results in compressive overloading, and it has been suggested that this overloading stimulates production of harmful oxidative radicals that are highly reactive and known to destroy hyaluronic acid, collagen, and proteglycans[96,97] (see chapter 7). Bruxism also has been suggested to be the causal factor for chondromalacia and subsequent internal derangements.[98] However, although bruxism is frequently associated with various TMDs, a causal relationship has not been demonstrated.[99]

Changes in Synovial Fluid and Joint Lubrication

Predisposition for the development of TMJ disc derangement is most probably associated with more than one etiologic factor. Whatever the etiologic factor (eg, trauma, bruxism, or otherwise), derangement of the TMJ disc seems to be associated with its inability to glide smoothly because of increased intra-articular friction.[38,40,100] This idea has recently been conceptualized by Nitzan.[101] Theoretically, the increase in friction may be caused by changes in the synovial fluid that affect the joint's lubrication and nutritional requirements and/or changes in the articulating surfaces.

The synovial membrane produces synovial fluid. This membrane lines the inner side of the joint capsule and disc, except the articulating surfaces. It consists of two layers: a discontinuous intima and the subsynovial tissue, which is richly supplied with blood vessels.[102] The synovial fluid provides the nutritional and metabolic needs for the articular tissues of the joint. It is also an important protector of the articular surfaces, largely by means of surface-active phospholipids.[103] The glycoprotein lubricin acts as a water-soluble carrier of surface-active phospholipids and contributes to the achievement of very low coefficients of friction.[104]

The hyaluronic acid in the synovial fluid has been assumed to keep the articular surfaces apart under low loads because of its high viscosity,[105] and degradation of hyaluronic acid likely reduces the viscosity of the synovial fluid. However, this does not appear to affect the efficiency of the synovial fluid as a lubricant.[106] Rather, it mainly impairs the protective function of the synovial fluid. Hyaluronic acid has recently been shown to adhere to the surface-active lipids and protect them from lysis by phospholipase A_2.[107]

The long-term health of a synovial joint depends on the effectiveness of the mechanisms that control stress in articular tissues and in which all joint structures are involved. The lubricating ability is dependent on the synovial membrane, the synovial fluid, the disc, and the fibrocartilage covering the bony joint components. Its ultrastructure indicates that fibrocartilage is a microporous tissue with a certain amount of permeability.[108] The synovial fluid can therefore move through the articular tissue of the condyle and eminence as well as the surface layer of the disc. The lower the permeability, the longer it takes for fluid exchange to occur and the stiffer the tissue is under compressive loads. Thus, the mechanical response of the articular tissues, including the disc, depends on the amount of permeability of these tissues.[109]

The combination of the surface structure of the articular and synovial tissues on the one hand, and an effective lubrication mechanism on the other, allows these tissue surfaces to move with negligible resistance; that is, the coefficient of friction is almost zero.[110] The lubrication mechanism is primarily dependent on the synovial fluid, of which hyaluronic acid is considered to be a major effective constituent.[111] Although the exact mechanism of joint lubrication remains to be established, a combination of weeping and boundary lubrication is the most reasonable model. *Weeping lubrication* is the process in which loading causes fluid to be squeezed out of the cartilage at the point of contact between the loaded surfaces.[112] As long as the cartilage is loaded, fluid continues to be squeezed out of the tissue. At low magnitudes of stress, however, the load is transferred to the phospholipid-glycoprotein *boundary lubricant* adhering to the cartilage surface.[113–115]

An important feature of weeping lubrication is the low initial friction, which increases with the duration of loading. With short-term loading (less than 2 minutes) and cyclic short-term loading, there is a high availability of fluid from the cartilage and this is accompanied by reduced friction.[116] However, a longer duration of loading increases the friction, because there is greater lateral fluid flow within the cartilage, leaving less fluid available to move to the surface where it can be used to recharge the "hydrostatic bearing."[117]

Another possible explanation is that the shear stress between the articular surfaces increases as the load increases,[27] because the frictional coefficient in the TMJ is presumably dependent on the shear behavior of the disc.[118] In a recent study, Tanaka et al[118] showed that the mean frictional coefficient in the TMJ after 5 seconds of loading with a compressive load of 50 N is 0.0145, which is within the range of frictional coefficients measured in other joints.[110,119] The frictional coefficient increased with an increase of the compressive load and with an increase of the period of stationary loading; after 60 minutes, the frictional coefficient was 1.25 to 1.50 times that measured after 5 seconds. After prolonged loading, lubrication by a fluid film between the articular surfaces is probably exhausted.

However, if the results reported by Tanaka et al[118] in the TMJ are compared with those reported in other synovial joints, the increase of the frictional coefficient with the increase in loading time in the TMJ is very small. This striking difference may be explained by the presence of the disc. The disc contains much water and is a viscoelastic structure, accounting for its flexibility and permitting it to function more or less as a fluid.[120] Tanaka et al,[118] therefore, suggest that the lubricating function in the TMJ is relatively stable, even with prolonged compression, compared to the lubricating function in joints without a disc.

Thus, the disc appears to be the principal factor in reducing surface friction. Friction on the surface of the condyle in the absence of the disc is at least three times greater than the friction measured with the disc in place.[37,116] The lubrication capabilities of the articular eminence are expected to be similar to those of the condyle but have not yet been established.

Mechanical Considerations

The surfaces of the articulating bones in the TMJ are highly incongruent. If the articular disc were absent, the contact area of the opposing articular surfaces would be very small. However, the disc is capable of deforming and adapting its shape to that of the condylar and temporal articular surfaces, and this ensures that TMJ loads are distributed over larger contact areas.[121,122]

During jaw movement, the disc moves along the articular surfaces of both the mandibular condyle and articular eminence with very low friction, thus minimizing shear stress along the disc.[123] However, when the synovial fluid degrades and its viscosity decreases, the boundary lubrication between the articular surfaces is reduced, resulting in an increase in the frictional coefficient.[101] Damage to the articulating surfaces influences the lubricating system and vice versa. As a consequence, knowledge of the frictional characteristics of the sliding surfaces and the synovial mechanism is of great importance for an understanding of the dynamics of the TMJ and of the onset of internal disc derangements.

Increased friction prevents the disc from sliding in conjunction with the condyle, which has been referred to as *disc hesitation*.[38] Repetitive disc hesitation gradually stretches the ligaments attaching the disc to the condyle, thus increasing disc mobility.[2,40] As explained in the previous section, the lubrication capacity becomes exhausted during sustained static loading, increasing friction considerably so that the disc adheres to the eminence.[124,125] However, because sustained static loading had only a relatively small effect on the frictional coefficient in the TMJ (owing to the presence of the disc),[118] other factors may be more likely to give rise to functional impairment.

The adaptive capacity of the joint structures is often exceeded by prolonged overloading, and the viscoelastic properties of the disc, which permit energy dissipation, are affected. While intermittent physiologic compressive loading has an anabolic effect on the joint structures, continuous compression of greater magnitude has a catabolic effect.[126] The subsequent change in the frictional characteristics of the articular surfaces induces increased shear stress in the disc, which in turn leads to fatigue and damage.

Osborn[24] formulated a hypothesis of disc failure based on an analysis of the biomechanical constraints in relation to the disc's shape, function, and stability. Without a disc, the articular tissues covering the bony joint components are distorted considerably when compressed because peak loads are increased. Thus, although the shape of the disc and its viscoelastic properties are important for stabilizing it on the condyle, an additional major function of the disc is to destabilize the condyle and in this way allow the disc-condyle assembly to slide under compressive loading.

Further, Osborn[24] showed that the disc is arguably squeezed off the condyle by compressive forces during jaw movements. When these forces cannot be resisted by the thickened edges of the disc, it prolapses; mechanically, this occurs in an anterior rather than in a posterior direction. Such compressive overloading generates free radicals, either directly or indirectly. This is due to the transient hypoxia that follows the increase of intra-articular pressure, disturbing synovial capillary perfusion, which is followed by reperfusion when stress is released.[127,128] If the adaptive capacity of the joint is intact, these radicals are controlled by the potent scavenging activity of the synovial joint fluid.[129] However, when the scavenging capacity is compromised or exceeded by increased production of free radicals, there are low levels of scavengers left in the synovial fluid.[130] As a result, the joint tissues and the lubrication mechanism are damaged.[97] For example, hyaluronic acid is degraded and its synthesis is inhibited by the action of free radicals. The resulting impairment of articular surface protection can result in both derangements and degeneration of the tissues involved (see chapter 7).

Clicking As the First Clinical Sign of Disc Derangement

Clicking is commonly accepted as the first clinical sign of TMJ disc derangement. At the same time, there is considerable controversy with regard to the diagnostic as well as the therapeutic aspects of clicking. It is striking that more joint sounds are detected clinically than are reported by patients.[131,132] Reducing disc derangement is the most common underlying cause of clicking. However, in about a quarter of patients with a clicking TMJ, magnetic resonance imaging shows a normal disc position.[133] Thus, there must be causes of clicking other than disc derangement. These include:

1. Clicking associated with condylar hypermobility[89]
2. Enlargement of the lateral pole of the condyle crossing the lateral ligament during movement,[134] causing a clicking sound at the same point of each active translatory movement, which diminishes when the same movement is carried out under compression
3. A structural irregularity on the articular eminence, eg, due to a developmental or growth disturbance, prior

trauma, or an abusive habit causing localized hypertrophy of the cartilage[4,5,8]

4. Loose intra-articular bodies other than the disc, such as in synovial chondromatosis

Conversely, about one third of asymptomatic patients have an anteriorly positioned disc.[12,18,84,87,133] Apparently, in these patients, the mandibular condyle slides off and back on the disc without any clicking.[135] These joints seem to be completely adapted and should, therefore, be considered a normal variant.[2,40]

Some forms of disc derangement can be associated with the formation of adhesions, most frequently occurring in the upper joint compartment.[70,136] As a compensatory mechanism, translation of the condyle frequently occurs in the lower compartment, which can be accompanied by clicking sounds. Adhesions that occur without disc derangement are recognized by a restriction of the protrusive range of movement.[137] Reproducibility of the previously mentioned clinical characteristics is a prerequisite for an accurate differential diagnosis.

Conclusion

It has been shown that the tissues in painful clicking TMJs can be viewed as quite similar to the tissues in normal joints.[29] This would imply that joints with reducing disc derangements usually do not display degenerative changes. However, Pereira et al,[5] among others, have shown that a considerable proportion of a group of young patients with normal TMJ disc position have degenerative changes on the articular surfaces. This indicates that causes of joint degeneration other than disc derangements play a role in such instances.

However, it cannot be denied that disc derangements can also be an important etiologic factor in degenerative joint disease. This is also supported by the observation that a sequence from painful clicking to closed lock is found in a smaller number of patients than is usually assumed.[57] Therefore, the conclusion can be drawn that patients with disc derangement are at risk of developing osteoarthritis. The factors that may play a role in determining the outcome of this risk have been discussed in this chapter.

Conversely, patients with degenerative changes in the joint's articular surfaces are at risk of developing disc derangements as a result of the changed frictional characteristics of the joint surfaces as well as insufficient joint lubrication. These risk factors have also been discussed in

this chapter. The common denominator seems to be the imbalance among such factors as joint loading (involving its magnitude, frequency, duration, and direction), the adaptive capacity of the tissues, and the adequacy of the joint's lubrication mechanism.

References

1. Kaplan AS. Classification. In: Kaplan AS, Assael LA. Temporomandibular Disorders. Diagnosis and Treatment. Philadelphia: Saunders, 1991.
2. Stegenga B. Osteoarthritis of the temporomandibular joint organ and its relationship to disc displacement. J Orofac Pain 2001;15:193–205.
3. de Bont LGM, Boering G, Liem RSB, Eulderink F, Westesson PL. Osteoarthrosis and internal derangement of the temporomandibular joint. A light microscopic study. J Oral Maxillofac Surg 1986;44:634–643.
4. Pereira FJ Jr, Lundh H, Westesson PL, Carlsson LE. Clinical findings related to morphologic changes in TMJ autopsy specimens. Oral Surg Oral Med Oral Pathol Oral Radiol Endod 1994;78:288–295.
5. Pereira FJ Jr, Lundh H, Westesson PL. Morphologic changes in the temporomandibular joint in different age groups. An autopsy investigation. Oral Surg Oral Med Oral Pathol Oral Radiol Endod 1994;78:279–287.
6. Adams JC, Hamblen DL. Outline of Orthopedics, ed 11. Edinburgh: Churchill Livingstone, 1990.
7. Stegenga B. Temporomandibular joint degenerative diseases: Clinical diagnosis. In: Stegenga B, de Bont LGM (eds). Management of Temporomandibular Joint Degenerative Diseases: Biologic Basis and Treatment Outcome. Basel: Birkhäuser, 1996.
8. Bell WE. Temporomandibular Disorders. Classification, Diagnosis, Management, ed 3. Chicago: Year Book, 1990.
9. Dijkgraaf LC, de Bont LGM, Otten E, Boering G. Three-dimensional visualization of the temporomandibular joint: A computerized multisectional autopsy study of disc position and configuration. J Oral Maxillofac Surg 1992;50:2–10.
10. Hellsing G, Holmlund A. Development of anterior disc displacement in the temporomandibular joint: An autopsy study. J Prosthet Dent 1985;53:397–401.
11. Turell J, Ruiz HG. Normal and abnormal findings in temporomandibular joints in autopsy specimens. J Orofac Pain 1987;1:257–275.
12. Kircos LT, Ortendahl DA, Mark AS, Arakawa M. Magnetic resonance imaging of the TMJ disc in asymptomatic volunteers. J Oral Maxillofac Surg 1987;45:852–854.
13. Westesson PL, Eriksson L, Kurita K. Reliability of a negative clinical temporomandibular joint examination: Prevalence of disc displacement in asymptomatic temporomandibular joints. Oral Surg Oral Med Oral Pathol Oral Radiol Endod 1989;68:551–554.

14. Drace JE, Enzmann DR. Defining the normal temporomandibular joint: Closed, partially open and open mouth MR imaging of asymptomatic subjects. Radiology 1990; 177:67–71.

15. Lundh H, Westesson PL. Clinical signs of temporomandibular joint internal derangement in adults. An epidemiologic study. Oral Surg Oral Med Oral Pathol Oral Radiol Endod 1991;72:637–641.

16. Tallents RH, Hatala M, Katzberg RW, Westesson PL. Temporomandibular joint sounds in asymptomatic volunteers. J Prosthet Dent 1993;69:298–304.

17. Romanelli GG, Harper R, Mock D, Pharoah MJ, Tenenbaum HC. Evaluation of temporomandibular joint internal derangement. J Orofac Pain 1993;7:254–262.

18. Tallents RH, Katzberg RW, Murphy W, Proskin H. Magnetic resonance imaging findings in asymptomatic volunteers and symptomatic patients with temporomandibular disorders. J Prosthet Dent 1996;75:529–533.

19. Morrow D, Tallents RH, Katzberg RW, Murphy WC, Hart TC. Relationship of other joint problems and anterior disc position in symptomatic TMD patients and in asymptomatic volunteers. J Orofac Pain 1996;10:15–20.

20. de Bont LGM, Liem RSB, Havinga P, Boering G. Fibrous component of the temporomandibular joint disc. Cranio 1985;3:368–373.

21. Nakano T, Scott PG. Changes in the chemical composition of the bovine temporomandibular joint disc with age. Arch Oral Biol 1996;41:845–853.

22. Minarelli AM, Del Santo Junior M, Liberti EA. The structure of the human temporomandibular joint disc: A scanning electron microscopic study. J Orofac Pain 1997;11:95–100.

23. Mizoguchi I, Scott PG, Dodd CM, et al. An immunohistochemical study of the localization of biglycan, decorin and large chondroitin-sulphate proteoglycan in adult rat temporomandibular joint disc. Arch Oral Biol 1998;43:889–898.

24. Osborn JW. The disc of the human temporomandibular joint: Design, function and failure. J Oral Rehabil 1985;12:279–293.

25. Tanaka E, Kawai N, Hanaoka K, et al. Shear properties of the temporomandibular joint disc in relation to compressive and shear strain. J Dent Res 2004;83:476–479.

26. Spirt AA, Mak AF, Wassell RP. Nonlinear viscoelastic properties of articular cartilage in shear. J Orthop Res 1989;7:43–49.

27. Zhu Q, Mow VC, Koob TJ, Eyre DR. Viscoelastic shear properties of articular cartilage and the effects of glycosidase treatments. J Orthop Res 1993;11:771–781.

28. Hamerman D. The biology of osteoarthritis. N Engl J Med 1989;320:1322–1330.

29. Paegle DI, Holmlund A, Hjerpe A. Matrix glycosaminoglycans in the temporomandibular joint in patients with painful clicking and chronic closed lock. Int J Oral Maxillofac Surg 2003;32:397–400.

30. Axelsson S, Holmlund A, Hjerpe A. Glycosaminoglycans in normal and osteoarthrtitic human temporomandibular joint discs. Acta Odontol Scand 1992;50:113–119.

31. Stegenga B, Vissink A, de Bont LGM. Mondziekten en kaakchirurgie. Assen, The Netherlands: Van Gorcum, 2000.

32. Rees LA. Structure and function of the mandibular joint. Br Dent J 1954;96:125–133.

33. Wilkinson TM, Crowley CM. A histologic study of retrodiscal tissues of the human temporomandibular joint in the open and closed position. J Orofac Pain 1994;8:7–17.

34. Roth TE, Goldberg JS, Behrents RG. Synovial fluid pressure determination in the temporomandibular joint. Oral Surg Oral Med Oral Pathol Oral Radiol Endod 1984;57:583–588.

35. Ward DM, Behrents RG, Goldberg JS. Temporomandibular joint synovial fluid pressure response to altered mandibular positions. Am J Orthod Dentofac Orthop 1990;98:22–28.

36. Nickel JC, McLachlan KR. An analysis of surface congruity in the growing human temporomandibular joint. Arch Oral Biol 1994;39:315–321.

37. Nickel JC, McLachlan KR. A comparison of the lubrication properties of the mandibular condyle and TMJ disc [abstract 1619]. J Dent Res 1994;73:304.

38. Ogus HD, Toller PA. Common disorders of the temporomandibular joint. Bristol: Wright, 1981.

39. Isberg AM, Isacsson G. Tissue reactions of the temporomandibular joint following retrusive guidance of the mandible. Cranio 1986;4:143–148.

40. Stegenga B, de Bont LGM, Boering G, van Willigen JD. Tissue responses to degenerative changes in the temporomandibular joint. J Oral Maxillofac Surg 1991;49:1079–1088.

41. Eriksson L, Westesson PL, Macher D, Hicks D, Tallents RH. Creation of disc displacement in human temporomandibular joint autopsy specimens. J Oral Maxillofac Surg 1992; 50:869–873.

42. Mills DK, Daniel JC, Herzog S, Scapino RP. An animal model for studying mechanisms in human temporomandibular joint disc derangement. J Oral Maxillofac Surg 1994;52:1279–1292.

43. Merlini L, Palla S. The relationship between condylar rotation and anterior translation in healthy and clicking temporomandibular joints. Schweiz Monatsschr Zahnmed 1988;98:1191–1199.

44. Ferrario VF, Sforza C, Miani A Jr, Serrao G, Tartaglia G. Open-close movements in the human temporomandibular joint: Does a pure rotation around the intercondylar hinge axis exist? J Oral Rehabil 1996;23:401–408.

45. Carpentier P, Yung JP, Bonnet S. Insertions of the lateral pterygoid muscle: An anatomical study of the temporomandibular joint. J Oral Maxillofac Surg 1988;46:477–482.

46. Luder HU, Bobst P. Wall architecture and disc attachment of the human temporomandibular joint. Schweiz Montsschr Zahnmed 1991;101:557–570.

47. Kurita K, Westesson PL, Tasaki M, Liedberg J. Temporomandibular joint: Diagnosis of medial and lateral disc displacement with anteroposterior arthrography. Correlation with cryosections. Oral Surg Oral Med Oral Pathol Oral Radiol Endod 1992;73:364–368.

48. Westesson PL, Larheim TA, Tanaka H. Posterior disc displacement in the temporomandibular joint. J Oral Maxillofac Surg 1998;56:1266–1273.

49. Rasmussen OC. Description of population and progress of symptoms in a longitudinal study of temporomandibular arthropathy. Scand J Dent Res 1981;89:196–203.

50. Wilkes CH. Internal derangement of the TMJ: Pathologic variations. Arch Otolaryngol Head Neck Surg 1989;115:39–54.

51. de Leeuw R, Boering G, Stegenga B, de Bont LGM. Temporomandibular joint osteoarthrosis: Clinical and radiographic characteristics 30 years after nonsurgical treatment. Cranio 1993;11:15–24.

52. Westesson PL, Bronstein SL, Liedberg J. Internal derangement of the temporomandibular joint: Morphologic description with correlation to joint function. Oral Surg Oral Med Oral Pathol Oral Radiol Endod 1985;59:323–331.

53. Lundh H, Westesson PL, Kopp S. A three-year follow-up of patients with reciprocal temporomandibular joint clicking. Oral Surg Oral Med Oral Pathol Oral Radiol Endod 1987;63:530–533.

54. Farrar WB, McCarty WJ. A Clinical Outline of Temporomandibular Joint Diagnosis and Treatment. Montgomery, AL: Normandie, 1982.

55. Lundh H, Westesson PL, Kopp S, et al. Anterior repositioning splint in the treatment of temporomandibular joints with reciprocal clicking: Comparison with a flat occlusal splint and an untreated control group. Oral Surg Oral Med Oral Pathol Oral Radiol Endod 1985;60:131–136.

56. Wänman A, Agerberg G. Temporomandibular joint sounds in adolescents: A longitudinal study. Oral Surg Oral Med Oral Pathol Oral Radiol Endod 1990;69:2–9

57. Könönen M, Waltimo A, Nyström M. Does clicking in adolescence lead to painful temporomandibular joint locking? Lancet 1996;347:1080–1081.

58. Sato S, Goto S, Nasu F, Motegi K. Natural course of disc displacement with reduction of the temporomandibular joint: Changes in clinical signs and symptoms. J Oral Maxillofac Surg 2003;61:32–34.

59. Westesson PL, Lundh H. Arthrographic and clinical characteristics of patients with disc displacement who progressed to closed lock during a six month period. Oral Surg Oral Med Oral Pathol Oral Radiol Endod 1989;67:654–657.

60. Kondoh T, Westesson PL, Takahashi T, Seto K. Prevalence of morphological changes in the surfaces of the temporomandibular joint disc associated with internal derangement. J Oral Maxillofac Surg 1998;56:339–343.

61. Kurita K, Westesson PL, Sternby NH, et al. Histologic features of the temporomandibular joint and posterior disc attachment: Comparison of symptom-free persons with normally positioned discs and patients with internal derangement. Oral Surg Oral Med Oral Pathol Oral Radiol Endod 1989;67:635–643.

62. Murakami S, Takahashi A, Nishiyama H, et al. Magnetic resonance evaluation of the temporomandibular joint disc position and configuration. Dentomaxillofac Radiol 1993;22:205–207.

63. Hamada Y, Kondoh T, Sekiya H, Seto K. Morphologic changes in the unloaded temporomandibular joint after mandibulectomy. J Oral Maxillofac Surg 2003;61:437–441.

64. Sato S, Sakamoto M, Kawamura H, et al. Long-term changes in clinical signs and symptoms and disc position and morphology in patients with nonreducing disc displacement in the temporomandibular joint. J Oral Maxillofac Surg 1999;57:23–29.

65. Ren YF, Isberg A, Westesson PL. Steepness of the articular eminence in the temporomandibular joint: Tomographic comparison between asymptomatic volunteers with normal disc position and patients with disc displacement. Oral Surg Oral Med Oral Pathol Oral Radiol Endod 1995;80:258–266.

66. Kurita K, Westesson PL, Yuasa H, Toyoma M, Machida J, Ogi N. Natural course of untreated symptomatic temporomandibular joint disc displacement without reduction. J Dent Res 1998;77:361–365.

67. Sato S, Goto S, Kawamura H, Motegi K. The natural course of nonreducing disc displacement of the TMJ: Relationship of clinical findings at initial visit to outcome after 12 months without treatment. J Orofac Pain 1997;11:315–320.

68. Sato S, Kawamura H, Nagasaka H, Motegi K. The natural course of anterior disc displacement without reduction in the temporomandibular joint: Follow-up at 6, 12 and 18 months. J Oral Maxillofac Surg 1997;55:234–239.

69. Minakuchi H, Kuboki T, Matsuka Y, Maekawa K, Yantani H, Yamashita A. Randomized controlled evaluation of non-surgical treatments for temporomandibular joint anterior disc displacement without reduction. J Dent Res 2001;80:924–928.

70. Bewyer DC. Biomechanical and physiological processes leading to internal derangement with adhesions. J Orofac Pain 1989;3:44–49.

71. Hamada Y, Kondoh T, Kamei K, Seto K. Disc mobility and arthroscopic condition of the temporomandibular joint associated with long-term mandibular discontinuity. J Oral Maxillofac Surg 2001;59:1002–1005.

72. Ellis E, Carlson DS. The effects of mandibular immobilization on the masticatory system. A review. Clin Plast Surg 1989;16:133–146.

73. Juniper RP. Temporomandibular joint dysfunction: A theory based upon electromyographic studies of the lateral pterygoid muscle. Br J Oromaxillofac Surg 1984;22:1–8.

74. Liu ZJ, Wang HV, Pu WY. A comparative electromyography of the lateral pterygoid muscle and arthrography in patients with TMJ disturbance syndrome sounds. J Prosthet Dent 1989;62:229–233.

75. Wilkinson TM. The relationship between the disc and lateral pterygoid muscle in the human temporomandibular joint. J Prosthet Dent 1988;60:715–724.

76. Naidoo LC, Juniper RP. Morphometric analysis of the insertion of the upper head of the lateral pterygoid muscle. Oral Surg Oral Med Oral Pathol Oral Radiol Endod 1997;83:441–446.

77. White LW. The lateral pterygoid muscle: Fact and fiction. J Clin Orthod 1985;19:584–587.

78. Moffett BC. Histologic aspects of temporomandibular joint derangements. In: Moffett BC, Westesson PL. Diagnosis of Internal Derangements of the Temporomandibular Joint. Vol 1: Double-Contrast Arthrography and Clinical Correlation. Seattle: University of Washington Continuing Dental Education, 1984:27.

79. Perry HT, Xu Y, Forbes DP. The embryology of the temporomandibular joint. Cranio 1985;3:125–132.

80. Eriksson PO, Eriksson A, Ringqvist M, Tornell LE. Special histochemical muscle-fibre characteristics of the human lateral pterygoid muscle. Arch Oral Biol 1981;26:495–507.

81. Mao J, Stein JW, Osborn JW. The size and distribution of fiber types in jaw muscles: A review. J Orofac Pain 1992;6:192–201.

82. Isberg A, Isacsson G, Johansson AS, Larson O. Hyperplastic soft tissue formation in the temporomandibular joint associated with internal derangement. Oral Surg Oral Med Oral Pathol Oral Radiol Endod 1986;61:32–38.

83. Isacsson G, Linde C, Isberg A. Subjective symptoms in patients with temporomandibular disc displacement versus patients with myogenic craniomandibular disorders. J Prosthet Dent 1989;61:70–71.

84. Katzberg RW, Westesson PL, Tallents RH, Drake CM. Anatomic disorders of the temporomandibular joint disc in asymptomatic subjects. J Oral Maxillofac Surg 1996;54:147–153.

85. Pressman BD, Shellock FG, Schames J, Schames M. MR imaging of temporomandibular joint abnormalities associated with cervical hyperextension/hyperflexion (whiplash) injuries. J Magn Reson Imaging 1992;2:569–574.

86. Garcia R Jr, Arrington JA. The relationship between cervical whiplash and temporomandibular joint injuries: An MRI study. Cranio 1996;14:233–239.

87. Tasaki MM, Westesson PL, Isberg AM, Ren YF, Tallents RH. Classification and prevalence of temporomandibular joint disc displacement in patients and symptom-free volunteers. Am J Orthod Dentofac Orthop 1996;109;249–626.

88. Bergman H, Andersson F, Isberg A. Incidence of temporomandibular joint changes after whiplash trauma: A prospective study using MR imaging. AJR Am J Roentgenol 1998;171:1237–1243.

89. Johansson AS, Isberg A. The anterosuperior insertion of the temporomandibular joint capsule and condylar mobility in joints with and without internal derangement: A double-contrast arthrotomographic investigation. J Oral Maxillofac Surg 1991;49:1142–1148.

90. Westling L. Temporomandibular joint dysfunction and systemic joint laxity. Swed Dent J Suppl 1992;81:1–79.

91. Pereira FJ, Lundh H, Eriksson L, Westesson PL. Microscopic changes in the retrodiscal tissues of painful temporomandibular joints. J Oral Maxillofac Surg 1996;54:461–468.

92. Dijkstra PU, de Bont LGM, van der Weele LT, Boering G. The relationship between temporomandibular joint mobility and peripheral joint mobility reconsidered. Cranio 1994;12:149–155.

93. Dijkstra PU. Temporomandibular Joint Osteoarthrosis and Joint Mobility [thesis]. Groningen, The Netherlands: University of Groningen, 1993.

94. Isberg A, Hágglund M, Paesani D. The effect of age and gender on the onset of symptomatic temporomandibular joint disc displacement. Oral Surg Oral Med Oral Pathol Oral Radiol Endod 1998;85:252–276.

95. LeResche L. Epidemiology of temporomandibular disorders: Implications for the investigation of etiologic factors. Crit Rev Oral Biol Med 1997;8:291–305.

96. Milam SB. Articular disc displacement and degenerative temporomandibular joint disease. In: Sessle BJ, Bryant PS, Dionne RS (eds). Temporomandibular Disorders and Related Pain Conditions. Progress in Pain Research and Management, vol 4. Seattle: IASP Press, 1995:89–112.

97. Milam SB, Zardeneta G, Schmitz JP. Oxidative stress and degenerative temporomandibular joint disease: A proposed hypothesis. J Oral Maxillofac Surg 1998;56:214–223.

98. Quinn JH. Pathogenesis of temporomandibular joint chondromalacia and arthralgia. Oral Maxillofac Surg Clin North Am 1989;1:47–57.

99. Lobbezoo F, Lavigne GJ. Do bruxism and temporomandibular disorders have a cause-and-effect relationship? J Orofac Pain 1997;11–23.

100. Ogus HD. The mandibular joint: Internal rearrangement. Br J Oral Maxillofac Surg 1987;25:218–226.

101. Nitzan DW. The process of lubrication impairment and its involvement in temporomandibular joint disc displacement: A theoretical concept. J Oral Maxillofac Surg 2001;59:36–45.

102. Dijkgraaf LC, de Bont LGM, Boering G, Liem RSB. The structure of the normal synovial membrane of the temporomandibular joint. A review of the literature and a study of synovial membrane of clinically normal TMJs of oncology patients. J Oral Maxillofac Surg 1996;54:332–338.

103. Hills BA, Thomas K. Joint stiffness and 'articular gelling': Inhibition of the fusion of articular surfaces by surfactant. Br J Rheumatol 1998;37:532–538.

104. Hills BA. Synovial surfactant and the hydrophobic articular surface. J Rheumatol 1996;23:1323–1325.

105. Mow VC, Ateshian GA. Lubrication and wear of diarthrodial joints. In: Mow VC, Hayes WC (eds): Basis Orthopedic Biomechanics, ed 2. Philadelphia, Lippincott-Raven, 1977.

106. Swann DA, Radin EL, Nazimiec M, et al. Role of hyaluronic acid in joint lubrication. Ann Rheum Dis 1974;33:318–326.

107. Nitzan DW, Nitzan U, Dan P, Yedgar S. The role of hyaluronic acid in protecting surface active phospholipids from lysis by exogenous phospholipase A_2. Rheumatology 2001;40:336–340.

108. de Bont LGM, Liem RSB, Boering G. Ultrastructure of the articular cartilage of the mandibular condyle: Aging and degeneration. Oral Surg Oral Med Oral Pathol Oral Radiol Endod 1985;60:631–641.

109. Beek M, Koolstra JH, van Ruijven LJ, van Eijden TM. Three-dimensional finite element analysis of the cartilaginous structures in the human temporomandibular joint. J Dent Res 2001;80:1913–1918.

110. Forster H, Fisher J. The influence of continuous sliding and subsequent surface wear on the friction of articular cartilage. Proc Inst Mech Eng 1999;213:329–345.

111. Mabuchi K, Tsukamoto Y, Obara T, Yamaguchi T. The effect of additive hyaluronic acid on animal joints with experimentally reduced lubricating ability. J Biomed Mater Res 1994;28:865–870.

112. McCutchen CW. Lubrication of and by articular cartilage. In: Hall BK (ed). Cartilage: Biomedical Aspects, ed 9. New York: Academic Press, 1983:87–107.

113. Swann DA, Hendren RB, Radin EL, Sotman SL, Duda EA. The lubricating activity of synovial fluid glycoproteins. Arthritis Rheum 1981;24:22–30.

114. Hills BA, Butler BD. Surfactants identified in synovial fluid and their ability to act as boundary lubricants. Ann Rheum Dis 1984;43:641–648.

115. Hatton MN, Swann DA. Studies on bovine temporomandibular joint synovial fluid. J Prosthet Dent 1986;56:635–638.

116. Nickel JC, McLachlan KR. In vitro measurement of the frictional properties of the temporomandibular joint disc. Arch Oral Biol 1994;39:323–331.

117. Nickel JC, Iwasaki LR, Feely DE, Stormberg KD, Beatty MW. The effect of disc thickness and trauma on disc surface friction in the porcine temporomandibular joint. Arch Oral Biol 2001;46:155–162.

118. Tanaka E, Kawai N, Tanaka M, et al. The frictional coefficient of the temporomandibular joint and its dependency on the magnitude and duration of joint loading. J Dent Res 2004;83:404–407.

119. Forster H, Fisher J. The influence of loading time and lubricant on the friction of articular cartilage. Proc Inst Mech Eng 1996;210:109–119.

120. Tanaka E, van Eijden T. Biomechanical behaviour of the temporomandibular joint disc. Crit Rev Oral Biol Med 2003;14:138–150.

121. Tanne K, Tanaka E, Sakuda M. The elastic modulus of the temporomandibular joint disc from adult dogs. J Dent Res 1991;70:1545–1548.

122. Scapino RP, Canham PB, Finlay HM, Mills DK. The behaviour of collagen fibers in stress relaxation and stress distribution in the jaw-joint disc of rabbits. Arch Oral Biol 1996;41:1039–1052.

123. Nickel JC, McLachlan KR. In vitro measurement of the stress-distribution properties of the pig temporomandibular joint disc. Arch Oral Biol 1994;39:439–448.

124. Rao VM, Liem MD, Farole A, Razek AA. Elusive 'stuck' disc in the temporomandibular joint: Diagnosis with MR imaging. Radiology 1993;189:823–827.

125. Nitzan DW, Marmary Y. The 'anchored disc phenomenon': A proposed etiology for sudden onset, severe and persistent closed lock of the TMJ. J Oral Maxillofac Surg 1997;55:797–802.

126. Burger EH, Klein-Nulend J, Veldhuijzen JP. Mechanical stress and osteogenesis in vitro. J Bone Miner Res 1992;7:S397–S401.

127. Nitzan DW. Intra-articular pressure in the functioning temporomandibular joint and its alterations by uniform elevation of the occlusal plane. J Oral Maxillofac Surg 1984;52:671–679.

128. Blake DR, Merry P, Unsworth J, et al. Hypoxic-reperfusion injury in the inflamed human joint. Lancet 1989;1(8633):289–293.

129. Sato H, Takahashi T, Ide H, et al. Antioxidant activity of synovial fluid, hyaluronic acid and two subcomponents of hyaluronic acid. Synovial fluid scavenging effect is enhanced in rheumatoid arthritis patients. Arthritis Rheum 1988;31:63–71.

130. Takahashi T, Kondo T, Kamei K, et al. Elevated levels of nitric oxide in synovial fluid from patients with temporomandibular disorders. Oral Surg Oral Med Oral Pathol Oral Radiol Endod 1996;82:505–509.

131. Sadowsky NA, Muhl ZF, Sakols EI, Sommerville JM. Temporomandibular joint sounds related to orthodontic therapy. J Dent Res 1985;64:1392–1395.

132. Hardison JD, Okeson JP. Comparison of three clinical techniques for evaluating joint sounds. Cranio 1990;8:307–311.

133. Davant TS, Greene CS, Perry HT, Lautenslager EP. A quantitative computer-assisted analysis of disc displacement in patients with internal derangement using sagittal view magnetic resonance imaging. J Oral Maxillofac Surg 1993;51:974–979.

134. Griffin CJ. The prevalence of the lateral subcondylar tubercle of the mandible in fossil and recent man with particular reference to Anglo-Saxons. Arch Oral Biol 1977;22:633–639.

135. Isberg A. Temporomandibular Joint Dysfunction. A Practitioner's Guide. London: Martin Dunitz, 2001.

136. Montgomery MT, Van Sickels JE, Harms SE, Trash WJ. Arthroscopic TMJ surgery: Effects on signs, symptoms and disc position. J Oral Maxillofac Surg 1989;47:1263–1271.

137. Holmlund AB, Axelsson S. Temporomandibular arthropathy: Correlation between clinical signs and symptoms and arthroscopic findings. Int J Oral Maxillofac Surg 1996;25:178–181.

Systemic Conditions Affecting the TMJ

Mauno Könönen and Bengt Wenneberg

More than 100 heterogenous acute and chronic conditions, some with multisystem involvement, can affect the musculoskeletal system. Clinically, the most important of these conditions that affect the temporomandibular joint (TMJ) complex are the systemic diseases of the musculoskeletal system and the systemic connective tissue disorders. This chapter focuses on the less common of these diseases and disorders: Sjögren syndrome (SS); ankylosing spondylitis (AS); psoriatic arthritis (PA); Reiter syndrome (RS), also known as *reactive arthritis*; systemic lupus erythematosus (SLE); scleroderma; mixed connective tissue disease (MCTD); gout; and calcium pyrophosphate deposition disease (CPDD). The more common systemic diseases affecting the TMJ, namely seropositive rheumatoid arthritis and juvenile rheumatoid arthritis, are discussed in chapter 15.

Sjögren Syndrome

Sjögren syndrome is a systemic autoimmune disease of unknown etiology and pathogenesis leading to xerostomia and dry eyes. These "sicca" ("dry") symptoms result from an autoimmune process that often may affect other organs, such as neural systems, skin, mucosa, lungs, and kidneys. SS also can develop as a secondary phenomenon, in which the sicca symptoms are associated with rheumatoid arthritis (RA), SLE, or scleroderma.

Epidemiology

The prevalence of primary SS, judging from blood donor subjects, has been estimated to be 0.08%.

TMJ Involvement

SS is sometimes associated with polyarthritis, and thus the TMJ may also be affected.

Spondyloarthritides

A group of five seronegative rheumatoid diseases are called *spondyloarthritides* or *spondyloarthropathies*: AS, PA, RS, spondylitis of inflammatory bowel disease, and undifferentiated spondyloarthropathy. These disorders can show close clinical, epidemiologic, and genetic relationships.[1–3] Consideration of these disorders as a nosologic family is based on their tendency to share a number of clinical, pathologic, and radiographic features. Thus, many patients at some time possess features of any or all of these seronegative rheumatic diseases.

The prevalence of the spondyloarthropathies varies in different populations in close relationship with the genetic marker of these diseases, HLA-B27 (Table 9-1). AS and RS in particular have been associated with HLA-B27;

| Table 9-1 | Frequency of the HLA-B27 phenotype* in different populations |

Population	Frequency (%) of HLA-B27
Western Canadian (Haida Indian)	50
Finnish	12–18
Northern Scandinavian	10–16
Central European (Slavic)	7–14
Western European	6–9
Southern European	2–6
Middle Eastern (Arab, Jewish, Iranian)	3–5
African American	3–4
African	1
Japanese	1

*Genetic marker of spondyloarthropathies.

whereas PA is associated with the presence of HLA-B27 only in those patients with spondylitis.

The spondyloarthropathies can also involve the TMJ and masticatory muscles, causing symptoms in the head, face, and jaws.[4]

Ankylosing Spondylitis

Ankylosing spondylitis is a rheumatic disease characterized by inflammatory stiffening of the spine and arthritis of the sacroiliac joints. It varies from episodes of back pain throughout life to a severe disease that attacks the spine and peripheral joints, resulting in severe joint and back stiffness, loss of motion, and deformity. AS is an ancient disease dating back to Egyptian mummies that show typical spinal calcifications.

Epidemiology

The prevalence of AS varies greatly in different populations investigated, ranging from less than 1% to 6%. In white populations, the prevalence of AS appears to be about 1%. A strong association between AS and HLA-B27 has been described and confirmed throughout the world. Previously it was believed that AS is predominantly a male disease, because in surveys the sex ratio varied from 10:1 to 3.3:1, but recent epidemiologic research suggests an almost even sex distribution. However, AS is more severe and more joints are affected in males.[5]

Sacroiliac and spinal disease develops around the age of 20 years in patients with "primary AS" (range, 15 to 40 years).

Etiology, pathology, and general features

The cause of AS is not known, but genetic factors are obvious, as shown by its association with HLA-B27. A gastrointestinal genesis is also suspected.[5]

In AS, the primary pathologic site is not the synovium but rather the site where the ligaments and the capsule insert into the bone (enthesopathy). AS is also characterized by fibrosis and ossification rather than joint destruction and instability. It is usually progressive, most often beginning in the sacroiliac joints and proceeding upward to involve the synovial joints of the spine. The peripheral joints are frequently involved in AS; the hips and shoulders are affected in about half of the patients. Knees, feet, and wrists may also be involved, but the fingers are rarely involved in AS, unlike in RA. The synovitis that occurs in patients with peripheral joint disease often resembles that seen in RA.

A number of extra-articular manifestations, such as prostatitis, iritis, pulmonary fibrosis, bowel disease, and cardiovascular disease, may also occur.[5]

TMJ involvement

AS has a tendency to affect fibrocartilaginous structures; thus the TMJ is of particular interest because these joint surfaces are fibrocartilaginous. However, the incidence of TMJ involvement in AS has been reported to be as low as 0% and as high as 32% in radiographic studies.[6,7] The variations in frequency are due to differences in examination techniques, in the patient populations, and in the criteria for classifying a joint as being involved.

Wenneberg and coworkers[8–11] examined 100 individuals with AS and compared them with an age- and sex-matched healthy control group with respect to subjective symptoms and clinical signs in the masticatory system and radiographic changes in the TMJ. Wenneberg[12] suggested a causal relationship between AS and temporomandibular involvement in at least 15% to 20% of individuals with AS. The most common subjective symptom from the masticatory system in patients with chronic AS is difficulty in opening the mouth wide.[8] In patients with AS who are in acute phases of TMJ arthritis, pain is a frequent complaint,[12] as it is in patients with other inflammatory joint diseases affecting the TMJ, such as RA and PA.[13–15] Clinical signs of significantly decreased maximal mouth opening capacity, palpatory tenderness of the TMJ, crepitation, and masticatory muscle tenderness are frequent in patients with AS.[9,13] Occlusal changes are probably caused by loss of TMJ tissue. However, in patients with AS, the loss of joint tissue generally does not lead to an anterior open bite, in contrast to those with RA, in whom it is quite a common feature.[12,15]

The most common radiographic changes in patients with AS are flattening of the mandibular condyle and erosion of the cortical outline,[10,16] as observed in patients with other inflammatory joint diseases[13,14,16,17] (see Fig 10-29). Ankylosis of the TMJ has been reported in surprisingly few cases,[18] despite the tendency for ankylosis in other fibrocartilaginous joints in AS patients.

Many subjective, clinical, and radiographic features found in the masticatory system of AS patients are more severe in males.[8–10] Subjective, clinical, and radiographic indices of this disorder in the masticatory system are correlated with the general extent and/or severity of AS.[12] Similar relationships have also been proposed in RA[15] and PA.[14] When AS affects the masticatory system, there is an average time lag of 8 years from the onset of the general disease to masticatory symptoms.[8]

Psoriatic Arthritis

Psoriatic arthritis is an inflammatory arthritis associated with psoriasis. Although most patients with PA have a benign course, a subgroup of patients has a severe, mutilating form of arthritis. The association of psoriasis and arthritis was first described by the French physician Alibert in the early 19th century.

Epidemiology

The prevalence of psoriasis has been estimated to be 1% to 2% in North American and northern European whites and much lower in blacks and American Indians. PA occurs in about 5% to 10% of the psoriatic population, and thus the general prevalence is about 0.1%. The sex ratio in PA is even, although males tend to have more severe joint symptoms.

A genetic predisposition to PA has been demonstrated in family and HLA studies. However, the association with the HLA system is not as strong as in AS.

Psoriasis often begins in the second and third decades, and the onset of PA is usually between the ages of 30 and 50 years. However, the mutilating form of PA may start before the age of 20 years.[3,19]

Etiology, pathology, and general features

The cause of PA remains unknown; however, heredity seems to play a major role. Microbiologic agents have been suspected to act as triggering factors for arthritis in genetically predisposed individuals. Synovitis is the basic pathologic lesion in the peripheral arthritis and is generally indistinguishable from RA. Five overlapping clinical PA groups have been recognized[19]:

1. Arthritis of the distal interphalangeal joints
2. Destructive (mutilans) arthritis
3. Symmetric polyarthritis indistinguishable from RA
4. Asymmetric oligoarthritis
5. Spondyolarthropathy

Variability in definitions regarding symmetry, arthritis type, and peripheral and axial overlap pattern has resulted in differences in the reported prevalence figures in different studies. In large-scale studies of PA, most patients have polyarthritis. Spondyloarthropathy develops in 20% to 40% of patients. This is rarely seen as a predominant feature at the onset of PA but begins later in its course and tends to affect men and older patients. The sacroiliac and spinal effects are usually asymmetric, in contrast to AS, which demonstrates bilateral involvement. Destructive (mutilans) arthritis occurs in less than 5% of patients with PA. It is primarily found in younger patients and is characterized by a severe destructive arthritis that principally affects the small joints of the hands and feet. Distal interphalangeal joint predominance is seen in about 5% of PA cases. However, all peripheral joints may be involved in PA. Moreover, the patterns of PA are not permanent; more than 60% of patients experience change from their initial pattern. This results in a heterogenous combination of joint diseases.[19]

Radiographic features characteristic of PA include bony ankylosis, destruction of the joints with narrowing of the spaces, bony proliferation, and erosion. Erosion in combination with tapering of a proximal phalanx and bony proliferation of the distal phalanx results in the typical "pencil-in-cup" deformity.

A number of extra-articular features, in addition to the psoriatic skin changes, may also be observed in patients with PA. In many cases, these features are similar to those described for AS.[3,19]

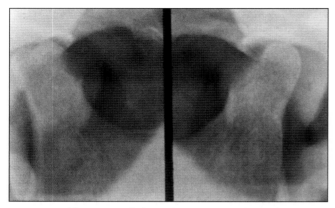

Fig 9-1 Mild erosion of the right condyle *(left)* and extensive erosion of the left condyle *(right)* in a patient with psoriatic arthritis. The patient has had the condition for several years. Other joints involved are the fingers, toes, wrists, ankles, and neck.

TMJ involvement

PA affecting the TMJ was first described by Lundberg[20] and Franks[21] in 1965. Different figures for radiographic TMJ involvement in patients with PA (ranging from 24% to 82%) have been reported.[14,16,20,22] Clinical involvement of the masticatory system is reported in about half of patients with PA.[14,22,23] The variations depend on differences in populations and examination techniques, as discussed earlier with regard to AS.

Könönen[23–26] examined 110 individuals with PA and compared them with a healthy control group matched for age, sex, and occlusal support. It was concluded that PA directly affects the masticatory system in about 20% to 30% of patients.[14] The most common subjective symptom affecting the masticatory system in patients with PA is pain from the TMJ area during function.[22,24] Difficulty in opening the mouth wide has been reported in selected patients,[16,20–22,27] but it is not typical in an unselected PA population.[24] Typical clinical signs frequently found in patients with PA are tenderness to palpation of the TMJs and masticatory muscles and TMJ crepitation.[23] Major occlusal changes are absent in individuals with PA.[23]

Radiographic changes in the TMJ are frequently observed,[16,22,26,27] and the most common finding is erosion of the cortical outline, which is a typical sign of

inflammatory TMJ involvement.[28] Flattening of the mandibular condyle, which is often found in patients with PA,[26] is also a common finding in those with RA,[29,30] AS,[10] and osteoarthrosis[31] (Fig 9-1; also see Figs 10-26 and 10-28). In patients with PA, significant associations have been found between the radiographic changes in the TMJ (especially cortical erosions) and the subjective symptoms and clinical signs, which also correlated with the severity and extent of the joint disorder.[25] The symptoms affecting the masticatory system start, on average, 7 years after the onset of PA.[24]

Reiter Syndrome

Reiter syndrome, or reactive arthritis, can be defined as an aseptic arthritis triggered by an infectious agent not present in the joint. Reiter syndrome usually includes a combination of urethritis, arthritis, and conjunctivitis, which occur either concurrently or sequentially. In addition to these major components, a variety of other signs and symptoms may occur. Hans Reiter first described RS in 1916, when a lieutenant in the Prussian army developed the three most typical features.[32]

Epidemiology

The prevalence of RS is unknown and difficult to assess for several reasons. First, other seronegative spondyloarthropathies can cause diagnostic difficulties because of overlapping symptoms. Second, the early manifestations of RS are often forgotten or suppressed by the patient and are easily overlooked by the physician. However, evidence exists that RS is a fairly common inflammatory joint disease. It is considered to be the most common cause of inflammatory arthritis in young males in western European-derived countries. The male-female ratio is difficult to assess because of the anatomic regions affected by the disease, but it has been estimated that RS is at least 10 times more frequent in males. RS usually develops in the third decade, although both earlier and later onsets have been reported.[32]

Etiology, pathology, and general features

The interrelationship between environmental and genetic factors is evident in RS. The etiology still remains unknown, but several infective agents and a specific genetic (HLA-B27) background are recognized. There are two forms of RS: the epidemic form that develops after an enteral infection caused by strains of *Shigella*, *Salmonella*, and *Yersinia*, and the endemic form that follows a postvenereal infection mainly associated with *Chlamydia,* *Mycoplasma,* or *Yersinia* infections. The co-occurrence of RS and AIDS also has been reported.[32]

In addition to the three classic features of urethritis, polyarthritis, and conjunctivitis, a variety of other signs and symptoms, such as balanitis circinata, vulvitis, stomatitis, keratoderma blennorrhagicum, psoriasis-like skin lesions, nail lesions, cardiovascular disease, spinal disease, and neurologic complications, may occur in RS. The urethritis or diarrhea often precedes the other features of RS, and the arthritis starts a few weeks after the onset of the infection.

The joint involvement is mainly asymmetric, most often affecting the weight-bearing joints of the lower limbs and the sacroiliac joints. Spinal involvement may also occur. Enthesopathy is characteristic in RS as it is in AS.

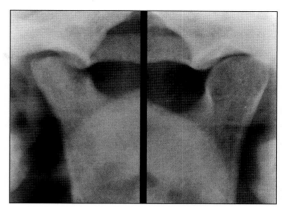

Fig 9-2 Patient with Reiter syndrome of 4 years' duration. The patient has the classic triad of urethritis, arthritis, and conjunctivitis. The right condyle *(left)* is eroded. The fingers, toes, knees, and neck are also affected. The patient is HLA-B27 positive.

TMJ involvement

In a controlled study of male patients with RS, one fourth of patients reported recurrent pain, swelling, and/or stiffness in the TMJ area, which was significantly more frequent than was reported by control subjects. The clinical signs also were significantly more frequent and severe in the RS patients than in the controls, especially tenderness to palpation of the TMJ and masticatory muscles as well as pain during mandibular movements. The most characteristic sign or symptom in patients with RS was pain in the TMJ during function. The severity of both the subjective symptoms and clinical signs correlated positively with the extent and severity of several RS features.[33] Similar relationships have been proposed in RA,[15] PA,[14] and AS.[12]

A controlled radiographic study of TMJ involvement in RS revealed that RS patients had more radiographic signs than controls. The most characteristic radiographic sign in the condyle in the RS group was unilateral erosion (12%)[34] (Fig 9-2). TMJ involvement occurs, on average, 6 years after the onset of RS.[33]

Comparison of Involvement of the TMJ and Masticatory System in RA and the Spondyloarthritides

Two studies[35,36] have evaluated the subjective, clinical, and radiographic features in the masticatory system and TMJs in patients with RA, PA, and AS and compared the findings to those in a healthy control group. Subjective symptoms such as stiffness or tiredness in the jaws, diffi-

culty in opening the mouth wide, and pain in the jaws at rest and function, as well as clinical findings of palpatory tenderness, crepitation of the TMJ, and decreased mouth-opening capacity, were more frequent in the disease groups than in the controls (Tables 9-2 and 9-3). Subjects with RA and PA showed more frequent and more severe signs than did subjects with AS.[36] In the radiographic study,[35] changes were more frequent in subjects with RA, PA, and AS than in the control group. Subjects with RA had these changes significantly more often than did subjects with PA and AS (Table 9-4).

According to these studies, RA is the most severe systemic joint disease affecting the masticatory system and TMJs, followed in severity by PA, while AS showed the least severe involvement. This is also in agreement with the clinical opinion that RA is the most severe of these inflammatory joint diseases, followed in severity by PA and AS. Two studies of RS patients using the same methods as the previous studies also showed that RS is not as severe as RA, PA, or AS.[33,34] However, none of the subjective symptoms, clinical signs, or radiographic changes in the masticatory system and TMJs seem to be pathognomonic for any of these general joint diseases.

Subjective symptom	RA (n = 61)	PA (n = 61)	AS (n = 61)	C (n = 61)	RS (n = 52)
Table 9-2 Distribution (%) of subjective symptoms related to masticatory system function in patients with RA, PA, and AS and a control group[†] (C) and, for comparison, patients with RS[‡]					
Morning stiffness or fatigue in jaws	20**	22**	15*	3	19
Noises from the TMJ	61	57	44	46	44
Difficulties in opening mouth wide	33**	17	20*	5	8
Pain in the face or jaws; headache at rest	33**	20*	12	2	NA[§]
Pain in the face or jaws on opening wide and/or chewing	25*	43*	13	5	15
TMJ locking or luxation	7	17	5	13	12

*$P < .05$; **$P < .01$. Statistical significances refer to separate tests between the C group and the RA, PA, and AS groups.

[†]Data from Könönen et al.[36]

[‡]Data from Könönen.[33]

[§]NA indicates not available.

Connective Tissue Diseases

Systemic Lupus Erythematosus

Systemic lupus erythematosus is a chronic autoimmune multisystem disease arising from a combination of genetic and environmental factors that interact to cause a state of immune hyperactivity. Systems that SLE commonly may affect include the brain and peripheral nervous system, skin, joints, kidneys, lungs, serous membranes, and components of the blood, but other organs of the body also may be affected. The characteristic immune response is caused by certain self-antigens and involves both T- and B-cell activity.

Epidemiology

The disease is more common in females, but there are no exact prevalence figures at the population level. The incidence of SLE varies from 1.8 to 7.6 subjects per 100,000 per year.

SLE is one of several forms of lupus. Although other forms have fewer systemic features, patients presenting with some features of lupus, but not sufficient to warrant such a diagnosis, are usually diagnosed as having undifferentiated connective tissue disease. Only 13% of those initially diagnosed with undifferentiated connective tissue disease evolve to a true diagnosis of SLE over the next 5 years.[37]

Etiology, pathology, and general features

The pathogenic events underlying SLE appear to be related to genetic susceptibility, which in a given subject results in the production of a sustained and injurious autoimmune response. Clinically, SLE often starts with fatigue, weight loss, and low-grade fever, resulting in diagnostic problems because these symptoms are often attributed to diseases other than SLE. The patient's condition is often misdiagnosed as RA, fever of unknown origin, fibromyalgia, or even a psychiatric disease. Further, illnesses in the patient's family such as multiple sclerosis, rheumatic fever, scleroderma, or other inflammatory diseases also may cause diagnostic problems.[37]

TMJ involvement

One of the most common symptoms of SLE is symmetric polyarthritis, most frequently occurring in the fingers, knees, and wrists. Other joints such as the TMJ and sacroiliac joint may be involved, suggesting RA, AS, or MCTD rather than SLE. TMJ involvement has been found in a few studies.[38,39] In a controlled study of SLE patients, one third had subjective TMJ symptoms, 22% had clinical signs, and 11% had radiographic changes.[39]

Table 9-3	Clinical findings related to masticatory system function in patients with RA, PA, and AS and a control group[†] (C) and, for comparison, patients with RS[‡]				
Clinical finding	RA (n = 61)	PA (n = 61)	AS (n = 61)	C (n = 61)	RS (n = 52)
Tenderness to palpation (%)					
Masticatory muscles	13**	67**	54	39	46
TMJ	18	48**	36*	15	27
TMJ clicking (%)	20	48	25	30	29
TMJ crepitation (%)	82**	65**	28	19	37
Painful mandibular movements (%)	18*	25*	13	5	15
Mean maximal mouth opening (mm)	45**	50**	50**	56	57
(range)	(26–61)	(36–67)	(29–67)	(42–68)	(39–73)

*P < .05; **P < .01. Statistical significances refer to separate tests between the C group and the RA, PA, and AS groups.
[†]Data from Könönen et al.[36]
[‡]Data from Könönen.[33]

Table 9-4	Distribution (%) of radiographic changes in the mandibular condyle in patients with RA, PA, and AS and a control group[†] (C) and, for comparison, patients with RS[‡]				
Radiographic change	RA (n = 61)	PA (n = 61)	AS (n = 61)	C (n = 77)	RS (n = 49)
Flattening	34**	23*	20*	8	14
Osteophytes	7	13**	3	1	6
Loss of condylar head	8*	2	6	0	0
Cortical erosions	56**	18**	18**	1	12
Subcortical cysts	13**	0	0	0	0

*P < .05; **P < .01. Statistical significances refer to separate tests between the C group and the RA, PA, and AS groups.
[†]Data from Wenneberg et al.[35]
[‡]Data from Könönen et al.[34]

Scleroderma

Systemic sclerosis is a generalized disorder of connective tissue recognized clinically by thickening and fibrosis of the skin (scleroderma) and specific forms of involvement of organs including the heart, lungs, kidneys, and gastrointestinal tract.

Epidemiology

Scleroderma occurs in all racial groups and in all geographic regions, showing the highest onset between the ages of 30 and 50 years. The disease is three to four times more frequent in women. Because better diagnostic techniques are now available, the prevalence may be higher than previously recognized. The precise incidence remains undefined, but most studies suggest between 4 and 12 subjects per million per year.[40]

Etiology, pathology, and general features

The etiology and pathogenesis are unknown. Progressive systemic sclerosis can be fatal when affecting visceral organs such as the heart, kidneys, or lungs.

TMJ involvement

There are no systematic studies regarding the oral manifestations of scleroderma. Characteristic oral manifestations that may complicate dental treatment include limited

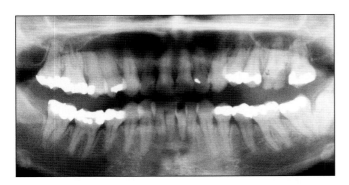

Fig 9-3 Typical widening of the periodontal ligaments in a patient with scleroderma.

mouth opening, TMJ dysfunction, mucogingival problems, xerostomia, telangiectasia, increased periodontal ligament width (Fig 9-3), and osseous resorption of the mandible.[41,42]

Mixed Connective Tissue Disease

Mixed connective tissue disease is a disorder showing overlapping features with a number of different connective tissue diseases. Because of the various overlapping features that have been reported, the existence of MCTD as a distinct disease entity has previously been considered controversial. Today, however, it is regarded as a distinct rheumatoid disease, although the exact prevalence is not known.[43]

Etiology, pathology, and general features

Clinical manifestations of MCTD often include concurrent development of features of SLE, scleroderma, polymyositis, dermatomyositis, and RA, but the overlapping features usually occur sequentially. Because of these overlapping features, it often takes several years to verify the most appropriate diagnosis. Early symptoms include fatigue, myalgia, arthralgia, and Raynaud's phenomenon. Nearly all patients have joint pain and stiffness.

TMJ involvement

Konttinen et al[44] examined 10 patients with MCTD for signs and symptoms in the masticatory system. The study included clinical, radiologic, histologic, and immunohistochemical examinations. All 10 patients showed symptoms or signs of temporomandibular disorders, and seven had radiographic changes in the TMJ. In five patients with normal-appearing mucosa, histologic examination revealed chronic inflammation.

Crystal-Induced Diseases

Gout

Gout is the traditional term for a heterogenous group of diseases found exclusively in human beings. The diseases may include: hyperuricemia, recurrent arthritides, sodium urate crystal deposition in and around joints (sometimes including deformity and crippling), renal disease, and uric acid urolithiasis.[45] Gout has been called both the "king of diseases" and the "disease of kings."

Epidemiology

The prevalence of gout varies worldwide, although it appears to be similar in Europe and North America (about 0.3%). The prevalence seems to increase with age and with increasing serum urate concentrations. The proposed relation between the incidence of gout and the magnitude of hyperuricemia has been confirmed in recent studies. Moreover, the fact that distinctive peak age incidences of gout in men and women occur about two to three decades after the respective sex-specific physiologic increments in serum urate suggests that, on average, hyperuricemia of many years' duration precedes the occurrence of symptomatic events. Gout is uncommon before the third decade.

More than 90% of patients with primary gout are men, and the onset in men is earlier than that in women, who rarely develop the disorder before menopause. In women the disease often presents as so-called secondary gout, complicated by renal disease or diuretic therapy. The fact that gout mainly affects men is in contrast to RA, OA, SLE, and most other connective tissue diseases.

Etiology, pathology, and general features

Only humans and the great apes excrete uric acid (weak organic acid) as the end product of purine metabolism, because of the lack of the enzyme uricase, which catalyzes the degradation of uric acid. The combination of a lack of uricase and the solubility properties of uric acid exposes subjects to the deposition of urate from supersaturated body fluids and the consequent risk of developing gout. The factors determining who will develop hyperuricemia, and among these subjects who will develop gout, are diverse and are best understood on the basis of purine metabolism and uric acid homeostasis. Gouty arthritis, recognized since antiquity, remains a common rheumatic disease. However, gout and RA rarely coexist; the reasons for this are not known.[45]

TMJ involvement

Gout rarely affects the TMJ alone. When it does, the disease is usually confined to the joint space and leads to pain and limitation of mouth opening in the acute phase.[46]

Calcium Pyrophosphate Deposition Disease

Calcium pyrophosphate deposition disease is characterized by the presence of crystal deposits in the affected joint. It is also called *pseudogout, chondrocalcinosis articularis*, or *pyrophosphate arthropathy* in the literature.

Epidemiology

In North America, the prevalence of calcium pyrophosphate deposition disease is estimated to be less than 1%.

Etiology, pathology, and general features

The presence of microcrystal deposits in the affected joint causes arthropathy, typically in the knees, but the hips, shoulders, hands, and feet also can be affected. It is particularly difficult to differentiate the disease from malignant tumors by the clinical and radiographic findings alone. A definitive diagnosis is based on histologic identification of the calcium pyrophosphate microcrystals. The crystals are weakly birefringent under a polarizing microscope, and radiographically they appear as asymptomatic deposits in fibrocartilaginous structures such as the TMJ (see Fig 10-43). The differential diagnosis is based on a quantitative analysis of the crystals or observation of the crystal structure in calcified sections.[47,48]

TMJ involvement

Only a few cases of TMJ involvement have been reported, but no systematic studies have been done.[4,47]

Conclusion

In many patients with systemic diseases, the TMJ and masticatory system also can be involved to varying degrees. When treating these patients, dentists and physicians should be aware of the natural history of these diseases and the problems they pose in the process of differential diagnosis. Regular functional examination of the masticatory system should be performed when there is a possibility that this system has been affected by a systemic condition, and adequate therapeutic measures should be taken when necessary.

References

1. Moll JMH, Haslock I, Macrae IF, et al. Association between ankylosing spondylitis, psoriatic arthritis, Reiter disease, the intestinal arthropathies and Behcet's syndrome. Medicine (Baltimore) 1974;53:343–361.
2. Wright V. Seronegative polyarthritis: A unified concept. Arthritis Rheum 1978;21:619–633.
3. Michet CJ, Conn DL. Psoriatic arthritis. In: Kelley WN, Harris ED Jr, Ruddy S, Sledge CB (eds). Textbook of Rheumatology, ed 3. Philadelphia: Saunders, 1989:1053–1063.
4. Wenneberg B. Other disorders. In: Zarb GA, Carlsson GE, Sessle BJ, Mohl ND (eds). Temporomandibular Joint and Masticatory Muscle Disorders, ed 2. Copenhagen: Munksgaard, 1994:367–388.
5. Calin A. Ankylosing spondylitis. In: Kelley WN, Harris ED Jr, Ruddy S, Sledge CB (eds). Textbook of Rheumatology, ed 3. Philadelphia: Saunders, 1989:1021–1037.
6. Crum RJ, Loiselle RJ. Temporomandibular joint symptoms and ankylosing spondylitis. J Am Dent Assoc 1971;83:630–633.
7. Maes HJ, Dihlman W. Befall der Temporomandibulargelenke bei der Spondylitis Ankylopoetica. Fortschr Roentgenstr 1968;109:513–516.
8. Wenneberg B, Kopp S. Subjective symptoms from the stomatognathic system in ankylosing spondylitis. Acta Odontol Scand 1982;40:215–222.
9. Wenneberg B, Kopp S. Clinical findings in the stomatognathic system in ankylosing spondylitis. Scand J Dent Res 1982;90:373–381.
10. Wenneberg B, Hollender L, Kopp S. Radiographic changes in the temporomandibular joint in ankylosing spondylitis. Dentomaxillofac Radiol 1983;12:25–30.
11. Wenneberg B, Kopp S, Hollender L. The temporomandibular joint in ankylosing spondylitis. Correlations between subjective, clinical, and radiographic features in the stomatognathic system and effects of treatment. Acta Odontol Scand 1984;42:165–173.
12. Wenneberg B. Inflammatory involvement of the temporomandibular joint. Diagnostic and therapeutic aspects and a study of individuals with ankylosing spondylitis. Swed Dent J Suppl 1983;20:1–54.
13. Carlsson GE, Kopp S, Öberg T. Arthritis and allied diseases of the temporomandibular joint. In: Zarb GA, Carlsson GE (eds). Temporomandibular Joint: Function and Dysfunction. Copenhagen: Munksgaard, 1979:269–320.
14. Könönen M. Craniomandibular Disorders in Psoriatic Arthritis. A Radiographic and Clinical Study [thesis]. Helsinki: University of Helsinki, 1987.
15. Tegelberg Å. Temporomandibular joint involvement in rheumatoid arthritis. A clinical study. Swed Dent J Suppl 1987;49:1–133.

16. Resnick D. Temporomandibular joint involvement in ankylosing spondylitis. Radiology 1974;112:587–591.

17. Åkerman S. Morphologic, radiologic and thermometric assessment of degenerative and inflammatory temporomandibular joint disease. An autopsy and clinical study. Swed Dent J Suppl 1987;52:1–110.

18. Sanders B. Temporomandibular joint ankylosis secondary to Marie-Strumpell disease. J Oral Surg 1975;33:784–786.

19. Gladman DD. Psoriatic arthritis. In: Kelley WN, Harris ED Jr, Ruddy S, Sledge CB (eds). Textbook of Rheumatology, ed 5, vol 2. Philadelphia: Saunders, 1997:999–1005.

20. Lundberg M. Röntgendiagnostik vid käkledsbesvär. Odontol Fören Tidskr 1965;29:209–240.

21. Franks AST. Temporomandibular joint arthrosis associated with psoriasis. Oral Surg 1965;19:301–303.

22. Rasmussen OC, Bakke M. Psoriatic arthritis of the temporomandibular joint. Oral Surg 1982;53:351–357.

23. Könönen M. Clinical signs of craniomandibular disorders in patients with psoriatic arthritis. Scand J Dent Res 1987;95:340–346.

24. Könönen M. Subjective symptoms from the stomatognathic system in patients with psoriatic arthritis. Acta Odontol Scand 1986;44:377–383.

25. Könönen M. Craniomandibular disorders in psoriatic arthritis. Correlations between subjective symptoms, clinical signs and radiographic changes. Acta Odontol Scand 1986;44:369–375.

26. Könönen M. Radiographic changes in the condyle of the temporomandibular joint in psoriatic arthritis. Acta Radiol 1987;28:185–188.

27. Lundberg M, Ericsson S. Changes in the temporomandibular joint in psoriasis arthropathica. Acta Derm Venereol 1967;47:354–358.

28. Kopp S, Wenneberg B, Clemensson E. Clinical, microscopical and biochemical investigation of synovial fluid from temporomandibular joints. Scand J Dent Res 1983;91:33–41.

29. Syrjänen S. The temporomandibular joint in rheumatoid arthritis. Acta Radiol Diagn 1985;26:235–243.

30. Uotila E. The temporomandibular joint in adult rheumatoid arthritis. A clinical and roentgenologic study. Acta Odontol Scand 1964;22(suppl 39):1–91.

31. Cassidy JT. Juvenile rheumatoid arthritis. In: Kelley WN, Harris ED Jr, Ruddy S, Sledge CB (eds). Textbook of Rheumatology, ed 3. Philadelphia: Saunders, 1989:1289–1311.

32. Calin A. Reiter's syndrome. In: Kelley WN, Harris ED Jr, Ruddy S, Sledge CB (eds). Textbook of Rheumatology, ed 3. Philadelphia: Saunders, 1989:1033–1046.

33. Könönen M. Signs and symptoms of craniomandibular disorders in men with Reiter disease. J Craniomandib Disord 1992;6:247–253.

34. Könönen M, Kovero O, Wenneberg B, Konttinen YT. Radiographic signs in the temporomandibular joint in Reiter disease. J Orofac Pain 2002;16:143–147.

35. Wenneberg B, Könönen M, Kallenberg A. Radiographic changes in the temporomandibular joint of patients with rheumatoid arthritis, psoriatic arthritis, and ankylosing spondylitis. J Craniomandib Disord 1990;4:35–39.

36. Könönen M, Wenneberg B, Kallenberg A. Craniomandibular disorders in rheumatoid arthritis, psoriatic arthritis, and ankylosing spondylitis. A clinical study. Acta Odontol Scand 1992;50:281–286.

37. Lahita RG. Clinical presentation of systemic lupus erythematosus. In: Kelley WN, Harris ED Jr, Ruddy S, Sledge CB. Textbook of Rheumatology, ed 5, vol 2. Philadelphia: Saunders, 1997:1028–1039.

38. Liebling MR, Gold RH. Erosions of the temporomandibular joint in systemic lupus erythematosus. Arthritis Rheum 1981;24:948–950.

39. Jonsson R, Lindvall AM, Nyberg G. Temporomandibular involvement in systemic lupus erythematosus. Arthritis Rheum 1983;26:1506–1510.

40. Seibold JR. Connective tissue diseases characterized by fibrosis. In: Kelley WN, Harris ED Jr, Ruddy S, Sledge CB. Textbook of Rheumatology, ed 5, vol 2. Philadelphia: Saunders, 1997:1133–1162.

41. Robbins JW, Craig RM Jr, Correll RW. Symmetrical widening of the periodontal ligament space in a patient with multiple systemic problems. J Am Dent Assoc 1986;113:307–308.

42. Tai CC, Lee P, Wood RE. Progressive systemic sclerosis in a child: Case report. Pediatr Dent 1993;15:275–279.

43. Bennett RM. Mixed connective tissue disease and other overlap syndromes. In: Kelley WN, Harris ED Jr, Ruddy S, Sledge CB. Textbook of Rheumatology, ed 5, vol 2. Philadelphia: Saunders, 1997:1065–1078.

44. Konttinen YT, Tuominen TS, Piirainen HI, et al. Signs and symptoms in the masticatory system in ten patients with mixed connective tissue disease. Scand J Rheumatol. 1990;19:363–373.

45. Kelley WN, Wortmann RL. Gout and hyperuricemia. In: Kelley WN, Harris ED Jr, Ruddy S, Sledge CB (eds). Textbook of Rheumatology, ed 5, vol 2. Philadelphia: Saunders, 1997:1313–1351.

46. Barthelemy I, Karanas Y, Sannajust JP, Emering C, Mondie JM. Gout of the temporomandibular joint: Pitfalls in diagnosis. J Craniomaxillofac Surg 2001;29:307–310.

47. Reginato AJ. Reginato AM. Diseases associated with deposition of calcium pyrophosphate or hydroxyapatite. In: Kelley WN, Harris ED Jr, Ruddy S, Sledge CB (eds). Textbook of Rheumatology, ed 5, vol 2. Philadelphia: Saunders, 1997:1352–1367.

48. Aoyama S, Kino K, Amagasa T, Kayano T, Ichinose S, Kimijima Y. Differential diagnosis of calcium pyrophosphate dihydrate deposition of the temporomandibular joint. Br J Oral Maxillofac Surg 2000;38:550–553.

PART II

Clinical Management

TMJ Imaging

Tore A. Larheim and Per-Lennart Westesson

Diagnostic Imaging Versus Clinical Examination

The clinical assessment of temporomandibular disorders (TMDs) provides relatively limited information with respect to the status of the temporomandibular joint (TMJ). Multiple studies have shown that the clinical diagnosis of conditions involving this joint is unreliable.[1] The lowest predictability of joint abnormalities in the two most frequent subgroups of disorders, namely internal derangement and osteoarthritis, has varied between 43% and 59%.[2,3] The accuracy of the clinical diagnosis of internal derangement related to reducing disc displacement was recently found to be 48%, when magnetic resonance imaging (MRI) was used as the "gold standard."[4]

Although clinical assessment is unreliable for determining the status of the joint, imaging should only be performed after a thorough physical examination that indicates the need for more information. The treatment decision must be based on a patient evaluation that integrates the imaging and the clinical findings, including the history and, in selected cases, other diagnostic data.

Magnetic resonance imaging is the preferred imaging modality for the heterogenous group of TMD patients. The standard imaging protocol consists of oblique sagittal and oblique coronal images of the TMJ that are obtained perpendicular and parallel to the long axis of the mandibular condyle.[5] The disc position and morphology, as well as the bone structures, are clearly visualized on closed-mouth images (Fig 10-1). The function of the disc and the condyle can usually be assessed on open-mouth images. The diagnostic accuracy of MRI on a fresh autopsy series of oblique sagittal and oblique coronal sections has been found to be 95% and 93% in determining the disc position and the bone status, respectively.[6]

Asymptomatic Volunteers

Disc Position and Function

The first MRI study of asymptomatic volunteers demonstrated disc displacement in about one third of the joints examined.[7] Later MRI studies of adults (mean age between 25 and 30 years) confirmed disc displacement in about one third of individuals with no symptoms.[8–10] The disc can be displaced in several directions.[9] Larheim et al[10] systematized the position of the disc in asymptomatic volunteers and patients and described 10 positions (Table 10-1), in addition to the position usually referred to as the *normal superior position* (see Fig 10-1). This detailed classification was made possible by an evaluation of both oblique sagittal and oblique coronal images using all sections throughout the entire joint. Three main categories of disc position could be distinguished (Table 10-2):

1. *Normal superior position*, assigned if this was the finding in every section (Fig 10-2)
2. *Partial disc displacement*, assigned if the disc was normally positioned in some oblique sagittal sections and displaced in other sections, whether or not there was also a lateral or a medial displacement (Fig 10-3)
3. *Complete disc displacement*, assigned if the disc was displaced in all sections, with or without a lateral or a medial displacement

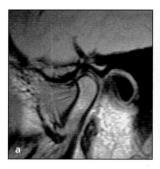
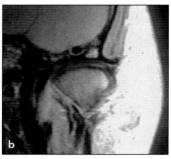
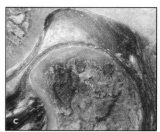
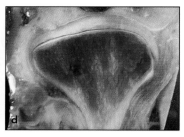

Fig 10-1 *(a)* Oblique sagittal and *(b)* oblique coronal MRIs of the TMJ in an asymptomatic volunteer in the closed-mouth position. The patient exhibits normal disc morphology (biconcave in oblique sagittal plane), normal disc position (posterior thick band located superior to the mandibular condyle), and normal bone (cortex and marrow). *(c)* Oblique sagittal and *(d)* oblique coronal sections from autopsy specimens, showing normal anatomy of the TMJ. Disc morphology, disc position, and bone are normal.

Table 10-1	Categories of TMJ disc position in MRIs taken in the closed-mouth position*
Category	**Disc position**
Normal superior	Normal on all oblique sagittal and coronal images
Partial anterior in lateral part	Anteriorly displaced on lateral images; otherwise normal
Partial anterior in medial part	Anteriorly displaced on medial images; otherwise normal
Complete anterior	Anteriorly displaced on all oblique sagittal images without lateral or medial displacement
Partial anterolateral	Anteriorly displaced on lateral images, with lateral displacement
Complete anterolateral	Anteriorly displaced on all oblique sagittal images, with lateral displacement
Partial anteromedial	Anteriorly displaced on medial images, with medial displacement
Complete anteromedial	Anteriorly displaced on all oblique sagittal images, with medial displacement
Lateral	Laterally displaced on oblique coronal images; otherwise normal
Medial	Medially displaced on oblique coronal images; otherwise normal
Posterior	Posteriorly displaced on all or some oblique sagittal images, with or without lateral or medial displacement

*From Larheim et al.[10] Reprinted with permission. Categories were modified from those used by Tasaki et al.[9]

The differentiation between partial and complete disc displacement with sagittal MRI was previously described and confirmed by surgery but was not systematically analyzed in volunteers and patients.[11]

In the asymptomatic volunteers, most joints showed normal superior disc position (see Table 10-2). Of the joints with disc displacement, almost all (90%) showed partial displacement in the closed-mouth position, routinely reducing to normal position during mouth opening.[10] These functional observations substantiate those of previous studies of asymptomatic volunteers in which only a few individuals had a displaced disc that did not reduce during mouth opening.[7–9]

In the series of asymptomatic volunteers studied by Larheim et al,[10] 35% had disc displacement, mostly as a unilateral finding. The high prevalence of disc displacement found in all MRI studies of asymptomatic volunteers has led to the suggestion that the condition might represent a congenital normal anatomic variant.[7,12] However, in a consecutive series of 30 infants and young children, aged

Table 10-2	Distribution of TMJ disc displacements according to main categories*	
	No. of joints (%)	
Main category	Patients[†] (n = 115)	Volunteers (n = 124)
Normal superior	43 (37.4)	94 (75.8)
Partial disc displacement[‡]	26 (22.6)	27 (21.8)
Complete disc displacement	46 (40.0)	3 (2.4)

*From Larheim et al.[10] Reprinted with permission.
[†]Patients had TMJ pain and dysfunction. Disc position could not be determined in one joint.
[‡]Lateral, medial, and posterior disc displacement were included in this main category.

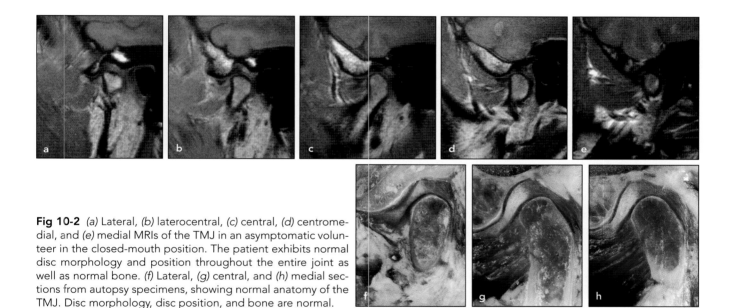

Fig 10-2 *(a)* Lateral, *(b)* laterocentral, *(c)* central, *(d)* centromedial, and *(e)* medial MRIs of the TMJ in an asymptomatic volunteer in the closed-mouth position. The patient exhibits normal disc morphology and position throughout the entire joint as well as normal bone. *(f)* Lateral, *(g)* central, and *(h)* medial sections from autopsy specimens, showing normal anatomy of the TMJ. Disc morphology, disc position, and bone are normal.

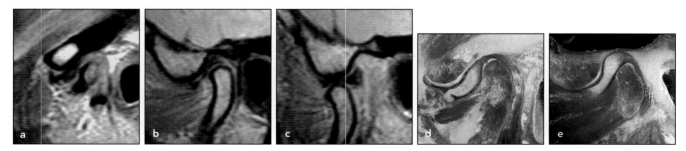

Fig 10-3 *(a)* Lateral and *(b)* centromedial MRIs of the TMJ in an asymptomatic volunteer in the closed-mouth position. The images reveal anterior disc displacement in the lateral part and normal disc position in the centromedial part of the joint. *(c)* Open-mouth image of the same TMJ, showing normal disc position and normal bone. (Figs 10-3a to 10-3c from Larheim et al.[10] Reprinted with permission.) *(d)* Lateral and *(e)* medial sections from autopsy specimens, showing partial disc displacement. The sections reveal anterior disc displacement in the lateral part and normal disc position in the medial part of the joint.

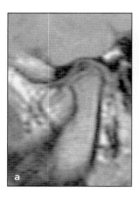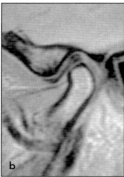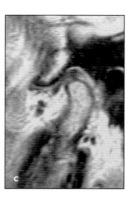

Fig 10-4 MRIs of the TMJ in asymptomatic (a) 11-year-old, (b) 40-year-old, and (c) 56-year-old volunteers, showing normal anatomy. (From Larheim et al.[10] Reprinted with permission.)

2 months to 5 years (mean, 2.5 years), who had been referred for brain imaging, normal superior disc position was found in all joints in all patients.[13] A study of volunteers aged 6 to 25 years showed that 11% of the individuals between the ages of 6 and 11 years had disc displacement.[14] Thus, TMJ disc displacement seems to be an acquired condition that may develop rather early in life.

Normal superior disc position does not necessarily mean an exact 12-o'clock position of the posterior band (see Figs 10-2 and 10-3),[15] and the normal disc morphology may vary considerably; the shape of the disc seems to be biconcave with the posterior band on "top" of the condyle at a wide range of ages (Fig 10-4).

Cortical Bone and Bone Marrow

In asymptomatic populations of volunteers, the prevalence of cortical bone abnormalities has been reported to vary from zero to fewer than 3% of the joints.[9,14,16] The osseous changes have consisted of condylar flattening and formation of small osteophytes found unilaterally, but otherwise there is a smooth cortical outline.[14] Such an osseous change should generally not be interpreted as osteoarthritis (discussed later in the chapter), because the bone changes most likely represent remodeling; ie, there is an intact surface layer. Bone remodeling, regarded as a functional adaptation of the joint, may be found in both asymptomatic and symptomatic individuals, particularly minimal flattening of the condyle and/or the articular eminence. This has been found unilaterally in 35% of the joints in asymptomatic volunteers.[16]

In studies of asymptomatic volunteers, the condylar bone marrow has been interpreted as normal in all joints of all individuals examined with MRI.[16,17] Normal bone marrow is defined as having a homogenous bright signal on proton density images and a homogenous intermediate signal on T2-weighted images (Fig 10-5). This has been demonstrated in a study comparing MRI and histologic observations of the mandibular condyle in patients selected for disc surgery in whom core biopsies were made of the condylar marrow, including those with a completely normal MRI signal.[18]

Joint Fluid

Joint fluid may appear as dots or lines of bright T2 signal along the articular surfaces in asymptomatic volunteers.[19] In a large study of volunteers,[17] it was demonstrated that more than half of the individuals had a small amount of fluid; in about one fifth of subjects, there was a moderate amount of fluid (Fig 10-6). The presence of a moderate amount of fluid was related to the disc displacement in that part of the joint.

Patients with TMDs

Internal Derangement Related to Displacement of the Disc

Internal derangement (ID) is a general orthopedic term implying a mechanical fault that interferes with the smooth action of a joint.[20] ID is thus a functional diagnosis, and for the TMJ the most common ID is displacement of the disc. A number of studies using different imaging modalities have demonstrated a high prevalence of disc displacement in TMD patients (for review, see Larheim[21] and Westesson

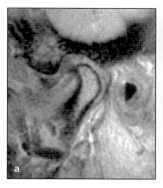
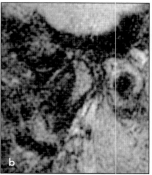
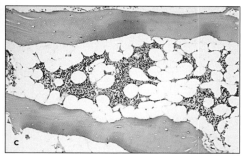

Fig 10-5 *(a)* Proton density and *(b)* corresponding T2-weighted MRIs of the TMJ in a TMD patient, showing normal bone marrow. There is a normal homogenous signal from the bone marrow, and the images reveal a slightly displaced disc and a small osteophyte on the condyle. *(c)* Histologic section of a bone marrow biopsy from the same mandibular condyle. Normal hematopoietic elements are interspersed with marrow fat and intact trabecular bone. (Hematoxylin-eosin stain; original magnification ×50. From Larheim et al.[18] Reprinted with permission.)

Fig 10-6 *(a)* Proton density and *(b)* corresponding T2-weighted MRIs of the TMJ in an asymptomatic volunteer, showing joint fluid. There is an increased T2 signal consistent with fluid in the superior compartment of the anterolateral recess. The disc is displaced in this part of the joint. This was the maximum amount of fluid observed among asymptomatic volunteers. (From Larheim et al.[17] Reprinted with permission.)

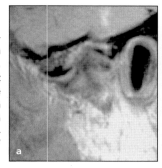
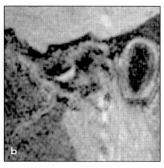

et al[1]). In most large MRI studies, about 80% of patients referred for diagnostic imaging of the TMJ will have an imaging diagnosis of disc displacement.[8,9,10,14,22]

Disc Displacement in Patients and Asymptomatic Volunteers

The differences in the MRIs of patients and asymptomatic volunteers, discussed by Larheim et al,[10] also included the type of disc displacement. The main category of disc displacement that was found frequently in patients and very seldom in asymptomatic volunteers was complete disc displacement (see Table 10-2). Partial disc displacement was equally frequent in patients and in volunteers. In joints with complete disc displacement, two categories were predominantly found: complete anterior displacement, ie,

anterior displacement without any lateral or medial component, and complete anterolateral displacement (Table 10-3). In 56% of the joints in these two categories of displacement, the disc did not reduce to a normal position during mouth opening (Fig 10-7). Of all the nonreducing discs in the total series of patients, 89% belonged to these two categories. Disc displacement with a lateral component was found more frequently than displacement with a medial component, supporting some previous MRI studies.[9,22]

The other categories of disc displacement did not show evident differences between patients and volunteers (see Table 10-3). Pure lateral or medial disc displacement can be clearly demonstrated only with oblique coronal imaging (Fig 10-8)[23,24] and seems to occur equally seldom in patients and in asymptomatic volunteers.[10] Posterior disc displacement (Fig 10-9) is also infrequently observed.[25]

Table 10-3	Distribution of TMJ disc displacements according to category*†

| Category | No. of joints (%) | |
	Patients‡ (n = 115)	Volunteers (n = 124)
Normal superior	43 (37.4)	94 (75.8)
Partial anterior in lateral part	4 (3.5)	8 (6.5)
Partial anterior in medial part	2 (1.7)	3 (2.4)
Complete anterior	18 (15.7)	2 (1.6)
Partial anterolateral	9 (7.8)	8 (6.5)
Complete anterolateral	27 (23.5)	0 (0.0)
Partial anteromedial	0 (0.0)	0 (0.0)
Complete anteromedial	1 (0.9)	1 (0.8)
Lateral	5 (4.3)	3 (2.4)
Medial	3 (2.6)	5 (4.0)
Posterior	3 (2.6)	0 (0.0)
Total	72 (62.6)	30 (24.2)

*From Larheim et al.[10] Reprinted with permission.
†See Table 10-1.
‡Patients had TMJ pain and dysfunction. Disc position could not be determined in one joint.

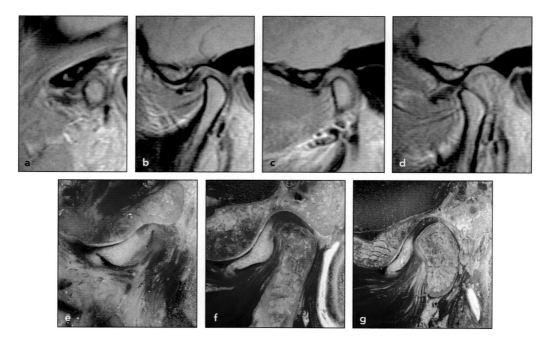

Fig 10-7 (a) Lateral, (b) central, and (c) medial MRIs of the TMJ in an ID patient in the closed-mouth position. (d) MRI of the same patient in the open-mouth position. The disc is anteriorly displaced in the closed-mouth position, but the bone is normal. (From Larheim et al.[10] Reprinted with permission.) (e) Lateral, (f) central, and (g) medial sections from autopsy specimens, showing complete anterior disc displacement in all sections and normal bone.

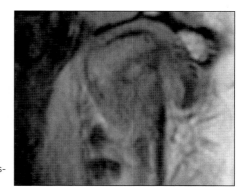

Fig 10-8 Oblique coronal MRI of the TMJ in an ID patient, showing a laterally displaced disc.

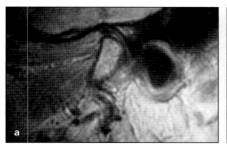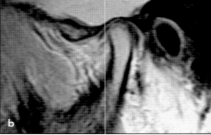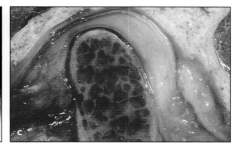

Fig 10-9 *(a and b)* Oblique sagittal MRIs of the TMJ in two ID patients. The posterior band of the disc is located posterior to the top of the condyle in these two patients. *(c)* Oblique coronal section from an autopsy specimen, showing posterior disc displacement. The posterior thick band is located at the posterior aspect of the condyle. (From Westesson et al.[25] Reprinted with permission.)

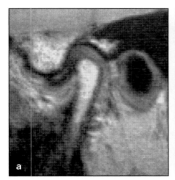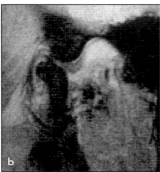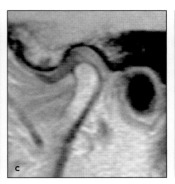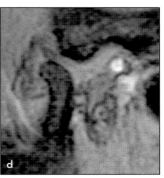

Fig 10-10 Patient with reducing disc displacement, followed for 10 years. MRIs taken in the *(a)* closed-mouth and *(b)* open-mouth positions at baseline. There is disc displacement with normalization during mouth opening. The bone is normal. Images taken in the *(c)* closed-mouth and *(d)* open-mouth positions at the 10-year follow-up, showing disc displacement without normalization during mouth opening. The bone is still normal.

Progression of Disc Displacement over Time

Clinical studies have indicated that a TMJ disc disorder such as a reducing disc displacement with normal condylar cortical bone may be stable for decades,[26] but there are no long-term longitudinal studies with soft tissue imaging documentation. In a series of patients followed for 10 to 15 years (Larheim, unpublished data, 2004), reducing disc displacement with normal condylar cortical bone either did not change during the observation period or developed into a nonreducing disc displacement that still exhibited normal cortical bone (Fig 10-10). A reducing disc disorder may be nonprogressive for many years, but it also can develop into a nonreducing condition. Short-term clinical studies and long-term studies have indicated that, although clicking

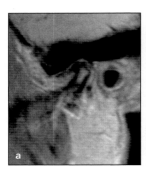
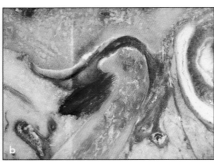

Fig 10-11 *(a)* Patient with osteoarthritis. There is an irregular cortical outline with sclerosis/osteophytosis of the condyle. The MRI also reveals anterior disc displacement and disc degeneration. *(b)* Autopsy specimen revealing osteophyte formation on the condyle and a displaced, degenerated disc.

sounds in the TMJ are fairly common, the progression to a more severe disc displacement, ie, without reduction, seems to be relatively uncommon.[26–29]

Osteoarthritis, Osteoarthrosis, and Degenerative Joint Disease

Osteoarthritis (osteoarthrosis or degenerative joint disease) has been extensively described as a noninflammatory focal degenerative disorder of synovial joints, primarily affecting the articular cartilage and subchondral bone.[30] Because inflammatory changes are not pronounced in most of the affected articulations, the suffix *–osis* appears to be more appropriate than *–itis*.[31] This condition frequently affects the TMJ, where it also is considered a noninflammatory condition.[32] However, internal TMJ derangement both with and without bone changes may have an evident inflammatory component, as can be observed on MRIs. Thus, *osteoarthritis* may be an appropriate term, although it is principally a degenerative rather than an inflammatory condition. In our experience, however, the same TMJ, when followed over time, may show either inflammatory or noninflammatory changes, as judged from MRIs.

Osteoarthritis is defined as deterioration of the articular soft tissue cover and exposure of the underlying bone. Radiologically, cortical bone erosion and/or productive bone changes such as sclerosis and/or osteophytosis must be observed before an imaging diagnosis of TMJ osteoarthritis can be made (Fig 10-11). If bone surface irregularities are not found, the differentiation between osteoarthritis with minimal sclerosis and osteophytosis and remodeling may be impossible. *Remodeling* is defined as changes in the form of the articular tissues with a remaining intact soft tissue cover; the TMJ has a capacity to proliferate and adapt morphologically to various mechanical stresses.[33]

Osteoarthritis is the common final pathway for a multitude of joint conditions. Several autopsy studies have found a high correlation with internal derangement (discussed later), but similar bone changes have also been found in joints with normal disc position.[34,35] Osteoarthritis may also occur as a result of trauma in which the disc position is often normal.[36] Thus, osteoarthritis is common in the TMJ.

Osteoarthritis is the most prevalent arthropathy in humans.[31] Single joints, frequently the knee, hip, and wrist, or multiple joints, known as *generalized osteoarthritis*, may be involved.[37] TMJ abnormalities in patients with generalized osteoarthritis have seldom been reported, but a comparison of such patients with those having generalized RA is available.[38] Both groups had TMJ pain and dysfunction, and tomography showed abnormalities in 80% of the osteoarthritis patients and in 71% of the RA patients. However, soft tissue imaging was not performed, and the prevalence of internal derangement was not estimated even clinically. (See chapters 3, 7, and 8 for further discussion.)

Internal Derangement and Osteoarthritis

A strong association between disc displacement, in particular without reduction, and osteoarthritis has been demonstrated both in autopsy studies[34,35,39] and in clinical studies.[40–45] Therefore, it is widely assumed that disc displacement can lead to osteoarthritis (see chapter 8). However, there is an obvious lack of longitudinal studies to prove this causal relationship. In a longitudinally followed patient series (Larheim TA. Unpublished data, 2004), five of seven joints showing nonreducing disc displacement with normal bone at baseline had developed osteoarthritis when examined 10 to 15 years later (Fig 10-12). Although the series is too small to indicate any frequency of this situation, long-standing nonreducing disc displacement can precede the development of osteoarthritis. If early osteoarthritis was present at baseline in the same series of patients, the condition tended to progress during the observation period (Fig 10-13).

Some authors have proposed that internal derangement may be a sign of osteoarthritis rather than its cause (see

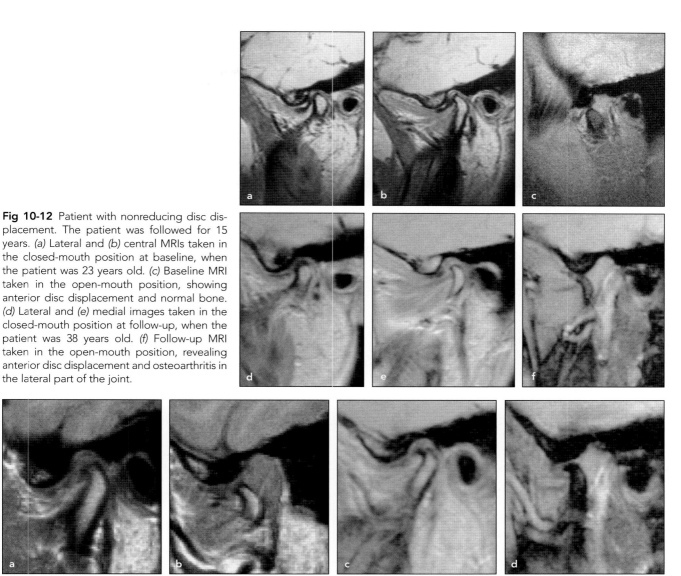

Fig 10-12 Patient with nonreducing disc displacement. The patient was followed for 15 years. (a) Lateral and (b) central MRIs taken in the closed-mouth position at baseline, when the patient was 23 years old. (c) Baseline MRI taken in the open-mouth position, showing anterior disc displacement and normal bone. (d) Lateral and (e) medial images taken in the closed-mouth position at follow-up, when the patient was 38 years old. (f) Follow-up MRI taken in the open-mouth position, revealing anterior disc displacement and osteoarthritis in the lateral part of the joint.

Fig 10-13 Patient with nonreducing disc displacement (contralateral joint of the patient shown in Fig 10-12). The patient was followed for 15 years. MRIs taken in the (a) closed-mouth and (b) open-mouth positions at baseline reveal condylar flattening and probable initial osteoarthritis. In images taken in the (c) closed-mouth and (d) open-mouth positions at the 15-year follow-up, osteoarthritis is evident. (See a more lateral image of this joint at follow-up in Fig 10-11a.)

chapter 8).[32] We are convinced that the most common cause of osteoarthritis in the TMJ is a permanently displaced disc. Despite the lack of documentation from longitudinal imaging studies, the progressive course that most likely occurs in many patients was described in detail by Wilkes as occurring in five different stages.[45] It should be stressed that Wilkes' series, although large, was highly selective because only surgically treated cases were included and retrospectively studied.

Disc Deformation, Pseudodisc, and Stuck Disc

It is generally accepted that the disc in a normal position has a biconcave shape, and usually the posterior band is the thickest part (see Figs 10-1 to 10-4). This disc morphology may obviously endure for decades even in joints with reducing disc displacement.[26] In joints with nonreducing disc displacement, it is well accepted that a deformation of the disc

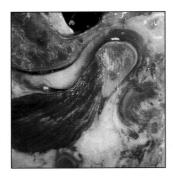 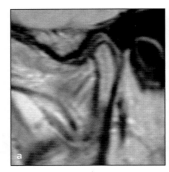 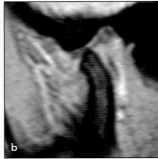

Fig 10-14 Autopsy specimen showing a pseudodisc and fibrosis of the posterior disc attachment.

Fig 10-15 Patient with a stuck disc following a whiplash injury. MRIs taken in the *(a)* closed-mouth and *(b)* open-mouth positions. The disc is positioned normally in the closed-mouth position and does not move with the condyle on mouth opening.

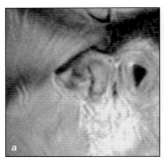 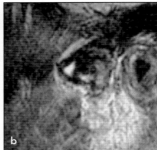

Fig 10-16 *(a)* Proton density and *(b)* corresponding T2-weighted MRIs of the TMJ in a patient, showing joint effusion, disc displacement, and disc deformation. The bone is normal. This amount of fluid was used as a reference image for the definition of joint effusion. (From Larheim et al.[17] Reprinted with permission.)

gradually occurs, including thickening of the posterior band and shortening of the disc (Fig 10-7), and the disc assumes a biconvex shape before osteoarthritis develops. During the further progression to osteoarthritis, the disc will degenerate and may perforate and actually diminish in size (see Figs 10-11 to 10-13). The disc also may be deformed in patients and asymptomatic volunteers with partial disc displacement, although to a smaller degree (see Fig 10-3).

Pseudodisc is an expression proposed by Manzione and Tallents[46] to describe another form of tissue alteration secondary to disc displacement (Fig 10-14). This condition was actually described previously in a histologic study showing that the posterior disc attachment can undergo adaptive change characterized by connective tissue hyalinization.[47] Such a fibrosis will appear on the MRI as a band-like structure of low signal intensity replacing the normally high signal from the posterior attachment.[48]

Stuck disc is defined as a disc, either in a normal or displaced position, that does not move together with the condyle on mouth opening, probably because of fibrous adhesions between the disc and the articular eminence.[49] Such a condition, even with a normally positioned disc, is an internal derangement by definition (Fig 10-15).

Internal Derangement and Joint Effusion

MRI evidence of joint effusion was recognized in one of the earliest TMJ studies using surface coil technology,[50] and later studies have shown a relationship between joint effusion and a displaced disc.[19,22,51–55] When a systematic correlation between the different stages of internal derangement and pain was made, an association between joint effusion and pain was found.[19] This association has been questioned by some[56] but confirmed by others.[53–55]

Because TMJ fluid is also frequently found in asymptomatic volunteers and is related to disc displacement,[17] it is necessary to define an abnormal amount of fluid. We have defined joint effusion as more fluid than the amount maximally found in volunteers, which was labeled *moderate fluid* (see Fig 10-6). Thus, to be considered an effusion, at least a large amount of fluid has to be found (Fig 10-16).[17] According to this definition, 70 patients (13.4%) in a consecutive series of 523 patients had TMJ effusion.[54] Almost all of these patients (96%) had an internal derangement, mostly bilateral (80%). The joint effusion was predominantly unilateral (61.4%) or there was less fluid in the con-

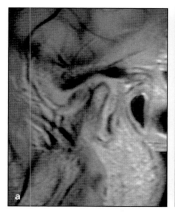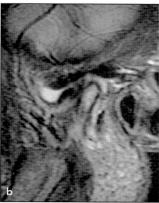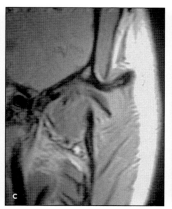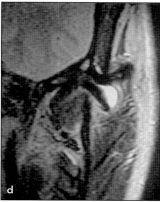

Fig 10-17 *(a)* Proton density (oblique sagittal view), *(b)* corresponding T2-weighted (oblique sagittal view), *(c)* proton density oblique coronal, and *(d)* corresponding T2-weighted oblique coronal MRIs of the TMJ in an ID patient, showing joint effusion. There is effusion in the upper compartment of the anterolateral recess.

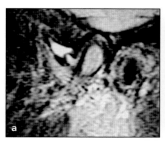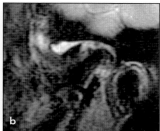

Fig 10-18 T2-weighted MRIs of the TMJ in a TMD patient, showing *(a)* joint effusion, normal cortical bone, normal bone marrow, and disc displacement and *(b)* joint effusion, osteoarthritis, abnormal bone marrow, and disc displacement. (Fig 10-18b from Larheim et al.[54] Reprinted with permission.)

tralateral joint (30%); only 6 patients (8.6%) had bilateral effusion. In 68% of the 76 joints with effusion, the fluid was found exclusively or predominantly in the anterolateral recess of the upper compartment (Fig 10-17), and it occurred more often in joints with normal cortical bone (59%) than in those with osteoarthritis (41%) (Fig 10-18).

Variations in Joint Effusion over Time

Joint effusion will vary over time in the same patient. This was illustrated in a patient with inflammatory TMJ disease and internal derangement. The patient was followed by MRI for about 16 months and demonstrated a variation of joint effusion and marrow edema reflecting exacerbation and subsidence of inflammation.[57] The cyclic changes corresponded well with the patient's pain experience. Recently, a longitudinal study of patients with internal derangement also showed variations in TMJ fluid and pain during the observation period.[55] More longitudinal studies in this field, with correlation to patients' symptoms, are necessary.

Internal Derangement and Bone Marrow Abnormalities

Studies based on alterations of the MRI signals similar to those found in the femoral head have suggested that osteonecrosis (avascular or aseptic necrosis) can affect the mandibular condyle.[51,58,59] However, this was a controversial subject until histologic documentation was published.[18] In a series of 50 TMJs in 44 patients in whom MRI and surgery were performed for painful internal derangements, a core biopsy specimen was obtained from the marrow of the mandibular condyle at the time of surgery. The biopsy was obtained whether or not abnormal MRI signals were observed in the marrow. Thus, joints with normal MRI signals and normal histology were also included (see Fig 10-5).

This highly selected material from surgically treated patients showed histologically that abnormal bone marrow was present in more than one third (36%) of the joints.[18] Half of these joints showed marrow edema without osteonecrosis, and half of the joints showed osteonecrosis, with or without marrow edema (Fig 10-19). For compari-

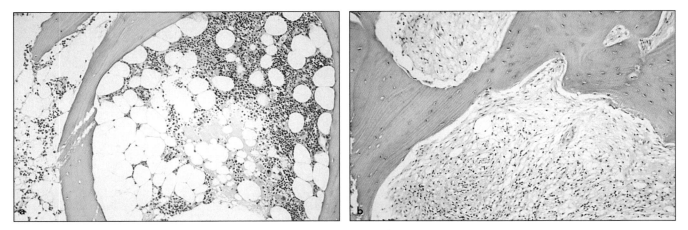

Fig 10-19 Histologic sections of the mandibular condyle from bone marrow biopsies of the TMJ in TMD patients. *(a)* Early marrow edema: a patchy focus with serum proteins within the marrow interstitium surrounded by areas of normal hematopoietic marrow. *(b)* Osteonecrosis: complete loss of hematopoietic marrow. There is evidence of an inflammatory cell infiltrate. (Hematoxylin-eosin stain; original magnification ×50. From Larheim et al.[18] Reprinted with permission.)

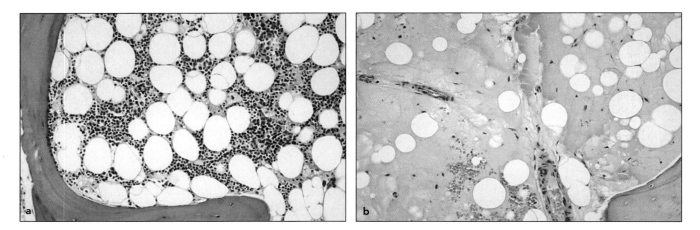

Fig 10-20 Histologic sections of a femoral head from bone marrow biopsies of a hip joint. *(a)* Normal bone marrow (compare with Fig 10-19a). *(b)* Avascular necrosis. There is complete loss of hematopoietic marrow (compare with Fig 10-19b). (Hematoxylin-eosin stain; original magnification ×50.)

son, normal bone marrow and osteonecrosis in the hip joint are shown in Fig 10-20. Table 10-4 shows the MRI classification of the mandibular condyle marrow and Table 10-5 shows the correlation of the MRI findings and the histologic evaluation of the core biopsy specimens.

Reliability of Bone Marrow Assessment with MRI

More than half of the joints with marrow edema were normal on MRI (see Table 10-5), probably because most edema involved only small areas of the condyle marrow (see Fig 10-19). MRI seems to be fairly insensitive for the detection of focal areas of marrow edema, as also experienced in an experimental study of the femoral head.[60] On the other hand, Table 10-5 shows a sensitivity of 78% for detecting osteonecrosis of the TMJ with MRI.[18] The most reliable MRI signs of osteonecrosis are a combination of edema and sclerosis of the bone marrow (Fig 10-21). However, cases with marrow sclerosis on MRI could either involve osteonecrosis (Fig 10-22) or advanced osteoarthritis histologically (Fig 10-23), giving a positive predictive value of only 54%. Thus, if all cases with marrow sclerosis on MRI were interpreted as osteonecrosis, there would be many false-positive diagnoses (see Table 10-5).

Table 10-4	MRI classification of bone marrow of mandibular condyles*	

MRI classification	Signal intensity patterns
I. Normal	Homogeneous bright signal on T1-weighted (proton density) images and homogenous intermediate signal on T2-weighted images
II. Edema	Decreased signal on T1-weighted (proton density) images and increased signal on T2-weighted images; edema pattern
III. Osteonecrosis	a. Decreased signal on T1-weighted (proton density) images and on T2-weighted images; sclerosis pattern
	b. Combination of edema (II) and sclerosis (IIIa) patterns

*From Larheim et al.[18] Reprinted with permission.

Table 10-5	Correlation of MRI interpretation and histologic evaluation of core biopsy specimens from 50 mandibular condyles*			

| | MRI diagnosis (No. of specimens) | | | |
Histologic diagnosis	Normal	Marrow edema	Osteonecrosis	Total
Normal	27	2	3	32
Marrow edema	5	1	3	9
Osteonecrosis	2	0	7	9
Total	34	3	13	50

*From Larheim et al.[18] Reprinted with permission.

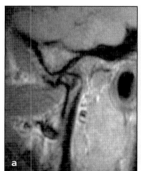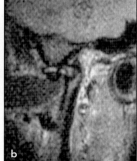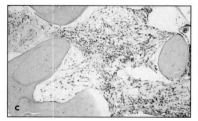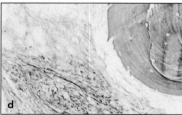

Fig 10-21 Osteonecrosis revealed in (a) proton density and (b) corresponding T2-weighted MRIs of the TMJ. There is a combination of marrow edema (decreased signal on the proton density image and increased signal on the T2-weighted image) and marrow sclerosis (decreased signals on the proton density and T2-weighted images) within the condylar head. Anterior disc displacement and osteoarthritis are evident. (c) Histologic specimen from the bone marrow of the same mandibular condyle. Osteonecrosis is revealed by the complete loss of hematopoietic marrow. There is evidence of inflammatory cell infiltrate. (Hematoxylin-eosin stain; original magnification ×50.) (d) Histologic specimen treated with reticulin fiberstain, showing a marked increase of reticulin fiber deposition. (Original magnification ×50. From Larheim et al.[18] Reprinted with permission.)

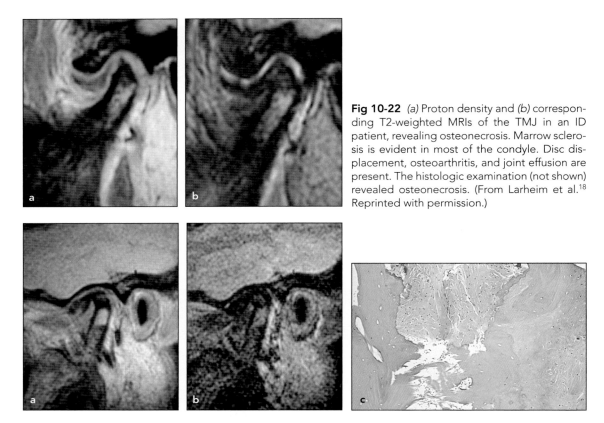

Fig 10-22 (a) Proton density and (b) corresponding T2-weighted MRIs of the TMJ in an ID patient, revealing osteonecrosis. Marrow sclerosis is evident in most of the condyle. Disc displacement, osteoarthritis, and joint effusion are present. The histologic examination (not shown) revealed osteonecrosis. (From Larheim et al.[18] Reprinted with permission.)

Fig 10-23 Patient with advanced osteoarthritis (a) proton density and (b) corresponding T2-weighted MRIs of the TMJ reveal sclerotic marrow in most of the condyle. Disc displacement and osteoarthritis are evident. (c) Histologic section of a bone marrow biopsy from the same mandibular condyle. The marrow space has been replaced by dense sclerotic bone and fibrous tissue, suggesting a reparative process and not osteonecrosis. (Hematoxylin-eosin stain; original magnification ×50. (From Larheim et al.[18] Reprinted with permission.)

Bone Marrow Abnormalities and Joint Effusion

Larheim et al[18] found that 39% of TMJs (7 of 18) with histologically documented marrow edema and/or osteonecrosis showed MRI signs of joint effusion (see Fig 10-22), ie, an amount of TMJ fluid not observed in asymptomatic volunteers.[17] This inflammatory reaction was observed in both early and late osteonecrosis[18] and is in accordance with MRI observations in the various stages of osteonecrosis of the hip.[61] In a clinical MRI study of TMJs selected for internal derangement and effusion, 40% showed abnormal bone marrow.[54] The association between abnormal bone marrow and TMJ effusion has also previously been observed in clinical MRI studies.[51,58,59]

Bone Marrow Abnormalities and Cortical Bone Integrity

Almost half (four of nine) of the TMJs with histologically documented marrow edema without evidence of necrosis showed normal cortical bone on MRI.[18] This has been substantiated in clinical MRI studies[54,62,63] (Fig 10-24). Obviously, bone marrow edema can occur in the mandibular condyle with no signs of either osteonecrosis or osteoarthritis. Normal cortical bone was found on MRIs of two patients with histologic evidence of osteonecrosis in the mandibular condyle[18] (Fig 10-25). This finding has also been substantiated in clinical MRI studies.[54,62,63] Thus, marrow edema, osteonecrosis, and osteoarthritis of the TMJ may be separate entities. This is known from the hip, where

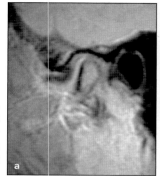
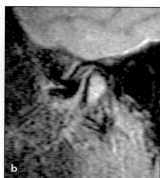

Fig 10-24 Marrow edema in the entire condyle, normal cortical bone, and disc displacement revealed in (a) proton density and (b) corresponding T2-weighted MRIs of the TMJ in an ID patient. (From Larheim et al.[54] Reprinted with permission.)

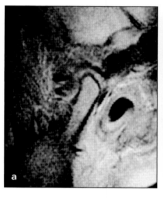
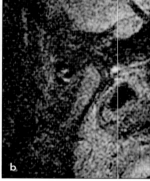
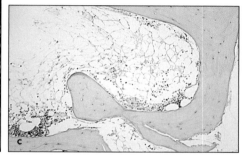

Fig 10-25 (a) Proton density and (b) corresponding T2-weighted MRIs of the TMJ in a patient with osteonecrosis. Cortical bone is normal, and there is a normal signal from the bone marrow. Disc displacement and deformation are evident. (c) Histologic specimen of a bone marrow biopsy from the same mandibular condyle, showing a focus of marrow necrosis, loss of hematopoietic elements, and breakdown of marrow fat. (Hematoxylin-eosin stain; original magnification ×50. From Larheim et al.[18] Reprinted with permission.)

osteoarthritis develops secondary to osteonecrosis after weakening of the subarticular bone with collapse and subarticular fracture.[64]

Pathogenesis of Abnormal Bone Marrow

The pathogenesis of osteonecrosis is in general poorly understood, but it is well known that marrow edema in the hip may be a precursor to osteonecrosis and that marrow edema may be transient.[60,65] In the hip, the predisposing factors for osteonecrosis include sickle cell disease, long-term steroid therapy, and alcoholism. Nontraumatic cases are frequently bilateral, whereas trauma can cause unilateral osteonecrosis.[66] None of these systemic factors were present in the TMJ patient group studied histologically, and all cases were unilateral including the two patients with bilateral histologic observations.[18] Therefore, the pathogenesis is probably different in the TMJ

than in other joints. Because most TMJ patients with histologic evidence of osteonecrosis showed MRI signs of osteoarthritis and all patients had an internal derangement, the etiology in this joint is probably related to local microtrauma from the internal derangement and/or osteoarthritis rather than vascular compromise. The relationship with internal derangement and osteoarthritis has also been suggested by others.[51,54,58,59,62,63,67]

The relationship between bone marrow alterations and osteoarthritis is not completely understood in other joints either.[18] Moreover, the distinction between primary osteonecrosis and necrosis secondary to osteoarthritis may be impossible based on core biopsy specimens. In advanced cases of osteoarthritis, microscopic foci of necrosis are frequently found immediately adjacent to the joint surface. Occasionally, small infarcts can occur, but again they are found at the joint surface and only in joints with advanced osteoarthritis.[68] Of course, the end stage of both of these pathologic processes is likely to be indistinguishable.

| Table 10-6 | Disc position categories in the closed-mouth position in 70 patients with TMDs examined with MRI*† |

MRI findings	Disc position category (No. of TMJs)‡							
	Normal superior	Partial anterior in lateral part	Complete anterior	Partial anterolateral	Complete anterolateral	Complete anteromedial	Lateral	Total
All joints with effusion	3	4	35	4	28	1	1	76
Disc displacement in open-mouth position	0	0	27	0	22	1	1	51
Bone marrow abnormalities	1	0	10	0	6	1	0	18
Cortical bone abnormalities	2	0	16	1	10	1	1	31

*From Larheim et al.[54] Reprinted with permission.
†Patients with previous TMJ surgery, systemic inflammatory joint disease, facial growth disturbances, direct traumas to or fractures of facial bones, condylar hyperplasia, or condylar tumor, as well as patients whose MRIs were of inferior quality, were excluded from the study.
‡See Table 10-1.

Clinical Meaning of Abnormal Bone Marrow

Osteonecrosis of the femoral head is a debilitating, progressive disease associated with severe pain, breakdown of bone, and loss of height that often requires total hip replacement. In the TMJ, the condition seems less aggressive and we have noted a few cases in which there was no or little progression over a 3-year period. However, the "natural course" of osteonecrosis in the mandibular condyle is unknown. In histologically documented material, the surgical TMJ treatment was based on the clinical findings and the MRI documentation of internal derangement, not on the abnormal bone marrow that occasionally occurred.[18] In this highly selected patient series, however, the frequency of bone marrow abnormalities (36%) was about four times higher than was found in a consecutive series of patients referred for TMJ imaging (8% to 10%)[17,62,69] and almost at the same level as that found in selected joints with effusion (40%).[54] Moreover, in a clinical study, an association of TMJ pain with abnormal bone marrow in the mandibular condyle was found in joints with the same status of internal derangement.[63] Presently, no documentation exists as to whether patients with bone marrow abnormalities should be treated differently than those without such abnormalities. This problem should be addressed in longitudinal studies focusing on the clinical significance of osteonecrosis of the mandibular condyle.

Summary

In patients with TMDs referred for diagnostic imaging, the predominant TMJ finding is an internal derangement related to disc displacement, which is significantly more frequent than in asymptomatic volunteers. Furthermore, complete disc displacement in the closed-mouth position, nonreducing disc displacement, joint effusion, and condylar marrow abnormalities are significantly more frequent in such patients.

In a detailed analysis of 70 patients with TMJ effusion,[54] almost all patients had disc displacement bilaterally. However, the joint effusion was mostly unilateral or there was a lesser amount of fluid in the contralateral joint. The abnormal bone marrow was mostly unilateral. Many patients had unilateral pain or more pain on one side, in accordance with the general opinion about pain experience in patients with TMDs. In a regression analysis, the self-reported within-patient difference in TMJ pain on the two sides was positively dependent on TMJ effusion and condylar marrow abnormalities but negatively dependent on cortical bone abnormalities. Of the 73 TMJs with ID and effusion in this study, 86% fell within two categories of disc displacement, complete anterior or complete anterolateral displacement. In these two categories, 78% had a nonreducing displacement, 25% had bone marrow abnormalities, and 41% had osteoarthritis (Table 10-6). Thus, this seems to be a subgroup of patients with TMDs showing severe intra-articular pathology, mostly without osteoarthritis, and probably before this condition develops.

It should be emphasized, however, that patients with effusion (and/or abnormal bone marrow) seem to constitute only a minor portion of patients (fewer than one fourth) referred for diagnostic TMJ imaging. The majority of patients have an internal derangement (specific types of disc displacement, usually not found in asymptomatic volunteers) but without accompanying joint abnormalities.

Patients with Systemic Inflammatory Joint Diseases (Arthritides)

General Pathologic and Radiologic Abnormalities

There are a number of systemic inflammatory diseases that are characterized by prominent inflammation of the synovial membrane. Rheumatoid arthritis (RA) is the most frequent, but other well-known diseases are the seronegative spondyloarthropathies, eg, ankylosing spondylitis and psoriatic arthropathy (see chapter 9).

Pathologically, edema and cellular accumulation result in a macroscopically evident thickened synovial membrane, with synovial villous formation and joint effusion. This "synovial" stage of RA is accompanied by four different types of radiographic abnormality[31]: soft tissue swelling, periarticular osteoporosis, loss of interosseous space because of cartilage destruction, and cortical erosions, which relate to the location of the aggressive inflammatory synovial tissue, pannus, in peripheral portions of the joint where bone does not possess protective cartilage. In advanced stages of the disease, more severe bone destruction may occur, corresponding to an intraosseous extension of the inflamed synovium. In long-standing disease, secondary osteoarthritis (occasionally with fragmentation and loose joint bodies) may be observed, and the end stage may become intra-articular fibrous ankylosis or, occasionally, bony ankylosis.[31]

Different imaging modalities (MRI, computerized tomography [CT], ultrasound, radionuclide imaging, etc), as well as conventional radiography, are used to study patients with arthritis.[70] Conventional radiography is probably still the most frequently used technique in the establishment of a specific diagnosis, when combined with the history, physical examination, and laboratory data. However, even the early reports of MRI indicated its diagnostic value in the examination of different joints.[70–72] In particular, MRI allows differentiation of inflammatory pannus

from effusion, first documented in the knee joint when gadopentetate dimeglumine was used for enhancement of the inflamed synovium and pannus formation.[73–75]

Diagnostic Imaging Versus Clinical Examination of the TMJ

Symptoms and signs in the TMJ of patients with arthritides such as RA, ankylosing spondylitis, and psoriatic arthropathy may be similar. Imaging examinations are therefore mandatory for differential diagnosis. However, in patients with RA, radiographic bone abnormalities may not correlate with the clinical findings. Joints with normal bone can be symptomatic, whereas joints with severe abnormalities may be silent.[76,77] Furthermore, the clinical assessment of joint function may not correlate with the radiographic assessment. A clinical mouth-opening capacity of more than 40 mm resulting from evident rotation of the condyle may be observed in patients in whom radiographs have indicated impaired translatory motion.[78,79] Anterior bite opening may be a characteristic clinical sign, predominantly occurring in patients with RA and severe bilateral destruction of the condyles.[78,80] Morning stiffness and swelling over the TMJ area are occasionally reported.

Radiographic Bone Destruction

Change in the radiologic joint space, especially narrowing, is a hallmark of most types of arthritis,[70] but this is an unreliable sign in the assessment of TMJ involvement, for several reasons: (1) the joint space may not be accurately visualized on certain types of radiographs, ie, transcranial or panoramic views; (2) the space is highly variable throughout the joint; and (3) dental occlusion with molar support may prevent the joint space from collapsing. Thus, of the four types of radiographic abnormalities considered classic manifestations of RA, only cortical erosion is of diagnostic value.

The frequency of radiographically visible TMJ destruction varies in the different diseases and seems to be greater in rheumatoid arthritis than in ankylosing spondylitis and psoriatic arthropathy.[76,81] However, the destructive bone abnormalities in the TMJ are similar in the different arthritides, although RA involvement seems to be bilateral more frequently. In one study of older patients (mean age, 58 years) with RA of long duration (more than 20 years), radiographic TMJ abnormalities were found in more than 80%,[78] sup-porting the results of a previous study.[82] The destructive bone changes were frequently accompanied by

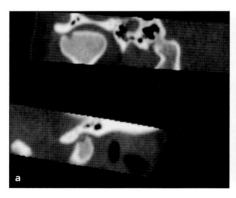
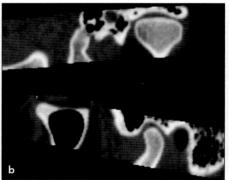
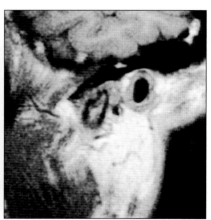

Fig 10-26 Computerized tomograms of the TMJ in a patient with psoriatic arthropathy. *(a)* Right joint. Oblique coronal, central section, and oblique sagittal, lateral section. Small, "punched-out" areas of cortical destruction are visible. *(b)* Left joint. The oblique coronal, central section, and oblique sagittal, central section, reveal normal bone.

Fig 10-27 MRI of the TMJ in a patient with rheumatoid arthritis. The image reveals complete destruction of the articular disc and cortical destruction of the lateral part of the condyle.

productive bone changes indicating secondary osteoarthritis in this age group, which could make it difficult to distinguish RA from osteoarthritis unrelated to the chronic systemic disease.

Comparison of Imaging Methods for Bone Evaluation

Tomography is superior to other conventional radiographic methods for depicting minor cortical erosions in the TMJ and may show progression of erosions during a 3-month period.[21,80] CT has been found to be particularly valuable for depicting TMJ erosions[83,84] and proved in a comparative study to be superior to conventional tomography for depicting subtle cortical changes.[85] Punched-out destructions typically may be found in various locations of the joint with CT (Fig 10-26). In cases complicated with bony ankylosis, CT is definitely the imaging method of choice.[80]

Soft Tissue and Bone Manifestations

Granulomatous synovial tissue (pannus) growing into the disc and bone has been documented in autopsy specimens of the TMJ,[86] in surgically treated patients,[87–90] by arthroscopy,[91] and by imaging.[36,88,92–94]

In 20 symptomatic TMJs of patients (mean age, 28 years) with RA, ankylosing spondylitis, or psoriatic arthropathy examined with arthrotomography,[92] irregularity in the outline of the contrast material, bone contour-contrast material gaps, and/or small joint compartments were found as indirect signs of synovial hyperplasia or pannus formation in 75%. Normal disc position was found in the majority of joints, but 40% showed perforation in the central thin portion of the disc. In most joints, both soft tissue abnormalities and cortical erosions were found. Larheim et al[36] published the first description of the MRI manifestations of RA (including patients with juvenile arthritis), ankylosing spondylitis, and psoriatic arthropathy in the TMJ. Of 36 TMJs in 28 symptomatic patients (mean age, 29 years), 78% were diagnosed as having rheumatic disease involvement. The most typical MRI findings were bone destruction or deformation and soft tissue abnormalities (normal disc position, abnormal disc structure [fragmentation, poor delineation, and severe flattening], and severely destroyed discs [Fig 10-27]). Only four joints showed joint effusion. Side-by-side comparison of MRI and tomographic images showed a high level of agreement concerning both cortical erosions and secondary osteoarthritis, but MRI demonstrated additional abnormalities, such as marrow edema and marrow sclerosis.[36]

In two studies comparing MRI, arthrotomography, CT, and conventional tomography with surgical observations,[88,93] MRI was found to be superior for the assessment of moderate or severe rheumatic TMJ involvement. However, CT was the superior method for assessing the bony details. MRI without contrast injection seemed to be of limited value in early diagnosis of the disease because of its inability to show the synovial thickening.

The value of contrast-enhanced MRI for the assessment of the pathologic synovial membrane in the TMJ involved by rheumatic disease was demonstrated by Smith et al,[94] indicating that the early "synovial stage" of

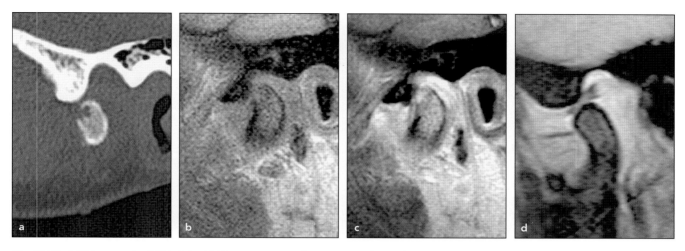

Fig 10-28 (a) Direct sagittal CT of the TMJ in a patient with psoriatic arthropathy (same patient as in Fig 10-26), revealing a punched-out area of destruction in the condyle. (b) T1-weighted precontrast and (c) T1-weighted postcontrast MRIs. The contrast medium enhances the visibility of both the pathologic synovial membrane and pannus in the joint compartments and the area of condylar destruction. (d) MRI taken in the open-mouth position, revealing a normal disc in the normal position.

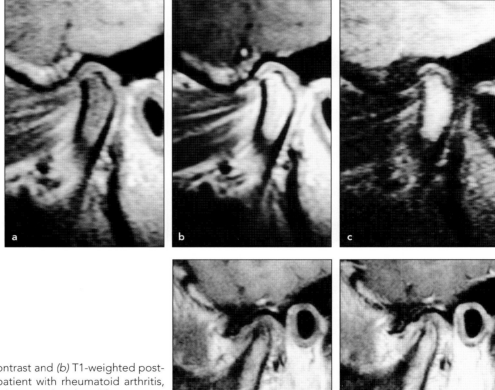

Fig 10-29 (a) T1-weighted precontrast and (b) T1-weighted postcontrast MRIs of the TMJ in a patient with ankylosing spondylitis. The abnormal, thin disc is in a normal position. The contrast medium enhances the visibility of the pathologic synovial membrane and pannus in both compartments, the cortical erosion of the condyle, and the marrow edema. (c) T2-weighted MRI. There is an increased signal from the bone marrow, consistent with edema.

Fig 10-30 (a) T1-weighted precontrast and (b) T1-weighted postcontrast MRIs of the TMJ in a patient with rheumatoid arthritis, showing severe destruction of the articular disc. The contrast medium enhances the visibility of the pathologic synovial membrane and pannus.

the disease, ie, before bone is involved, also may be detected. MRI manifestations in the TMJ with varying severity of rheumatic involvement are illustrated with three patients: one with psoriatic arthropathy (Fig 10-28),

another with ankylosing spondylitis (Fig 10-29), and the third with RA (Fig 10-30). These subgroups of patients cannot be distinguished based on the abnormalities revealed by TMJ MRI.

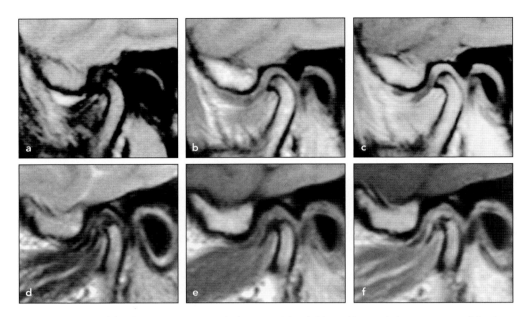

Fig 10-31 MRIs of the TMJ in a patient with rheumatoid arthritis and internal derangement of the *(a to c)* right and *(d to f)* left joints. *(a)* T2-weighted image, revealing joint effusion in the anterior recess of the upper compartment. *(b)* T1-weighted precontrast image. *(c)* T1-weighted postcontrast image, enhancing the visibility of the pathologic synovial membrane in the periphery of the effusion, around the displaced disc, and in the posterior attachment. *(d)* T2-weighted image. There is no fluid. *(e)* T1-weighted precontrast image. *(f)* T1-weighted postcontrast image, enhancing the visibility of the pathologic synovial membrane and pannus around the displaced disc and in the posterior attachment.

Internal Derangement

A patient with generalized inflammatory joint disease and symptomatic TMJs does not necessarily have rheumatic TMJ involvement. Some patients obviously have internal derangement unrelated to their generalized disease.[36,88,92,93] It should be emphasized, however, that patients with systemic disease involving the TMJ may also have disc displacement, probably complicating the condition for the patient. A patient with bilateral disc displacement and RA involving both TMJs is illustrated in Fig 10-31.

Value of Longitudinal Examinations

In one patient with psoriatic arthropathy and unilateral TMJ symptoms followed with MRI during a 1-year-and-4-month period, a normally positioned disc developed into a disc displacement. The question was raised whether there could be a causal relationship between this displacement and the rheumatic involvement of the TMJ due to destruction of the posterior attachment.[57] This patient also demonstrated joint effusion and marrow edema, indicating an inflammatory process with high activity. At follow-up, neither joint effusion nor marrow edema could be visualized. This longitudinal study thus demonstrated the capability of MRI to depict exacerbation and subsidence of inflammation.[57] Surgical TMJ treatment was planned both for this patient and the patient illustrated in Fig 10-31, but was not performed because their inflammatory disease deactivated. This clinical picture is in accordance with the experience with the arthritides in general. Great variations, with exacerbations and remissions, are observed clinically, although a progressive disease course is typical.

Juvenile Arthritis—General Aspects

The true frequency of juvenile arthritis is not known, but about 3% to 5% of all patients with RA are historically reported to experience onset before 16 years of age.[95] Juvenile arthritis differs in many respects from RA in adults. It is a heterogenous disease with different subgroups, depending on the different classifications used. Whereas rheumatoid factor seropositivity is common in adults, it is seldom found in patients with juvenile arthritis.

Three sets of diagnostic criteria, with different disease names, have been used for this condition: juvenile rheumatoid arthritis, chronic arthritis, or idiopathic arthritis.[95] There are generally two peak ages of onset, between 1 and 3 years of age and around 9 years of age. At onset, large joints, such as knees, wrists, and ankles, are more prominently involved than the small peripheral joints that are typically involved in adult RA. Bony ankylosis in the cervical spine is particularly characteristic of juvenile arthritis as well as mandibular growth disturbances such as facial asymmetry or micrognathia (Fig 10-32).

Although conventional radiographic methods for imaging the different joints are routinely used as an adjunct to the clinical examination of these patients, MRI was recognized early to be of diagnostic value for evaluating both synovial hyperplasia and the status of the articular cartilage, as well as the occurrence of avascular necrosis, none of which can be evaluated with conventional radiography.[96,97]

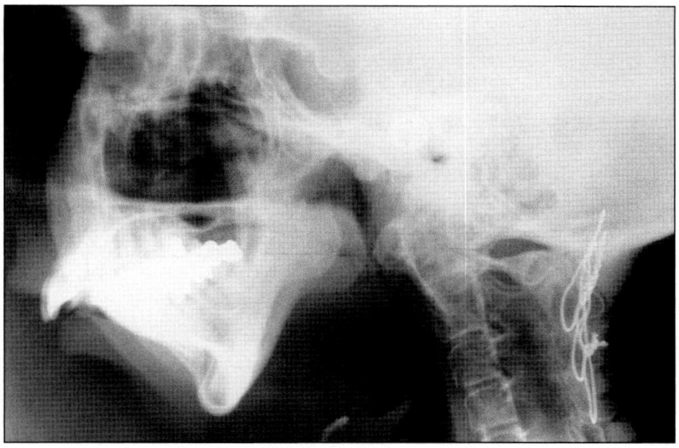

Fig 10-32 Lateral cephalogram of the facial skeleton of a 28-year-old woman with juvenile rheumatoid arthritis. Micrognathia is evident, and there is bony ankylosis of the cervical spine (which has been surgically fixed).

Juvenile Arthritis of the TMJ

The TMJ is frequently involved in patients with juvenile arthritis, depending on different parameters such as disease duration, the patient's age, and the disease type at onset.[21,98,99] In particular, patients with a polyarticular disease course will develop TMJ abnormalities. Of 29 patients with pauciarticular onset who had developed polyarticular disease at data registration, 62% showed radiographic TMJ involvement, compared to 25% of 36 patients whose disease remained pauciarticular from onset.[100] Because clinical symptoms such as pain may not be as dominant in children as in adults with RA, radiographic examinations are mandatory for the diagnostic assessment of TMJ involvement in children.[98]

Panoramic radiographic examinations have been used and found valuable for screening of condylar deformities such as flattening. However, typical imaging findings in this patient group also include a flat fossa and eminence, which can be diagnosed with transcranial radiography or a tomographic method.[21,99,101] The TMJ in children with severe juvenile arthritis has been noted to resemble the normal infantile TMJ in appearance. It has therefore been postulated that the changes observed in affected TMJs are due to lack of normal joint development rather than joint destruction by the inflammatory process.[102,103] Later MRI findings in this disease have not resolved this issue, and further prospective studies are needed.[104]

The fact that TMJ arthritis may be found even without cortical erosions, paralleling findings in other joints such as the knee, is important to know for the diagnostic assessment of this disease. Reparative changes in previous bone

erosions and "normalization" or even "overgrowth" of the mandibular condyle may occur, because of extensive remodeling in patients with low disease activity.[21,99] On the other hand, progressive bone destruction in the TMJ during a 6-month period has been demonstrated in longitudinal studies of children with high disease activity.[105]

In patients with juvenile arthritis, MRI has proved to be valuable for the diagnostic assessment of TMJ involvement, as first described by Larheim et al[36] and later confirmed by Taylor et al.[104] Contrast-enhanced MRI may reveal the inflamed synovium and pannus formation as in adult RA, ie, before the bone structures are involved.[94,106] In 15 children (mean age, 12 years) with a short generalized disease history, 87% had TMJ involvement on contrast-enhanced MRI.[106]

Typically, MRI reveals both bone abnormalities (bone destruction or bone deformation without cortical erosions or a combination of bone destruction and deformation) and soft tissue abnormalities (flat disc in a normal position or poorly delineated or destroyed disc). Joint effusion is not frequently reported, probably because the patients were not in a very active phase when imaged. A 14-year-old patient with high disease activity and unilateral TMJ involvement is shown in Fig 10-33. A 12-year-old patient, referred by an orthodontist because of an anterior open bite and flattened condyles revealed on a panoramic image, is shown in Fig 10-34. In this previously undiagnosed patient, CT and MRI manifestations of juvenile arthritis are evident in both TMJs (Fig 10-35). In this age group, internal TMJ derangement also may be found.[107] Thus, internal derangement may occasionally

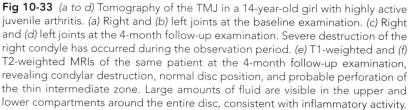

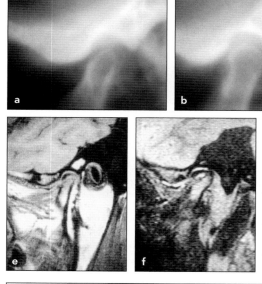

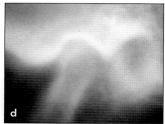

Fig 10-33 *(a to d)* Tomography of the TMJ in a 14-year-old girl with highly active juvenile arthritis. *(a)* Right and *(b)* left joints at the baseline examination. *(c)* Right and *(d)* left joints at the 4-month follow-up examination. Severe destruction of the right condyle has occurred during the observation period. *(e)* T1-weighted and *(f)* T2-weighted MRIs of the same patient at the 4-month follow-up examination, revealing condylar destruction, normal disc position, and probable perforation of the thin intermediate zone. Large amounts of fluid are visible in the upper and lower compartments around the entire disc, consistent with inflammatory activity.

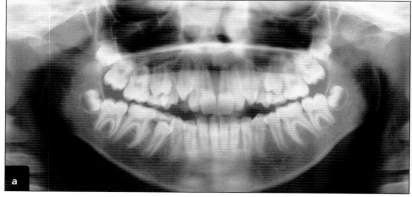

Fig 10-34 *(a)* Panoramic radiograph and *(b)* lateral cephalogram of a 12-year-old girl with flattened condyles and anterior open bite without a known cause.

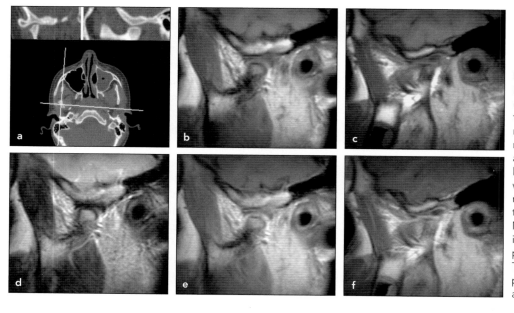

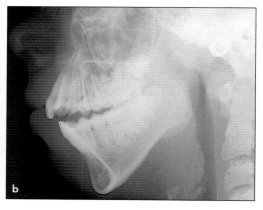

Fig 10-35 Same patient as in Fig 10-34. *(a)* CT of the right TMJ. *(b and c)* T1-weighted precontrast MRIs of the left TMJ. Abnormalities are similar in both the right and left joints: a flat fossa and eminence and a flat condyle located anteriorly in the fossa when the patient is in the closed-mouth position. The disc position is normal. *(d)* T2-weighted MRI of the left TMJ. No joint fluid is visible. *(e and f)* T1-weighted postcontrast MRIs of the left TMJ, enhancing the view of the pathologic synovial membrane and pannus.

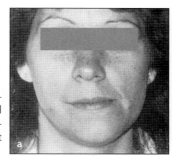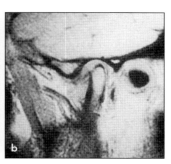

Fig 10-36 Mandibular asymmetry secondary to internal derangement and condylar hypoplasia. (a) Photograph, revealing facial asymmetry. (b) Oblique sagittal MRI, revealing internal derangement, osteoarthritis, and a hypoplastic condyle. (From Westesson et al.[1] Reprinted with permission.)

be visible as the only imaging abnormality in children with juvenile arthritis.[21,99]

Unilateral TMJ involvement is rather frequent; about 40% was reported by Larheim et al.[98] Unilateral involvement may result in jaw asymmetry and underdevelopment on the affected side.[100] However, unilateral TMJ abnormality may seldom lead to micrognathia, which is typically observed in patients with severe bilateral TMJ abnormalities.[108] Depending on different parameters, the TMJ involvement will not always have an evident impact on mandibular growth.

Patients with Other Conditions

Facial (Mandibular) Asymmetry

Asymmetry of the mandible, and thus the face, is generally due to diminished or increased condylar growth. Many causes are obvious and generally accepted. Jaw fractures, juvenile arthritis, and congenital anomalies (eg, hemifacial microsomia) can lead to mandibular underdevelopment, and condylar hyperplasia and tumors can lead to mandibular overgrowth. However, in many cases, the cause of the mandibular growth disturbance is unclear, and an association with internal derangement has received increasing attention in the literature (Fig 10-36).

In 1985, 3 of 31 patients aged 8 to 16 years were reported to have an obvious growth deficit and internal derangement of the TMJ with accompanying degenerative bone changes, condylar hypoplasia, and a short mandibular neck.[107] All three patients had previously sustained trauma to the mandible, and at least two of them had experienced fractures.

A series of patients with mandibular asymmetry and even micrognathia, mostly adults up to 69 years of age, was reported in 1990.[59] It was claimed that this was due to internal derangement and bony abnormalities of the

TMJ, mostly osteoarthritis, osteochondritis dissecans, and avascular necrosis. However, patients with previous implant surgery, as well as those who had intra-articular fractures or systemic inflammatory joint diseases, were included; furthermore, no statistical analyses were performed on this large series of patients.

In another study of orthodontic and orthognathic surgery patients with a wide range of ages, the definition of mandibular asymmetry was clearly based on posteroanterior cephalograms, and a statistically significant association with a history of prepubertal trauma was found.[109]

Another study reported the findings in 11 patients aged 12 to 32 years with prominent mandibular asymmetry; they were part of a series of about 300 seeking treatment for TMJ pain and dysfunction.[110] Condylar hyperplasia leading to mandibular overgrowth was identified as the cause of asymmetry in 5 of the 11 patients. The other six patients had an internal derangement and deformed, degenerative, and hypoplastic condyles and short mandibular necks. Five of these were unilateral and one had a more pronounced TMJ abnormality on the affected side. None of these patients had a history of mandibular fracture.

From these studies, it appears that internal derangement and joint degeneration, leading to hypoplasia of the condyle and mandibular neck, may have an effect on the entire ramus. This is supported by earlier studies on inhibited mandibular growth associated with *arthrosis deformans juvenilis*, a term introduced by Boering in 1966.[111] In this series of 400 patients, about one fourth were aged 20 years or younger. Many had mandibular growth disturbances and no history of trauma. Although this was before the advent of soft tissue imaging, a number of the patients had an obvious internal derangement.

MRI studies have shown that disc displacement frequently occurs in preorthodontic adolescents, supporting previous studies.[112] Nebbe and Major[112] have used statistical methods to systematically analyze the relationship between TMJ internal derangement visible on MRI and

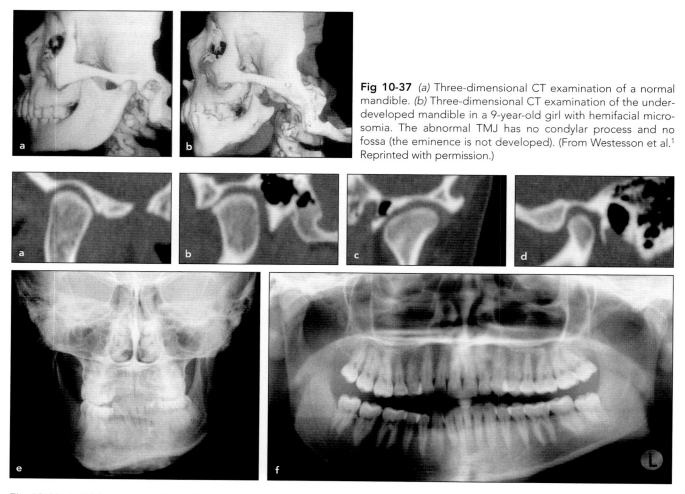

Fig 10-37 *(a)* Three-dimensional CT examination of a normal mandible. *(b)* Three-dimensional CT examination of the underdeveloped mandible in a 9-year-old girl with hemifacial microsomia. The abnormal TMJ has no condylar process and no fossa (the eminence is not developed). (From Westesson et al.[1] Reprinted with permission.)

Fig 10-38 *(a)* Oblique coronal and *(b)* oblique sagittal CT sections of the enlarged condyle in a 23-year-old patient with condylar hyperplasia, revealing a normal fossa. Corresponding *(c)* oblique coronal and *(d)* oblique sagittal CT sections of the contralateral normal joint for comparison. *(e)* Posteroanterior cephalogram, revealing facial asymmetry. *(f)* Panoramic radiograph, revealing mandibular asymmetry and overdevelopment of the right condylar process.

craniofacial asymmetry in orthodontic patients and concluded that there is a correlation with mandibular morphology and position.[113] The frequency and severity of the mandibular growth disturbances caused by TMJ internal derangement, and thus the clinical implications, should be the subject of future studies.

Congenital Anomalies

These are rare and very heterogenous. A bifid condyle may be detected randomly on panoramic radiographs and is usually of no clinical significance. Hemifacial microsomia is characterized by pronounced facial asymmetry. The TMJ is always underdeveloped but may have a disc in a normal position on the underdeveloped side.[1] In more severe cases, the entire joint may be absent; three-dimensional CT is the preferred imaging evaluation (Fig 10-37).

Condylar Hyperplasia and Osteochondroma

Condylar hyperplasia is the most common postnatal growth abnormality of the TMJ, usually detected in the third decade when the mandible continues to grow unilaterally and the patient develops evident facial asymmetry (Fig 10-38). Bone scintigraphy is widely advocated as a method to assess growth activity presurgically.[114] Benign tumors such as osteochondroma and osteoma may be diffi-

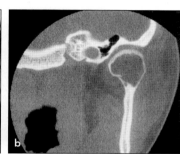

Fig 10-39 Patient with osteochondroma. *(a)* MRI and *(b)* CT of the TMJ reveal an enlarged mandibular condyle with an irregular outline and mineralization. The temporal component is normal. The disc is normal and located in a normal position. (Courtesy of Dr Donald Macher, Rochester, NY.) (From Westesson et al.[1] Reprinted with permission.)

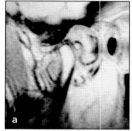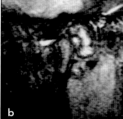
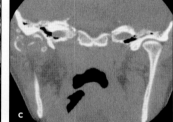

Fig 10-40 *(a)* MRI and *(b)* CT of the TMJ in a patient with a simple bone cyst. The mandibular condyle is enlarged, and there is thinning of the intact cortex. The temporal component is normal, and the disc is normal and located in a normal position. (From Westesson et al.[1] Reprinted with permission.)

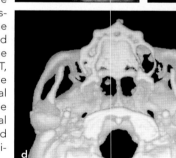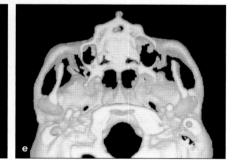

Fig 10-41 *(a)* T1-weighted and *(b)* T2-weighted MRIs of the TMJ in a patient with synovial chondromatosis. The expansive process posterior to the condyle has displaced the condyle out of the fossa (in the closed-mouth position). Joint effusion and excessive amounts of fluid are present. The condyle and disc are normal. *(c)* Coronal CT, revealing calcifications posterior to the condyle. *(d)* Preoperative three-dimensional CT. A large mass is located posterior to the condyle. *(e)* Postoperative three-dimensional CT. The mass was surgically removed together with a number of smaller cartilaginous elements.

cult to differentiate from this condition, but osteochondroma is usually more irregular in outline and may be more sclerotic (Fig 10-39).

Simple Bone Cyst

Simple bone cysts are most frequently found in the body of the mandible but may even occur in the condyle (Fig 10-40).

Synovial Chondromatosis

This is probably the most frequently reported benign lesion in the TMJ. It is expansive and can be locally aggressive; the first case with extension through the base of the skull into the middle cranial fossa was reported in 1987.[115] This aggressive behavior has also been documented in later published cases. The lesion usually is monoarticular and characterized by severe synovitis in addition to other abnormalities, such as multiple calcifications within the joint arising

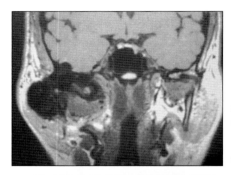

Fig 10-42 T1-weighted MRI of the TMJ in a patient with pigmented villonodular synovitis. A large mass of very low signal also penetrates the skull base. The T2-weighted images also showed an extremely low signal, and there was no enhancement on postcontrast images. (Courtesy of Dr Tim Larsson, Seattle, WA.) (From Westesson et al.[1] Reprinted with permission.)

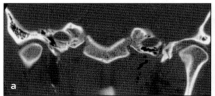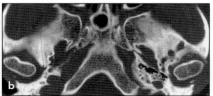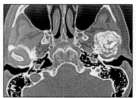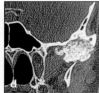

Fig 10-43 (a) Coronal and (b) axial CTs of a patient with early calcium pyrophosphate dehydrate deposition disease (pseudogout) in the left TMJ, characterized by subtle calcifications in the joint space. (c) Axial and (d) coronal CTs of a patient with advanced calcium pyrophosphate dehydrate deposition disease, showing extensive soft tissue calcifications.

from cartilaginous metaplasia of the synovial membrane (Fig 10-41). The disc and the condyle may be completely intact. The relative merits of CT and MRI for depicting the bone and soft tissue abnormalities have been beautifully demonstrated by Herzog and Mafee.[116]

Pigmented Villonodular Synovitis

Like synovial chondromatosis, pigmented villonodular synovitis may extend through the base of the skull.[117] The bony joint components are usually eroded,[1] as is the skull base in extensive cases (Fig 10-42). This expansive tumor or tumorlike condition is characterized by nodular synovial proliferation and hemarthrosis.[118] Due to the presence of blood by-products, T2-weighted MRIs show an extremely low signal.[1] As is the case with synovial chondromatosis,[21] pigmented villonodular synovitis is not enhanced on postcontrast MRIs.[1]

Crystal Deposition Diseases

Three common crystal deposition diseases affect joints in general, of which calcium pyrophosphate dehydrate crystal deposition disease (pseudogout) is the most common.[31] The deposition diseases can mimic a variety of conditions, including RA and osteoarthritis. Several cases also have been reported in the TMJ, and symptoms may mimic those of other TMDs. Extensive cases present with enlarged masses. In such cases, erosive changes of the bony joint components are usually found. They are all characterized by subtle or severe calcifications within the joint space, and these are best demonstrated on CT images[1] (Fig 10-43).

Coronoid Hyperplasia

Restricted mouth opening can have several causes, most frequently related to the masticatory muscles (trismus) and/or an internal derangement (nonreducing disc displacement or closed lock). However, one cause of restricted mouth opening that may be overlooked because the examination is generally focused on joint abnormalities is elongation of the coronoid process. In a series of 163 consecutive patients referred for radiographic examination of the TMJ, 5% had restricted mouth opening caused by coronoid process hyperplasia.[119] For detailed evaluation of the impingement between the malar bone and the coronoid process, three-dimensional CT is highly valuable[120] (Fig 10-44).

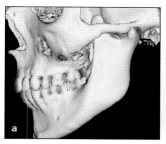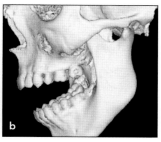

Fig 10-44 Three-dimensional CTs of patients with coronoid hyperplasia, taken in the *(a)* closed-mouth and *(b)* open-mouth positions. Movement of the mandible is impeded by contact of the enlarged coronoid process with the zygomatic process of the maxilla during mouth opening.

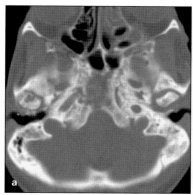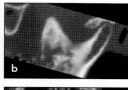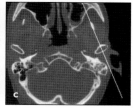

Fig 10-45 *(a)* Axial CT of the TMJ in a patient with osteoradionecrosis, revealing destruction of the right mandibular condyle and skull base. *(b)* Reformatted oblique sagittal CT of the TMJ in another patient with osteoradionecrosis. Destructive changes of the coronoid process are visible. *(c)* Axial view of patient in Fig 10-45b.

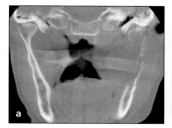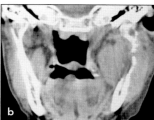

Fig 10-46 *(a)* Bone and *(b)* soft tissue CTs of the TMJ and mandible in a patient with a metastasis from lung cancer. There is severe destruction of the left mandibular ramus and condyle, and a large soft tissue mass is present.

Osteoradionecrosis

Osteoradionecrosis of the mandible may develop after radiotherapy in the oropharyngeal region, and CT has proved to be excellent to assess the amount of bone destruction.[121] Even the mandibular condyle may be involved, leading to impaired mandibular function (Fig 10-45).

Malignant Tumors

Malignant tumors rarely affect the TMJ, but there have been reports of patients treated for various TMDs in whom the underlying cause of the pain was an undiagnosed malignant tumor.[122,123] The need for diagnostic imaging and reimaging when the clinical symptoms do not correlate with the clinical signs has been emphasized.[123] A patient with restricted mouth opening and deviation caused by a malignant tumor involving the TMJ is shown in Fig 10-46.

References

1. Westesson P-L, Yamamoto M, Sano T, Okano T. Temporomandibular joint. In: Som PM, Curtin HD (eds). Head and Neck Imaging, ed 4. St Louis: Mosby, 2003:995–1053.
2. Paesani D, Westesson PL, Hatala MP, et al. Accuracy of clinical diagnosis for TMJ internal derangement and arthrosis. Oral Surg Oral Med Oral Pathol 1992;73:360–363.
3. Roberts C, Katzberg RW, Tallents RH, et al. The clinical predictability of internal derangements of the temporomandibular joint. Oral Surg Oral Med Oral Pathol 1991;71:412–504.
4. Emshoff R, Brandlmaier I, Bosch R, et al. Validation of the clinical diagnostic criteria for temporomandibular disorders for the diagnostic subgroup—Disc derangement with reduction. J Oral Rehabil 2002;29:1139–1145.
5. Musgrave MT, Westesson PL, Tallents RH, Manzione JV, Katzberg RW. Improved magnetic resonance imaging of the temporomandibular joint by oblique scanning planes. Oral Surg Oral Med Oral Pathol 1991;71:525–528.
6. Tasaki MM, Westesson PL. Temporomandibular joint: Diagnostic accuracy with sagittal and coronal MR imaging. Radiology 1993;186:723–729.

7. Kircos LT, Ortendahl DA, Mark AS, Arakawa M. Magnetic resonance imaging of the TMJ disc in asymptomatic volunteers. J Oral Maxillofac Surg 1987;45:852–854.

8. Katzberg RW, Westesson PL, Tallents RH, Drake CM. Anatomic disorders of the temporomandibular joint disc in asymptomatic subjects. J Oral Maxillofac Surg 1996;54:147–153.

9. Tasaki MM, Westesson PL, Isberg AM, Ren Y-F, Tallents RH. Classification and prevalence of temporomandibular joint disk displacement in patients and symptom-free volunteers. Am J Orthod Dentofac Orthop 1996;109:249–262.

10. Larheim TA, Westesson PL, Sano T. Temporomandibular joint disk displacement: Comparison in asymptomatic volunteers and patients. Radiology 2001;218:428–432.

11. Kerstens HCJ, Golding RP, valk J, Van der Kwast WAM. Magnetic resonance imaging of partial temporomandibular disc displacement. J Oral Maxillofac Surg 1989;47:25–29.

12. De Bont LG, Dijkgraaf LC, Stegenga B. Epidemiology and natural progression of articular temporomandibular disorders. Oral Surg Oral Med Oral Pathol Oral Radiol Endod 1997;83:72–76.

13. Paesani D, Salas E, Martinez A, Isberg A. Prevalence of temporomandibular joint disk displacement in infants and young children. Oral Surg Oral Med Oral Pathol Oral Radiol Endod 1999;87:15–19.

14. Ribeiro RF, Tallents RH, Katzberg RW, et al. The prevalence of disc displacement in symptomatic and asymptomatic volunteers aged 6 to 25 years. J Orofac Pain 1997;11:37–47.

15. Drace JE, Enzmann DR. Defining the normal temporomandibular joint: closed-, partially open-, and open-mouth MR imaging of asymptomatic subjects. Radiology 1990;177:67–71.

16. Brooks SL, Westesson P-L, Eriksson L, Hansson LG, Barsotti JB, Arbor A. Prevalence of osseous changes in the temporomandibular joint of asymptomatic persons without internal derangement. Oral Surg Oral Med Oral Pathol 1992;73:118–122.

17. Larheim TA, Katzberg RW, Westesson PL, Tallents RH, Moss ME. MR evidence of temporomandibular joint fluid and condyle marrow alterations: Occurrence in asymptomatic volunteers and symptomatic patients. Int J Oral Maxillofac Surg 2001;30:113–117.

18. Larheim TA, Westesson PL, Hicks DG, Eriksson L, Brown DA. Osteonecrosis of the temporomandibular joint: Correlation of magnetic resonance imaging and histology. J Oral Maxillofac Surg 1999;57:888–898.

19. Westesson PL, Brooks SL. Temporomandibular joint: Relationship between MR evidence of effusion and the presence of pain and disk displacement. AJR Am J Roentgenol 1992;159:559–563.

20. Adams JC, Hamblen DL. Outline of Orthopedics, ed 13. London: Churchill Livingstone, 2001:135.

21. Larheim TA. Current trends in temporomandibular joint imaging. Oral Surg Oral Med Oral Pathol Oral Radiol Endod 1995;80:555–576.

22. Paesani D, Westesson PL, Hatala M, Tallents RH, Kurita K. Prevalence of temporomandibular joint internal derangement in patients with craniomandibular disorders. Am J Orthod Dentofacial Orthop 1992;101:41–47.

23. Katzberg RW, Westesson PL, Tallents RH, et al. Temporomandibular joint: MR assessment of rotational and sideways disk displacements. Radiology 1988;169:741–748.

24. Brooks SL, Westesson PL. Temporomandibular joint: Value of coronal MR images. Radiology 1993;88:317–321.

25. Westesson PL, Larheim TA, Tanaka H. Posterior disc displacement in the temporomandibular joint. J Oral Maxillofac Surg 1998;56:1266–1273.

26. De Leeuw R, Boering G, Stegenga B, de Bont LG. TMJ articular disc position and configuration 30 years after initial diagnosis of internal derangement. J Oral Maxillofac Surg 1995;53:234–241.

27. Pullinger AG, Seligman D. TMJ osteoarthrosis: A differentiation of diagnostic subgroups by symptom history and demographics. J Craniomandibular Disord 1987;1:251–256.

28. Lundh H, Westesson PL, Kopp S. A three year follow-up of patients with reciprocal temporomandibular joint clicking. Oral Surg Oral Med Oral Pathol 1987;63:530–533.

29. Greene CS, Laskin DM. Long-term status of TMJ clicking in patients with myofascial pain and dysfunction. J Am Dent Assoc 1988;117:461–465.

30. Sokoloff L. The pathology of osteoarthrosis and the role of ageing. In: Nuki G (ed). The Aetiopathogenesis of Osteoarthrosis. London: Pitman Medical, 1980:1–15.

31. Resnick D. Common disorders of synovium-lined joints: pathogenesis, imaging abnormalities, and complications. AJR Am J Roentgenol 1988;151:1079–1093.

32. Stegenga B, de Bont LG, Boering G, Van Willigen JD. Tissue responses to degenerative changes in the temporomandibular joint: A review. J Oral Maxillofac Surg 1991;49:1079–1088.

33. Moffett BC Jr, Johnson LC, McCabe JB, Askew HC. Articular remodeling of the adult temporomandibular joint. Am J Anat 1964;115:119–142.

34. Scapino RP. Histopathology associated with malposition of the human temporomandibular joint disk. Oral Surg Oral Med Oral Pathol 1983;55:382–397.

35. De Bont LG, Boering G, Liem RS, Eulderink F, Westesson PL. Osteoarthritis and internal derangement of the temporomandibular joint: A light microscopic study. J Oral Maxillofac Surg 1986;44:634–643.

36. Larheim TA, Smith HJ, Aspestrand F. Rheumatic disease of the temporomandibular joint: MR imaging and tomographic manifestations. Radiology 1990;175:527–531.

37. Peyron JG, Altman RD. The epidemiology of osteoarthritis. In: Moskowitz RW, Howell DS, Goldberg VM, Mankin HJ (eds). Osteoarthritis: Diagnosis and Medical/Surgical Management, ed 2. Philadelphia: Saunders, 1992:15–37.

38. Gynther GW, Tronje G, Holmlund AB. Radiographic changes in the temporomandibular joint in patients with generalized osteoarthritis and rheumatoid arthritis. Oral Surg Oral Med Oral Radiol Endod 1996;81:613–618.

39. Westesson PL, Rohlin M. Internal derangement related to osteoarthrosis in temporomandibular joint autopsy specimens. Oral Surg Oral Med Oral Pathol 1984;57:17–22.

40. Eriksson L, Westesson PL. Clinical and radiological study of patients with anterior disk displacement of the temporomandibular joint. Swed Dent J 1983;7:55–64.

41. Katzberg RW, Keith DA, Guralnick WC, Manzione JV Jr, Ten Eick WR. Internal derangements and arthritis of the temporomandibular joint. Radiology 1983;146:107–112.

42. Westesson PL. Structural hard-tissue changes in temporomandibular joints with internal derangement. Oral Surg Oral Med Oral Pathol 1985;59:220–224.

43. Anderson QN, Katzberg RW. Pathologic evaluation of disc dysfunction and osseous abnormalities of the temporomandibular joint. J Oral Maxillofac Surg 1985;43:947–951.

44. Brand JW, Whinery JG Jr, Anderson QN, Keenan KM. The effects of temporomandibular joint internal derangement and degenerative joint disease on tomographic and arthrotomographic images. Oral Surg Oral Med Oral Pathol 1989; 67:220–223.

45. Wilkes CH. Internal derangements of the temporomandibular joint: Pathological variations. Arch Otolaryngol Head Neck Surg 1989;115:469–477.

46. Manzione JV, Tallents RH. "Pseudomeniscus" sign: Potential indicator of repair or remodeling in temporomandibular joints with internal derangements. Presented to the Radiologic Society of North America. Radiology 1992;185(suppl):175.

47. Isacsson G, Isberg A, Johanson AS, Larson D. Internal derangement of the temporomandibular joint: Radiographic and histologic changes associated with severe pain. J Oral Maxillofac Surg 1986;44:771–778.

48. Paesani D, Westesson P-L. MR imaging of the TMJ: Decreased signal from the retrodiscal tissue. Oral Surg Oral Med Oral Pathol 1993;76:631–635.

49. Rao VM, Liem MD, Farole A, Razek AA. Elusive "stuck" disk in the temporomandibular joint: Diagnosis with MR imaging. Radiology 1993;189:823–827.

50. Harms SE, Wilk RM, Wolford LM, Chiles DG, Milam SB. The temporomandibular joint: Magnetic resonance imaging using surface coils. Radiology 1985;157:133–136.

51. Schellhas KP, Wilkes CH. Temporomandibular joint inflammation: Comparison of MR fast scanning with T1- and T2-weighted imaging techniques. AJR Am J Roentgenol 1989;153: 93–98.

52. Carlos GA, Florencio M, Muñoz M, Martin-Granizio R. Effusion in magnetic resonance imaging of the temporomandibular joint: A study of 123 joints. J Oral Maxillofac Surg 1998;56:314–318.

53. Rudisch A, Innerhofer K, Bertram S, Emshoff R. Magnetic resonance imaging findings of internal derangement and effusion in patients with unilateral temporomandibular joint pain. Oral Surg Oral Med Oral Pathol Oral Radiol Endod 2001;92:566–571.

54. Larheim, TA, Westesson PL, Sano T. MR grading of temporomandibular joint fluid: Association with disk displacement categories, condyle marrow abnormalities and pain. Int J Oral Maxillofac Surg 2001;30:104–112.

55. Yano K, Sano T, Okano T. A longitudinal study of magnetic resonance (MR) evidence of temporomandibular joint (TMJ) fluid in patients with TMJ disorders. Cranio 2004;22: 64–71.

56. Murakami K, Nishida M, Bessho K, Iizuka T, Tsuda Y, Konishi J. MRI evidence of high signal intensity and temporomandibular arthralgia and relating pain. Does the high signal correlate to the pain? Br J Oral Maxillofac Surg 1996;34: 220–224.

57. Larheim TA, Smith HJ, Aspestrand F. Rheumatic disease of temporomandibular joint with development of anterior disk displacement as revealed by magnetic resonance imaging. A case report. Oral Surg Oral Med Oral Pathol 1991;71: 246–249.

58. Schellhas KP, Wilkes CH, Fritts HM, Omlie MR, Lagrotteria LB. MR of osteochondritis dissecans and avascular necrosis of the mandibular condyle. AJR Am J Roentgenol 1989;152: 551–560.

59. Schellhas KP, Piper MA, Omlie MR. Facial skeleton remodeling due to temporomandibular joint degeneration: An imaging study of 100 patients. AJR Am J Roentgenol 1990;155: 373–383.

60. Nakamura T, Matsumoto T, Nishino M, Tomita K, Kadoya M. Early magnetic resonance imaging and histologic findings in a model of femoral head necrosis. Clin Orthop Relat Res 1997;334:68–72.

61. Mitchell DG, Steinberg ME, Dalinka MK, Rao VM, Fallon M, Kressel HY. Magnetic resonance imaging of the ischemic hip: Alterations within the osteonecrotic, viable, and reactive zones. Clin Orthop Relat Res 1989;244:60–77.

62. Sano T, Westesson PL, Larheim TA, Rubin SJ, Tallents RH. Osteoarthritis and abnormal bone marrow of the mandibular condyle. Oral Surg Oral Med Oral Pathol Oral Radiol Endod 1999;87:243–252.

63. Sano, T, Westesson PL, Larheim TA, Tahagi R. The association of temporomandibular joint pain with abnormal bone marrow in the mandibular condyle. J Oral Maxillofac Surg 2000;58:254–257.

64. Sweet DE, Madewell JE. Pathogenesis of osteonecrosis. In Resnick D, Niwayama G (eds). Diagnosis of Bone and Joint Disorders, ed 2, vol 5. Philadelphia: Saunders, 1988: 3188–3237.

65. Plenk H Jr, Hofmann S, Eschberger J, et al. Histomorphology and bone morphometry of the bone marrow edema syndrome of the hip. Clin Orthop Relat Res 1997;334:73–84.

66. Hauzeur JP, Pasteels JL, Orloff S. Bilateral non-traumatic aseptic osteonecrosis in the femoral head. An experimental study of incidence. J Bone Surg Am 1987;69:1221–1225.

67. Reiskin AB. Aseptic necrosis of the mandibular condyle: A common problem? Quintessence Int 1979;2:85–89.

68. Milgram JW. Radiologic and Histologic Pathology of Nontumorous Diseases of Bone and Joints. Northbrook, IL: Northbrook Publishing, 1990:959.

69. Lieberman JM, Gardner CL, Motta AO, Schwartz RD. Prevalence of bone marrow signal abnormalities observed in the temporomandibular joint using magnetic resonance imaging. J Oral Maxillofac Surg 1996;54:434–439.

70. Kaye JJ. Arthritis: Roles of radiography and other imaging techniques in evaluation. Radiology 1990;177:601–608.

71. Beltran J, Caudill JL, Herman LA, et al. Rheumatoid arthritis: MR imaging manifestations. Radiology 1987;165:153–157.

72. Aisen AM, Martel W, Ellis JH, McCune WJ. Cervical spine involvement in rheumatoid arthritis: MR imaging. Radiology 1987;165:159–163.

73. Reiser MF, Bongartz GP, Erlemann R, et al. Gadolinium-DTPA in rheumatoid arthritis and related diseases: First results with dynamic magnetic resonance imaging. Skeletal Radiol 1989;18:591–597.

74. König H, Sieper J, Wolf KJ. Rheumatoid arthritis: Evaluation of hypervascular and fibrous pannus with dynamic MR imaging enhanced with Gd-DTPA. Radiology 1990;176:473–477.

75. Kursunoglu-Brahme S, Riccio T, Weisman MH, et al. Rheumatoid knee: Role of gadopentetate-enhanced MR imaging. Radiology 1990;176:831–835.

76. Larheim TA, Johannessen S, Tveito L. Abnormalities of the temporomandibular joint in adults with rheumatic disease: A comparison of panoramic, transcranial, and transpharyngeal radiography with tomography. Dentomaxillofac Radiol 1988;17:109–113.

77. Åkerman S, Kopp S, Nilner M, Petersson A, Rohlin M. Relationship between clinical and radiologic findings of the temporomandibular joint in rheumatoid arthritis. Oral Surg Oral Med Oral Pathol 1988;66:639–643.

78. Larheim TA, Storhaug K, Tveito L. Temporomandibular joint involvement and dental occlusion in a group of adults with rheumatoid arthritis. Acta Odontol Scand 1983;41:301–309.

79. Larheim TA, Flöystrand F. Temporomandibular joint abnormalities and bite force in a group of adults with rheumatoid arthritis. J Oral Rehabil 1985;12:477–482.

80. Larheim TA. Rheumatoid arthritis and related joint diseases. In: Katzberg RW, Westesson PL (eds). Diagnosis of the Temporomandibular Joint. Philadelphia: Saunders, 1993:303–326.

81. Wenneberg B, Könönen M, Kallenberg A. Radiographic changes in the temporomandibular joint of patients with rheumatoid arthritis, psoriatic arthritis, and ankylosing spondylitis. J Craniomandib Disord 1990;4:35–39.

82. Ericsson S, Lundberg M. Alterations in the temporomandibular joint at various stages of rheumatoid arthritis. Acta Rheumatol Scand 1967;13:257–274.

83. Avrahami E, Segal R, Solomon A, et al. Direct coronal high resolution computed tomography of the temporomandibular joints in patients with rheumatoid arthritis. J Rheumatol 1989;16:298–301.

84. Guipille P, Fouquet B, Cotty P, Goga D, Mateu J, Valat JP. The temporomandibular joint in rheumatoid arthritis. Correlations between clinical and computed tomography features. J Rheumatol 1990;17:1285–1291.

85. Larheim TA, Kolbenstvedt A. Osseous temporomandibular joint abnormalities in rheumatic disease: Computed tomography versus hypocycloidal tomography. Acta Radiol 1990;31:383–387.

86. Blackwood HJJ. Arthritis of the mandibular joint. Br Dent J 1963;115:317–326.

87. Haanæs HR, Larheim TA, Nickerson JW, Pahle JA. Discectomy and synovectomy of the temporomandibular joint in the treatment of rheumatoid arthritis: Case report with three-year follow-up study. J Oral Maxillofac Surg 1986;44:905–910.

88. Larheim TA, Bjørnland T, Smith HJ, Aspestrand F, Kolbenstvedt A. Imaging temporomandibular joint abnormalities in patients with rheumatic disease. Comparison with surgical observations. Oral Surg Oral Med Oral Pathol 1992;73:494–501.

89. Bjørnland T, Larheim TA, Haanæs HR. Surgical treatment of temporomandibular joints in patients with chronic arthritic disease: Preoperative findings and one-year follow-up. Cranio 1992;10:205–210.

90. Bjørnland T, Refsum SB. Histopathologic changes of the temporomandibular joint disk in patients with chronic arthritic disease. A comparison with internal derangement. Oral Surg Oral Med Oral Pathol 1994;77:572–578.

91. Holmlund AB, Gynther G, Reinhold FP. Rheumatoid arthritis and disk derangement of the temporomandibular joint. A comparative arthroscopic study. Oral Surg Oral Med Oral Pathol 1992;73:273–277.

92. Larheim TA, Bjørnland T. Arthrographic findings in the temporomandibular joint in patients with rheumatic disease. J Oral Maxillofac Surg 1989;47:780–784.

93. Larheim TA, Smith HJ, Aspestrand F. Temporomandibular joint abnormalities associated with rheumatic disease: Comparison between MR imaging and arthrotomography. Radiology 1992;183:221–226.

94. Smith HJ, Larheim TA, Aspestrand F. Rheumatic and non-rheumatic disease in the temporomandibular joint: Gadolinium-enhanced MR imaging. Radiology 1992;185:229–234.

95. Cassidy JT, Petty RE. The juvenile idiopathic arthritides. In: Cassidy JT, Petty RE (eds). Textbook of Pediatric Rheumatology, ed 4. Philadelphia: Saunders, 2001:214–321.

96. Yulish BS, Lieberman JM, Newman AJ, Bryan PJ, Mulopulos GP, Modic MT. Juvenile rheumatoid arthritis: Assessment with MR imaging. Radiology 1987;165:149–152.

97. Senac MO, Deutsch D, Bernstein BH, et al. MR imaging in juvenile rheumatoid arthritis. AJR Am J Roentgenol 1988;150:873–878.

98. Larheim TA, Höyeraal HM, Stabrun AE, Haanæs HR. The temporomandibular joint in juvenile rheumatoid arthritis: Radiographic changes related to clinical and laboratory parameters in 100 children. Scand J Rheumatol 1982;11:5–12.

99. Larheim TA. Imaging of the temporomandibular joint in juvenile rheumatoid arthritis. In: Westesson P-L, Katzberg RW (eds). Imaging of the Temporomandibular Joint, vol 1. Cranio Clinics International. Baltimore: Williams and Wilkins, 1991:155–172.

100. Stabrun AE, Larheim TA, Höyeraal HM, Rösler M. Reduced mandibular dimensions and asymmetry in juvenile rheumatoid arthritis: Pathogenetic factors. Arthritis Rheum 1988;31:602–611.

101. Larheim TA, Dale K, Tveito L. Radiographic abnormalities of the temporomandibular joint in children with juvenile rheumatoid arthritis. Acta Radiol Diagn (Stockh) 1981;22:277–284.

102. Larheim TA. Radiographic appearance of the normal temporomandibular joint in newborns and small children. Acta Radiol Diagn (Stockh) 1981;22:593–599.

103. Resnick D, Niwayama G. Juvenile chronic arthritis. In: Resnick D, Niwayama G (eds). Diagnosis of Bone and Joint Disorders, ed 2, vol 2. Philadelphia: Saunders 1988:1069–1102.

104. Taylor DB, Babyn P, Blaser S, et al. MR evaluation of the temporomandibular joint in juvenile rheumatoid arthritis. J Comput Assist Tomogr 1993;17:449–454.

105. Kvien TK, Larheim TA, Hoyeraal HM, Sandstad B. Radiographic temporomandibular joint abnormalities in patients with juvenile chronic arthritis during a controlled study of sodium aurothiomalate and D-penicillamine. Br J Rheumatol 1986;25:59–66.

106. Kuseler A, Pedersen TK, Herlin T, Gelineck J. Contrast enhanced magnetic resonance imaging as a method to diagnose early inflammatory changes in the temporomandibular joint in children with juvenile chronic arthritis. J Rheumatol 1998;25:1406–1412.

107. Katzberg RW, Tallents RH, Hayakawa K, Miller TL, Goske MJ, Wood BP. Internal derangements of the temporomandibular joint: Findings in the pediatric age group. Radiology 1985;154:125–127.

108. Larheim TA, Haanæs HR. Micrognathia, temporomandibular joint changes and dental occlusion in juvenile rheumatoid arthritis of adolescents and adults. Scand J Dent Res 1981;89:329–338.

109. Skolnick J, Iranpour B, Westesson PL, Adair S. Prepubertal trauma and mandibular asymmetry in orthognathic surgery and orthodontic patients. Am J Orthod Dentofacial Orthop 1994;105:73–77.

110. Westesson PL, Tallents RH, Katzberg RW, Guay JA. Radiographic assessment of asymmetry of the mandible. AJNR Am J Neuroradiol 1994;15:991–999.

111. Nickerson JW, Boering G. Natural course of osteoarthrosis as it relates to internal derangement of the temporomandibular joint. Oral Maxillofac Surg Clin North Am 1989;1:27–45.

112. Nebbe B, Major PW. Prevalence of TMJ disc displacement in a pre-orthodontic adolescent sample. Angle Orthod 2000;70:454–463.

113. Nebbe B, Major PW, PraSad NG. Male adolescent facial pattern associated with TMJ disk displacement and reduction in disk length: Part II. Am J Orthod Dentofacial Orthop 1999;116:301–307.

114. Gray RJ, Horner K, Testa HJ, Lloyd JJ, Sloan P. Condylar hyperplasia: Correlation of histologic and scintigraphic features. Dentomaxillofac Radiol 1994;23:103–107.

115. Nokes SR, King PS, Garcia R Jr, Silbiger ML, Jones JD III, Castellano ND. Temporomandibular joint chondromatosis with intracranial extension: MR and CT contributions. AJR Am J Roentgenol 1987;148:1173–1174.

116. Herzog S, Mafee M. Synovial chondromatosis of the TMJ: MR and CT findings. AJNR Am J Neuroradiol 1990;11:742–745.

117. Eisig S, Dorfman HD, Cusamano RJ, Kantrowitz AB. Pigmented villonodular synovitis of the temporomandibular joint. Case report and review of literature. Oral Surg Oral Med Oral Pathol 1992;73:328–333.

118. Rickert RR, Shapiro MJ. Pigmented villonodular synovitis of the temporomandibular joint. Otolaryngol Head Neck Surg 1982;90:668–670.

119. Isberg A. Isacsson G, Nah K-S. Mandibular coronoid process locking: A prospective study of frequency and association with internal derangement of the temporomandibular joint. Oral Surg Oral Med Oral Pathol 1987;63:275–279.

120. Takahashi A, Hao-Zong W, Murakami S, Kondoh H, Fujishita M, Fuchihata H. Diagnosis of coronoid process hyperplasia by three-dimensional computed tomographic imaging. Dentomaxillofac Radiol 1993;22:149–154.

121. Störe G, Larheim TA. Mandibular osteoradionecrosis: A comparison of computed tomography with panoramic radiography. Dentomaxillofac Radiol 1999;28:295–300.

122. Christiansen EL, Thompson JR, Appleton SS. Temporomandibular joint pain/dysfunction overlying more insidious diseases: Report of two cases. J Oral Maxillofac Surg 1987;45:335–337.

123. Drum RK, Fornadley JA, Schnapf DJ. Malignant lesions presenting as symptoms of craniomandibular dysfunction. J Orofac Pain 1993;7:294–299.

Analysis of TMJ Synovial Fluid

Regina Landesberg and Linda L. Huang

Laboratory testing is valuable for diagnosing disease, assessing risk, predicting prognosis, and monitoring treatment. Although a number of serum laboratory tests are currently used in the diagnosis and treatment of rheumatoid arthritis (RA), no such tests are clinically available for other temporomandibular disorders (TMDs) (see chapter 15). However, many cytokines, enzymes, and tissue breakdown products that have been identified in synovial fluid could potentially serve as diagnostic markers of pathologic changes. In this chapter, these biomarkers will be described and their possible future use as laboratory tests for the diagnosis of various TMDs will be discussed.

Osteoarthritis and the TMJ

Significant evidence indicates that the pathologic process associated with the majority of TMDs is osteoarthritis (OA). Histologic as well as arthroscopic studies have shown changes in the later stages of certain TMDs that are consistent with those observed in OA of other synovial joints.[1,2] In the early stages of OA, microscopic breakdown of the articular surface occurs and chondrocyte clustering is seen. As the disease progresses, further matrix depletion occurs, first affecting the proteoglycans and then altering collagen fiber architecture. The articular surface subsequently undergoes vertical and horizontal splitting, fibrillation, and thinning; the end result is a denuding of the subchondral bone.[1–9] In this process, synovial alterations include both proliferation and inflammation.[10–13]

The role that the disc plays in this scenario is controversial. Although initially it was postulated that disc displacement preceded the onset of osteoarthritic changes in the joint, the increased association of disc malpositioning with articular degeneration has prompted some investigators to suggest that the degenerative process predisposes the disc to displacement[10,11] (see chapter 8).

The initiation of the osteoarthritic process in the TMJ is thought to be triggered by certain traumatic events. Several investigators have suggested that such mechanical stress leads to oxidative stress and the generation of free radicals within the temporomandibular joint (TMJ)[14,15] (see chapter 7). These free radicals possess vast capacity to modify the cellular milieu, both directly, by engagement of signaling pathways such as p21[ras] and activation of the pleiotropic transcription factor nuclear factor κB (NFκB), and indirectly, by causing oxidation of sugars and lipids, ultimately resulting in the chemical modification of proteins and lipids.[16–23] One consequence of such events is the generation of advanced glycation end products (AGEs). AGEs themselves exert distinct cellular effects by both direct and indirect means.   AGEs have the capacity to directly modify basement membranes and components of the extracellular matrix as well as the ability to engage specific cellular receptors.[27–30]

The best studied of these receptors is the receptor for AGE (RAGE), a multiligand signaling receptor of the immunoglobulin superfamily of cell surface molecules. One of the most prevalent AGEs found in vivo, N^{ϵ}-carboxymethyllysine (CML) adducts, specifically engages RAGE. Recent investigations have strongly suggested that CML-AGEs may form in multiple inflammatory states.[31–38] Recent studies have demonstrated the presence of CML-AGEs in the synovial tissue of nondiabetic human subjects with OA, supporting the contention that these modified adducts may form, at least initially, in affected joints because of the impact of mechanical stress.[37]

RAGE also serves as a signaling receptor for S100/calgranulin polypeptides produced by activated leukocytes and mononuclear phagocytes. Although long associated with chronic inflammation, a mechanism linking S100/calgranulin proteins to perturbation of key inflammatory effector cells, including macrophages and lymphocytes, had not been identified until it was recently shown that a member of this family (extracellular newly identified RAGE-binding protein [EN-RAGE], also known as *S100A12*) bound to and activated RAGE. In fact, RAGE is a receptor capable of interacting with a broad range of S100/calgranulins (both S100A and S100B polypeptides).[38] Importantly, previous studies have demonstrated that synovial fluid levels of S100/calgranulins are markers of disease activity in disorders such as juvenile RA.[39]

Cytokines and the TMJ

It is well established that tumor necrosis factor α (TNF-α) and interleukin 1β (IL-1β) are inflammatory cytokines critically important to the pathogenesis of joint injury (see chapter 7). These cytokines are produced by a number of different cell types, including macrophages and synovial cells. Both cause induction of fever and directly stimulate resorption of bone. Furthermore, both cytokines up-regulate and activate several extracellular matrix–degrading enzymes, such as the matrix metalloproteinases (MMPs), in chondrocytes, synovial cells, and fibroblasts.[40–48]

The association of cytokines and inflammatory mediators with certain TMDs has been suggested by numerous clinical studies. Shafer and colleagues[49] described a relationship between the extent of elevation of TNF- in TMJ synovial fluid and the degree of pain and surgical outcome. This study, however, did not include a control group. Uehara and colleagues[50] studied soluble tumor necrosis factor receptors (sTNF-I and sTNF-II) in synovial fluid aspirates from patients who exhibited both anterior disc displacement without reduction and radiographically demonstrable osteoarthritic changes. These soluble receptors inhibit the biologic activity of TNF by binding to the cytokine and making it unavailable to cell surface receptors. The levels of both receptors were significantly greater in patients than in controls. Although the levels of sTNF-I did not correlate with the clinical symptoms, sTNF-II had a negative correlation with joint pain.[50]

Suzuki and colleagues[51] have identified a correlation between the levels of IL-1β in the synovium and both the degree of pain and the extent of clinical synovitis. Their study included controls from two cadaver specimens. Kubota and colleagues[52] reported that synovial fluid levels of IL-1β in patients with internal derangement or OA were greater than levels in fluid from 15 asymptomatic joints. Alstergren and colleagues[53] showed a correlation between synovial fluid levels of IL-1β and pain or tenderness on palpation. However, all of the patients in this study had systemic diseases (RA, psoriatic arthritis, etc), and the majority were taking nonsteroidal anti-inflammatory drugs and/or glucocorticoids.[53,54] Furthermore, several studies have demonstrated an increase in synovial fluid levels of IL-6 in certain TMD patients that correlated with the degree of clinically determined synovitis.[55,56] It is important to note, however, that some studies failed to show a relationship between the levels of synovial fluid cytokines and the extent of pain or synovitis.[56]

Recently, Kaneyama and colleagues[57] performed a comprehensive study that examined TNF-α, IL-6, IL-1β, sTNF-I, sTNF-II, IL-6 soluble receptor (IL-6sR), IL-1 soluble receptor type II (IL-1sRII), and IL-1 receptor antagonist (IL-1RA) in the synovial fluid of 55 patients with various TMJ diseases, including OA. The study included five asymptomatic male controls. The total protein concentration was significantly higher in patients with internal derangements than in the control group. The patients with OA had significantly higher synovial fluid protein levels than did the group with internal derangement. TNF-α was detected in only 40% of patients and was undetectable in the controls. sTNF-I was detected in both patients and controls, but levels were significantly higher in patients. There was no difference between the levels found in patients with internal derangement and those with OA.

IL-6 was detected in 67% of patients and was absent in the control fluid samples. However, there was no difference in IL-6 levels between patients with internal derangement and patients with OA. IL-6sR was high in all groups, and there was no difference between them. IL-1β was detected in 71% of patients but was not found in the control group. There was no difference in the levels of IL-1β between the patients with internal derangement and the patients with OA.

The level of IL-1sRII was significantly greater in osteoarthritic patients than in control subjects. The synovial fluid levels of IL-1sRII in patients with internal derangement were higher than those in control subjects; however, the differences were not statistically significant. The levels of IL-1sRII in patients with internal derangement were not significantly different from levels found in the patients with OA. There were no differences among the groups in IL-1RA levels.[57]

The failure to find differences in IL-1RA levels is in sharp contrast to the findings of Fang et al.[58] They studied synovial fluid from 14 joints with internal derangement and 17 joints in patients with OA. Seven samples from four asymptomatic patients served as controls. IL-1RA was significantly elevated in those with internal derangement or OA. Control fluid was negative and there was no difference in levels between the two patient groups. They also examined transforming growth factor β (TGF-β) in the synovial fluid. It was absent in the control samples and significantly elevated in patients' synovial fluid. There were also significantly higher amounts of TGF-β in the osteoarthritic group than in the patients with internal derangement.[58]

Several other inflammatory mediators have been shown to be elevated in TMD patients. Alstergren and Kopp[59] studied prostaglandin E_2 (PGE$_2$) in 24 patients (30 joints) and four healthy controls (six joints). PGE$_2$ was detectable in 20 of 30 synovial fluid samples from patients with inflammatory TMJ disorders and absent from control fluid. The PGE$_2$ levels correlated with pain associated with joint movement. All of the patients included in this study had systemic arthritic diseases.[59]

Quinn and colleagues[60] investigated cyclooxygenase-2 (COX-2) in synovial tissue and fluid from 12 patients with internal derangement using the polymerase chain reaction (PCR). COX-2 was found in 16 of 17 tissue samples and 12 of 16 fluid samples. No control group was used in this study.[60] Seki et al[61] examined synovial tissues from 10 patients with internal derangement or OA for COX-1 and COX-2. Their control group consisted of five patients being treated for condylar fractures. COX-2 expression was strong in 11 of 13 TMD patients and weak or absent from the control subjects. COX-1 expression was similar in the patient and the control groups. COX-2 expression was correlated with the severity of synovitis.[61]

Chang and Israel[62] examined synovial fluid aspirates from 20 symptomatic TMD patients and 13 controls for β-glucuronidase, immunoglobulin A (IgA), and immunoglobulin G (IgG) using enzyme-linked immunosorbent assay (ELISA). Both β-glucuronidase and IgG levels were significantly elevated in the patient group, while IgA levels were not statistically elevated. The researchers concluded that these inflammatory mediators are the result of serum exudate as well as the infiltration of chronic inflammatory cells into the joint space.

All these studies, taken together, highlight the concept that cytokines are present in the synovial fluid of patients with certain TMDs and most likely contribute to the pathogenesis of joint damage. However, it is important to note that the majority of studies had no control subjects or had a control population that was small and not age- or sex-matched to the study subjects.

Proteolytic Enzymes and the TMJ

In addition to cytokines, the MMPs are key molecules linked to tissue injury in the inflamed joint. The MMPs are a group of proteases that are capable of degrading extracellular matrix components, particularly collagen, gelatin, and proteoglycans. The MMP family consists of 20 zinc-dependent enzymes that have a high degree of similarity. However, the differences in their substrate specificity and expression following cellular stimulation suggest that each of these proteases has distinct functions. Enzyme activity is controlled at three levels: transcriptional regulation, activation of latent precursor molecules, and regulation by specific inhibitory molecules (tissue inhibitors of metalloproteinases [TIMPs]). Transcription of several MMP genes is upregulated by various cytokines (TGF-β, basic fibroblast growth factor [bFGF], IL-1, and TNF-α) and is repressed by steroid hormones.[45,47,63–66]

Of the 20 MMPs, three are collagenases: fibroblast type (MMP-1), neutrophil type (MMP-8), and collagenase 3 (MMP-13). These collagenases are known to degrade collagen types I, II, III, VII, and X; gelatin; and proteoglycan core protein. These are the only MMPs that can degrade intact fibers of type I and type II collagen. It has recently been demonstrated that MMP-8 and MMP-13 are produced by articular chondrocytes from osteoarthritic cartilage. Stromelysin-1 (MMP-3), stromelysin-2 (MMP-10), and stromelysin-3 (MMP-11) break down proteoglycan core protein; fibronectin; laminin; collagen types IV, V, IX, and X; elastin; and proteoglycan core protein. Although the two gelatinases (MMP-2 and MMP-9) cannot degrade native type I and type II collagen, once the collagen trimers are denatured by acidic conditions or by other proteolytic enzymes, the gelatinases can cleave these fibrillar collagens. MMP-2 and MMP-9 are up-regulated by TGF-β, as well as by IL-1 and TNF-α, while other MMPs are unaffected by TGF-β. The potential role of the MMPs in degradative disease processes is apparent; however, the details as to their specific regulation, as well as where they fall in the overall disease cascade, must be evaluated.[63–66]

Multiple studies have examined the levels of MMPs in synovial fluid from TMD patients. Kanyama and colleagues[67] showed higher levels of MMP-1, -2, -3, and -9 in synovial fluid from patients with TMJ OA than in fluid from a control population. Ishimaru and colleagues[68] found an increase in levels of MMP-3 in synovial fluid from TMD patients who reported pain. However, they failed to shown any differences in levels of MMP-1 or TIMP-1.[68] Kubota and colleagues[52] demonstrated an increase in MMP-3 in the synovial fluid from two of seven patients with disc displacement without reduction. Although other investigators have shown detectable levels of MMP-1, -2, -3, -8, and -13 in the synovial fluid of certain TMD patients, no control groups were included in these studies.[69] Taken together, these findings strongly suggest that cytokines, such as IL-1, IL-6, and TNF-α, and the MMPs play significant roles in the processes linked to inflammation and tissue destruction associated with OA and other TMDs.

Proteoglycan Breakdown Products and the TMJ

Proteoglycans and their components (aggrecan, keratan sulfate, and chondroitin sulfate) are major structural elements of the articular cartilage of the knee, hip, and TMJ. The cartilage degradation that occurs in RA and OA results in the release of several matrix components into the synovial fluid. Lark and colleagues[70] identified aggrecan metabolic fragments generated by MMPs and aggrecanase in the articular cartilage from patients with OA and RA.[70] Additionally, several studies have shown proteoglycan fragments in synovial fluid aspirates from the knee following acute injury and OA.[71–77] Researchers examined synovial fluid keratan sulfate epitopes in patients undergoing arthroscopic TMJ procedures.[78,79] They found the levels of keratan sulfate were highest in patients with OA only and

in patients with OA and synovitis. Patients with synovitis (without OA) or patients without obvious arthroscopically detectable inflammatory changes had significantly lower but detectable levels of keratan sulfate. Normal controls were not included in these studies.[78,79] A proposed cascade of events, based on currently available data, is depicted in Fig 11-1.

Osteoarthritis in Joints Other Than the TMJ

Osteoarthritis is an age-related progressive disease that is characterized by degradation of articular cartilage and bone in synovial joints. The destruction of the cartilage matrix components, primarily collagen and proteoglycans, alters the structure and ultimately the function of the joint. The joints most commonly involved are the hands, feet, knee, hip, and spine.

The pathogenesis of OA is multifactorial, but the process appears to be initiated by biomechanical stress on the cartilage surface. Once the pathologic sequence commences, net cartilage degradation is a balancing act of cytokines, matrix-degrading proteases, and protease inhibitors; chondrocytes play a central role (Fig 11-2, Table 11-1, and Boxes 11-1 and 11-2).[80,81] Three collagenases, collagenase 1 (MMP), collagenase 2 (MMP-8), and collagenase 3 (MMP-13), are increased in osteoarthritic synovial fluid. MMP-2 and MMP-3 (gelatinase A and stromelysin-1) have also been shown to be elevated in osteoarthritic knees. Although numerous cytokines are elevated in the synovial fluid from the knee joints of patients with OA, IL-1, IL-6, IL-8, and TNF-α appear to be the most relevant.[80]

In addition to the previously mentioned cytokines and proteases, several cartilage-degrading molecules may prove to be useful clinical markers for the diagnosis and monitoring of OA. As previously discussed, aggrecan fragments are elevated in the synovial fluid of knee joints with OA.[70] Additionally, the recently described ELISA for crosslinked peptides from type II collagen (CTX-II) has shown a strong correlation between synovial fluid levels and the prevalence and progression of radiographic findings in the knee and the hip.[82,83] Garnero and colleagues[84] demonstrated increased urinary CTX-II in patients with rapidly destructive hip OA compared to patients with slowly progressive disease and healthy controls. Future research will determine the clinical utility of this assay in identifying osteoarthritic patients who are at high risk of rapid joint destruction.

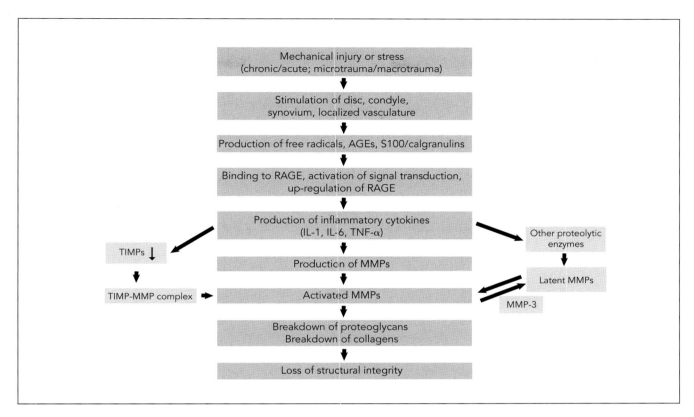

Fig 11-1 Biochemical cascade involved in pathologic changes in the TMJ. (AGE) advanced glycation end product; (RAGE) receptor for AGE; (IL) interleukin; (TNF) tumor necrosis factor; (MMP) matrix metalloproteinase; (TIMP) tissue inhibitor of metalloproteinase.

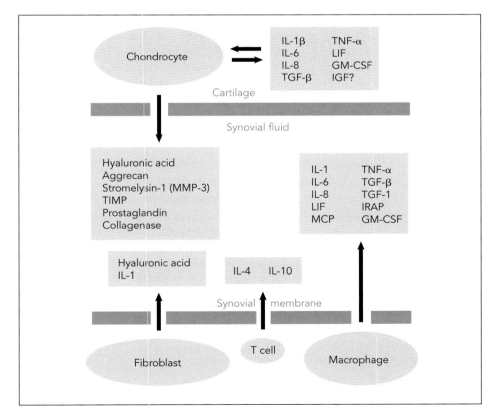

Fig 11-2 Chondrocyte, fibroblast, macrophage, and T-cell interactions with cytokines and proteases in synovial fluid during degradation of cartilage. (IL) Interleukin; (TNF) tumor necrosis factor; (LIF) leukemia inhibitory factor; (GM-CSF) granulocyte-macrophage–colony-stimulating factor; (TGF) transforming growth factor; (IGF) insulin-like growth factor; (MMP) matrix metalloproteinase; (TIMP) tissue inhibitor of metalloproteinase; (IRAP) insulin-regulated aminopeptidase; (MCP) monocyte chemoattractant protein.

Table 11-1	Cytokines present in knee joints, cell types from which they originate, and their principal effects on other cytokines and cellular processes during joint degradation*	

Cytokine	Main cell source	Principal effects in arthropathies
IL-1	M, L, F, other cells	**Up-regulate:** ACR, other cytokines, MMPs, PGE$_2$, COX-2, NO, endothelial adhesion molecules, angiogenesis, osteoclast activation, procoagulant activity
IL-2	T$_H$1 cells	**Increase:** T- and B-cell growth and activation **Up-regulate:** TNF-α, IFN-γ
IL-4	T$_H$2 cells	**Increase:** Growth, B, T, and mast cells **Up-regulate:** IL-1RA **Down-regulate:** IL-1, TNF, IL-6, IL-8, IFN-γ
IL-6	M, T$_H$2 cells, other cells	**Increase:** ACR (protein synthesis), B- and T-cell proliferation and activation **Up-regulate:** Fibroblast proliferation
IL-7		**Up-regulate:** IgG synthesis, adhesion molecules **Down-regulate:** Lymphocyte death
IL-8	M, F, other cells	**Increase:** Neutrophil activation and chemotaxis, angiogenesis
IL-10	T$_H$2 cells	**Increase:** B-cell differentiation and Ig synthesis **Decrease:** Class II HLA expression **Up-regulate:** IL-1RA **Down-regulate:** IL-1, IL-2, TNF, IL-6, IL-8, IFN-γ **Decrease:** Adhesion molecules, PGE$_2$, NO, MMPs
IL-11		**Increase:** ACR (protein synthesis) **Down-regulate:** IL-1, TNF-α, IFN-γ, IL-12
IL-12	M, other cells	**Up-regulate:** IL-1, TNF-α, IFN-γ, IL-18
IL-13	T$_H$2 cells	**Increase:** B-cell division and differentiation, IL-1RA **Down-regulate:** IL-1, TNF, IL-6, IL-8, IFN-γ, PGE$_2$
IL-15		**Increase:** T-cell proliferation **Up-regulate:** Chemokines, TNF-α
IL-16	CD8+ T cells	**Increase:** Eosinophil chemotaxis, T-cell infiltration
IL-17	T cells	**Increase:** Osteoclast activation, PGE$_2$, NO, chemokines
IL-18		**Up-regulate:** IL-1, TNF-α, IFN-γ **Increase:** Adhesion molecules
MCP-1 family	M, F, other cells	**Increase:** Mononuclear cell activation and chemotaxis
TGF-β family	M, F, other cells	**Increase:** Matrix and collagen synthesis **Up-regulate:** IL-1RA **Down-regulate:** IL-1, IL-2, TNF
TNF-α	M, L, F, other cells	**Increase:** ACR, endothelial adhesion molecules, procoagulant activity **Up-regulate:** MMPs, PGE$_2$, COX-2, NO, other cytokines

*IL = Interleukin; M = monocyte/macrophage; L = lymphocyte; F = fibroblast; ACR = acute phase response; MMP = matrix metalloproteinase; PGE$_2$ = prostaglandin E$_2$; COX = cyclooxygenase; NO = nitric oxide; TNF = tumor necrosis factor; IFN = interferon; IL-1RA = interleukin 1 receptor antagonist; IgG = immunoglobulin G; MCP = monocyte chemoattractant protein.

Box 11-1	Cytokines* present in diseased temporomandibular and knee joints and their status: Up-regulated (UR), down-regulated (DR), or no change (NC)				

Cytokines in diseased TMJs		Cytokines in diseased knee joints			
IL-1β—UR	COX-1—NC	IL-1—UR	COX-1—UR	LIF—UR	
IL-6—UR	COX-2—UR	IL-2—UR	COX-2—UR	IRAP—UR	
IL-8—UR	PGE₂—UR	IL-4—UR	PGE₂—UR	MCP-1—UR	
IL-10—NC	BMPs—UR	IL-6—UR	FLIP—UR	VCAM-1—UR	
	RANTES—UR	IL-7—UR	MIP-1α—UR	IFN-γ—UR	
	IFN-γ—UR	IL-8—UR	MIP-1β—UR	PDGF—UR	
	TGF-β family—UR	IL-10—UR	SCF—UR	VEGF—UR	
	TNF-α—UR	IL-11—UR	GRO-α—UR	EGF—UR	
		IL-12—UR	BMPs—UR	FGF—UR	
		IL-13—UR	RANTES—UR	IGF—DR	
		IL-15—UR	RANKL—UR	TGF-β family—UR	
		IL-16—UR	GM-CSF—UR	TNF-α—UR	
		IL-17—UR	Mac-1—UR	Osteopontin—UR	
		IL-18—UR	LFA-1—UR		

*IL = Interleukin; COX = cyclooxygenase; PGE₂ = prostaglandin E₂; FLIP = FLICE-like inhibitory protein; MIP = macrophage inflammatory protein; SCF = stem cell factor; GRO = growth-related gene product; BMPs = bone morphogenetic proteins; RANTES = regulated upon activation normal T cell expressed and secreted; RANKL = receptor activator of nuclear factor κB ligand; GM-CSF = granulocyte-macrophage colony-stimulating factor; Mac = macrophage; LFA = lymphocyte function–associated antigen; LIF = leukemia inhibitory factor; IRAP = insulin-regulated aminopeptidase; MCP = monocyte chemoattractant protein; VCAM = vascular cell adhesion molecule; IFN = interferon; PDGF = Platelet-derived growth factor; VEGF = vascular endothelial growth factor; EGF = endothelial growth factor; FGF = fibroblast growth factor; IGF = insulin-like growth factor; TGF = transforming growth factor; TNF = tumor necrosis factor.

Box 11-2	Proteases* present in diseased temporomandibular and knee joints and their status: Up-regulated (UR), down-regulated (DR), or no change (NC)			

Proteases in diseased TMJs		Proteases in diseased knee joints	
Tryptases—UR	MMP-9—UR	Tryptases—UR	MMP-9—UR
MMP-1—UR	MMP-13—UR	MMP-1—UR	MMP-13—UR
MMP-2—UR	TIMP-1—NC	MMP-2—UR	TIMP-1—DR
MMP-3—UR	TIMP-2—NC	MMP-3—UR	TIMP-2—DR
MMP-8—UR		MMP-8—UR	Plasminogen—UR

*MMP = matrix metalloproteinase; TIMP = tissue inhibitor of metalloproteinase.

Rheumatoid Arthritis

Rheumatoid arthritis is a chronic systemic inflammatory disease that targets the synovial joints. It is a relatively common disorder; approximately 1% of adults are affected worldwide. RA is characterized by a constellation of symptoms including fatigue, low-grade fevers, anemia, neuropathy, Sjögren syndrome, vasculitis, and renal disease.[84] No specific laboratory tests exist for the diagnosis and monitoring of disease progression in RA. The diagnosis of RA is based on clinical signs and symptoms as well as supporting serologic findings. Rheumatoid factor (RF), an antibody (most commonly immunoglobulin [IgM]) that recognizes IgG as an antigen, is the most characteristic serum laboratory abnormality seen in RA. Patients who are positive for

RF have more aggressive joint disease that is often accompanied by more severe extra-articular joint manifestations than are found in RF-negative patients.[85,86] Increased incidence of RF is also associated with a number of other diseases, such as systemic lupus erythematosus and primary Sjögren syndrome. Furthermore, RA is associated with other autoantibodies such as antinuclear antibodies.[85,86]

Anti–citrilline-containing peptide (anti-CCP) antibodies, particularly when used in conjunction with RF, may be useful in the diagnosis of polyarthritis.[87] Citrilline is a posttranscriptionally modified arginine residue. Studies suggest that an increased risk of progressive joint damage may be associated with anti-CCP–positive early RA patients.[88] Anti-CCP antibody testing is approved by the US Food and Drug Administration, and its use for the diagnosis of RA appears to be increasing.

C-reactive protein (CRP) has been used for many years to monitor disease activity in RA. Irrespective of RF seropositivity, when the CRP and erythrocyte sedimentation rate are both elevated, patients are more likely to exhibit radiographically visible progression of their disease. Cumulative CRP production also correlates with the extent of destruction observed on radiographs in RA.[89,90]

Several potential biologic markers for RA are currently under investigation. Anti-perinuclear factor (APF) and anti-keratin antibodies (AKA) may precede clinical RA and/or indicate a higher relative risk for the development of RA.[91] Other markers have been proposed for laboratory diagnosis of RA: antineutrophil cytoplasmic antibodies (ANCA), anti-RA33 antibodies, anti-Sa antibodies, and anti-p68 (BiP) antibodies.[92–94] Furthermore, polymorphisms in the promoter region for the MMP-3 gene, as well as the IL-10 promoter gene, have also been shown to be associated with severe disease.[95,96]

Serum hyaluronan, a product of the synovium, is elevated in joint disease and correlates with disease activity. MMP-1 and MMP-3, products of diseased synovium, are also elevated in the serum of patients with RA and appear to correlate with radiographically demonstrated joint damage.[97,98] High serum levels of cartilage oligomeric matrix protein (COMP), a marker of cartilage metabolism, are found in patients with early RA and appear to correlate with rapid hip joint destruction.[99,100] Similar to the findings in patients with OA, increased levels of urinary CTX-II appear to correlate with radiographic progression of rheumatoid joint disease.[84,101]

Synovial fluid from rheumatic joints is abundant in IL-17, a T-cell–derived cytokine that regulates cartilage metabolism. IL-1, IL-6, IL-18, TNF-α, and granulocyte-macrophage–colony-stimulating factor are also present in large amounts in the joint fluid.[102] Elevated synovial fluid aggrecan content is predictive of knee and hip joint destruc-

tion.[100] Serum levels of vascular endothelial growth factor are also greater in synovial fluid from patients with RA than in fluid from healthy controls and OA patients.[103–105]

Conclusion

The pathologic cascade that takes place in the majority of patients appears to be similar to that observed with OA in other synovial joints. The relevant cytokines, particularly IL-β, IL-6, and TNF-α, are up-regulated in the synovial fluid. In addition, the matrix-degrading enzymes, specifically the MMPs, appear to have similar profiles in certain TMDs and OA, although MMPs in the synovial fluid from patients with these TMDs have not been as extensively characterized as have MMPs associated with OA. These cytokines and MMPs could be candidates to serve as potential biomarkers.

A promising biomarker, the crosslinked peptide from type II collagen, is elevated in both the synovial fluid and urine of OA patients with cartilage degeneration. CTX-II is derived from type II collagen breakdown of the articular cartilage in the knee and hip joint. The articular surface of the mandibular condyle is covered with fibrocartilage that is composed of type I collagen. Assays for crosslinked peptides of type I collagen (NTX) have been available for several years and are routinely used for the diagnosis and monitoring of treatment of osteoporosis. This assay could be used to evaluate collagen degradation in the synovial fluid of TMD patients.

In contrast to the knee joint, where synovial fluid has access to all joint surfaces, the TMJ is separated into upper and lower compartments by the disc. The lower joint space is not routinely accessed during arthrocentesis and arthroscopy. The extent of diffusion between the two joint spaces has not been reported, making it difficult to predict if breakdown products from the condylar surface will be detectable in synovial fluid aspirates from the upper joint space. Keratan sulfate breakdown products have been detected in synovial fluid from the superior joint space; while this suggests that a significant amount of diffusion takes place between compartments, it is possible that the breakdown products were derived from the disc, which also contains keratan sulfate.

The unique anatomic properties of the TMJ may present specific difficulties in analyzing biomarkers in TMD patients. Thus, while it is clear that there are multiple candidates for biomarkers in the synovial fluid that could be useful in the diagnosis and treatment of various TMDs, intensive research will be required before these are available as tests for use in patient care.

References

1. De Bont LGM, Boering G, Liem RSB, Eulderink F, Westesson PL. Osteoarthritis and internal derangement of the temporomandibular joint: A light microscopic study. J Oral Maxillofac Surg 1986;44:634–643.

2. De Bont LGM, Boering G, Liem RSB, Havinga RT. Osteoarthritis of the temporomandibular joint: A light microscopic and scanning electron microscopic study of the articular condyle. J Oral Maxillofac Surg 1985;43:481–488.

3. Clark GT. Diagnosis and treatment of painful temporomandibular disorders. Dent Clin North Am 1987;31:645–674.

4. Clark GT, Mulligan R. A review of the prevalence of temporomandibular dysfunction. Gerodontology 1984;3:321–326.

5. Bonacci CE, Syrop SB, Gold N, Israel H. Temporomandibular/facial pain. NY State Dent J 1992;58:30–33.

6. Abubaker AO. Differential diagnosis of arthritis of the temporomandibular joint. Oral Surg Clin North Am 1995;7:1–21.

7. Howerton D, Zysset M. Anatomy of the temporomandibular joint and related structure with surgical anatomic considerations. Oral Surg Clin North Am 1989;1:229–246.

8. De Bont LGM, Liem RSB, Havinga R, Boering G. Fibrous component of the temporomandibular joint disk. Cranio 1985;3:368–373.

9. Haskin CL, Milam SB, Cameron IL. Pathogenesis of degenerative joint disease in the human temporomandibular joint. Crit Rev Oral Biol Med 1995;6:248–277.

10. Stegenga B, De Bont LGM, Boering G. Osteoarthritis as a cause of craniomandibular pain and dysfunction: A unifying theory. J Oral Maxillofac Surg 1989;47:249–256.

11. Stegenga B, De Bont LGM, Boering G, Van Willigen JD. Tissue responses to degenerative changes in the temporomandibular joint: A review. J Oral Maxillofac Surg 1991;49:1079–1088.

12. De Bont LGM, Boering G, Havinga P, Liem RSB. Spatial arrangement of collagen fibrils in the articular cartilage of the mandibular condyle: A light microscopic and scanning electron microscope study. J Oral Maxillofac Surg 1984;42:306–313.

13. Dijgraaf LC, De Bont LGM, Boering G, Liem RSB. The structure, biochemistry, and metabolism of osteoarthritic cartilage: A review of the literature. J Oral Maxillofac Surg 1995;53:1182–1192.

14. Milam SB, Zardeneta G. Oxidative stress and degenerative temporomandibular joint disease: A proposed hypothesis. J Oral Maxillofac Surg 1998;56:214–223.

15. Haskin CL, Milam SB, Cameron IL. Pathogenesis of degenerative joint disease in the human temporomandibular joint. Crit Rev Oral Biol Med 1995;6:248–277.

16. Lander HM, Tauras JM, Ogiste JS, Hori O, Moss RA, Schmidt AM. Activation of the receptor for advanced glycation end products triggers a p21ras-dependent mitogen-activated protein kinase pathway regulated by oxidant stress. J Biol Chem 1997;272:17810–17814.

17. Sundaresan M, Yu ZX, Ferrans VJ, Irani K, Finkel T. Requirement for generation of H_2O_2 for platelet-derived growth factor signal transduction. Science 1995;270:296–299.

18. Lo YYC, Cruz TF. Involvement of reactive oxygen species in cytokine and growth factor induction of c-fos expression in chondrocytes. J Biol Chem 1995;270:11727–11730.

19. Stevenson MA, Pollock SS, Coleman CN, Calderwood SK. X-irradiation, phorbol esters, and H_2O_2 stimulate mitogen-activated protein kinase activity in NIH-3T3 cells through the formation of reactive oxygen intermediates. Cancer Res 1994;54:12–15.

20. Fialkow L, Chan CK, Rotin D, Grinstein S, Downey GP. Activation of the mitogen-activated protein kinase signaling pathway in neutrophils. Role of oxidants. J Biol Chem 1994;269:31234–31242.

21. Anderson MT, Staal FJT, Gitler C, Herzenberg LA, Herzenberg LA. Separation of oxidant-initiated and redox-regulated steps in the NF-κB signal transduction pathway. Proc Natl Acad Sci U S A 1994;91:11527–11531.

22. Staal FJI, Anderson MT, Staal GE, Herzenberg LA, Herzenberg LA. Redox regulation of signal transduction: Tyrosine phosphorylation and calcium influx. Proc Natl Acad Sci U S A 1994;91:3619–3622.

23. DeForge LE, Fantone JC, Kenney JS, Remick DG. Oxygen radical scavengers selectively inhibit interleukin 8 production in human whole blood. J Clin Invest 1992;90:2123–2129.

24. Ikeda K, Higashi T, Sano H, et al. Carboxymethyllysine protein adduct is a major immunological epitope in proteins modified with AGEs of the Maillard reaction. Biochem 1996;35:8075–8083.

25. Reddy S, Bichler J, Wells-Knecht K, Thorpe SR, Baynes JW. Carboxymethyllysine is a dominant AGE antigen in tissue proteins. Biochem 1995;34:10872–10878.

26. Ahmed MU, Brinkmann FE, Degenhardt TP, Thorpe SR, Baynes JW. N-epsilon-(carboxymethyl) lysine, a product of proteins by methylglyoxal. Biochem J 1997;324:565–570.

27. Tanaka S, Avigad G, Brodsky B, Eikenberry EF. Glycation induces expansion of the molecular packing of collagen. J Mol Biol 1988;203:495–505.

28. Haitoglou CS, Tsilbary EC, Brownlee M, Charonis AS. Altered cellular interactions between endothelial cells and nonenzymatically glycosylated laminin/type IV collagen. J Biol Chem 1992;267:12404–12407.

29. Giardino I, Edelstein D, Brownless M. Nonenzymatic glycosylation in vitro and in bovine endothelial cells alters basic fibroblast growth factor activity. A model for intracellular glycosylation in diabetes. J Clin Invest 1994;94:110–117.

30. Bucala R, Tracey K, Cerami A. AGEs quench nitric oxide and mediate defective endothelium-dependent vasodilation in experimental diabetes. J Clin Invest 1991;87:432–438.

31. Schmidt AM, Yan SD, Yan SF, Stern DM. The multiligand receptor RAGE as a progression factor amplifying immune and inflammatory responses. J Clin Invest 2001;108:949–955.

32. Smith MA, Taneda S, Richey P, et al. Advanced Maillard reaction end products are associated with Alzheimer disease pathology. Proc Natl Acad Sci U S A 1994;91:5710–5714.

33. Sousa MM, Du Yan S, Fernandes R, Guimaraes A, Stern D, Saraiva MJ. Familial amyloid polyneuropathy: Receptor for advanced glycation end products–dependent triggering of neuronal inflammatory and apoptotic pathways. J Neurosci 2001;21:7576–7586.

34. Schleicher E, Wagner E, Nerlich A. Increased accumulation of glycoxidation product carboxymethyllysine in human tissues in diabetes and aging. J Clin Invest 1997;99:457–468.

35. Kislinger T, Fu C, Huber B, et al. N$^\varepsilon$-(carboxymethyl) lysine modifications of proteins are ligands for RAGE that activate cell signaling pathways and modulate gene expression. J Biol Chem 1999;274:31740–31749.

36. Anderson MM, Requena JR, Crowley JR, Thorpe SR, Heinecke J. The myeloperoxidase system of human phagocytes generates N-(carboxymethyl) lysine on proteins: A mechanism for producing advanced glycation endproducts at sites of inflammation. J Clin Invest 1999;104:103–113.

37. Drinda S, Franke S, Canet CC, et al. Identification of the advanced glycolation end products N-carboxymethyllysine in the synovial tissue of patients with rheumatoid arthritis. Ann Rheum Dis 2002;61:488–492.

38. Hoffman MA, Drury S, Fu C, et al. RAGE mediates a novel proinflammatory axis: A central cell surface receptor for S100/calgranulin polypeptides. Cell 1999;97:899–901.

39. Frosch M, Strey A, Vogl T, et al. Myeloid-related proteins 8 and 14 are specifically secreted during interaction of phagocytes and activated endothelium and are useful markers for monitoring disease activity in pauciarticular-onset juvenile rheumatoid arthritis. Arthritis Rheum 2000;43:628–637.

40. Martel-Pelletier J, Clouthier JM, Pelletier JP. Cytokines, interleukin-1, and tumor necrosis factor in human osteoarthritic tissues [abstract]. Trans Orthop Res Soc 1990;15:111.

41. Pelletier JP, Martel-Pelletier J. Evidence for involvement of interleukin-1 in human osteoarthritic cartilage degradation: Protective effect of NSAID. J Rheumatol 1989;16:19–27.

42. Vilcek J, Lee TH. Tumor necrosis factor: New insights into the molecular mechanisms of its multiple actions. J Biol Chem 1991;266:7314–7316.

43. Saklatvala J. Tumour necrosis factor α stimulates resorption and inhibits synthesis of proteoglycan in cartilage. Nature 1986;322:547–549.

44. Dinarello CA. Biology of interleukin-1. FASEB J 1988;2:108–115.

45. Birkedal-Hansen W, Moore GI, Bodden MK, et al. Matrix metalloproteinases: A review. Crit Rev Oral Biol Med 1993;4:197–250.

46. Woessner JF Jr. Matrix metalloproteinases and their inhibitors in connective tissue remodeling. FASEB J 1991;5:2145–2154.

47. Konttinen YT, Ainola M, Valleala H, et al. Analysis of 16 different matrix metalloproteinases (MMP-1 to MMP-20) in the synovial membrane: Different profiles in trauma and rheumatoid arthritis. Ann Rheum Dis 1999;58:691–697.

48. Kaneko O, Tomita T, Nakase T, et al. Expression of proteinases and inflammatory cytokines in subchondral bone regions in the destructive joint of rheumatoid arthritis. Rheumatology 2001;40:247–255.

49. Shafer DM, Assael L, White LB, Rossomando EF. Tumor necrosis factor-α as a biochemical marker of pain and outcome in temporomandibular joints with internal derangements. J Oral Maxillofac Surg 1994;52:786–791.

50. Uehara J, Kuboki T, Fujisawa T, Kojima S, Maekawa K, Yatani H. Soluble tumour necrosis factor receptors in synovial fluids from temporomandibular joints with painful anterior disc displacement without reduction and osteoarthritis. Arch Oral Biol 2004;49:133–142.

51. Suzuki T, Segami N, Kaneyama K, Nishimura M, Nojima T. Specific expression of interleukin-1β; in temporomandibular joints with internal derangements. Oral Surg Oral Med Oral Pathol 1999;88:413–417.

52. Kubota E, Imamura H, Kubota T, Shibata T, Murakami KI. Interleukin 1β and stromelysin (MMP3) activity of synovial fluid as possible markers of osteoarthritis in the temporomandibular joint. J Oral Maxillofac Surg 1997;55:20–27.

53. Alstergren P, Kopp S, Theodorsson E. Synovial fluid sampling from the temporomandibular joint: Sample quality criteria and levels of interleukin-1β and serotonin. Acta Odontol Scand 1999;57:16–22.

54. Alstergren P, Ernberg M, Kvarnstrom M, Kopp S. Interleukin-1β in synovial fluid from the arthritic temporomandibular joint and its relation to pain, mobility, and anterior open bite. J Oral Maxillofac Surg 1998;56:1059–1065.

55. Kubota E, Kubota T, Matsumoto J, Shibata T, Murakami KI. Synovial fluid cytokines and proteinases as markers of temporomandibular joint disease. J Oral Maxillofac Surg 1998;56:192–198.

56. Nishimura M, Segami N, Kaneyama K, Suzuki T, Miyamaru M. Proinflammatory cytokines and arthroscopic findings of patients with internal derangement and osteoarthritis of the temporomandibular joint. Br J Oral Maxillofac Surg 2002;40:68–71.

57. Kaneyama K, Segami N, Sun W, Sato J, Fujimura K. Analysis of tumor necrosis factor-α, interleukin-6, interleukin-1β, soluble tumor necrosis factor receptors I and II, interleukin-6 soluble receptor, interleukin-1 soluble receptor type II, interleukin-1 receptor antagonist, and protein in the synovial fluid of patients with temporomandibular joint disorders. Oral Surg Oral Med Oral Pathol Oral Radiol Endod 2005;99:276–284.

58. Fang PK, Ma XC, Ma DL, Fu KY. Determination of interleukin-1 receptor antagonist, interleukin-10, and transforming growth factor-β1 in synovial fluid aspirates of patients with temporomandibular disorders. J Oral Maxillofac Surg 1999;57:922–928; discussion 928–929.

59. Alstergren P, Kopp S. Prostaglandin E$_2$ in temporomandibular joint synovial fluid and its relation to pain and inflammatory disorders. J Oral Maxillofac Surg 2000;58:180–186; discussion 186–188.

60. Quinn JH, Kent JH, Moise A, Lukiw WJ. Cyclooxygenase-2 in synovial tissue and fluid of dysfunctional temporomandibular joints with internal derangement. J Oral Maxillofac Surg 2000;58:1229–1232; discussion 1232–1233.

61. Seki H, Fukuda M, Iino M, Takahashi T, Yoshioka N. Immuno-histochemical localization of cyclooxygenase-1 and -2 in synovial tissues from patients with internal derangement or osteoarthritis of the temporomandibular joint. Int J Oral Maxillofac Surg 2004;33:687–692.

62. Chang H, Israel HA. Analysis of inflammatory mediators in TMJ synovial fluid lavage samples of symptomatic patients and asymptomatic controls. J Oral Maxillofac Surg 2005;63: 761–765.

63. Matrisian L. The matrix-degrading metalloproteinases. Bioassays 1992;14:455–463.

64. Cole AA, Chubinskaya S, Schumacher B, et al. Chondrocyte matrix metalloproteinase-8. J Biol Chem 1996;271:11023–11026.

65. Mitchell PG, Magna HA, Reeves LM, et al. Cloning, expression, and type II collagenolytic activity of matrix metalloproteinase-13 from human osteoarthritic cartilage. J Clin Invest 1996; 97:761–768.

66. Huhtala P, Tuuttila A, Chow LT, Lohi J, Keski-Oja J, Tryggvason K. Complete structure of the human gene for 92-kDa type IV collagenase. Divergent regulation of expression for the 92- and 72-kilodalton enzyme genes in HT-1080 cells. J Biol Chem 1991;266:16485–16490.

67. Kanyama M, Kuboki T, Kojima S, et al. Matrix metalloproteinases and tissue inhibitors of metalloproteinases in synovial fluids of patients with temporomandibular joint osteoarthritis. J Orofac Pain 2000;14:20–30.

68. Ishimaru JI, Oguma Y, Goss AN. Matrix metalloproteinase and tissue inhibitor of metalloproteinase in serum and lavage synovial fluid of patients with temporomandibular joint disorders. Br J Oral Maxillofac Surg 2000;38:354–259.

69. Srinivas R, Sorsa T, Tjäderhane L, et al. Matrix metalloproteinases in mild and severe temporomandibular joint internal derangement synovial fluid. Oral Surg Oral Med Oral Pathol 2001;91:517–525.

70. Lark MW, Bayne EK, Flanagan J, et al. Aggrecan degradation in human cartilage. Evidence for both matrix metalloproteinase and aggrecanase activity in normal, osteoarthritic, and rheumatoid joints. J Clin Invest 1997;1;100:93–106.

71. Dahlberg L, Friden T, Roos H, Lark MW, Lohmander LS. A longitudinal study of cartilage matrix metabolism in patients with cruciate ligament rupture—Synovial fluid concentrations of aggrecan fragments, stromelysin-1 and tissue inhibitor of metalloproteinase-1. Br J Rheumatol 1994;33:1107–1111.

72. Lohmander LS, Dahlberg L, Ryd L, Heinegard D. Increased levels of proteoglycan fragments in knee joint fluid after injury. Arthritis Rheum 1989;32:1434–1442.

73. Lohmander, LS Roos, H Dahlberg, L Hoerrner, LA Lark, MW. Temporal patterns of stromelysin-1, tissue inhibitor, and proteoglycan fragments in human knee joint fluid after injury to the cruciate ligament or meniscus. J Orthop Res 1994;12:21–28.

74. Ratcliffe A, Doherty M, Maini RN, Hardingham TE. Increased concentrations of proteoglycan components in the synovial fluids of patients with acute but not chronic joint disease. Ann Rheum Dis. 1988;47:826–832.

75. Ratcliffe A, Grelsamer RP, Kiernan H, Saed-Nejad F, Visco D. High levels of aggrecan aggregate components are present in synovial fluids from human knee joints with chronic injury or osteoarthrosis. Acta Orthop Scand Suppl 1995;266: 111–115.

76. Lohmander LS, Ionescu M, Jugessur H, Poole AR. Changes in joint cartilage aggrecan after knee injury and in osteoarthritis. Arthritis Rheum 1999;42:534–544.

77. Ratcliffe A, Flatow EL, Roth N, Saed-Nejad F, Bigliani LU. Biochemical markers in synovial fluid identify early osteoarthritis of the glenohumeral joint. Clin Orthop Relat Res 1996; 330:45–53.

78. Ratcliffe A, Israel HA, Saed-Nejad F, Diamond B. Proteoglycans in the synovial fluid of the temporomandibular joint as an indicator of changes in cartilage metabolism during primary and secondary osteoarthritis. J Oral Maxillofac Surg 1998;56:204–208.

79. Israel HA, Diamond BE, Saed-Nejad F, Ratcliffe A. Correlation between arthroscopic diagnosis of osteoarthritis and synovitis of the human temporomandibular joint and keratan sulfate levels in the synovial fluid. J Oral Maxillofac Surg 1997;55:210–217; discussion 217–218.

80. Punzi L, Calo L, Plebani M. Clinical significance of cytokine determination in synovial fluid. Crit Rev Clin Lab Sci 2002; 39:63–88.

81. Lee DM, Kiener HP, Brenner MB. Synoviocytes. In: Harris ED, Budd R, Firestein G, et al (eds). Kelley's Textbook of Rheumatology, ed 7. Philadelphia: Saunders, 2004:175–188.

82. Lohmander LS, Atley LM, Pietka TA, Eyre DR. The release of crosslinked peptides from type II collagen into human synovial fluid is increased soon after joint injury and in osteoarthritis. Arthritis Rheum 2003;48:3130–3139.

83. Reijman M, Hazes JM, Bierma-Zeinstra SM, et al. A new marker for osteoarthritis: Cross-sectional and longitudinal approach. Arthritis Rheum 2004;50:2471–2478.

84. Garnero P, Conrozier T, Christgau S, Mathieu P, Delmas PD, Vignon E. Urinary type II collagen C-telopeptide levels are increased in patients with rapidly destructive hip osteoarthritis. Ann Rheum Dis 2003;62:939–943.

85. O'Dell J. Rheumatoid arthritis. In: Goldman L, Ausiello D (eds). Cecil Textbook of Medicine, ed 22. Philadelphia: Saunders, 2004:1644–1653.

86. Taylor PC, Maini RN. Biological markers in the diagnosis and assessment of outcome in rheumatoid arthritis. UpToDate [serial online] 2003. Available at: http://www.uptodate.com. Accessed 17 Dec 2004.

87. Bas S, Genevay S, Meyer O, Gabay C. Anti-cyclic citrullinated peptide antibodies, IgM and IgA rheumatoid factors in the diagnosis and prognosis of rheumatoid arthritis. Rheumatology (Oxford) 2003;42:677–680.

88. Meyer O, Labarre C, Dougados M, et al. Anticitrullinated protein/peptide antibody assays in early rheumatoid arthritis for predicting five year radiographic damage. Ann Rheum Dis 2003;62:120–126.

89. Combe B, Dougados M, Goupille P, et al. Prognostic factors for radiographic damage in early rheumatoid arthritis: A multiparameter prospective study. Arthritis Rheum 2001; 44:1736–1743.

90. Amos RS, Constable TJ, Crockson RA, Crockson AP, McConkey B. Rheumatoid arthritis: Relation of serum C-reactive protein and erythrocyte sedimentation rates to radiographic changes. Br Med J 1977;1(6055):195–197.

91. Sebbag M, Simon M, Vincent C, et al. The antiperinuclear factor and the so-called antikeratin antibodies are the same rheumatoid arthritis-specific autoantibodies. J Clin Invest 1995;95:2672–2679.

92. Blass S, Union A, Raymackers J, et al. The stress protein BiP is overexpressed and is a major B and T cell target in rheumatoid arthritis. Arthritis Rheum 2001;44:761–771.

93. Hassfeld W, Steiner G, Graninger W, Witzmann G, Schweitzer H, Smolen JS. Autoantibody to the nuclear antigen RA33: A marker for early rheumatoid arthritis. Br J Rheumatol 1993; 32:199–203.

94. Hassfeld W, Steiner G, Studnicka-Benke A, et al. Autoimmune response to the spliceosome. An immunologic link between rheumatoid arthritis, mixed connective tissue disease, and systemic lupus erythematosus. Arthritis Rheum 1995;38:777–785.

95. Constantin A, Lauwers-Cances V, Navaux F, et al. Stromelysin 1 (matrix metalloproteinase 3) and HLA-DRB1 gene polymorphisms: Association with severity and progression of rheumatoid arthritis in a prospective study. Arthritis Rheum 2002;46:1754–1762.

96. Lard LR, van Gaalen FA, Schonkeren JJ, et al. Association of the -2849 interleukin-10 promoter polymorphism with autoantibody production and joint destruction in rheumatoid arthritis. Arthritis Rheum 2003;48:1841–1848.

97. Yamanaka H, Matsuda Y, Tanaka M, et al. Serum matrix metalloproteinase 3 as a predictor of the degree of joint destruction during the six months after measurement, in patients with early rheumatoid arthritis. Arthritis Rheum 2000; 43:852–858.

98. Green MJ, Gough AK, Devlin J, et al. Serum MMP-3 and MMP-1 and progression of joint damage in early rheumatoid arthritis. Rheumatology (Oxford) 2003;42:83–88.

99. Forslind K, Eberhardt K, Jonsson A, Saxne T. Increased serum concentrations of cartilage oligomeric matrix protein. A prognostic marker in early rheumatoid arthritis. Br J Rheumatol 1992;31:593–598.

100. Mansson B, Carey D, Alini M, et al. Cartilage and bone metabolism in rheumatoid arthritis. Differences between rapid and slow progression of disease identified by serum markers of cartilage metabolism. J Clin Invest 1995;95: 1071–1077.

101. Landewe R, Geusens P, Boers M, et al. Markers for type II collagen breakdown predict the effect of disease-modifying treatment on long-term radiographic progression in patients with rheumatoid arthritis. Arthritis Rheum 2004; 50:1390–1399.

102. Gravallese EM. Synovial pathology in rheumatoid arthritis. 2. UpToDate [serial online] 2003. Available at: http://www.uptodate.com. Accessed 17 Dec 2004.

103. Harada M, Mitsuyama K, Yoshida H, et al. Vascular endothelial growth factor in patients with rheumatoid arthritis. Scand J Rheumatol 1998;27:377–380.

104. Ballara S, Taylor PC, Reusch P, et al. Raised serum vascular endothelial growth factor levels are associated with destructive change in inflammatory arthritis. Arthritis Rheum 2001;44:2055–2064.

105. Nagashima M, Wauke K, Hirano D, et al. Effects of combinations of anti-rheumatic drugs on the production of vascular endothelial growth factor and basic fibroblast growth factor in cultured synoviocytes and patients with rheumatoid arthritis. Rheumatology (Oxford) 2000;39:1255–1262.

The Role of Technology in TMD Diagnosis

Charles S. Greene

The classic approach to diagnosis of temporomandibular disorders (TMDs) has been based on the medical model of listening to chief complaints, recording subjective histories, and obtaining physical findings from direct examination (see chapter 17). The most common complaint of TMD patients is pain of musculoskeletal origin, which can be localized or diffuse and usually is exacerbated by jaw function. Because the temporomandibular joint (TMJ) complex is located in the head, which is by far the most richly innervated part of the human body, distinguishing between the pain of TMDs and other types of craniofacial pain conditions can be quite challenging. To put this in perspective, the International Headache Society in 1988 developed diagnostic criteria,[1] revised in 2004,[2] for labeling more than 150 types of craniofacial pain disorder,[3] and there are several overlapping characteristics among some of them. Therefore, it is not surprising that many clinicians find it difficult at times to achieve a differential diagnosis of these conditions. They would like to have proven technologic assessment procedures that could help them to discriminate among various problems.

Historically, the technology that has been most widely used to evaluate TMD patients is imaging, originally with simple radiographs and later with tomography, computed tomography, arthrography, scintigraphy, and magnetic resonance imaging. The value and limitations of these techniques are discussed in chapter 10. Chapter 11 discusses the value of various laboratory tests that sometimes are used for the diagnosis of TMDs. The present chapter examines the potential value of other technologies that have been proposed for the diagnosis of TMDs, with special emphasis on devices that assess jaw movements (jaw-tracking devices), devices that measure jaw muscle activity (electromyography [EMG]), and devices that record TMJ sounds (sonography). The term *adjunctive diagnostic devices* is used throughout this chapter to describe these instruments, because this is the terminology contained in the product approval statements distributed by both the US Food and Drug Administration (FDA) and the American Dental Association (ADA).

Researchers in dentistry have improved our understanding of both normal and abnormal functioning of the masticatory system through the use of jaw tracking, sonography, and EMG in groups of TMD patients as well as in normal subjects.[3–5] As a result, the dental literature is filled with substantial information describing the mechanisms of human jaw functions in these various groups (see chapters 1 and 2). In other biomedical disciplines, clinicians have used similar devices to assess the health or illness status of patients, so there is some precedent for the clinical application of such technologies.

The important question, however, is whether clinicians can use these specific technological devices as diagnostic modalities to assess presumptive TMD patients or to screen normal populations for the presence of undiagnosed TMD problems. Some clinicians have claimed that these devices can be used to determine which treatment modalities should be provided for these patients. Because most of the experimental studies conducted with these technological devices have examined only groups of TMD patients and compared them to control subjects, the crucial issue is whether it is appropriate to use the techniques on one individual to reach a conclusion about his or her diagnosis.[6] Obviously, any valid, reliable, and meaningful objective data that could be obtained from technologic assessments would be a welcome addition to the information obtained from a direct clinical examination. On the other hand, any invalid, unreliable, or otherwise incorrect findings from such assessments could lead to errors in diagnosis and subsequent improper selection of treatment. In addition, healthy people might be considered to have a subclinical or hidden problem if certain findings on technologic assessments during routine medical or dental examinations were incorrectly interpreted as pathologic.

Evaluating Adjunctive Diagnostic Devices

General Issues

In addition to questions about the validity and reliability of various diagnostic devices, there is one central issue that must be addressed for all proposed diagnostic tests or procedures—their sensitivity and specificity.[7–9] *Sensitivity* refers to the ability of the test to correctly detect the presence of a condition in patients with a confirmed case of the disorder (true positives); failure to detect such conditions in patients are considered false negatives. *Specificity* refers to the ability to correctly confirm the absence of a condition in patients without the disorder (true negatives); healthy patients who are reported to have a problem based on testing are considered false positives.

The real presence or absence of a disease or a disorder is determined by the traditional "gold standard." ie, the diagnostic procedure or finding that is accepted as the best currently available indicator of the problem. As with other musculoskeletal disorders (and most headaches), the current gold standard for a positive diagnosis of a TMD is based on interpretation of the findings obtained from a history and clinical examination of the patient.[10–11]

A diagnostic procedure that yields a sensitivity ratio of 1.0 when compared with the gold standard is one that correctly identifies 100% of the cases established by the standard. A value of 0.5 (50%), on the other hand, means the accuracy of case detection is no better than chance alone. Similarly, a diagnostic test that finds 100% of a normal population to be healthy is ideally in alignment with the gold standard. Because perfect scores of this kind rarely occur with any diagnostic tests, the scientific and clinical communities have somewhat arbitrarily settled on a 70%

accuracy rate as being clinically acceptable for both sensitivity and specificity. However, in the case of more serious medical conditions that may have high rates of morbidity or mortality, it is important that the sensitivity standard be very high to avoid missing real patients, even if it ends up including many false-positive patients, who can be eliminated later through secondary testing.[12]

The field of TMDs generally is dealing with conditions of low morbidity, so it is more important that individuals not be diagnosed falsely and subjected to unnecessary treatments. Therefore, the specificity standard should be set higher in diagnostic testing for these conditions.[12] Although electromyography, sonography, and jaw tracking are all helpful research tools that have provided information leading to a better understanding of jaw function and dysfunction, they have not been proven to be as clinically useful or necessary as some of their advocates believe. This is largely due to their low specificity scores, ie, their tendency to "detect" TMDs in people who do not have a clinically significant jaw problem involving either pain or dysfunction (false-positive individuals).[12,13] Although the positive findings from these devices are described as quantitative and objective, clinicians still have to determine what constitutes a "real" TMD patient. As Mohl et al[14] point out, even with agreed-upon signs and symptoms of TMDs, patient complaint and treatment-seeking behavior remains an important issue. Does the label "TMD patient" apply, for example, to an individual with a palpably tender masseter muscle or an unusual jaw movement pattern if there is no patient complaint? Their conclusion is that establishment of a clinical diagnosis of TMD must be based initially on patients' symptomatic complaints and only subsequently on physical signs and other findings, because reversing this order may cause a healthy individual to be classified as a TMD patient. Until the advocates for TMD diagnostic devices can prove that positive findings obtained from their assessments either predict future symptomatic jaw problems or successfully detect hidden cases of TMD, the clinical use of such devices is not indicated for screening of random populations.[15]

Specific Issues

Before each device is discussed separately, some general points must be made about the potential value of adjunctive diagnostic devices as part of a TMD diagnostic process. Because TMDs are essentially orthopedic conditions involving joints and muscles, it would seem that precise measurement of jaw motion, muscle activity, or joint sounds would be very helpful—perhaps even indispensable. However, the danger of false-positive findings has become a serious concern; in addition, the issue of redundancy of findings raises questions about the necessity for certain tests.[6] For example, is it more helpful to the clinician to have a computer printout of a TMJ sound pattern than to use direct auscultation of the joint? Is it better to see that mandibular opening is limited by using a straight ruler, or should a jaw-tracking device be used to record this phenomenon? Likewise, is it valuable to see the mandible deviate to the left on a jaw-tracking printout, rather than observe it clinically, in a patient who has either a muscle-induced limitation or a disc interference problem on the left side? Furthermore, can the machine output help the clinician discriminate between these two possibilities?

The answers to these questions depend mainly on understanding that the output from these devices is being compared to some arbitrary concept of normal function. The major problem with the clinical application of any adjunctive biomedical test is that the standards for "normality" for each morphologic or functional variable have to be clearly established beforehand. In the case of the TMJ complex, the experimental studies done with all of the so-called adjunctive diagnostic devices have shown that the normal range of human jaw function varies widely from one individual to another.[15] When the performances of TMD patients and normal subjects on any particular test are compared, the group means may show statistically significant differences on one or more parameters. However, the broad range of individual findings in both groups often results in considerable overlap between the two groups, and therefore no individual diagnostic conclusions can be drawn.

In one example presented by Lund et al[12] (based on data from Dworkin et al[16]), the mean jaw-opening measurements of female TMD patients and matched asymptomatic females were 36.4 and 45.0 mm, respectively; this was a statistically significant difference. However, when these data were plotted on a graph, a considerable amount of overlap was found between the two curves, indicating that this measurement alone could not separate symptomatic patients from normal subjects.

A formal review and assessment of adjunctive diagnostic devices was carried out between 1989 and 1990 by Mohl and colleagues[14,17,18] at the request of the Council on Dental Materials, Instruments, and Equipment of the American Dental Association. In addition, a major review article by Lund and colleagues[12] on the diagnosis and monitoring of TMD patients with adjunctive devices was published in 1995. Greene[6] and Laskin and Greene[15] also examined these issues a few years earlier. The following descriptions and evaluations of the adjunctive diagnostic devices for TMDs[5] are drawn from these articles and other literature cited within them.

Jaw Tracking

Because impairment of jaw mobility and function are often among the main signs or symptoms of TMDs, it is not surprising that various parameters of jaw movement have been considered to be of diagnostic value. In addition to pantography and axiography devices that track jaw movement at the condylar level, several types of recording machines have been developed to track the movement of the entire mandible relative to the maxilla. A detailed discussion of the capabilities as well as the limitations of such machines is presented in chapter 4.

Using various machines to study mandibular movements in TMD patients, several investigators have examined jaw movement parameters that are considered to be of potential diagnostic value. These include amplitude of jaw movement in all three planes of space, reproducibility or consistency of jaw movements, and velocity as well as smoothness of jaw trajectories.

Cooper and Rabuzzi[19] believed that the amplitude and path of closure from rest position, as well as the form of voluntary opening and closing, had diagnostic importance. However, when Feine et al[20] tested the diagnostic criteria provided by the manufacturer of the device used by Cooper and Rabuzzi, they were unable to show significant differences between normal subjects and TMD patients. Chewing patterns also were supposed to be "poor" in TMD patients, but when dentists were asked to classify the printouts from jaw-tracking devices as good, fair, or poor according to the manufacturer's criteria, the outcomes were mixed for both normal subjects and TMD patients.[20] In addition, there was poor interobserver agreement, so no individual clinician's judgment could be relied on to classify normal (good) versus TMD (poor) results.

In other studies that investigated chewing patterns,[21,22] investigators reported a difference between normal subjects and TMD patients. However, these articles did not present criteria for judging the chewing patterns, and no statistical testing was done; in fact, it seemed that the chewing pattern was expected to be abnormal in the patient group simply because the patients were experiencing symptomatic jaw problems.

There have been reports that the velocity of voluntary jaw movements is less in TMD patients. Cooper and Rabuzzi[19] stated that a maximum vertical velocity of less than 300 mm/sec is "not healthy," but Feine et al[20] found that all of their healthy subjects had measurements below this limit (as did 80% of Cooper and Rabuzzi's asymptomatic subjects). Once again, the mean scores for TMD patients were somewhat lower than in normal individuals, but not at a significant level. As usual, there were wide variations in individual performances.

McCall et al[23] used phase plane modeling to quantify the irregularity of closing movements. Although dysfunctional patients had the highest scores, findings from the work of Naeije and Honee[24] suggest that this may be a function of velocity, because smoothness increases with speed. Neither of these articles suggested that there is diagnostic value in assessing this variable with a complex jaw-tracking system. Other investigators have studied the reproducibility of horizontal jaw movements in TMD patients compared to normal subjects, and some group differences were found in "accuracy scores." More severe symptoms correlated to lower scores.[5,25] However, these authors concluded that such tests would not be useful in the dental office because of high intersubject variability.

In two other studies evaluating the reliability and accuracy of jaw-tracking devices, Balkhi and Tallents[26] reported measurement errors in the range of 1% to 66%, while Tsolka et al[27] reported errors in the range of 9% to 30%. They also showed that these instruments consistently underestimated large mandibular movements, which inevitably will lead to the false-positive diagnosis of limited mandibular movement and the potential overtreatment of healthy people. Therefore, as Mohl et al[14] concluded in their first review article, "At the present time, the claim that jaw-tracking devices have diagnostic value for TMD is not well supported by the scientific evidence." This conclusion still seems to be valid 15 years later, but unfortunately the advocacy for using such devices has not disappeared.

Electromyography

Surface electromyography of the muscles of mastication has been advocated by some dentists as a "modern scientific approach" to the diagnosis and treatment of TMD patients, because the output from such devices is presumed to be both "quantitative" and "objective."[28] The use of EMG devices is based on the assumption that certain pathologic or dysfunctional conditions can be identified by abnormal activity of the masticatory muscles. These conditions include postural hyperactivity,[19,29–32] abnormal occlusal positions,[22,33–35] functional hyperactivity and hypoactivity,[31,36–38] muscle spasm,[36,37,39,40] muscle fatigue,[41,42] and muscle imbalance.[30,33,43,44] In addition, EMG recordings taken before and after certain treatments have been used to document changes in muscle function, which have been cited as "proof" that the treatment was successful.[39,41,42]

The original application of EMG devices in dentistry was mainly to study jaw and facial muscle functions under experimental conditions in various morphologic groups of human subjects, as well as to draw comparisons between dentate and edentulous subjects.[45–47] Similar devices have been used for many years to study the biomechanics of jaw function in various animals.[48,49] Clinically, they also were used to look for possible muscular differences between asymptomatic subjects and TMD pain-dysfunction patients.[50–52]

A large body of literature describes the outcomes of all these studies. However, an analysis of that literature, conducted by Mohl and colleagues,[17] uncovered several major deficiencies in a large percentage of the clinical trials, and these severely limit the interpretation of the results. Among their major criticisms were the lack of adequate control groups, the lack of studies showing reliability and validity of the methods, the inadequacy or nonexistence of statistical comparisons, and the declaration of conclusions that were not supported by the study results. The most significant problem, however, was the large interindividual variability in both normal and patient groups, resulting in considerable overlap between them.

Based on their own analysis, plus an earlier major review of the EMG literature by Lund and Widmer,[53] Mohl et al[17] concluded that "there is no evidence to support the use of EMG for the evaluation or diagnosis of TMD." They recommended that well-controlled clinical studies be conducted in the future to determine whether there are any objective, valid, repeatable, and diagnostically useful EMG differences between patient groups and normal subjects.

In the review articles by Lund and colleagues,[12,53] a number of specific methodologic problems are described to explain why EMG results cannot be taken at face value and then simply interpreted as demonstrating normal or abnormal muscle behaviors. There must be experimental controls for age, sex, facial form, skin thickness, electrode positioning, and a history of bruxism or other parafunctions before absolute EMG levels can be compared.[54–58] In addition, the researchers emphasized that the muscles of facial expression are a source of confounding signals when jaw muscles are being recorded with surface electrodes.[59,60] It has been shown that the faces of chronic pain patients express not only their emotional burden (for example, depression), but also their somatic burden of pain; this can increase the EMG signals coming from the facial muscles that lie between the surface electrodes and the masseter or temporal muscles.[61–63] Yet, despite all of these complicating factors, the manufacturers of surface EMG devices to be used for diagnosing and monitoring TMDs provide purchasers with cutoff values for "normal" resting muscle activity that are the same for all masticatory muscles in all people.

Lund et al[12] also discussed the combined use of muscle-stimulating devices and EMG machines. Presumably, these stimulators can relax hyperactive jaw muscles and then cause them to contract in a more physiologic way than when they are controlled by the brain. Because the occlusal relationship between the maxillary and mandibular teeth is the primary determinant of where the mandible will be located relative to the maxilla when the mouth is fully closed, the teeth are seen as "being in the way" of attaining an ideal maxillomandibular relationship.[28,64] Therefore, direct stimulation to the masticatory muscles can bypass this habitual jaw closure.

At least two major lines of evidence have been produced in recent years that refute this line of thinking. First, it has been shown that these devices do not stimulate muscle spindle afferents in the masseteric nerve, as originally claimed by Jankelson et al[65]; instead, they stimulate the superficial masseter muscle directly, producing a simple muscular twitch.[66] Second, recent EMG research in several other areas of the body has shown rather conclusively that neither myogenous TMDs nor related conditions, such as fibromyalgia, lower back pain, and tension-type headache, are caused by abnormal patterns of muscular activity.[60,67] All of these conditions had traditionally been described as muscular tension or spasm disorders, but EMG results did not confirm this concept. The specific issue of masticatory muscle hyperactivity and myogenous TMD pain is addressed by Lund in chapter 6.

Some advocates for using this combination of instruments have assumed that TMD patients have a mandibular rest position that is outside the normal range,[68] but there is no real evidence of this. Instead, two studies conducted by the same lead investigator[19,69] showed that about 40% of TMD patients fell outside this "normal" range, but the same was true for about the same number of asymptomatic subjects. When repetitive stimulation was used to suppress normal postural activity in these studies, about 80% of both groups were found to have an "abnormal freeway space."[19,69] Another so-called diagnostic application of these devices is to compare habitual and stimulated jaw closure to see if they coincide. Using the manufacturer's diagnostic criteria, it again was found that 80% of a randomly selected group had a "positive" diagnosis of myofascial TMD[19,69] but in fact these were false positives, because none of these subjects had masticatory pain or dysfunction.

As is the case with jaw-tracking instruments, the clinical utility of EMG devices appears to be severely limited by all sorts of technical problems, methodologic concerns, questions of data interpretation, and overlap between normal and patient groups. It has been more

than 20 years since Majewski and Gale[70] reported not only that EMG results failed to discriminate between these two groups but also that there was no consistent difference between symptomatic and asymptomatic sides in patients with unilateral myofascial pain. One might expect that these and other widely reported negative findings would have dampened the enthusiasm of advocates for the clinical use of EMG machines. Instead, they continue to be manufactured and sold to practicing dentists in several countries.

Sonography and Vibratography

Sonography is the technique of recording and graphically displaying sound. Various authors have attempted to demonstrate that certain TMJ sounds are an objective sign of various pathologic conditions within the joint. For example, simultaneous recordings of TMJ sounds and fluoroscopy,[71] cinematography,[72] or cineradiography[73] have demonstrated that clicking can occur during reduction of an anteriorly displaced articular disc. However, clicking can also occur if the disc and condyle "jump" during mouth opening or closing, presumably because of an obstacle or deformity on the articular surface. These *deviations in form* (DIF) have been described by Hansson and Oberg[74] as being potentially present on all four articulating surfaces (condyle, eminence, and top and bottom of the disc). Other sources of clicking-type sounds in the TMJ include fluid cavitation[75] as well as sudden movements of ligaments.[76]

Crepitation in the TMJ has usually been regarded as a sign of degenerative joint disease.[77] Although this noise is probably related to some type of intracapsular change, it is not clear whether it is pathognomonic for arthritis.[78,79] Other sources of TMJ crepitation also should be considered, such as lack of synovial fluid or translatory movement of the condyle over the retrodiscal tissues that are interposed between condyle and fossa in internal derangement cases.[80]

Some investigators have used more sophisticated methods for detection and analysis of TMJ sounds; these include spectral analysis and Doppler ultrasound. The use of spectral analysis is based on the concept that different sound sources produce specific frequency distributions of sound energy, and this can be used to discriminate among various intracapsular problems.[71,81–83] However, these studies have been limited by either lack of controls or lack of statistical analyses to prove whether specific TMJ conditions produce characteristic sounds. Gay and Bertolami,[80,83] for example, found no consistent differences in frequency spectra among patients with three different types of intracapsular problem (arthritis, reducing disc displacement, or nonreducing disc displacement).

Doppler ultrasound techniques, which have been used in clinical medicine as vascular and obstetric diagnostic procedures,[84] also have been suggested for analysis of TMJ sounds. They have been promoted as having the ability not only to differentiate among various sounds but also to identify posterior ligament hyperemia as well as adhesions between the disc and eminence.[85] All of these interpretations are supposed to be based on characteristic waveforms produced on the hardcopy printout. However, as one investigator has noted,[86] "Quite often, dissimilar sounds resembled one another graphically."

Joint sounds of all types are commonly found in random populations (estimates range from 15% to 65%).[16,87] Furthermore, many internally deranged and/or degenerated TMJs (15% to 30%) do not consistently produce any noises at all.[79,88]

A number of methodologic problems also must be considered in reference to the possible usefulness of sonography devices. These include the high variability of TMJ sounds from day to day in the same patient[89] as well as poor interobserver agreement in the interpretation of either tape recordings or graphic pictures of joint sounds.[89,90] In addition, it is difficult to separate pertinent TMJ sounds from artifacts such as room noise, respiration, skin and hair noise, blood flow, and crossover noises from the opposite TMJ. Gallo et al[91] were able to detect sounds with a microphone over the TMJ even without movement of the subject's mandible. Another source of contamination is the inner ear: otoacoustic emissions of 10 to 20 db have been recorded in about 50% of females and 25% of males.[92]

All of the aforementioned problems with sonography led Mohl et al[17] to conclude that, "there is insufficient evidence to warrant the use of special devices for the detection and analysis of TMJ sounds in the differential diagnosis of TMD." They also noted that the solution of technical problems to enable more accurate sound recording still would not assure the value of such devices, because there is no clear evidence that specific sound patterns represent specific TMJ conditions. Therefore, the use of TMJ sonography devices offers no particular advantage over a conventional stethoscope and direct auscultation.[12,16]

Conclusion

The three types of so-called adjunctive diagnostic devices for TMDs that were discussed in this chapter have been available for many years. Although the combination of electronic recording devices with computer technology

has made them easier to use and enhanced their quantitative properties, they still do what they did before: track the movements of the jaw; record the activities of the muscles; and record the sounds produced by the TMJ. The literature cited in this chapter seems to have stopped in the middle 1990s, mainly because the scientific controversy over the use of these devices had run its course by that time.[93] At least two major scientific position statements had been published by then, both of which condemned the clinical use of adjunctive diagnostic devices for TMD. The first came in 1989 from 11 Canadian neuroscientists[94] who said, "Thus, in our opinion, these instruments do not yet have a proven value in the diagnosis and treatment of TMD, and their uses for purposes other than research could lead to misdiagnosis and overtreatment of patients." These thoughts were echoed in a Scientific Information Statement published by the American Association for Dental Research in 1996, based on information submitted by the Neuroscience Group of that organization.[95]

Both the US FDA and the ADA also had been embroiled in this controversy for several years, but ultimately they both took similar actions in "approving" these instruments for clinical usage. These organizations classified the instruments as "measurement devices" because they do measure something. Both groups placed the burden of responsibility for the use and interpretation of the results squarely on the individual practitioner. The FDA's current statement[96] concludes:

> FDA has identified the following risks to health associated with [these] devices as follows: . . .) Improper treatment. There is no general consensus or established standard of care regarding the interpretation of the output of these devices. Therefore, a misdiagnosis of temporomandibular joint disorders and associated orofacial pain may lead to improper treatment.

The ADA's most recent statement[97] says:

> [Product Name] is accepted as a measurement device for the evaluation of the temporomandibular musculoskeletal complex. Responsibility for the proper selection of patients for testing and the interpretation of test results rests with the dentist.

In the end, the entire question of appropriate use (or nonuse) of adjunctive diagnostic devices revolves around their ability either to discover new patients who were previously unrecognized or to add clinically valuable information to what we can learn from direct examination of existing TMD patients. It is well known in the dental community that many patients over the years have consulted dentists about a wide variety of nonspecific head, neck, and upper body complaints. The main reason for this has been advertising in the popular media and teaching at various dental institutions or academies that suggests that such symptoms may be due to "TMJ." These patients have, in many cases, been subjected to a "TMJ diagnostic workup" involving radiographs, occlusodental analyses, and a variety of technologic assessments. Similar analyses have been performed for asymptomatic patients presenting for routine dental examinations. Despite having no clinical history of jaw pain or dysfunction, patients in both of these groups have been told they had a TMD, based solely on the results obtained from such testing.

In one study, 81% of a random population was found to have "covert" TMJ problems, based on findings from a jaw-tracking system.[19] As Feine et al[20] have pointed out, this is practically definitive proof that such machines are incapable of discriminating between sick and healthy people. It seems clear that the advocates for these "discovery" applications of TMD devices have failed to recognize the significant methodologic problems that make the analysis of one patient so different from research assessments done on groups of normal individuals or patients. As both the FDA's and the ADA's statements make clear, none of these devices can be even considered for use in the absence of clinical information, so they cannot be used to make a blind reading in which the test results by themselves establish a clinical diagnosis (unlike, for example, an electrocardiogram).

The more that results from testing match the clinical diagnosis already established, the more unnecessary the tests become. For example, is it really useful to have a jaw-tracking device confirm that a person with left-side jaw pain is deviating to the left upon opening? Considering that most clicking TMJs cannot readily be treated just to eliminate the noise (nor do they need to be), is it helpful to have a complex waveform analysis of that click from a sonography machine?

All clinicians hope to see future technological advances that will improve the understanding of the TMD phenomena and the diagnosis of patients with craniofacial pain. The profession has learned much from imaging technologies such as arthrography, magnetic resonance imaging, and, more recently, positron emission tomography of the brain in patients with pain. Analyses of synovial fluid and changes in the articular surface of the TMJ have led to a greater understanding of both pain and diseases of the TMJ, while molecular studies have improved the understanding of muscle pathophysiology.

There is little doubt that these and other discoveries will lead in time to more objective diagnostic procedures, which will have to be clinically validated. In the meantime, a posture of caution must be maintained about unproved technologies, and energy must be focused on good clinical diagnostic techniques that will lead to reasonable and effective treatments for patients with TMD patients but avoid the mislabeling of healthy subjects. This is the true meaning of evidence-based patient care.

References

1. Headache Classification Committee of the International Headache Society. Classification and diagnostic criteria for headache disorders, cranial neuralgia, and facial pain. Cephalgia 1988;8(suppl 7):1–96.
2. Headache Classification Subcommittee of the International Headache Society. The International Classification of Headache Disorders, ed 2. Cephalgia 2004;24(suppl 1):1–150.
3. Clark GT, Lynn P. Horizontal plane jaw movements in controls and clinic patients with temporomandibular dysfunction. J Prosthet Dent 1986;55:730–735.
4. McCall WD Jr, Rohan EA. Linear position transducer using a magnet and Hall effect devices. IEEE Trans Inst Meas 1977;26:133–136.
5. Jemt T, Hedegard GT. Reproducibility of chewing rhythm and of mandibular displacement during chewing. J Oral Rehabil 1982;9:531–537.
6. Greene CS. Can technology enhance TM disorder diagnosis? Calif Dent Assoc J 1990;18:21–24.
7. Begg CB. Statistical methods in medical diagnosis. Crit Rev Med Inform 1986;1:1–22.
8. McNeil B, Keeler E, Adelstein S. Primer on certain elements of medical decision making. N Engl J Med 1975;293:211–215.
9. Swets JA. Measuring the accuracy of diagnostic systems. Science 1988;240:1285–1293.
10. Mohl ND, Dixon DC. Current status of diagnostic procedures for temporomandibular disorders. J Am Dent Assoc 1994;125:56–64.
11. Widmer CG, Lund JP, Feine JS. Evaluation of diagnostic tests for TMD. Calif Dent Assoc J 1990;18:53–60.
12. Lund JP, Widmer CG, Feine JS. Validity of diagnostic and monitoring tests used for temporomandibular disorders. J Dent Res 1995;74:1133–1143.
13. Mohl ND. Temporomandibular disorders: The role of occlusion, TMJ imaging, and electronic devices. A diagnostic update. J Am Coll Dent 1991;58:4–10.
14. Mohl ND, McCall WD, Lund JP, Plesh O. Devices for the diagnosis and treatment of temporomandibular disorders. 1. Introduction, scientific evidence, and jaw tracking. J Prosthet Dent 1990;63:198–201.

15. Laskin DM, Greene CS. Technological methods in the diagnosis and treatment of temporomandibular disorders. Int J Technol Assess Health Care 1990;6:558–568. Reprinted in Quintessence Int 1992;23:95–102.

16. Dworkin SF, Huggins KH, LeResche L, Von Korff MR, Howard J, Truelove E. Epidemiology of signs and symptoms in temporomandibular disorders: Clinical signs in cases and controls. J Am Dent Assoc 1990;173:273–281.

17. Mohl ND, Lund JP, Widmer CG, McCall WD. Devices for the diagnosis and treatment of temporomandibular disorders. 2. Electromyography and sonography. J Prosthet Dent 1990;63:332–336.

18. Mohl ND, Ohrbach RK, Crow HC, Gross AJ. Devices for the diagnosis and treatment of temporomandibular disorders. 3. Thermography, ultrasound, electrical stimulation, and electromyographic biofeedback. J Prosthet Dent 1990;63: 472–477.

19. Cooper BC, Rabuzzi DD. Myofacial [sic] pain dysfunction syndrome: A clinical study of asymptomatic patients. Laryngoscope 1984;94:68–75.

20. Feine JS, Hutchins MO, Lund JP. An evaluation of the criteria used to diagnose mandibular dysfunction with the mandibular kinesiograph. J Prosthet Dent 1988;60:374–380.

21. Mongini F, Tempia-Valente G. A graphic and statistical analysis of the chewing movements in function and dysfunction. Cranio 1984;2:125–134.

22. Michler L, Moller E, Bakke M, Andreasen S, Heningsen E. On-line analysis of natural activity in muscles of mastication. J Craniomandib Disord 1988;2:65–82.

23. McCall WD Jr, Bailey JO Jr, Ash MM Jr. A quantitative measure of mandibular joint dysfunction: Phase plane modeling of jaw motion in man. Arch Oral Biol 1976;21:685–689.

24. Naeije M, Honee GLJ. The reproducibility of movement parameters of the empty open-close-clench cycle in man, and their dependency on the frequency of movements. J Oral Rehabil 1979;6:405–415.

25. Monteiro AA, Clark GT, Pullinger AG. Relationship between mandibular movement accuracy and masticatory dysfunction symptoms. J Craniomandib Disord 1987;1:237–242.

26. Balkhi KM, Tallents RH. Error analysis of a magnetic jaw-tracking device. J Craniomandib Disord 1991;5:51–56.

27. Tsolka P, Woelful JB, Man WK, Preiskel HW. A laboratory assessment of recording reliability and analysis of the K6 diagnostic system. J Craniomandib Disord 1992;6:273–280.

28. Cooper BC. The role of bioelectric instrumentation in the documentation and management of temporomandibular disorders. Oral Surg Oral Med Oral Pathol Oral Radiol Endod 1997;83:91–100.

29. Lous I, Sheik-ol-Eslam A, Moller E. Postural activity in subjects with functional disorders of the chewing apparatus. Scand J Dent Res 1970;78:404–410.

30. Dohrmann RJ, Laskin DM. An evaluation of electromyographic biofeedback in the treatment of myofascial pain-dysfunction. J Am Dent Assoc 1978;96:656–662.

31. Sheik-ol-Eslam A, Moller E, Lous I. Postural and maximum activity in elevators of mandible before and after treatment of functional disorders. Scand J Dent Res 1982;90:37–46.

32. Dolan EA, Keefe FJ. Muscle activity in myofascial pain-dysfunction patients: A structured clinical evaluation. J Craniomandib Disord 1988;2:101–105.

33. Moyers RE. Some physiologic considerations of centric and other jaw relations. J Prosthet Dent 1956;6:183–194.

34. Franks AST. Masticatory muscle hyperactivity and temporomandibular joint dysfunction. J Prosthet Dent 1965;15: 1122–1131.

35. Funakoshi M, Fujita N, Takehana S. Relations between occlusal interference and jaw muscle activities in response to changes in head position. J Dent Res 1976;55:684–689.

36. Moller E, Sheik-ol-Eslam A, Lous I. Response of elevator activity during mastication to treatment of functional disorders. Scand J Dent Med 1984;92:64–83.

37. Moller E. Muscle hyperactivity leads to pain and dysfunction: Position paper. In: Klineberg I, Sessle BJ (eds). Orofacial Pain and Neuromuscular Dysfunction. Oxford: Pergamon, 1985:69–92.

38. Yemm R. A neurophysiological approach to the pathology and aetiology of temporomandibular dysfunction. J Oral Rehabil 1985;12:343–353.

39. Ramfjord SP. Bruxism, a clinical and electromyographic study. J Am Dent Assoc 1961;62:21–44.

40. Gordon TE. The influence of the herpes simplex virus on jaw muscle function. Cranio 1983;2:31–38.

41. Von Boxtel A, Goudswaard P, Janssen K. Absolute and proportional resting EMG levels in muscle contraction and migraine headache patients. Headache 1983;23:223–228.

42. Naeije M, Hansson TL. Electromyographic screening of myogenous and arthrogenous TMJ dysfunction patients. J Oral Rehabil 1986;13:433–441.

43. Jankelson B, Pulley ML. Electromyography in Clinical Dentistry. Seattle: Myotronics Research, 1984.

44. Festa F. Joint distraction and condyle advancement with a modified functional distraction appliance. Cranio 1985;3: 344–350.

45. Moyers RE. An electromyographic analysis of certain muscles involved in temporomandibular movement. Am J Orthod 1950;36:481–515.

46. Pruzansky S. Application of electromyography to dental research. Am J Orthod 1952;44:49–58.

47. Hannam AG, Wood WW. Medial pterygoid muscle activity during the closing and compressive phases of human mastication. Am J Phys Anthropol 1981;55:359–367.

48. Hylander WL, Johnson KR. Temporalis and masseter function in humans and macaques during incision. Int J Primatol 1985;6:289–322.

49. Hiiemae KM. Mammalian mastication: A review of the activity of the jaw muscles and the movement they produce in chewing. In: Joysey KA, Butler PM (eds). Development, Function and Evolution of Teeth. London: Academic Press, 1978:359–398.

50. Perry HT. Muscular changes associated with temporomandibular joint dysfunction. J Am Dent Assoc 1957;54:614.

51. Jarabak JR. An electromyographic analysis of muscular and temporomandibular joint disturbances due to imbalances in occlusion. Angle Orthod 1956;26:170–190.

52. Stohler CS, Ashton-Miller JA, Carlson DS. The effects of pain from the mandibular joint and muscles on masticatory motor behavior in man. Arch Oral Biol 1988;33:175–182.

53. Lund JP, Widmer CG. An evaluation of the use of surface electromyography in the diagnosis, documentation, and treatment of dental patients. J Craniomandib Disord 1989;3:125–137.

54. Carlson KE, Alston W, Feldman DJ. Electromyographic study of aging in skeletal muscle. Am J Phys Med 1964;43:141–145.

55. Visser SL, De Rijk W. Influence of sex and age on EMG contraction pattern. Eur Neurol 1974;12:229–235.

56. Throckmorton GS, Finn RA, Bell WH. Biomechanics of differences in lower facial height. Am J Orthod Dentofac Orthop 1980;77:410–420.

57. Sherman RA. Relationships between jaw pain and jaw muscle contraction level: Underlying factors and treatment effectiveness. J Prosthet Dent 1985;54:114–118.

58. Newton JP, Abel RW, Robertson EM, Yemm R. Changes in human masseter and medial pterygoid muscles with age: A study by computed tomography. Gerodontics 1987;3:151–154.

59. Large RG, Lamb AM. Electromyographic (EMG) biofeedback in chronic musculoskeletal pain: A controlled trial. Pain 1983;17:167–177.

60. Lund JP, Stohler CS, Widmer CG. The relationship between pain and muscle activity in fibromyalgia and similar conditions. In: Vaeroy H, Merskey H (eds). Progress in Fibromyalgia and Similar Conditions. Amsterdam: Elsevier, 1993:307–323.

61. Schwartz GE, Fair PL, Salt P, Mandel MR, Klerman GL. Facial muscle patterning to affective imagery in depressed and nondepressed subjects. Science 1976;192:489–491.

62. Schwartz GE, Fair PL, Salt P, Mandel MR, Klerman GL. Facial expression and imagery in depression: An electromyographic study. Psychosomat Med 1976;38:337–347.

63. Tassinary LG, Caccioppo JT, Geen TR. A psychometric study of surface electrode placements for facial electromyographic recording. 1. The brow and cheek muscle regions. Psychophysiology 1989;26:1–16.

64. Jankelson RR. Neuromuscular Dental Diagnosis and Treatment. St Louis: Ishiyaku EuroAmerica, 1990.

65. Jankelson B, Sparks S, Crane PF, Radke JC. Neural conduction of the myo-monitor stimulus: A quantitative analysis. J Prosthet Dent 1975;34:245–253.

66. Dao TTT, Feine JS, Lund JP. Can electrical stimulation be used to establish a physiologic occlusal position? J Prosthet Dent 1988;60:509–514.

67. Lund JP, Widmer CG, Schwartz G. What is the link between myofascial pain and dysfunction? In: Van Steenberghe D, De Laat A (eds). Electromyography of Jaw Reflexes in Man. Belgium: Leuven University Press 1991:427–444.

68. Manns A, Zuazoia RV, Sirnan R, Quiroz M, Rocabado M. Relationship between the tonic elevator mandibular activity and the vertical dimension during the states of vigilance and hypnosis. Cranio 1990;8:163–170.

69. Cooper BC, Alleva M, Cooper DL, Lucente FE. Myofacial [sic] pain dysfunction: An analysis of 476 patients. Laryngoscope 96:1099–1106.

70. Majewski RF, Gale EN. Electromyographic activity of anterior temporal area pain patients and non-pain subjects. J Dent Res 1984;63:1228–1231.

71. Oster C, Katzberg R, Tallents R, Morris T, Bartholomew J, Hayakawa K. Characterization of temporomandibular joint sounds. Oral Surg Oral Med Oral Pathol 1984;58:10–16.

72. Isberg-Holm AM, Westesson PL. Movement of disc and condyle in temporomandibular joints with and without clicking: A high speed cinematographic and dissection study on autopsy specimens. Acta Odontol Scand 1982;40:165–177.

73. Isberg-Holm AM, Westesson PL. Movement of disc and condyle in temporomandibular joints with clicking: An arthrographic and cineradiographic study on autopsy specimens. Acta Odontol Scand 1982;40:151–164.

74. Hansson T, Oberg T. Arthrosis and deviations in form in the human temporomandibular joint. A macroscopic study on a human autopsy material. Acta Odontol Scand 1977;35:167–174.

75. Unsworth A, Dowson D, Wright V. "Cracking joints"—A bioengineering study of cavitation in the metacarpophalangeal joint. Ann Rheum Dis 1971;30:348–358.

76. Watt DM. Temporomandibular joint sounds. J Dent 1980;8:119–127.

77. Hansson T, Nilner MA. A study of the occurrence of symptoms of the temporomandibular joint masticatory musculature and related structures. J Oral Rehabil 1975;2:313–324.

78. Schiffman E, Anderson GC, Fricton J, Burton K, Schellhas K. Diagnostic criteria for intra-articular TM disorders. Community Dent Oral Epidemiol 1989;17:252–257.

79. Westesson PL, Eriksson L, Kurita K. Reliability of a negative clinical temporomandibular joint examination: Prevalence of disk displacement in asymptomatic temporomandibular joints. Oral Surg Oral Med Oral Pathol 1989;68:551–554.

80. Gay T, Bertolami CN. The acoustical characteristics of the normal temporomandibular joint. J Dent Res 1988;67:56–60.

81. Drum R, Litt M. Spectral analysis of temporomandibular joint sounds. J Prosthet Dent 1987;58:485–494.

82. Gay T, Bertolami CN, Donoff RB, Keith DA, Delly JP. The acoustical characteristics of the normal and abnormal temporomandibular joint: Diagnostic implications. J Oral Maxillofac Surg 1987;45:397–407.

83. Gay T, Bertolami CN. The spectral properties of temporomandibular joint sounds. J Dent Res 1987;66:1189–1194.

84. Burns PN, Jaffe CC. Quantitative flow measurements with Doppler ultrasound. Techniques, accuracy, and limitations. Radiol Clin North Am 1985;23:641–657.

85. Hutta JL, Morris TW, Katzberg RW, Tallents RH, Espeland MA. Separation of internal derangements of the temporomandibular joint using sound analysis. Oral Surg Oral Med Oral Pathol 1987;63:151–157.

86. Davidson SL. Doppler auscultation: An aid in temporomandibular joint diagnosis. J Craniomandib Disord 1988;2:128–132.

87. Gross AJ, Gale EN. A prevalence study of the clinical signs associated with mandibular dysfunction. J Am Dent Assoc 1983;107:932–936.

88. Kircos LT, Ortendahl DA, Mark AS, Arakawa M. Magnetic resonance imaging of the TMJ disc in asymptomatic volunteers. J Oral Maxillofac Surg 1987;45:852–854.

89. Widmer CG. Temporomandibular joint sounds: A critique of techniques for recording and analysis. J Craniomandib Disord 1989;4:213–217.

90. Eriksson L, Westesson PL, Sjoberg H. Observer performance in describing temporomandibular joint sounds. Cranio 1987;5:32–35.

91. Gallo, LM, Airoldi R, Ernst B, Palla S. TMJ sounds: Quantitative spectral analysis of asymptomatic subjects [abstract]. J Dent Res 1991;70:371.

92. McFadden D. A speculation about the parallel ear asymmetries and sex differences in hearing sensitivity and otoacoustic emissions. Hearing Res 1993;68:143–151.

93. Greene CS, Lund JP, Widmer CG. Clinical diagnosis of orofacial pain: Impact of recent FDA ruling on electronic devices. J Orofac Pain 1995;9:7–8.

94. Lund JP, Lavigne G, Feine JS, et al. The use of electronic devices in the diagnosis and treatment of temporomandibular disorders. J Can Dent Assoc 1989;55:747–750.

95. American Association of Dental Research: Scientific Information Statement on Temporomandibular Disorders. AADR Reports 1996;18(4).

96. Food and Drug Administration, Department of Health and Human Services. Medical Devices: Classification of the Dental Sonography Device and Jaw Tracking Device. Final rule. Fed Regist 2003 Dec 2;68(231):67365–67367. Available at: http://frwebgate1.access.gpo.gov/cgi-bin/waisgate.cgi?WAISdoc228275484422+0+0+0&WAISaction=retrieve. Accessed 1 July 2005.

97. Council on Scientific Affairs, American Dental Association. Acceptance Program Guidelines: Devices for Evaluation of Temporomandibular Musculoskeletal Complex (TMSC). Adopted May 1997. Available at: http://www.ada.org/prof/resources/positions/standards/guide_TMSC.pdf. Accessed 1 July 2005.

Psychological and Psychosocial Assessment

Samuel F. Dworkin

While psychological and psychosocial assessment is strongly advocated as an essential component of evaluating the patient with a temporomandibular disorder (TMD), formal psychiatric diagnosis is not essential to the activities of the primary TMD health care provider; hence this chapter focuses on psychological assessment and classification of the TMD patient, but does not engage methods and measures for achieving differential psychiatric diagnosis, as might be deemed essential for the therapeutic goals of a psychiatrist or clinical psychologist. The objectives of this chapter are to:

1. Offer a brief rationale for why a psychological and psychosocial assessment should be conducted for TMD patients, whether by a TMD–orofacial pain specialist or a non-TMD specialist dentist or physician.
2. Describe the methods and measures that may be useful for conducting such an assessment, based on the best available scientific evidence and widespread clinical judgment.
3. Provide guidelines for obtaining and using biobehavioral data from psychological and psychosocial assessment of TMD patients.

Rationale

The scientific and clinical rationale for conducting a psychological and psychosocial assessment of TMD patients rests on four well-substantiated premises:

1. Many of the TMDs result in chronic pain.
2. Chronic pain is associated with psychological and psychosocial disturbance.

3. Increased levels of psychological and psychosocial impairment are often associated with poor treatment outcomes.
4. A multidimensional understanding of chronic pain improves diagnosis and treatment.

Chronic Pain in TMD Patients

The chief clinical characteristic of most TMDs is pain; for a significant number of patients, the pain is chronic or persistent. Persistent pain is almost exclusively the reason patients present for treatment of musculoskeletal disorders.[1] Therefore, it is the relief of pain that is the major treatment objective for both the patient and the clinician, and the elimination or reduction of such chronic pain is the major criterion by which the success of TMD treatment is judged in the overwhelming majority of cases.[2]

Chronic Pain, Psychological Disturbance, and Psychosocial Impairment

All of the most important chronic pain conditions, including back pain, common "tension" headache, fibromyalgia, and the TMDs have been repeatedly shown to include many patients with at least transient psychological and psychosocial upset.[3] A considerable minority of patients within each condition also manifest clinically significant depression, anxiety, somatization, high utilization of health services, and frequent use of a wide range of pain medications; in addition, they exhibit a significantly impacted lifestyle, which diminishes their capacity to work productively and/or to anticipate an optimistic future.[4–6]

Impaired Psychological and Psychosocial Functioning Among TMD Patients

Appreciable psychological and psychosocial upset has been shown to interact negatively with all forms of therapy, from medicines to surgery. Moreover, it has been repeatedly demonstrated that psychosocial factors are consistently better predictors of long-term treatment outcome than the physical findings, the diagnosis, or the amount of treatment sought.[7,8] It is therefore recommended that the level of psychological functioning in TMD patients be routinely assessed as one means of developing a better integrated, more rational, and more comprehensive approach to managing the problem.

Enhanced Diagnosis and Assessment and Increased Treatment Options

It is a universally accepted concept that conditions in which chronic pain is a critical clinical feature require a multidisciplinary approach for their differential diagnosis and assessment. Unfortunately, it is not universally recognized that psychological assessment can point clinicians toward a broader range of evidence-based effective biobehavioral therapies for managing TMD. This is especially true for the chronic pain component so frequently associated with TMDs (see chapter 26 for biobehavioral treatments, including those most dentists can deliver, that are complementary to the biobehavioral assessment methods and measures to be described).

The integrated, multidimensional approach to assessing and managing patients with TMD pain is best conceptualized through use of a biopsychosocial model, which allows the simultaneous consideration of physical and pathophysiologic *bio*logic processes, the higher order *psycho*logical (ie, cognitive and emotional) information processing that give rise to the patient's meaning and motivation in seeking treatment, and the *social* or behavioral impact on the life of the patient with chronic TMD-related pain.[9] A review of the wide-ranging topics presented in this book is adequate testimony to the need for such a multidisciplinary approach to TMD patients.

Another important issue to be considered is whether psychological upset precedes the onset of pain with certain TMDs, ie, psychological disturbance as a *cause* of the pain, or whether the psychological disturbance results from the chronic and persistent pain and other unwanted symptoms that may accompany the problem, ie, psychological disturbance as a *result* of the condition.

Both views are entirely appropriate and tenable and are probably valid at one time or another for many patients in the course of chronic TMD pain. However, there is insufficient evidence to support either view at the expense of the other. From a realistic clinical and therapeutic perspective, the issue of etiology with regard to psychological and psychosocial factors may be largely irrelevant, given the still limited information on the issue. A critical aspect of the biopsychosocial approach prevalent in chronic pain management is the increased opportunity it provides for simultaneously considering therapeutic interventions aimed at both the biologic (physical) dimensions of the problem as well as the psychological and psychosocial dimensions. This is based on the fundamental observation that both factors are simultaneously contributing to the current situation, independent of which came first. Finally, in this regard, if biobehavioral treatments are considered rational options for at least some TMD patients, then psychological and psychosocial assessment is mandatory to provide essential data around which to conduct such treatments.

Methods and Measures

The methods and measures for assessing the psychological and psychosocial status of TMD patients to be discussed in the following sections do not represent a comprehensive review of the large array of available methods and measures. Rather, the focus is on those that have been proven reliable and valid and have been shown to be useful to the clinician because they are easy to administer and the findings are easy to interpret.

Although the approach recommended in this chapter is that psychological and psychosocial assessment with standardized self-report questionnaires be routinely included when a pain history is gathered from TMD patients, some dentists may prefer a more informal initial approach. The following guidelines are offered to assist these clinicians in the determining whether or not to pursue a more detailed psychological and psychosocial assessment. Table 13-1 offers some specific questions clinicians may ask such patients.

The following are clinical indications for conducting psychological and psychosocial evaluation of TMD patients:

1. When the pain persists beyond the normal expected healing time without clear evidence of ongoing nociception from a physical defect and it significantly disrupts normal functioning in one or more of the following areas: ambulation; self-care; work; home care;

Table 13-1	Suggested questions for determining importance of behavioral factors in a chronic pain problem
What to Ask	**What to Look For**
What activities are you doing more of compared with before your pain began?	Increases in pleasurable activities
What activities are you doing less of compared with before your pain began?	Decreases in aversive/stressful activities
What effect has the pain had on your ability to work? How have things been going at work?	Inability to work because of pain, stresses at work, prior poor work history
What body movements do you avoid because of fear of increased pain?	Guarding, phobic avoidance, belief that pain equals damage
How can others tell when your pain is bad?	Others can easily tell when pain is bad
What do significant others do when your pain is bad?	Expressions of concern/sympathy; cautions to avoid activity; offers to take over tasks, suggestions to call doctor or take medications or "time outs" from stress or conflict
Are you involved in litigation related to your pain? Are you receiving or have you applied for disability compensation?	Financial implications of continued disability versus return to normal functioning
What kinds of stresses have you had recently besides your pain problem? Have you had any problems, such as the death or serious illness of someone close to you, marital problems, problems with your children, financial problems, or just a lot of "hassles"?	Major life stresses or "daily hassles"

recreational activities; and marital, family, or social relationships

2. When the patient exhibits signs or symptoms of significant psychological distress (eg, depression, anxiety)
3. When the disability greatly exceeds that expected on the basis of the physical findings
4. When the patient excessively uses the health care system or when the patient persists in seeking tests or treatments that are not indicated on the basis of the physical findings
5. When there is excessive or prolonged use of opioid or sedative hypnotic medications, alcohol, or other substances for pain control

Research Diagnosis Criteria for TMD Axis II Assessment Domains

The discussion of the methods and measures in this chapter is organized around measures included in the Research Diagnostic Criteria for TMD (RDC/TMD), developed by an international team of expert clinician-researchers.[10,11] The RDC/TMD, consistent with the multidimensional biopsychosocial model on which it is based, uses a dual-axis system to yield both a physical diagnosis and a psychological assessment. Axis I provides a standardized method for conducting a physical examination and history as well as diagnostic algorithms to yield a reliable diagnosis of the most common muscle, disc displacement, and degenerative joint disorders subsumed under the umbrella of TMDs.

Axis II of the RDC/TMD provides methods and measures for assessing psychological, behavioral, and psychosocial factors across four domains potentially useful in the clinical management of TMD patients: pain, mandibular function and behavior, psychological disturbance, and psychosocial disability.

Table 13-2 summarizes the domains and measures included within each domain of the RDC/TMD Axis II. The RDC/TMD does not assess certain psychological domains that nevertheless may be highly relevant to fully understand TMD patients, especially the more complex chronic pain patients. These additional domains that are not included in the RDC/TMD but are valuable to assess include anxiety; substance abuse; physical or sexual abuse; sleep disturbance; quality of life; and, possibly, posttraumatic stress disorder (PTSD). Table 13-3 summarizes these additional domains and relevant assessment measures useful to the clinician.

| Table 13-2 | Research Diagnostic Criteria (RDC) psychological and psychosocial domains and RDC and non-RDC assessment measures*† |

RDC domain	RDC measure		Non-RDC measure	
	Measure	**Description**	**Measure**	**Description**
Pain	VAS	0–10 linear scale	MPQ	Multiple descriptor items
Mandibular function	History questionnaire	Items to assess jaw function	MFIQ	Multiple subscales to assess jaw function
Psychological disturbance				
Depression	Symptom checklist	Screen for depression Values available for normal, moderate, severe	BDI	Self-report measure to assess depression severity
			CES-D	Self-report measure to assess depression severity
Somatization	Symptom checklist	Screen for nonspecific physical symptoms Values available for normal, moderate, severe	NA	
Psychosocial functioning	Graded Chronic Pain Scale	Index of pain severity and TMD pain-related psychosocial interference	MPI	Identifies adequate copers, interpersonally distressed and dysfunctional pain patients; uses multiple scales to assess pain impact, responses of others, activities

*The reader can find the actual items included in each of the Axis II measures included in RDC/TMD Axis II at the website for the RDC/TMD international research consortium.[11] The site provides instructions and/or algorithms for scoring and normative cutoff scores for differing levels of disturbed psychological and psychosocial functioning. Additional references provided in this chapter offer scientific evidence regarding these measures and outcomes associated with their use.

†VAS = visual analog scale; MPQ = McGill Pain Questionnaire; BDI = Beck Depression Inventory; CES-D = Center for Epidemiologic Studies Depression Scale; NA = not applicable; MFIQ = Mandibular Function Impairment Questionnaire; MPI = Multidimensional Pain Inventory.

Pain

Visual analog scales

The assessment of the patient's subjective (self-reported) TMD pain level is one of the first steps in developing a clinical picture of how the patient is experiencing the problem. Pain is most commonly assessed through the use of visual analog scales (VAS) or verbal descriptor scales (VDS), which ask for the patient's subjective rating of TMD pain intensity on a 0 to 10 scale.[12] The RDC/TMD Axis II includes such pain scales. The VAS is a 10-cm line, labeled at one end with "no pain" and at the other end with terms such as "most unbearable pain," "worst pain possible," etc. VDS scales are similar, except that they contain a graded series of labels generally equally spaced along the 10-cm line, with such verbal descriptors as "mild," "moderate," "highly painful," or "intolerable."

These types of easily administered and interpreted pain scales have been in worldwide use for decades, and virtually all reports concerning pain in the scientific literature contain this type of measure as a minimum means for assessing the patient's initial and follow-up pain levels.

Other measures of pain report

The McGill Pain Questionnaire (MPQ)[13] is a widely used scale for assessing the perceptual qualities of pain and has been used extensively in TMD research but is not included in the RDC/TMD Axis II. The patient is asked to select one word in each of several groupings of pain-related terms that best describe the pain being experienced. For example, *dull, aching,* and *throbbing* are some terms commonly selected by chronic TMD pain patients, while terms such as *lancinating, electric shock,* and *burning* are less frequently selected. The MPQ yields several subscale scores reflecting

Table 13-3	Assessment of non-Research Diagnostic Criteria (non-RDC) psychological and psychosocial domains using various psychometric measures	

Non-RDC domain	Measure*	Description
Anxiety	Spielberger State-Trait Anxiety Scale	Scales for assessing current anxiety states and more enduring anxiety traits
Substance abuse	AUDIT-C TICS	Screen for heavy alcohol use and/or dependence Brief assessment of drug and alcohol abuse
Sleep disturbance	PSQI	Commonly used measure to assess quality of sleep; can be supplemented with a single-item question (see text)
Quality of life	Oral Health–Related Quality of Life[ ]	Several measures available for assessing quality of life related to pain and other aspects of oral health
Posttraumatic stress disorder	CAPS	Clinician-administered to assess for common posttraumatic stress disorder diagnostic subcategories
Physical/sexual abuse	AVDR questions	General approach to document suspected physical/sexual abuse (see text)
Overall measures designed for medical patients	Prime-MD PHQ	Screens for major depressive and anxiety disorders, alcohol abuse/dependence, and somatoform disorders

*AUDIT-C = Alcohol Use Disorders Identification Test; TICS = two-item conjoint screening; PSQI = Pittsburgh Sleep Quality Inventory; CAPS = Clinician Administered PTSD

subjective assessment of pain intensity, sensory quality, and emotional charge, in addition to providing overall scale scores based on the number of words chosen and the weight given by the MPQ to each chosen word. Whether clinicians choose VAS-like scales or the MPQ probably will reflect personal preference and eventual ease of comparability with the kind of pain intensity reports prevalent in the literature or needed by third-party payers.

Mandibular function and behavior

Mandibular function is included in the RDC/TMD Axis II (and it has an equally justifiable place in Axis I as well) because jaw function is influenced by behavioral factors such as bruxism, pernicious oral habits, and, of course, the patient's self-report of subjective discomfort and pain experienced while eating, talking, smiling, etc. Assessment of mandibular function as measured by an objective performance, eg, physical assessment of chewing efficiency, would be an example of measuring an Axis I component of mandibular function. Both Axis I and Axis II perspectives are equally valid, because each measurement provides important information about different aspects of mandibular function and how the patient is able to accomplish that function.

Not surprisingly, measures of self-reported performance and objective assessment of clinical findings are often poorly correlated.[14] Maximum unassisted mouth opening, for example, is a clinical measure of jaw function that seems fairly objective. The dentist asks the patient to open the mouth as wide as possible without pain. Both the extent of mobility and any pain associated with that mobility provide important information about the state of anatomic structures involved. Depending on the nature of the accompanying pain report, the clinician also can determine whether psychological and/or psychosocial factors may be important in terms of how the subjective experience of pain imposes limitations on how the anatomic structures function.

The term *impairment* has been suggested by the Institute of Medicine (IOM)[15] to refer to that component of limitation in mandibular (or any organ system) function resulting from organic pathologic conditions. For example, if the mandible is impaired by underdevelopment of a condyle. This form of impairment is distinguished from *functional limitation*, defined as changes imposed on the person by the impairment; ie, the person may be prevented from chewing hard foods. At a global (or psychosocial) level, the person may exhibit a *handicap* or *dysfunction*, for example, reporting himself or herself unemployable because the jaw impairment does not allow communication with fellow workers.

The following summarizes the IOM approach to categorizing impairment, functional limitation, and dysfunction or handicap:

1. The *organ system* has an impairment.
2. The *person* exhibits functional limitation associated with that organ system.
3. *Psychochosocial interaction* with the world is dysfunctional or handicapped.

The relevance of such categorization to certain TMDs is that mandibular limitation may reflect varying degrees of impairment of the jaw and/or disability and dysfunction of the person. As is the case with every chronic pain condition, the extent of impairment is poorly correlated with the extent of disability and dysfunction. The clinician's task is to determine whether or not the reported performance is consistent with other clinical findings regarding expected system performance. For this reason, a biopsychosocial assessment of mandibular function is required.

A simple set of items describing common oral behaviors (eg, chewing hard food, yawning) is included in the RDC/TMD Axis II as a jaw function checklist (but not as a formal measurement scale). In the RDC/TMD Axis II scale at present, these oral behaviors are assessed in either positive or negative terms as being related to TMD pain. Unfortunately, the jaw function checklist of the RDC/TMD Axis II is the only RDC/Axis II component that has not been examined for reliability and validity (no data were available at the time the RDC/TMD was created). Although the scale is clinically helpful, it is likely to be replaced with different measures whose psychometric properties have been fully examined and found adequate for assessing jaw impairment, disability, and dysfunction.

In addition to RDC/TMD Axis II, an alternative scale, the Mandibular Functional Impairment Questionnaire (MFIQ),[16] is available and has attractive items in terms of commonly valued jaw behaviors that dentists want to know about. The present author has used the MFIQ in a research setting with helpful results, but its underlying scale characteristics are complex; among other things, it combines several levels of jaw behavior into a single domain. This makes interpretation of the levels of involvement in terms of the widely used IOM model more complicated and less useful clinically.

A scale currently still under development is based on the present Axis II items. Ohrbach and colleagues[17,18] have developed a psychometrically sound measurement instrument, the Jaw Functional Limitation Scale (JFLS), for three

domains presumably important in how individuals might regard their capacity in using the jaw: chewing performance, extent of vertical mobility, and ability to use the jaw system for verbal (and emotional) expression. Jaw functioning has been assessed in diverse diagnostic groups of TMD patients and has been compared to the clinical findings as well as to the more global disability psychosocial status, and the JFLS has shown good psychometric properties of reliability and validity as well as clinical usefulness.

Psychological status

The RDC/TMD Axis II assesses two critical areas of psychological functioning in TMD patients: depression and the presence of nonspecific physical symptoms, or somatization, using measures that are embedded within the Axis II questionnaire and that have established reliability, validity, and clinical utility. The RDC/TMD Axis II measures of depression and somatization also have been standardized with large population studies in the northwestern United States. Resulting norms for mild, moderate, and severe levels of depression and somatization are available in the RDC/TMD Axis II manual.

Depression
Screening of TMD patients for depression is highly recommended. Rates of clinically diagnosable depression in a primary medical care situation approximate 10%, and it has been amply demonstrated that not only do the rates of depression increase in tertiary care situations but also the risk of a major depressive disorder is increased substantially in patients with chronic TMD pain.[5,19] Most important, depression is a highly disabling condition, estimated to be perhaps the second-leading cause of disability worldwide (next to heart disease). In addition, it has been shown that profound depression is associated with the highest rates of suicide and suicide attempts. The US Surgeon General has suggested that all health providers, especially family practitioners, routinely screen patients for profound depression and its most important sequelae, suicidal behavior. Alerting patients to the well-established benefits of treating depression may provide dentists with an opportunity for introducing a lifesaving intervention.[20]

Depression is highly treatable and, according to clinical trials at the National Institutes of Health, all but the most profound cases of major depressive disorder are about equally treatable with medications as with several forms of psychotherapy. Treatment of depression need not, indeed should not, await resolution of the presenting condition but should be managed concurrently with required TMD treatment. However, to be treated, depression must be detected, but most physicians and dentists are not familiar enough to recognize the common signs and symptoms. Dentists, in particular, seem reluctant to inquire into such personal matters as depression and suicidal ideation, although depression is, regrettably, a too-regular concomitant of persistent TMD pain.

It is important to emphasize that it is appropriate for dentists to assess depression for the purpose of screening, but not for establishing a formal psychiatric diagnosis. The RDC/TMD Axis II measure of depression contains 20 items and assesses the cognitive, vegetative, and affective aspects of depression. It is based on the depression scale of the Symptom Checklist-90 (SCL-90), which is well-established and simple to administer and interpret as part of the RDC/TMD Axis II questionnaire battery. As used in the RDC/TMD Axis II, it shows the psychometric properties of high sensitivity but lower specificity for detecting depression, which fulfills the criteria for a useful screening instrument—that is, to err on the side of detecting someone who reports symptoms but who may not, on further investigation, yield a formal psychiatric diagnosis of depression.[21]

There are several measures of depression that have been reported in conjunction with the assessment of TMD and other chronic pain patients and for which normative values are available for comparison with patient scores. The most widely used of these measures are the Beck Depression Inventory (BDI)[22] and the Center for Epidemiologic Studies Depression Scale (CES-D).[23] Evidence suggests that both questionnaires have good predicative validity among chronic pain patients. The BDI is probably the most commonly used. It comes in several forms, the most popular being the scale form containing 21 items; scores of 12 to 14 have been recommended to separate chronic pain patients with low versus high levels of depressive symptoms.[24] The BDI includes assessment of cognitive (eg, worry), affective (eg, sadness), and neurovegetative (eg, sleep and appetite) symptoms of depression, as does the RDC/TMD Axis II measure of depression. The CES-D is a 20-item self-report inventory, with a total possible score ranging from 0 to 60, reflecting primarily both the number and frequency of depressive symptoms. These scales are also relatively easy to administer, score, and interpret. When choosing among pain assessment measures, clinicians may have their own preference for one over another of these well-established measures with regard to ease of administration, scoring, interpretation, and intended use.

Somatization

The RDC/TMD Axis II questionnaire battery includes a measure of somatization based on 11 scale items derived from the widely used somatization scale of the SCL-90.[25]

This measure is used to assess the presence of nonspecific physical symptoms (eg, hot or cold spells, faintness, or lump in the throat) and, on a scale of 0 to 4, to determine the extent to which they are appraised as troublesome. Five items assess the presence of different kinds of pain. It has proven useful in some instances to perform an additional analysis of scale responses, treating the pain items separately, making clearer the extent to which some TMD patients may experience a wide variety of physical symptoms separate from the widely dispersed pain symptoms many patients with chronic TMD pain concurrently report. While the formal psychiatric diagnosis of somatization disorder is rare, there is a fairly high prevalence of numerous physical symptoms and ailments together with inevitable psychiatric comorbidity among chronic TMD pain patients. This relationship eludes the patient's awareness and the awareness of health care providers not prepared to view chronic TMD pain from a biopsychosocial perspective.[26]

As with the measure of depression, the measure of somatization embedded in the RDC/TMD Axis II shows good reliability and clinical utility, and normative scores are available for a US population. Especially relevant, and supporting the contention that somatization should be assessed in TMD patients, elevated scores on this scale have been repeatedly shown to be highly correlated with the number of muscles tender to palpation,[27] and elevated somatization has been shown to be a predictor of poor outcome of TMD treatment.[8]

The term *somatization* continues to suggest for some an unwarranted yet pejorative implication about the presence of physical symptoms nonspecific to TMDs. The risk for patients is that the clinician may believe that the physical symptoms are somehow "psychological"—that is, mental phenomena with no basis in altered somatic signaling, which are to be taken only as an indication of the possible instability of the patient's psychological state. This unfortunate view, held by more than a few physicians and dentists, places an unfair burden on the patient of being one who is "making up" the symptoms—saying things that are not true or not important to the doctor.

Current evidence supports an alternative, biologically plausible view that is also more reconcilable to an explanatory model acceptable to most TMD patients with chronic pain and other subjective symptoms. Although definitive evidence is not yet available, it nevertheless seems useful to consider that a number of TMD patients may be significantly stressed about a wide variety of physical health, personal, interpersonal, and economic issues.[28] A generalized inability of the person and/or the body to cope may result in dysregulation of higher order information processing, which is related to maintaining homeostasis of ongoing bodily functions. Viewed in this light, those chronic TMD pain patients burdened with significant depression, anxiety, multiple pains, and other persistent symptoms may be best understood as patients unable to cope with disruptive factors in the physical, psychological, and psychosocial environments they occupy. It is prudent to be able to identify such patients, if for no other reason than to spare them the additional burden of unnecessary extensive diagnostic and treatment interventions to uncover the "real" causes of their TMD pain. For some, it may very well be that whatever is maintaining their chronic pain is also maintaining their other physical and psychological symptoms.

Psychosocial level of function

A critical aspect of chronic pain states is the toll they take on the patient's ability to maintain a productive life and rewarding interpersonal relationships and activities at home, work, or school. The terms *chronic pain behavior* and *dysfunctional chronic pain* were introduced to describe the psychosocial disability that emerges for a significant minority of chronic pain patients, including those with certain TMDs.

Chronic pain grade

The RDC/TMD Axis II assesses psychosocial disability using the Graded Chronic Pain (GCP) scale (grades 0 to IV).[29] The scale consists of seven 0 to 10 numeric rating scales embedded in the Axis II questionnaire that integrate assessment of TMD pain severity with assessment of TMD pain-related interference in activities of daily living (eg, days unable to go to work or school, attend to household responsibilities, or socialize with others). Thus, the Graded Chronic Pain scale not only provides a meaningful quantitative index of the extent to which pain is perceived as mild or severe, but it also captures the extent to which the pain is psychosocially disabling.

Through an easily applied scoring algorithm whose reliability and validity have been established, a chronic TMD pain grade can be obtained for each patient. Grade I is defined as pain of low intensity, averaging less than 5 on a 10-point scale and associated with little pain-related interference in daily living. Grade II is defined as high-intensity pain, equal to or greater than 5 on a 10-point scale, with moderate amounts of pain-related psychosocial disability. Grades III and IV are associated with increasing levels of pain-related psychosocial disability, regardless of the pain level. For most clinical and research purposes, functional TMD patients, ie, individuals not significantly disabled by their condition, are defined as grades I and II. In contrast, patients with chronic pain of

grades III and IV are defined as dysfunctional or revealing significant psychosocial disability and impairment.

Examination of the relationship between chronic pain grade and functional status demonstrates the utility of assessing patients in terms of their profile of psychosocial function. Functional patients (that is, RDC/TMD Axis II, grades I and II) show scores for both depression and somatization that are at or near the population mean for these measures. Dysfunctional TMD pain patients, grades III and IV, score significantly higher, in the top 15% to 25% of scores on measures of depression and on the presence of nonspecific physical symptoms, including other pains. However, the level of TMD pain-related dysfunction is not significantly associated with commonly assessed signs from the RDC/TMD Axis I clinical examination, such as range of mandibular motion and number of joint sounds.[30]

Analysis of baseline RDC/TMD data for TMD clinic patients appearing for care revealed that only about 11% of functional patients previously sought treatment from five or more providers, while about four times as many psychosocially dysfunctional patients (approximately 45%) had previously seen five or more health care providers. Support for conducting psychological and psychosocial assessment of TMD patients is provided by a parallel analysis of RDC/TMD somatization scores from these same patients. It was observed that about 50% of those scoring in the top quartile for somatization level also had seen as many as five or more providers, while only about 18% of those in the lowest quartile for somatization had sought care from so many providers.[27]

While recognizing the important role of psychosocial disability in patients with chronic TMD pain, the clinician must also maintain a perspective on the extent of psychosocial impairment in the TMD population. Studies using the GCP scale, replicated on totally independent samples in large population-based studies several years apart, indicate that of those reporting chronic TMD pain, about 35% to 40% are grade I, 35% to 40% are grade II, 15% to 18% are grade III, and 3% to 6% are grade IV.[29] However, in TMD specialty clinic settings, higher rates for grades III and IV are observed; it seems reasonable to estimate that in clinical settings where TMD patients are treated by dentist-specialists, chronic pain grades III and IV combined might comprise about one third of cases. In other words, even in a tertiary care setting, the majority of TMD pain cases are psychosocially functional, showing minimal or only moderate interference with their daily lives. However, the remaining more heavily disabled (ie, grades III and IV) chronic TMD pain patients require a disproportionate number of clinic visits, use much more medication, seek treatment from many more providers, and experience at least moderately high levels of somatization and depression. Moreover, their treatment outcomes are not related to how much treatment they have reported seeking.

The GCP scale was first applied to TMD patients and has been subsequently applied to assess psychosocial disability in a wide range of other pain conditions.[31] Most recently, the clinical utility of the GCP was demonstrated in two randomized clinical trials that tailored treatment for TMD patients solely according to RDC/TMD Axis II GCP status, independent of their RDC/TMD Axis I clinical diagnoses. Psychosocially functional TMD patients (ie, grades I and II) were distinguished from those showing significant TMD pain–related psychosocial interference with activities of daily living (ie, grades III and IV), and the two groups were exposed to very different management approaches. The functional TMD patients received only a self-management program delivered by registered dental hygienists, in lieu of usual specialty care delivered by dentists. One year after treatment was completed, this group showed significantly greater reduction in TMD pain level and ability to control their pain than did their counterpart control group, who received customary care from TMD specialists.[32]

In contrast, the psychosocially impaired group was randomly divided into those receiving customary care and those receiving a tailored intervention that integrated six sessions of cognitive-behavior therapy for chronic TMD-related pain (delivered by clinical psychologists) in addition to the customary care by dentist-specialists. The findings were much more complex for this group of TMD patients than in those showing low levels of psychosocial disability. In brief, the grade III and grade IV patients receiving the integrated care program did significantly better in terms of pain reduction and lowering of psychosocial disability, but the significant differences between them and the control group of patients receiving "treatment as usual" lasted only as long as the integrated treatment. One year after treatment, both groups were comparable in all the important study measures.

However, the reduction in pain reported after 1 year by all the patients in the grade III and grade IV dysfunctional group still left them with significantly high pain levels, averaging 5 on a 10 point scale. These scores were higher than the baseline pain levels reported by functional TMD patients before their treatment began. The same pattern was observed for depression and somatization scores; functional patients ended up with scores that dropped to the mean of the non-TMD population as a whole, while the depression and somatization scores of the dysfunctional group after treatment remained resistant to appreciable change from baseline levels.[33]

In summary, there is substantial evidence that psychosocial disability is prevalent in patients with chronic TMD pain, which is also associated with an elevated incidence of depression, anxiety, and somatization. High levels of psychosocial impairment are associated with increased numbers of treatment visits, increased use of pain medications, and resistance to change with treatment.

Other measures of psychosocial level of function

An important and widely used instrument to assess psychosocial function in patients with chronic pain is the Multidimensional Pain Inventory (MPI).[34] The MPI is much longer than the simple GCP scale but provides more information for those who find it helpful to have a more detailed measure of psychosocial function. The MPI assesses pain impact (severity and interference), responses of others, and activities and enables patients to be classified into dysfunctional, interpersonally distressed, and adaptive coper subgroups.

Such categorization has also proven useful in treatment planning. In one study, dysfunctional patients improved more when treatment of depression was added to standard appliance and biofeedback therapy.[35] Others working with the MPI have reported that patients with acute TMD pain who are dysfunctional and distressed on the MPI are more likely to develop chronic TMD pain; in addition, the dysfunctional profile predicted treatment failure.[36]

Domains Not Included in the RDC/TMD Axis II

Anxiety

Until the early 1970s, anxiety was considered the major psychological concomitant of acute and chronic pain, stemming from Sigmund Freud's initial formulations postulating an intimate relationship between pain and anxiety. The formulation that began to emerge in the 1970s was to differentiate between anxiety, as the major emotional concomitant of acute pain, and depression, as more importantly associated with chronic pain. This dichotomy has been borne out and proven clinically useful. However, the decades-long, almost total neglect of anxiety as a psychological condition of significance to patients with chronic pain was unfortunate. In recent years, researchers have begun to correct this oversight.[37]

The RDC/Axis II does not include a measure of anxiety. The decision was a pragmatic one to reduce the burden on patients of yet another psychological test that was mainly intended for epidemiologic and clinical research. Nevertheless, it seems reasonable to recommend that screening for the presence of anxiety be included in the psychological assessment of all patients with chronic pain, including those with TMDs.

Fortunately, there are several easy-to-use measures, including the anxiety scale of the SCL-90[25] and the Spielberger State-Trait anxiety scale.[38] Because these anxiety scales are, for the most part, symptom checklists, they are easy to administer and easy to interpret as screening measures. Although the evidence for the role that anxiety may play in the TMD pain experience is not nearly as abundant as the evidence for depression (and even for somatization), it is clear from the emerging scientific literature that anxiety will be receiving much more attention from researchers and clinicians in the immediate future.

Substance abuse

The RDC/TMD Axis II does not assess excessive use of alcohol, opiates, benzodiazepines, or other substances. Substance abuse, principally with alcohol and narcotics, is frequently reported in the literature to be more common in patients with chronic pain and TMDs than in the general population.[39] Dentists may wish to consider the Alcohol Use Disorders Identification Test (AUDIT-C)[40] as a brief screen for these problems. It uses three questions: *(1)* "How often do you have a drink containing alcohol?" *(2)* "How many drinks containing alcohol do you have on a typical day when you are drinking?" *(3)* "How often do you have six or more drinks on one occasion?"

An even briefer screen for both alcohol and drug abuse is the two-item conjoint screening test (TICS)[41]: *(1)* "In the last year, have you ever drunk or used drugs more than you meant to?" *(2)* "Have you felt you wanted or needed to cut down on your drinking or drug use in the last year?" These brief measures have been shown to have good sensitivity and specificity for detecting current substance abuse disorders.

Substance abuse is more likely in psychosocially disabled chronic TMD pain patients; through the use of these simple screening measures, the dentist may be uniquely situated to guide more heavily impaired patients toward more constructive methods for coping with their condition while simultaneously offering them an opportunity to significantly enhance their overall health and quality of life.

Sleep disturbance

Disturbed sleep is a potent dysregulator of homeostatic bodily processes, and sleep disturbances are consistently reported to be more frequent among patients with chronic pain than in the population at large. The Pittsburgh Sleep Quality Inventory[42] is a widely used measure of sleep disturbance. This inventory, supplemented with a single question ("How is your sleep overall?"), may serve as an adequate screen to detect the possible presence of a sleep disturbance warranting further pursuit. Once the problem is acknowledged by the patient, therapeutic modalities are available to enhance sleep hygiene. These range from medications to brief cognitive-behavioral therapy interventions. Although disturbed sleep is present in many TMD patients,[43] as yet there is little evidence directly linking sleep disturbance per se to the physical findings in such patients, although sleep disturbance is readily acknowledged to be part of the clinical picture with anxiety, depression, and substance abuse.

Quality of life, post-traumatic stress disorder, and physical and sexual abuse

In addition to the more commonly assessed psychological and psychosocial factors previously discussed, a number of other issues seem to have direct relevance for at least some patients with chronic TMD pain.

Quality of life

Quality of life measures cover a broad spectrum of personal and interpersonal functions and indicate how the person is coping with illness or other challenges to well-being. The available evidence supports the benefits of obtaining a better understanding of this broadly conceived approach to quality of life[44] than is implicitly present in the RDC/TMD Axis II screening assessment measures. However, it is not yet clear whether such measures are useful in a pragmatic sense to the clinician. The data are simply not in available, although quality of life measures seem most promising and are receiving attention in the literature. One excellent example is the Short Form-36 Survey (SF-36),[45] which is a well-established measure (abbreviated versions of the same measure, SF-20 and SF-12, are also available) with excellent psychometric properties that includes pain as an aspect of quality of life that is measured.

Post-traumatic stress disorder

PTSD is a psychiatric disorder that can occur following the experience or witnessing of life-threatening events, such as military combat, natural disasters, serious accidents, or violent personal assaults such as rape. People who suffer from PTSD often relive the experience through nightmares and flashbacks, have difficulty sleeping, and feel detached or estranged. These symptoms can be severe enough and last long enough to significantly impair the person's daily life. PTSD is marked by clear biologic changes as well as psychological symptoms. However, PTSD is complicated by the fact that it frequently occurs in conjunction with related disorders such as depression, substance abuse, problems of memory and cognition, and other problems of physical and mental health. The disorder is also associated with impairment of the person's ability to function in social or family life, including occupational instability and family discord.

There is good evidence supporting a synergy between chronic pain, including chronic TMD pain, and PTSD, but what remains unknown to date is the predictive value of routinely assessing PTSD in patients with TMD pain. However, it seems reasonable that screening measures be used in cases where PTSD is suspected. This can be accomplished with the Clinician Administered PTSD Scale (CAPS),[46] which has good psychometric properties.[47]

Physical and sexual abuse (domestic violence)

The literature contains numerous accounts of the frequent history of physical and sexual abuse in patients with chronic TMD pain.[48] The prevalence of such domestic violence is estimated to be about 16% of the American population. Although women are the most common target of such abuse, the very young and the elderly are also targets. Moreover, the epidemiologic studies increasingly show a trend for more men to be self-reported victims of domestic violence.

The consequences of abuse can be grave, and the overwhelming tendency is for victims to hide or deny any experience of abuse. Therefore, it is appropriate, after a secure doctor-patient relationship has been established, to recommend that dentists undertake sensitive screening for issues of physical and sexual abuse with patients in whom persistent pain is a dependable part of the clinical picture. The recommended assessment process in the so-called AVDR model: *a*sk about abuse; provide *v*alidating messages; *d*ocument presenting signs and symptoms; and *r*efer victims to specialists who treat victims of domestic violence.[49]

Psychological and Psychosocial Assessment in Primary Care

There is a burgeoning interest in alerting primary care physicians to the potential for common mental disorders, including anxiety, depression, somatization, and substance abuse, because these conditions generally include multiple physical symptoms that compel patients to seek primary medical care more frequently than they seek mental health services. It seems reasonable to suggest that dentists, most of whom are in effect also primary care providers, might also incorporate similar minimal screening approaches for their patients with chronic TMD pain (as well as their non-TMD patients). Toward this end, a brief, valid, self-administered screening questionnaire has been developed that is equally suited to the interest of dentists and physicians. The Primary Care Evaluation of Mental Disorders Patient Health Questionnaire (PRIME-MD PHQ,[48] typically referred to simply as *PRIME-MD*) screens for eight common mental disorders (major depressive disorders, panic disorders, other anxiety disorders, bulimia nervosa, other depressive disorders, probable alcohol abuse or dependence, and somatoform and binge-eating disorders). Research shows good agreement between PHQ diagnoses and those of mental health professionals.[50] The average time to review a patient's completed PHQ is less than 3 minutes.

Guidelines for Obtaining and Using Biobehavioral Assessment Data

It is recommended that biobehavioral assessments be conducted for screening purposes on all TMD patients presenting with pain, especially persistent pain, as part of their clinical picture. When such psychological and psychosocial measures are incorporated into a routinely administered battery of history questionnaires, it is unusual to find resistance to these inquiries. Instead many patients express gratitude for the clinician's interest in getting a comprehensive understanding of their total pain-related experiences.

As a general rule, biobehavioral assessment is conducted before the clinician encounters the patient, through the use of baseline history questionnaires. When resistance is met ("Why are you asking me such personal questions?" or "Why do you need to know that?"), the clinician should accept the patient's hesitancies and allow him or her not to answer any or all questions deemed sensitive or irrelevant. This rarely occurring resistance is best responded to with empathy and support, together with a brief explanation of how the desired information allows the clinician to better understand how patients are coping with their condition and assurance that such questions do not imply that the cause of the problem is psychologically related. Figures 13-1 and 13-2 offer some concrete guidelines with regard to patients for whom biobehavioral assessment seems especially indicated as well as guidelines to probes and actions for obtaining the relevant information.

Figures 13-1 and 13-2 also offer some clinically useful guidelines in the form of assessment algorithms for deciding whether or not to make biobehavioral management recommendations based on RDC/TMD Axis II findings. These algorithmic decision trees rely mainly on GCP scale scores and criterion scores assigned to patients after

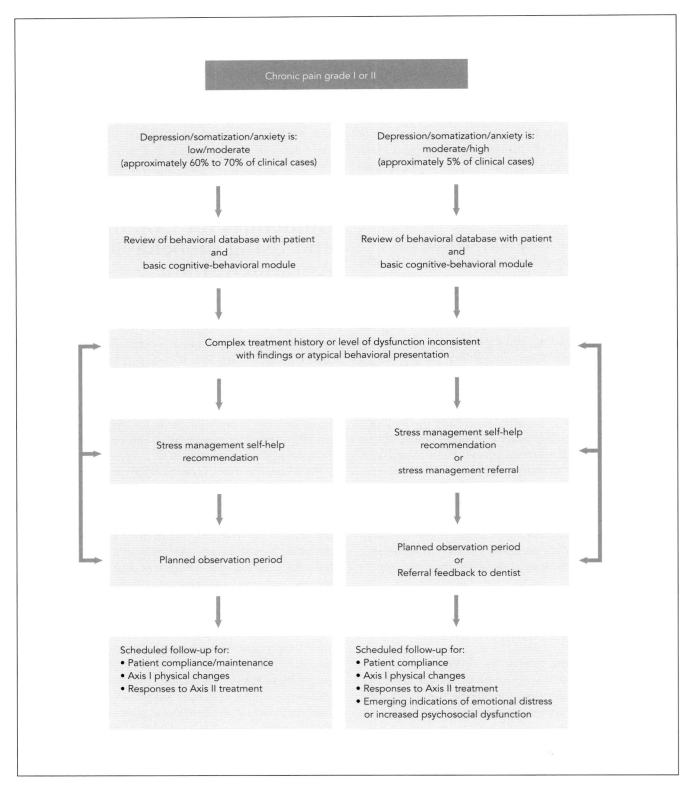

Fig 13-1 Biobehavioral assessment algorithm for making biobehavioral treatment recommendations in patients with a TMD and chronic pain grade I or II.

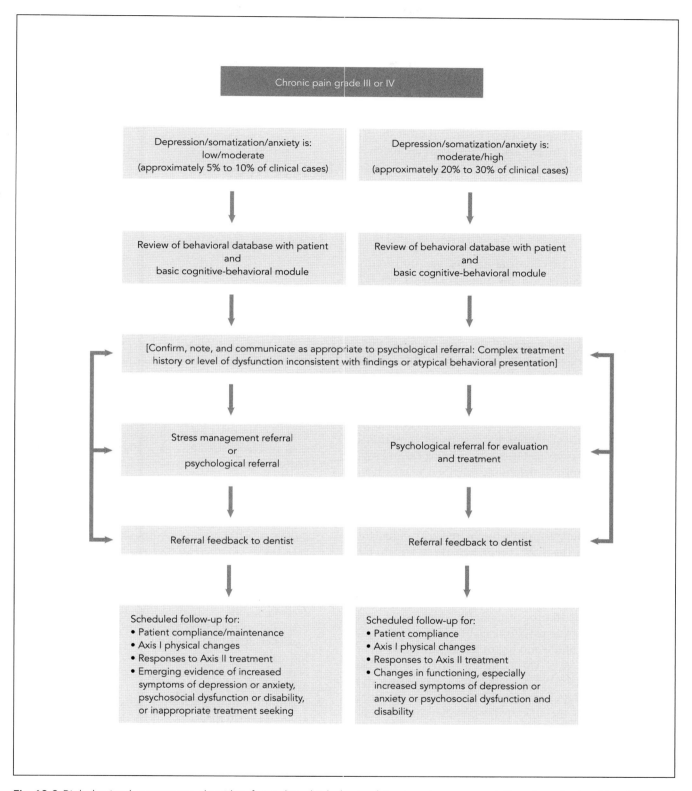

Fig 13-2 Biobehavioral assessment algorithm for making biobehavioral treatment recommendations in patients with a TMD and chronic pain grade III or IV.

RDC/TMD assessment of depression and somatization. These are offered as practical guides, the utility of which is supported by clinical studies[21,32,33] together with the author's clinical experience. The recommendations offered in Figs 13-1 and 13-2 should be considered a bridge between the approach to assessment presented in this chapter and the approaches to clinical management presented in other chapters of this book. It is most specifically relevant to the biobehavioral treatment approaches offered in chapter 26.

Summary

Psychological and psychosocial factors are universally accepted as prominent features among patients seeking treatment for amelioration of the pain associated with TMDs. Indeed, for a significant number of patients with chronic TMD pain, these pain-related emotional and behavioral factors may represent the major burden their condition imposes, putting an important stamp on the clinical presentation. While definitive information is not yet available regarding whether such emotional and behavioral factors are causes or effects of TMD pain, it is nevertheless widely accepted that comprehensive management of such patients requires attention to these issues. In practical terms, this means assessing levels of psychological and psychosocial disturbance to determine whether or not treatment decision-making should also include recommendations for incorporating psychological and/or behavioral management into comprehensive TMD treatment.

In terms of clinical utility for biomedical clinicians seeking to provide the most comprehensive treatment for their patients with chronic TMD pain, four domains of psychological and psychosocial assessment are recommended: (1) pain; (2) mandibular function and behaviors; (3) psychological status—principally, depression and somatization; and (4) psychosocial level of function as related to quality of life and use of health care services or medications. The RDC/TMD offers a battery of reliable and valid measures that have gained wide acceptance and use. Psychological domains worthy of assessment but not incorporated into the RDC/TMD include anxiety, substance abuse, and sleep disturbance. Additional domains relevant to a comprehensive assessment of the TMD patient include physical or sexual abuse, PTSD, and other related quality of life measures. For this last group, there is not yet sufficient evidence to confirm their utility as universal assessment screening measures, but there is evidence of their relevance in many patients with chronic TMD pain.

Finally, the major thrust of this chapter has been to persuade the reader that a biopsychosocial approach—the model system that guides all major multidisciplinary pain centers—should be used by all clinicians treating TMD patients. Current scientific evidence overwhelmingly confirms that this approach enhances both the understanding and the management of these complex disorders.

References

1. Rollman GB, Gillespie JB. The role of psychosocial factors in temporomandibular disorders. Curr Rev Pain 2000;4:71–78.
2. Dworkin SF, Huggins KH, LeResche L, et al. Epidemiology of signs and symptoms in temporomandibular disorders: Clinical signs in cases and controls. J Am Dent Assoc 1990;120: 273–281.
3. Drangsholt M, LeResche L. Temporomandibular disorder pain. In: Crombie I, Croft PR, Linton SJ, et al (eds). Epidemiology of Pain. Seattle: IASP Press, 1999:203–233.
4. Epker J, Gatchel RJ. Coping profile differences in the biopsychosocial functioning of patients with temporomandibular disorders. Psychosom Med 2000;62:69–75.
5. Keefe FJ, Rumble ME, Scipio CD, et al. Psychological aspects of persistent pain: Current state of the science. J Pain 2004; 5:195–211.
6. Katon W, Lin E, Von Korff M, et al. Somatization: A spectrum of severity. Am J Psychiatry 1991;148:34–40.
7. Ohrbach R, Dworkin SF. Five-year outcomes in TMD: Relationship of changes in pain to changes in physical and psychological variables. Pain 1998;74:315–326.
8. McCreary CP, Clark GT, Oakley ME, et al. Predicting response to treatment for temporomandibular disorders. J Craniomandib Disord Facial Oral Pain 1992;6:161–169.
9. Dworkin SF, Von Korff M, LeResche L. Epidemiologic studies of chronic pain: A dynamic-ecologic perspective. Ann Behav Med 1992;14:3–11.
10. Dworkin SF, LeResche L. Research Diagnostic Criteria for Temporomandibular Disorders: Review, criteria, examinations and specifications, critique. J Craniomandib Disord Facial Oral Pain 1992;6:301–355.
11. International Consortium for RDC/TMD-Based Research [website]. Available at http://www.rdc-tmdinternational.org. Accessed 1 July 2005.
12. Jensen MP, Karoly P. Self-report scales and procedures for assessing pain in adults. In: Turk DC, Melzack R (eds). Handbook of Pain Assessment. New York: Guilford Press, 1992:15–34.
13. Melzack R. The McGill Pain Questionnaire: Major properties and scoring methods. Pain 1975;1:277–299.
14. Wittink H, Rogers W, Gascon C, Sukiennik A, Cynn D, Carr AB. Relative contribution of mental health and exercise-related pain increment to treadmill test intolerance in patients with chronic low back pain. Spine 2001;26:2368–2374.

15. Osterweis M, Kleinman A, Mechanic D. Pain and Disability: Clinical, Behavioral and Public Policy Perspectives. Washington, DC: National Academy Press, 1987.

16. Stegenga B, de Bont LGM, de Leeuw R, et al. Assessment of mandibular function impairment associated with temporomandibular joint osteoarthrosis and internal derangement. J Orofac Pain 1993;7:183–195.

17. Ohrbach R, List T. Relationship of limitation and disability in TMD and other oral conditions [abstract]. J Dent Res 2003;82(special issue A):1023.

18. Ohrbach R, Dworkin SF, Granger CV. Cross-validation of a disability scale for chronic temporomandibular disorder pain [abstract]. Presented at the 9th World Congress on Pain, International Association for the Study of Pain, Vienna, Austria, 1999:228.

19. Turner JA, Dworkin SF. Screening for psychosocial risk factors in patients with chronic orofacial pain: Recent advances. J Am Dent Assoc 2004;135:1119–1125.

20. US Public Health Service. The Surgeon General's Call to Action to Prevent Suicide. Washington, DC: US Public Health Service, 1999.

21. Dworkin SF, Sherman J, Ohrbach R, et al. Reliability, validity and clinical utility of RDC/TMD Axis II scales: Depression, non-specific physical symptoms and graded chronic pain. J Orofac Pain 2002;16:207–220.

22. Beck AT, Ward CH, Mendelson M, et al. An inventory for measuring depression. Arch Gen Psychiatry 1961;4:561–571.

23. Radloff L. The CES-D scale: A self-report depression scale for research in the general population. J Appl Psychol Meas 1977;1:3385–3401.

24. Turk DC, Flor H. Pain > pain behaviors: The utility and limitations of the pain behavior construct. Pain 1987;31:277–295.

25. Derogatis LR, Cleary PA. Confirmation of the dimensional structure of the SCL-90: A study in construct validation. J Clin Psychol 1977;33:981–989.

26. Dworkin SF, Wilson L, Massoth DL. Somatizing as a risk factor for chronic pain. In: Grzesiak RC, Ciccone DS (eds). Psychologic Vulnerability to Chronic Pain. New York: Springer, 1994:28–54.

27. Wilson L, Dworkin SF, Whitney C, et al. Somatization and pain dispersion in chronic temporomandibular pain. Pain 1994;57:55–61.

28. Katon W, Lin E, Von Korff M, et al. Somatization: A spectrum of severity. Am J Psychiatry 1991;148:34–40.

29. Von Korff M, Ormel J, Keefe FJ, et al. Grading the severity of chronic pain. Pain 1992;50:133–149.

30. Dworkin SF. Perspectives on the interaction of biologic, psychologic and social factors in TMD. J Am Dent Assoc 1994;125:856–863.

31. Von Korff M. Epidemiologic and survey methods: Assessment of chronic pain. In: Turk DC, Melzack R (eds). Handbook of Pain Assessment. New York: Guilford Press, 2001:603–618.

32. Dworkin SF, Huggins KH, Wilson L, et al. A randomized clinical trial using Research Criteria for Temporomandibular Disorders-Axis II to target clinic cases for a tailored self-care treatment program. J Orofac Pain 2001;16:48–63.

33. Dworkin SF, Turner JA, Mancl L, et al. A randomized clinical trial of a tailored comprehensive care treatment program for temporomandibular disorders. J Orofac Pain 2002;16:259–276.

34. Kerns RD, Turk DC, Rudy TE. The West Haven-Yale multidimensional pain inventory (WHYMPI). Pain 1985;23:345–356.

35. Zaki H, Turk D, Rudy T. A comparison of splint and biofeedback treatments for TMJ pain [abstract 1230]. J Dent Res 1992;71(special issue):259.

36. Turk DC, Rudy TE, Kubinski JA, et al. Dysfunctional patients with temporomandibular disorders: Evaluating the efficacy of a tailored treatment protocol. J Consult Clin Psychol 1996;64:139–146.

37. McWilliams LA, Cox BJ, Enns MW. Mood and anxiety disorders associated with chronic pain: An examination in a nationally representative sample. Pain 2003;106:127–133.

38. Spielberger C, Gorsuch RL, Lushene RE. Manual for the State-Trait Anxiety Inventory. Palo Alto, CA: Consulting Psychological Press, 1970.

39. Marcus DA. Treatment of nonmalignant chronic pain. Am Fam Physician 2000;54:1331–1338,1345–1346.

40. Bush K, Kivlahan D, McDonell M, et al. The AUDIT alcohol consumption questions: An effective brief screening test for problem drinking. Arch Intern Med 1998;158:1789–1795.

41. Brown RL, Leobard T, Saunders L, et al. A two-item conjoint screen for alcohol and other drug problems. J Am Board Fam Pract 2001;14:95–106.

42. Buysse D, Reynolds CI, Monk T, et al. Pittsburgh Sleep Quality Index (PSQI). In: Schutte N, Malouff J (eds). Sourcebook Adult Assessment. New York: Plenum Press, 1995:193–213.

43. Yatani H, Studts J, Cordova M, et al. Comparison of sleep quality and clinical and psychologic characteristics in patients with temporomandibular disorders. J Orofac Pain 2002;16:221–228.

44. Kowalski C, Stohler C. Quality of Life and Pain: Methodology in Theory and Practice. In: Inglehart M, Bagramian R (eds). Oral Health–Related Quality of Life. Chicago: Quintessence, 2002:169–182

45. Ware J. The MOS 36-item short-form health survey (SF-36). Med Care 1992;30:473–480.

46. Blake D, Weathers F, Nagy L, et al. A clinician rating scale for assessing current and lifetime PTSD: The CAPS-1. Behav Res Ther 1990;13:187–188.

47. Shipherd J, Beck G, Hamble J, et al. A preliminary examination of treatment for posttraumatic stress disorder in chronic pain patients. J Trauma Stress 2003;16:451–457.

48. Sherman JJ, Carlson CR, Wilson JF, Okeson JP, McCubbin JA. 2005. Post-traumatic stress disorder among patients with orofacial pain. J Orofac Pain 2005;19:309–317.

49. Love C, Gerbert B, Caspers M, et al. Dentist's attitudes and behaviors regarding domestic violence. J Am Dent Assoc 2001;132:85–93.

50. Spitzer RL, Kroenke K, Williams J. Validation and utility of a self-report version of PRIME-MD: The PHQ Primary Care Study. JAMA 1999;282:1734–1737.

Concepts of TMD Etiology: Effects on Diagnosis and Treatment

Charles S. Greene

Various chapters in this book have discussed what is known currently about the pathophysiologic mechanisms underlying various temporomandibular disorders (TMDs). These mechanisms generally are described in terms of anatomic or biochemical changes—sometimes at the gross (macro) level, sometimes at the histologic (micro) level, and often at the molecular or genetic level. However, with the exception of the traumatic etiologies discussed in chapter 18, the exact causes of most TMDs remain either largely unknown or speculative. This fact has important implications for the selection of appropriate therapies for each patient. This chapter reviews the current knowledge about the etiologies of various TMDs, focusing mainly on the three most common conditions: myofascial pain and dysfunction (MPD), symptomatic disc derangements of the temporomandibular joint (TMJ), and painful inflammatory and degenerative conditions of the TMJ. A framework in which clinicians can still provide rational care for individual patients, despite limited certainty about the etiology of the TMD, also is discussed.

Despite the limitations previously mentioned, there has been significant scientific progress over the past 40 years, both in the understanding of the etiologic factors associated with various TMDs and in the rational treatment of patients with these conditions. The problems lie in the assumptions that frequently are made at the clinical level about "finding" the etiology of an individual patient's problem, followed by "selection" of an appropriate antietiologic treatment strategy. It is the purpose of this chapter to deal with these issues by raising the following questions:

1. What do we actually know with some degree of certainty about the role of various putative etiologic factors in causing subgroups of TMD patients to develop clinical problems?
2. What do we know about the host resistance or susceptibility factors that ultimately determine who develops TMDs when exposed to various etiologic factors?
3. Can this knowledge be transferred from the group level and applied to the individual patient in a reliable manner?
4. Are currently recommended treatment protocols, even at the highest scientific level, based on suppressing or eliminating etiologic factors?
5. If not, then what is the basis for these currently recommended protocols, most of which are quite successful for the vast majority of patients?

Semantics of Etiology

Before any discussion about etiology, some common semantic problems must be identified (Box 14-1). Clinicians often speak of finding the *cause* of a patient's pain, but they really mean the *source* (an anatomic structure producing the pain), which may not always be the same as the *site* (an area of referred or heterotopic pain). Other common expressions include *mechanism of pain*, which really means a description of the pathophysiologic process occurring in the anatomic structures, and *pathogenesis*, which refers to the origins and progression of a pathologic process.

Box 14-1	Semantics of orofacial pain "etiology"

- Site of pain (**location**) = Where does the patient feel pain?
- Source of pain (**tissue**) = Where does the pain originate?
- Mechanism of pain (**how**) = What is the pathophysiologic process of pain?
    - Primary = Inflammatory, neuropathic, myofascial, vascular
    - Secondary = Neuroplasticity → heterotopic and referred pain
        - Central sensitization
        - Sympathetically maintained pain
- Cause of pain (**why**) = What is the etiology or pathogenesis of the pain?

Most confusing of all are references to *diagnosing the etiology*, which usually describes a mental process within the clinician's mind. In this chapter, the term *etiology* is defined in both the simplest and the strictest way: We want to know *why* a particular patient began to have both the biology and the perception of his or her pain (in the absence of frank trauma).

Historical Review of Etiologic Theories

The evolution of etiologic concepts in the field of TMDs has been thoroughly discussed in the literature,[1,2] so only a brief review of some older and some more recent concepts will be offered. This field began as a lateral transfer of responsibility from otolaryngologists to dentists in the early 1930s. Although some articles had appeared in the dental literature before that time,[3–5] it was the pronouncements of J. B. Costen[6] that established the TMJ as a separate source of facial pain and about 11 other symptoms (most of which turned out to be impossible to connect anatomically with the TMJ).[7,8] It is not important to belabor the details of Costen's concepts,[6] but their main impact was to lay the foundation for two propositions that dominated the field for years:

1. These so-called TMJ problems were the result of structural malalignments between the mandible and the cranium.
2. Only dentists could take care of TMJ problems because of the structural corrections that would be required.

Terms such as *overclosed vertical dimension*,[9] *condylar malposition*,[10] *trapped mandibles*,[11] *occlusal disharmony*,[12] and *neuromuscular imbalance*[13] all were variants of this initial conceptual framework, and the treatments to correct all of them became part of the lexicon of dental therapies for many years. Whatever one may think of these concepts, it is clear that they were the basis for an etiologic viewpoint and that the related therapies were seen as being antietiologic; indeed, the word *definitive* often was used to describe the curative value of these treatment approaches.

During this same general time period, the orthodontic profession developed its own version of structural disharmony concepts as the basis for TMD problems, and corrective treatments were proposed to prevent or eliminate symptoms. These orthodontic concepts have been discussed in detail in other publications.[14,15] However, it is important to note that the orthodontic viewpoint recently has converged considerably toward the traditional prosthodontic/occlusal viewpoint,[16] as more and more members of both groups have become devotees of using mechanical and electronic instrumentation to analyze and treat their patients.[17,18] Although some have argued that such an approach is helpful in providing good orthodontic or prosthodontic care, such concepts and instrumentation have not been shown to be of specific value in diagnosing or treating patients who have TMDs[19–22] (see chapter 12).

Another structural concept of TMD etiology has been proposed by various physical therapists, chiropractors, and dentists,[23,24] based on the notion that "bad" craniocervical relationships may cause certain TMDs. Although this etiologic theory has enjoyed some popularity in the past (and is still popular in some regions of the world), several studies have demonstrated that there are no consistent postural findings that differentiate TMD patients from normal subjects.[25,26]

In more recent years, other etiologic factors besides structural ones have been recognized and discussed as a result of large studies of patient populations.[27,28] For example, trauma at both the macro and micro levels[29] has been observed in the history of certain patients, with rather clear relationships to onset of symptoms in many cases. The most significant changes in etiologic theorizing, however, began in the 1950s and 1960s when the Columbia University group[30–32] as well as the University of Illinois group[33–35] proposed a psychophysiologic theory of etiology for many TMDs, especially those involving MPD. Again, these concepts arose from studies of large TMD patient populations, in which a variety of psychometric approaches were used to assess personality characteristics as well as various state-trait variables.[36–38] In addition, a large number of experimental stress provocation studies showed that TMD/MPD patients differed from normal subjects in many of their responses, and several psychophysical measurement studies demonstrated other significant physiologic differences between the groups.[39–46]

Although Laskin's classic article about the etiology of MPD[33] served as the basis for much of this experimental and analytical work, eventually his psychophysiologic theory proved to be incomplete as an etiologic explanation for the development of myofascial pain. Based on their research findings as well as those from other centers, the University of Illinois group published an important article in 1982 to express these reservations.[47] Today, the importance of psychological factors in the onset, progression, treatment, and persistence of various TMDs is recognized as foundational knowledge in this field (see chapters 13 and 26).[48] However, the reasons why some patients exhibit TMD symptoms while others do not remain unexplained by the psychophysiologic theory of etiology.

Finally, no historical review of etiologic concepts in the field of TMDs is complete without at least a brief consideration of the unorthodox and pseudoscientific theories that have been proposed. This is a topic that also has been discussed previously.[49,50] Many of these ideas originated outside of the dental profession (eg, craniosacral therapy from osteopathy, applied kinesiology or jaw malalignment theories from chiropractic, and nutritional theories), only to be warmly embraced by dentists.[50] Other theories have originated within the profession, such as the notion that TMJ malalignment causes whole-body symptoms,[51] or that neuromuscular imbalance in the face causes widespread problems with other muscles or even in various organs.[52] These peculiar concepts have only served to muddy the TMD waters further, but fortunately each one seems to have died a deserved natural death within a reasonable period of time.

Hybrid Theories

Most of the previously discussed etiologic concepts could be described as unicausal, implying a simplicity of cause and effect that became increasingly untenable as more was learned about TMDs. In the past 25 years, various hybrid concepts of etiology have emerged. The earliest was Ramfjord and Ash's proposal[53,54] that a combination of stress and occlusal disharmonies was responsible for the onset of TMD symptoms in previously asymptomatic persons with "bad" occlusions. Rather than focus on the psychological component, however, they advocated occlusal correction as the primary treatment. This type of lip service to the concepts of psychobiology has been repeated by many others who have claimed that they appreciate the importance of psychological factors but who emphasized mainly mechanical treatments in their clinical approaches to patients with TMDs.

Most recently, the combination of biologic and psychological perspectives in etiologic theories about TMD has been given the name *biopsychosocial*,[55,56] and this concept is discussed extensively in chapters 13 and 26.

Another approach to describing the complicated nature of etiologies is to invoke the word *multifactorial*,[57,58] thereby indicating an awareness that many extrinsic factors in the environment as well as various intrinsic factors within the patient might be involved in the development of symptomatic TMDs. This is intellectually attractive in the sense that it suggests an appreciation of complexity, but does it indicate a deeper understanding of what is actually happening to patients with TMDs?

Obviously, it is important to consider the true meaning of the words *biopsychosocial* and *multifactorial* as expressions of etiologic thinking in the TMD field. In doing so, the reader should question their application at two levels of patient analysis: *(1)* How do they help us understand *groups* of TMD patients? and *(2)* How do they help us understand *individual* patients?

A reasonable answer to these questions, adapted from the discussion of this issue by Okeson,[56] is as follows: The word *biopsychosocial* is actually a combination of three words, producing an excellent descriptor of the world that most patients with pain (and especially patients with chronic pain) are living in from day to day. They have a *biological* problem (ie, activation of pain pathways, with or without a demonstrable pathologic condition) that may have *psychological* antecedents as well as behavioral consequences. This situation exists in a *social* framework that includes interpersonal relationships with friends, families, and health providers, which almost always produces major negative experiences for the patients as well as their immediate families. How can we assess all of these variables at the individual patient level with the crude physical and psychometric tools that are currently available? At this time it is not possible to do so with any degree of precision or certainty, and therefore this concept is valuable only at the group level.

The word *multifactorial* is in many ways even worse in these respects. Of course we know that very complicated assortments of extrinsic physical and psychological factors are acting on the intrinsic host factors of physical susceptibility and mental healthiness. Behavioral issues including stress, anxiety, interpersonal relationships, and oral habits are potentially significant in such an etiologic matrix, and physical issues of joint anatomy, loading, and pathology, as well as muscle physiology, are undeniably important— but how are we supposed to assess all of this in an individual patient? Once again, it appears that this concept is both correct and valuable at the group level, but it cannot be specifically applied to any one patient sitting in a clinician's office.

Idiopathic Concept of Etiology

The central thesis of this chapter is that there is a set of musculoskeletal disorders affecting the stomatognathic system about which a lot is known in general, thanks to nearly 40 years of systematic research, but about which little is known regarding the etiology at the *individual patient* level. In fact, as the old joke goes, we used to know a lot more about TMD etilogies before we submitted them to so much systematic research! Some doctors seem to be discouraged that these negative conclusions about TMD etiology leave clinicians with nothing solid to hang their hats on, and so the profession ends up using the term *idiopathic* (a disease of unknown origin or for which no cause is known) to describe the current state of knowledge about the etiology of most TMDs.[59–63]

However, any dissatisfaction about the relative ignorance regarding specific etiologies should be greatly mitigated by the enormous amount of specific knowledge that does exist, thanks again to the extensive research of the past 40 years. An assessment of the traditional triad of diagnosis, etiology, and treatment indicates that the profession has vastly improved its ability to recognize and classify patients with TMDs and that logical, sensible, and successful methods have been developed for treating most of these patients. This conclusion is strongly supported by the widely reported treatment success rates of 75% to 90% from around the world.[64–74]

Despite the current gaps in the profession's knowledge, as well as the ability to measure etiologic factors, most TMDs can be managed clinically based entirely on the application of research-based treatment protocols to specific TMD diagnostic categories—an approach that requires little or no attention to individual etiologic factors. Although some clinicians may disagree, current scientific evidence suggests that this is what most of them really are doing when they provide treatment for most of their TMD patients, regardless of protestations to the contrary (Table 14-1). Even in the face of known etiologies, many TMD patients cannot be treated "antietiologically" simply because the causative factor or event cannot be undone (eg, traumatic injuries to the mandible or spontaneous displacements of the articular disc), or because the disease process is irreversible (eg, arthritis). Therefore, clinicians must have an intellectual framework that enables them to provide good care for their TMD patients while recognizing the limitations of the current state of knowledge.

Primary Care for TMD Patients

Almost all of the current authoritative review articles and guidelines for treating the most common TMDs (masticatory muscle pain, disc derangements, and osteoarthritis) suggest a conservative, reversible approach to initial therapy.[57,75–80] This approach includes the use of well known and widely accepted treatment modalities, including various medications, oral appliances, physical therapies, and home care procedures, as well as a cognitive-behavioral information program that teaches patients about their condition and how it should be managed.

Unfortunately, some people have created a false dichotomy between this initial phase I therapy and a so-called phase II regimen that requires irreversible dental and skeletal changes to be made.[54,81,82] Under this concept, the use of oral appliances to reposition the mandible in phase I often intentionally produces an unavoidable phase II.[83] Alternatively, some have argued that phase I is merely a palliative approach that is fine if it works but that in many cases the clinician must be prepared to "escalate" to more aggressive treatments.[84,85] Under this concept, treatment failure becomes the excuse to perform invasive therapies, rather than a sign of the possibility of nonresponding chronic pain (with all of its psychological implications) (see chapter 26).

In a 1992 article on initial therapy for TMDs,[86] it was argued that good primary care should not be viewed as merely a first phase of treatment. Instead, it is the actual

Standard	Diagnosis	Etiology	Treatment	Current situation
Ideal	Clear and correct Measurable Demonstrable	Specific Measurable Treatable	Antietiologic Definitive Successful	Not achievable at this time
Acceptable	Presumptive Probably correct Categorical labels	Unclear Complex Reversible	Empirically validated Matched to diagnosis Conservative	Frequently achievable; represents best current practice
Wrong/bad	Parochial specialty labeling Technologic diagnosis Possibly correct	Favorite theory Morphofunctional analysis Mechanical concept	Prolonged appliance wear Bite-changing procedures Jaw repositioning	Most common current practice, despite lack of scientific foundation
Outrageous	Misdiagnosis of pain Neglect of serious pathologic conditions Neglect of chronicity	Guru/cult concepts Quackery concepts Parochial specialty concepts	Whole-body procedures Quackery procedures Extreme dental procedures	All too common; represents fringe of current practice

Table 14-1 Relationships among diagnosis, etiology, and treatment in TMDs

treatment program that most TMD patients require and one that will be quite successful for many of them. In that article, the dangers of various irreversible treatment approaches and improper escalation of therapy were described. Many other researchers in this field have proposed a similar viewpoint,[75–80] and the long-term research on clinical outcomes from around the world supports the use of conservative and reversible treatments as the *only* appropriate way to treat the vast majority of TMD patients.[64–74] This important conclusion is represented most clearly and concisely in the American Academy of Orofacial Pain's *Orofacial Pain: Guidelines for Assessment, Diagnosis, and Management.*[57] It is interesting that the same concepts are echoed in a major review article dealing with the management of lower back pain.[87]

Treating TMDs in a Biopsychosocial Framework

Most researchers in the TMD field have observed that the primary symptom that determines treatment-seeking behavior is the facial and head pain experienced by these patients. Because it is well known that both acute and chronic pain have psychological associations, a responsible clinician must take that fact into account while treating all patients with TMDs. The literature supporting that

conclusion and endorsing that approach to TMD treatment goes back more than 40 years, beginning with the early studies of Schwartz,[30,88] Moulton,[32,89] Laskin,[33] and others.[34–36,47] These ideas were advanced greatly by the work of Rugh and Solberg[37,90] in the 1970s and 1980s as well as the work of Turk et al[91,92] in the past 15 years.

Perhaps the strongest focus on psychological issues has come from the diverse investigations directed by Dworkin et al[93–95] for many years, and their use of the term *biopsychosocial* has become widely recognized as a most appropriate label for the TMD patient population (see chapter 13). Along with Turk et al,[91] they have recommended the use of a cognitive-behavioral approach to educating and treating TMD patients, and they have clearly demonstrated its effectiveness.[93–95] This approach offers the dual benefit of teaching patients how to self-manage many of their symptoms while enhancing the feeling of empowerment (locus of control) that comes from such skills.

As pointed out earlier, this is not an etiologic issue, but rather a tactical one. Good clinicians need to be sensitive to the psychological ramifications of pain in both patients with acute TMDs and those with chronic TMDs, and they must expect to encounter significant psychological issues such as anxiety and depression more frequently in the latter group.[92] Only by developing this kind of awareness can clinicians avoid the mistakes of escalation to either surgery or major dental treatment instead of referring their nonresponding patients for the kind of complex chronic pain management that is much more likely to be appropriate. In the end, it is this awareness that defines the biopsychosocial approach to the diagnosis and treatment of patients with TMDs.

A False Dichotomy: Palliative Versus Definitive Treatments

The arguments in medical circles about palliative versus definitive treatments are as old as Greek and Roman times, when healers debated bloodletting and amputations as alternatives to poultices, herbs, and incantations. The implication always has been the same: A good doctor must not settle for mere palliation when a definitive cure is available. However, as Stohler and Zarb[75] pointed out in their excellent article advocating a low-technology, high-prudence approach to TMD therapy, the word *cure* cannot be used in the absence of knowledge of causal mechanisms and especially without the availability of biotechnologies that interfere with those mechanisms. Therefore, this argument becomes a false dichotomy in those conditions where it cannot be properly applied—for example, low back pain, headaches, and TMDs.

In the TMD field, this argument is best understood by considering the phase I versus phase II controversy.[96–99] Several important articles addressing this controversy have appeared in the TMD literature during the past 25 years, and all of these have reached similar conclusions: TMD patients treated with conservative and reversible modalities on the whole responded as well as patients treated with more aggressive regimens, in both the short-term and long-term assessment of outcomes.[64–74] In other words, phase I therapy alone, or combined with phase II, produces similar overall results in large populations of TMD patients. Because, by definition, phase II treatment involves irreversible procedures, these outcomes strongly suggest that phase II represents unnecessary overtreatment in most cases.[83,86,100]

Thus, the distinction between palliative and definitive treatment has little meaning in the management of these benign musculoskeletal disorders. Instead, the profession can now speak more rationally about TMD treatment in terms of three clinically and intellectually important considerations:

1. The natural history of each of the major TMDs, especially the intracapsular diseases and derangements, is now fairly well understood. In general, the course of these conditions is characterized by positive tissue

adaptations and recovery from episodes of pain and dysfunction (see chapters 7, 8, 30, 32, and 33).

2. The objective of TMD treatment generally should be to make patients more comfortable (palliation) while the previously mentioned healing and adaptations are occurring and to enhance the amount of recovery as much as possible. These treatments should be selected on the basis of the clinical subdiagnoses of myogenous and/or arthrogenous conditions, as defined by the American Academy of Orofacial Pain's guidelines[57] and by Dworkin and LeResche (Research Diagnostic Criteria/TMD).[101] In addition, the psychological distress associated with being sick, as well as worry about the illness itself, must be addressed, which means that simple behavioral management techniques should be incorporated in every treatment protocol (see chapter 26).

3. Successful TMD treatment, therefore, should be defined as a return to a more normal biopsychosocial existence, in which pain is either greatly diminished or gone and in which patients have been educated to self-manage most recurrences of the problem, if any arise.

These conclusions about treatment are further supported by the official *Scientific Information Statement on Temporomandibular Disorders*, published by the American Association of Dental Research in 1996[102]:

Based on the evidence from clinical trials [of TMDs], . . . it is strongly recommended that, unless there are specific and justifiable indications to the contrary, treatment be based on the use of conservative and reversible therapeutic modalities. While no specific therapies have been proven to be uniformly effective, *many of the conservative modalities have provided at least palliative relief from symptoms without producing harm* [emphasis added].

Future Perspectives

Most research articles as well as book chapters end with calls for future scientists to continue searching for more answers to the main topical issue—in this case, to learn more about the etiology of the various TMDs so that better treatments can be provided. Although all clinicians should endorse that sentiment, it is more likely that most of the future progress in understanding TMDs will come from intensive studies of the pathophysiologic mechanisms underlying all kinds of muscle and joint pain as well a deeper understanding of the phenomena of neuroplasticity that lead to chronic pain. Some of these kinds of studies already are either completed or under way (for a review, see Greene[103]), and several examples are discussed in other chapters of this book. Eventually such studies should provide the scientific basis for developing tissue-targeted therapies that will reverse the pathologic processes rather than merely palliating the associated symptoms.

Finally, the enormous impact that neuroplasticity has on the pain experiences reported by patients with chronic pain must be considered (see chapters 4 and 5). The research by Dubner,[104] Sessle,[105,106] and many others in this field has demonstrated how in some individuals normal peripheral sensitization of receptors even by disease or trauma can lead to the amplification and persistence of pain that go far beyond "normal."[107] Long-term changes in nerve cell activity at the level of the spinal cord and higher centers in the brain (central sensitization) are a frequent result of nerve excitation or injury. The mechanisms that determine whether the body suppresses or facilitates this sensitization are still largely unknown, but significant work is proceeding in these areas.

Hopefully, these diverse scientific investigations will lead ultimately to specific therapies for each kind of TMD. Even patients with chronic orofacial pain problems can look forward to more specific treatments, as the perpetuating mechanisms of chronic pain become better understood. Until then, the limits of professional knowledge about both etiologies and mechanisms must be recognized. Fortunately, enough scientific information is already available to enable clinicians to provide the majority of TMD patients with what they want most—relief from pain, return to more normal function, and avoidance of iatrogenic harm.

References

1. Greene CS. Myofascial pain-dysfunction syndrome: The evolution of concepts. In: Sarnat BG, Laskin DM (eds). The Temporomandibular Joint, ed 3. Springfield, IL: Thomas, 1980:277–288.
2. Greene CS. Temporomandibular disorders: The evolution of concepts. In: Sarnat BG, Laskin DM (eds). The Temporomandibular Joint: A Biologic Basis for Clinical Practice, ed 4. Philadelphia: Saunders, 1992:298–315.
3. Wright WH. Deafness as influenced by malposition of the jaws. J Natl Dent Assoc 1920;7:979–992.
4. Monson GS. Occlusion as applied to crown and bridge work. J Natl Dent Assoc 1920;7:399–413.
5. Decker JC. Traumatic deafness as a result of retrusion of condyles of mandible. Ann Otol Rhinol Laryngol 1925;34:519–527.
6. Costen JB. A syndrome of ear and sinus symptoms dependent upon disturbed function of the temporomandibular joint. Ann Otol Rhinol Laryngol 1934;43:1–15.
7. Sicher H. Temporomandibular articulation in mandibular overclosure. J Am Dent Assoc 1948;36:131–139.
8. Zimmerman AA. Evaluation of Costen's syndrome from an anatomic point of view. In: Sarnat BG (ed). The Temporomandibular Joint. Springfield, IL: Thomas, 1951:82–110.
9. Block LS. Diagnosis and treatment of disturbances of the temporomandibular joint, especially in relation to vertical dimension. J Am Dent Assoc 1947;34:253–260.
10. Weinberg LA. Role of condylar position in TMJ dysfunction-pain syndrome. J Prosthet Dent 1979;41:636–643.
11. Thompson JR. Temporomandibular disorders: Diagnosis and treatment. In: Sarnat BG (ed). The Temporomandibular Joint, ed 2. Springfield, IL: Thomas, 1964:146–184.
12. Posselt U. The temporomandibular joint and occlusion. J Prosthet Dent 1971;25:432–438.
13. Jankelson B. Neuromuscular aspects of occlusion. Dent Clin North Am 1979;23:157–168.
14. Greene CS. Orthodontics and the temporomandibular joint. Angle Orthod 1982;55:166–172.
15. Greene CS. Orthodontics and temporomandibular disorders. Dent Clin North Am 1988;32:529–538.
16. Roth RH. Temporomandibular pain-dysfunction and occlusal relationships. Angle Orthod 1973;43:136–153.
17. Crawford SD. Condylar position, as determined by the occlusion and measured by the CPI instrument, and signs and symptoms of temporomandibular dysfunction. Angle Orthod 1999;69:103–116.
18. Greene CS. Clinical research. Studying relationships between occlusion and TM disorders [letter]. Angle Orthod 1999;69:391–392.
19. Mohl ND, McCall WD, Lund JP, Plesh O. Devices for the diagnosis and treatment of temporomandibular disorders. 1. Introduction, scientific evidence, and jaw tracking. J Prosthet Dent 1990;63:198–201.
20. Mohl, ND, Lund JP, Widmer CG, McCall WD. Devices for the diagnosis and treatment of temporomandibular disorders. 2. Electromyography and sonography. J Prosthet Dent 1990;63:332–336.
21. Mohl ND, Ohrbach RK, Crow HC, Gross AJ. Devices for the diagnosis and treatment of temporomandibular disorders. 3. Thermography, ultrasound, electrical stimulation, and electromyographic feedback. J Prosthet Dent 1990;63:472–477.
22. Lund JP, Widmer CG, Feine JS. Validity of diagnostic and monitoring tests used for temporomandibular disorders. J Dent Res 1995;74:1133–1143.
23. Rocabado M, Tapia V. Radiographic study of the craniocervical relation in patients under orthodontic treatment and the incidence of related symptoms. Cranio 1987;5:36–42.
24. Mannheimer JS, Rosenthal RM. Acute and chronic postural abnormalities as related to craniofacial pain and temporomandibular disorders. Dent Clin North Am 1991;35:185–208.

25. Hackney J, Bade D, Clawson A. Relationship between forward head posture and diagnosed internal derangement of the temporomandibular joint. J Orofac Pain 1993;7:386–390.

26. Darlow LA, Pesco J, Greenberg MS. The relationship of posture to myofascial pain dysfunction syndrome. J Am Dent Assoc 1987;114:73–75.

27. Seligman DA, Pullinger AG. The role of functional occlusal relationships in temporomandibular disorders: A review. J Craniomandib Disord 1991;5:265–279.

28. Carlsson GE, Droukas B. Dental occlusion and the health of the masticatory system—A literature review. J Craniomandib Pract 1984;2:142–147.

29. Pullinger AG, Seligman DA. Trauma history in diagnostic subgroups of temporomandibular disorders. Oral Surg Oral Med Oral Pathol 1991;71:529–534.

30. Schwartz L. Conclusions of the TMJ Clinic at Columbia. J Periodontol 1958;29:210–212.

31. Marbach JJ, Lipton JA. Aspects of illness behavior in patients with facial pain. J Am Dent Assoc 1978;96:630–638.

32. Moulton RE. Emotional factors in non-organic temporomandibular joint pain. Dent Clin North Am 1966;Nov:609–620.

33. Laskin DM. Etiology of the pain-dysfunction syndrome. J Am Dent Assoc 1969;79:147–153.

34. Laskin DM, Greene CS. Influence of the doctor-patient relationship on placebo therapy for patients with myofascial pain-dysfunction (MPD) syndrome. J Am Dent Assoc 1972;85:892–894.

35. Lupton DE. Psychological aspects of temporomandibular joint dysfunction. J Am Dent Assoc 1969;79:131–136.

36. Schwartz RA, Greene CS, Laskin DM. Personality characteristics of patients with myofascial pain-dysfunction (MPD) syndrome unresponsive to conventional therapy. J Dent Res 1979;58:1435–1439.

37. Rugh JD, Solberg WK. Psychological implications in temporomandibular pain and dysfunction. In: Zarb GA, Carlsson GE (eds). Temporomandibular Joint Function and Dysfunction. Copenhagen: Munksgaard, 1979:239–268.

38. Malow RM, Olson RE, Greene CS. Myofascial pain-dysfunction syndrome: A psychophysiological disorder. In: Golden C, Alcaparras S, Strider F, Graber B (eds). Applied Techniques in Behavioral Medicine and Medical Psychology. New York: Grune & Stratton, 1981:101–133.

39. Mercuri LG, Olson RE, Laskin DM. The specificity of response to experimental stress in patients with myofascial pain-dysfunction syndrome. J Dent Res 1979;58:1866–1871.

40. Malow RM, Grimm L, Olson RE. Differences in pain perception between myofascial pain dysfunction patients and normal subjects: A signal detection analysis. J Psychosom Res 1980;24:303–309.

41. Curran SL, Carlson CR, Okeson JP. Emotional and physiologic responses to laboratory challenges: Patients with temporomandibular disorders versus matched control subjects. J Orofac Pain 1996;10:141–150.

42. Fillingim RB, Maixner W, Kincaid S, Sigurdsson A, Harris MB. Pain sensitivity in patients with temporomandibular disorders: Relationship to clinical and psychosocial factors. Clin J Pain 1996;12:260–269.

43. Flor H, Birbaumer N, Schulte W, Roos R. Stress-related electromyographic responses in patients with chronic temporomandibular pain. Pain 1991;46:145–152.

44. Kapel L, Glaros AG, McGlynn FD. Psychophysiological responses to stress in patients with myofascial pain-dysfunction syndrome. J Behav Med 1989;12:397–406.

45. Katz JO, Rugh JD, Hatch JP, Langlais RP, Terezhalmy GT, Borcherding SH. Effect of experimental stress on masseter and temporalis muscle activity in human subjects with temporomandibular disorders. Arch Oral Biol 1989;34:393–398.

46. Maixner W, Fillingim R, Booker D, Sigurdsson A. Sensitivity of patients with painful temporomandibular disorders to experimentally evoked pain. Pain 1995;63:341–351.

47. Greene CS, Olson RE, Laskin DM. Psychological factors in the etiology, progression, and treatment of MPD syndrome. J Am Dent Assoc 1982;105:443–448.

48. Rugh JD, Davis SE. Temporomandibular disorders: Psychological and behavioral aspects. In: Sarnat BG, Laskin DM (eds). The Temporomandibular Joint: A Biologic Basis for Clinical Practice, ed 4. Philadelphia: Saunders, 1992:329–345.

49. Greene CS. A critique of nonconventional treatment concepts and procedures for temporomandibular disorders. In: Laskin DM, Greenfield W, Gale E, et al (eds). President's Conference on Examination, Diagnosis, and Management of Temporomandibular Disorders. Chicago: American Dental Association, 1983:177–181.

50. Greene CS. An evaluation of unconventional methods of diagnosing and treating temporomandibular disorders. Oral Maxillofac Surg Clin North Am 1995;7:167–173.

51. Gelb H (ed). Clinical Management of Head, Neck, and TMJ Pain and Dysfunction. Philadelphia: Saunders, 1977.

52. Goodheart GJ. Kinesiology and dentistry. J Am Soc Prev Dent 1976;6:16–18.

53. Ramfjord. SP. Dysfunctional temporomandibular joint and muscle pain. J Prosthet Dent 1961;11:353–374.

54. Ramfjord SP, Ash MM. Occlusion, ed 3. Philadelphia: Saunders, 1983.

55. Dworkin SF, Burgess JA. Orofacial pain of psychogenic origin: Current concepts and classification. J Am Dent Assoc 1987;115:565–571.

56. Okeson JP. Bell's Orofacial Pains, ed 5. Chicago: Quintessence, 1995:475–479.

57. American Academy of Orofacial Pain, Okeson JP (ed). Orofacial Pain: Guidelines for Assessment, Classification, and Management. Chicago: Quintessence, 1996:119–127.

58. Fricton JR, Kroening RJ, Hathaway KM (eds). Temporomandibular Disorders and Craniofacial Pain: Diagnosis and Management. St Louis: Ishiaku EuroAmerica, 1988.

59. Woda A, Pionchon P. Focus Paper: A unified concept of idiopathic orofacial pain: Clinical features. J Orofac Pain 1999;13:172–184.

60. Fricton JR. Critical commentary. 1. A unified concept of idiopathic orofacial pain: Clinical features. J Orofac Pain 1999;13:185–189.

61. Okeson JP. Critical commentary. 2. A unified concept of idiopathic orofacial pain: Clinical features. J Orofac Pain 1999;13:189–191.

62. Van der Waal I. Critical commentary. 3. A unified concept of idiopathic orofacial pain: Clinical features. J Orofac Pain 1999;13:192–194.

63. Harris M. Idiopathic orofacial pain: Idiopathic facial pain. In: Campbell JN (ed). Pain: An Updated Review. Seattle: IASP Press, 1996:403–412.

64. Zarb GA, Thompson GW. Assessment of clinical treatment of patients with temporomandibular joint dysfunction. J Prosthet Dent 1970;24:542–554.

65. Greene CS, Laskin DM. Long-term evaluation of conservative treatment for myofascial pain-dysfunction syndrome. J Am Dent Assoc 1974;89:1365–1368.

66. Greene CS, Markovic M. Response to nonsurgical treatment of patients with positive radiographic findings in the temporomandibular joints. J Oral Surg 1976;34:692–697.

67. Cohen SR. Follow-up evaluation of 105 patients with myofascial pain-dysfunction syndrome. J Am Dent Assoc 1978;97:825–828.

68. de Leeuw R, Boering G, Stegenga B, de Bont LG. Symptoms of temporomandibular joint osteoarthrosis and internal derangement 30 years after non-surgical treatment. Cranio 1995;13:81–88.

69. Mjersjo C, Carlsson GE. Long-term results of treatment for temporomandibular joint pain-dysfunction. J Prosthet Dent 1983;49:809–815.

70. Greene CS, Laskin DM. Long-term evaluation of treatment for myofascial pain-dysfunction syndrome: A comparative analysis. J Am Dent Assoc 1983;107:235–238.

71. Mjersjo C, Carlsson GE. Analysis of factors influencing the long-term effects of treatment of TMJ pain-dysfunction. J Oral Rehabil 1984;11:289–297.

72. Okeson JP, Hayes DK. Long-term results of treatment for temporomandibular disorders: An evaluation by patients. J Am Dent Assoc 1986;112:473–478.

73. Greene CS, Laskin DM. Long-term status of clicking in patients with myofascial pain and dysfunction. J Am Dent Assoc 1988;117:461–465.

74. Garafis P, Grigoriadu E, Zarafi A, et al. Effectiveness of conservative treatment for craniomandibular disorders: A 2-year longitudinal study. J Orofac Pain 1994;8:309–314.

75. Stohler CS, Zarb GA. On the management of temporomandibular disorders: A plea for a low-tech, high-prudence therapeutic approach. J Orofac Pain 1999;13:255–261.

76. de Bont LG, Dijkgraaf LC, Stegenga B. Epidemiology and natural progression of articular temporomandibular disorders. Oral Surg Oral Med Oral Pathol Oral Radiol Endod 1997;83:72–76.

77. Clark GT, Seligman DA, Solberg WK, Pullinger AG. Guidelines for the examination and diagnosis of temporomandibular disorders. J Craniomandib Disord 1989;3:7–14.

78. Clark GT, Seligman DA, Solberg WK, Pullinger AG. Guidelines for the treatment of temporomandibular disorders. J Craniomandib Disord 1990;4:80–88.

79. Zarb GA, Carlsson GE, Sessle BJ, Mohl ND. Temporomandibular Joint and Masticatory Muscle Disorders. Copenhagen: Munksgaard, 1994.

80. Clark GT. A diagnosis and treatment algorithm for common TM disorders. J Jpn Prosthodont Soc 1996;40:1029–1043.

81. Cooper BC. The role of bioelectronic instrumentation in the documentation and management of temporomandibular disorders. Oral Surg Oral Med Oral Pathol Oral Radiol Endod 1998;83:91–100.

82. Dawson PE. Evaluation, Diagnosis, and Treatment of Occlusal Problems, ed 2. St Louis: Mosby, 1989.

83. Moloney F, Howard JA. Internal derangements of the temporomandibular joint. 3. Anterior repositioning splint therapy. Aust Dent J 1986;31:30–39.

84. McCarty WL, Farrar WB. Surgery for internal derangements of the temporomandibular joint. J Prosthet Dent 1979;42:191–196.

85. Nickerson JW, Veaco NS. Condylotomy in surgery of the temporomandibular joint. Oral Maxillofac Surg Clin North Am 1989;1:303–327.

86. Greene CS. Managing TMD patients: Initial therapy is the key. J Am Dent Assoc 1992;123:43–45.

87. Flor H, Turk DC. Etiologic theories and treatments for chronic back pain. 1. Somatic models and interventions. Pain 1984;19:105–121.

88. Schwartz L. The pain-dysfunction syndrome. In: Schwartz L, Chayes CM (eds). Facial Pain and Mandibular Dysfunction. Philadelphia: Saunders, 1968:140–155.

89. Moulton R. Psychiatric considerations in maxillofacial pain. J Am Dent Assoc 1955;51:408–414.

90. Rugh JD, Solberg WK. Psychological implications in temporomandibular pain and dysfunction. Oral Sci Rev 1976;7:3–30.

91. Turk DC, Rudy TE, Kubinski JA, Zaki HS, Greco CM. Dysfunctional patients with temporomandibular disorders: Evaluating the efficiency of a tailored treatment protocol. J Consult Clin Psychol 1996;64:139–146.

92. Turk DC, Zaki HS, Rudy TE. Effects of intraoral appliances and biofeedback/stress management alone and in combination in treating pain and depression in patients with temporomandibular disorders. J Prosthet Dent 1993;70:158–164.

93. Dworkin SF. Behavioral and educational modalities. Oral Surg Oral Med Oral Pathol Oral Radiol Endod 1997;83:128–133.

94. Wilson L, Dworkin SF, Whitney C, LeResche L. Somatization and pain dispersion in chronic temporomandibular disorder pain. Pain 1994;57:55–61.

95. Dworkin SF, Turner JA, Wilson L, et al. Brief group cognitive-behavioral intervention for temporomandibular disorders. Pain 1994;59:175–187.

96. Stohler CS. Occlusal therapy in the treatment of temporomandibular disorders. Oral Maxillofac Surg Clin North Am 1995;7:129–139.

97. Okeson JP. Long-term treatment of disk-interference disorders of the temporomandibular joint with anterior repositioning occlusal splints. J Prosthet Dent 1988;60:611–616.

98. Clark GT. Interocclusal appliance therapy. In: Mohl ND, Zarb GA, Carlsson GE, Rugh JD (eds). A Textbook of Occlusion. Chicago: Quintessence, 1988:271–284.

99. Magnusson T, Carlsson GE. Treatment of patients with functional disorders in the masticatory system: A survey of 80 consecutive patients. Swed Dent J 1980;4:145–153.

100. Joondeph DR. Long-term stability of orthopedic repositioning. Angle Orthod 1999;69:201–209.

101. Dworkin SF, LeResche L. Research diagnostic criteria for temporomandibular disorders: Review, criteria, examination and specifications, critique. J Craniomandib Disord 1992;6:301–355.

102. American Association of Dental Research: Scientific Information Statement on Temporomandibular Disorders. AADR Reports 1996;18(4).

103. Greene CS. Focus Paper: The etiology of temporomandibular disorders: Implications for treatment. J Orofac Pain 2001;15:93–105.

104. Dubner R. Neuronal plasticity and pain following peripheral tissue inflammation or nerve injury. In: Bond MR, Charlton JE, Woolf CJ (eds). Proceedings of the Sixth World Congress on Pain. Amsterdam: Elsevier, 1991:264–276.

105. Sessle BJ. The neural basis of temporomandibular joint and masticatory muscle pain. J Orofac Pain 1999;13:238–245.

106. Sessle BJ. Acute and chronic craniofacial pain: Brainstem mechanisms of nociceptive transmission and neuroplasticity, and their clinical correlates. Crit Rev Oral Biol Med 2000;11:57–91.

107. Ren K, Dubner R. Focus Paper: Central nervous system plasticity and persistent pain. J Orofac Pain 1999;13:155–163; discussion 164–171.

TMJ Arthritis

A. Omar Abubaker

Arthritis is an important public health problem among all age groups in the United States, with an overall prevalence of 8% among women and 5% among men. More than 40 million people suffer from some form of arthritis; among these, 12 million have osteoarthritis (OA) and 8 million have rheumatoid arthritis (RA).[1,2] Because of the many variants of arthritis, and because the temporomandibular joint (TMJ) is susceptible to many of these forms, clinicians involved in the management of temporomandibular disorders (TMDs) often face a significant diagnostic challenge in delineating these conditions from other causes of TMD symptoms. They therefore must be familiar with the signs and symptoms of each of these entities and be able to assign to them a relative clinical significance. This process represents the core of differential diagnosis and is the key to successful management of these diseases.

The diagnosis of arthritis of the TMJ should involve an orderly and systematic review of the patient's history and a thorough physical examination. The information obtained from the history and physical examination should then be combined with preliminary radiographic studies to develop a working differential diagnosis. Based on this working diagnosis, additional procedures such as advanced imaging studies (magnetic resonance imaging [MRI], computerized tomography [CT] scan, and bone scans) and specific laboratory tests may be necessary to make the final diagnosis. This diagnostic approach is cost effective and protects patients from being subjected to a battery of unnecessary tests.

This chapter examines the significance of the various components involved in establishing a diagnosis of arthritis in the TMJ (history, physical examination, imaging studies, and laboratory tests). This discussion is followed by a review of the important features of each of these components as they relate to the different arthritic diseases that may affect this joint.

Patient Evaluation

History

Basic information obtained from the history, such as age, sex, and family history, may be beneficial in the differential diagnosis of arthritic diseases that have an age, gender, or familial predilection. For example, in a child with pain in the TMJ area, parotitis or mumps should be considered; in a teenager with a painful TMJ and a history of fever, both juvenile rheumatoid arthritis (JRA) and septic arthritis should be considered. JRA affects girls three times more often than it does boys and rarely affects patients beyond the age of 18 to 20 years. Ankylosing spondylitis (AS), on the other hand, most frequently occurs in patients between the ages of 20 and 40 years, while infectious arthritis, gonococcal arthritis, and Reiter syndrome normally affect the TMJ in sexually active men. Gout also affects mainly men, usually those older than 40 years, and it rarely affects women before menopause.[3]

Information regarding the onset, nature, and severity of the pain and the duration of the symptoms can be used to delineate the rate of progression of the disease and provide a basis for differentiation among arthritic conditions. The duration of morning stiffness may serve as a measure of the inflammatory activity and therefore provide a basis for differentiation between OA, which involves less than 30 minutes of stiffness, and RA, which involves more than 30 minutes. Associated features such as motor or sensory nerve symptoms and rapidly progressive destruction of the mandibular condyle may be more indicative of a malignancy than of an arthritic condition. Similarly, patients presenting with incidental findings of bony changes in the TMJ and a past history of malignancy should be carefully evaluated for metastatic disease.

Information regarding involvement of other joints or other systems, or a history of other joint surgery, is also important in the diagnosis of arthritic diseases of the TMJ. A history of trauma or symptoms of metabolic disease may be helpful in the diagnosis of traumatic and metabolic arthritis. A history of previous TMJ surgery should also be noted, because certain postoperative TMJ changes may mimic the clinical and radiographic presentations of arthritis. The family history may provide relevant data for the diagnosis of those forms of arthritis that have some genetic basis, such as AS, RA, and gout.[4]

The review of systems may also provide additional information important in the differential diagnosis of arthritis, because RA, JRA, OA, gout, and pseudogout all may have polyarticular and systemic manifestations. Therefore, the presence of articular signs and symptoms in other joints, including the characteristic monoarticular features of certain forms of arthritis as well as related systemic changes, should be investigated. For example, psoriatic arthritis (PA) has unique associated dermatologic findings on the extensor surface of the joints and the scalp, while gout has a characteristic involvement of the great toe, causing pain and swelling. Similarly, small pustules on the palms of the hands in the presence of a painfully swollen TMJ are suggestive of gonococcal arthritis. Red patches on the face, loss of demarcation of the vermilion border, restricted mouth opening, and pitted nails are all signs of scleroderma and other collagen diseases. Finally, although swelling and redness may also be present in gout and Reiter syndrome, fever is most frequently associated with infectious arthritis.[1]

Physical Examination

The physical examination of the TMJ should include inspection, palpation, and auscultation. Inspection detects swelling and erythema, the degree and pattern of joint movement, and the presence of overlying lesions. For example, if the joint and the adjacent region are swollen, erythematous, and warm, gout, septic arthritis, and RA should be included in the differential diagnosis. When erythema and swelling are associated with joint trauma, septic and traumatic arthritis are more likely. Reiter syndrome and PA may also cause warmness of the joint, but not to the same degree as gout. When the joint is tender to palpation but cold, OA or a connective tissue disease should be suspected. Finally, reduced interincisal opening, deviation on opening, and the presence of a newly developed anterior open bite may be indicators of the degree of joint involvement, whether the disease is unilateral or bilateral, and if there is bilateral condylar resorption.

Palpation of the joint may also help determine if there is swelling and tenderness, as well as if there are joint sounds and their type. However, auscultation is a more sensitive method than palpation for determining the presence and type of joint sounds. Crepitation is generally an indication of advanced joint disease, whereas clicking is usually indicative of disc deformity or disc position abnormalities.

Imaging Studies

In the evaluation of arthritic diseases of the TMJ, most clinicians obtain an initial screening view such as a panoramic radiograph. If bony changes are noted, additional imaging studies should be done. Depending on the working diagnosis, these studies may include MRI, CT, linear tomography, and radionuclide bone scans. These imaging modalities provide more detailed information about involvement of the hard and soft tissues of the joint and the extension of any lesions into the adjacent tissues. MRI can be used to detect early arthritic changes, determine disc position, and note joint effusion or other forms of fluid collection[5] (see chapter 10).

Radionuclide scans, although nonspecific, are quite sensitive for detecting reactive osteoblastic processes even in the absence of conventional radiographic changes. These scans can detect a variety of bone diseases including neoplasia, fibrous dysplasia, and arthritis.[6,7] They can also be helpful in assessing bone repair and in the staging of OA of the TMJ.[8]

Ultrasonography is also able to detect certain pathologic changes in the TMJ and may be considered as a diagnostic tool for rheumatoid arthritis and psoriatic arthritis of the TMJ.[9]

Laboratory Tests

Laboratory tests are usually obtained in the final phase of the diagnostic process, but occasionally are requested at the same time as the advanced imaging studies or after their completion. Although the diagnosis of the different forms of arthritis of the TMJ is generally made from the history and physical and imaging examinations, certain laboratory tests occasionally provide information that may lead to confirmation of the diagnosis. However, laboratory tests should be used with caution in the diagnosis of arthritic disease because of their lack of specificity, the degree of overlap in such tests among these diseases, and the possibility of false-positive tests. Accordingly, the laboratory tests should only be interpreted in light of a through history and physical examination.

Table 15-1	Signs and symptoms useful in the differential diagnosis of arthritis*		
Sign or symptom	**Degenerative**	**Inflammatory**	**Psychogenic**
Stiffness (duration)	Few minutes; "gelling"	Hours; often pronounced after rest	Little or no variation in intensity with rest or activity
Pain	Follows activity Relieved by rest	Even at rest; nocturnal pain may interfere with sleep	Little or no variation in intensity with rest or activity
Weakness	Present, usually localized and not severe	Often pronounced	Often a complaint; neurasthenia
Fatigue	Unusual	Often severe with onset in afternoon	Often in morning upon arising
Emotional depression and lability	Unusual	Common, coincides with fatigue; often disappears if disease remits	Often present
Tenderness localized over afflicted joint	Usually present	Almost always present; the most sensitive indication of inflammation	Tender "all over," doesn't want to be touched, tendency to push away or grasp examiner's hand
Swelling	Effusion common; little synovial reaction	Effusion common; often synovial proliferation and thickening	None
Heat and erythema (skin)	Unusual but may occur	More common	None
Crepitation	Coarse to medium	Medium to fine	None, except with coexistent arthritis
Bony spurs	Common	Sometimes found; usually with antecedent osteoarthritis	None, except with coexistent osteoarthritis

*Adapted from McCarthy.[3]

Because many of the arthritic diseases share an immunologic abnormality to a variable degree, most of the laboratory tests that are used in the diagnosis of such diseases are immunologically based. The most commonly used tests are *(1)* rheumatoid factor (RF), which is usually positive in 70% to 80% of patients with RA, and may also be positive in lower titers in other forms of arthritis, including gout, JRA, and PA; *(2)* antinuclear antibody (ANA) test, which is positive in 50% of patients with RA, some patients with JRA, and most patients with collagen diseases; *(3)* C-reactive protein, which is elevated mostly in RA, Reiter syndrome, and collagen diseases; *(4)* erythrocyte sedimentation rate (ESR), which, although nonspecific, is elevated in various inflammatory states, including RA and its variants; and *(5)* serum uric acid, which is typically elevated in gouty arthritis, although PA and AS are also occasionally associated with such an elevation. Other laboratory studies that are occasionally useful include serum chemistry, hematologic testing, urinalysis, blood culture, and synovial fluid Gram stain, culture, and polarizing microscopy examination.[1,3,4,10,11] For more information about laboratory tests, see chapter 11.

Classification of Arthritis

Although some degree of similarity and overlap exists in the signs and symptoms of the different arthritic diseases, the clinician must be able to distinguish between the individual conditions. One form of classification is to divide the diseases into those of inflammatory, degenerative, or psychogenic origin based on their signs and symptoms (Table 15-1).[3] However, a more clinically useful classification, based on cause, further subdivides arthritic diseases into the following groups:

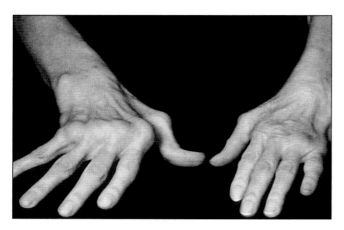

Fig 15-1 Ulnar deviation and subluxation of metacarpophalangeal joints in the right hand of a patient with rheumatoid arthritis. (©1972–2004 American College of Rheumatology Clinical Slide Collection. Used with permission.)

1. Inflammatory arthritis:
   a. Rheumatoid arthritis
   b. Juvenile rheumatoid arthritis
   c. Psoriatic arthritis
   d. Ankylosing spondylitis
   e. Reiter syndrome
2. Degenerative (osteo)arthritis
3. Infectious arthritis:
   a. Gonococcal arthritis
   b. Syphilitic arthritis
   c. Tuberculous arthritis
   d. Lyme disease–associated arthritis
4. Metabolic arthritis:
   a. Gout
   b. Pseudogout
5. Traumatic arthritis

Other conditions that may produce symptoms similar to those arising from primary arthritis should occasionally be included in the differential diagnosis. These entities include arthritis associated with chronic inflammatory bowel disease, reflex sympathetic dystrophy, sarcoidosis, systemic lupus erythematous, and scleroderma. Review of the specific signs and symptoms of these conditions is beyond the scope of this chapter.

Inflammatory Arthritis

Rheumatoid Arthritis

Rheumatoid arthritis is a chronic inflammatory disease that primarily affects the periarticular structures such as the synovial membrane, capsule, tendons, tendon sheaths, and ligaments. It secondarily involves the articular cartilage and subchondral bone. The prevalence of RA among the general population is about 2% to 2.5%, with a female to male predilection ratio of 2.5 to 3.0:1 and a peak onset of the disease between the patient ages of 40 and 60 years.[2,12] Approximately 50% to 75% of patients with RA have involvement of the TMJ during the course of the disease.[13–16]

Clinical findings

The disease often has an insidious onset and runs a slow, chronic course with progressive destruction of the articular soft tissues and eventual destruction of the cartilage and bone. It has a symmetric, polyarticular involvement, and the small peripheral joints are affected first (wrists, elbows, and ankles). It then progresses symmetrically toward the central skeleton, involving the knee, shoulders, and cervical spine. In the advanced stages, when the inflammatory tissue infiltrates the articular cartilage and bone, erosion and destruction of the articular disc, cartilage, and subchondral bone result.

Such total destruction causes joint deformity and loss of joint function. Joint deformity may also result, in part, from involvement of the tendons, muscles, and ligaments.[3] In the hands, such deformity may be in the form of the characteristic ulnar deviation (Fig 15-1), and swan neck and boutonniere deformities of the fingers. In larger joints, such deformities cause limitation of motion, flexion contraction, genu valgus, and genu varus.[3,4]

RA also has characteristic extra-articular and systemic features that include ocular involvement such as episcleritis, iritis, and keratoconjunctivitis; pulmonary features such as pleurisy, pleural effusion, and fibrosis; cardiac features such as pericarditis and cardiac arrhythmias; vasculitis causing skin ulcerations and osteoporosis; and the presence of subcutaneous nodules in pressure and friction areas in 20% to 25% of patients. Systemic signs and symptoms of RA include fatigue, weight loss, fever, and anemia.[4] When RA is present in combination with anemia, neutropenia, thrombocytopenia, and hypersplenism, the condition is called *Felty syndrome.*[17]

A close relationship exists between involvement of the TMJ and the severity of the systemic disease. When the TMJ is involved, it is bilateral in 34% to 75% of those patients.[15] Signs and symptoms of the TMJ involvement include deep, dull, aching pain in the preauricular area, especially during function; muscle tenderness with decreased bite force; limited range of motion; crepitation or clicking; and morning joint stiffness.[18–21] The pain is occasionally referred to the temporal region and angle of the mandible. As the disease progresses, the condylar bone is resorbed and scar tissue is formed between the joint surfaces and within the joint capsule. This causes further limitation of movement of the jaw.[22]

Mandibular movement may be severely limited in the late stages of the disease. This is usually caused by fibrous ankylosis and rarely by bony ankylosis.[23] Perhaps the most striking feature of advanced RA affecting the TMJ is development of a progressive class II malocclusion and anterior open bite deformity with impairment of chewing and phonation. This deformity is caused by loss of normal ramus height secondary to destruction of the mandibular condyles.

Imaging findings

Because RA is primarily a soft tissue disease, the early stages are characterized by the absence of radiographic changes. Even when these changes are present, they lack specificity and are difficult to interpret. However, with the use of MRI, changes such as disc destruction and/or displacement, condylar cortical bone erosion, joint effusion, and cartilage irregularity and thinning can be seen.[9,24] Once bone is involved in the later stages of the disease, radiographic changes in the TMJ occur in 19% to 84% of patients[13,19]; the incidence and severity of these changes are related to the duration of the disease.

The radiographic features of RA of the TMJ include loss of joint space, condylar destruction, and flattening and anterior positioning of the condyle (see Fig 10-30). This may be accompanied by flattening and anterior positioning of the condyle as well as flattening of the articular eminence and erosion of the glenoid fossa.[25–28] In advanced stages of the disease, the radiographic changes may include a sharp, pointed condyle, osteophyte formation, lipping, shortened posterior ramus length causing premature posterior occlusion, an anterior open bite, and deepening of the antegonial notch.[29]

Laboratory findings

The preliminary diagnosis of RA is frequently based on the clinical and radiographic findings, and the laboratory tests are used to confirm the diagnosis. The most commonly used test is for RF, which is positive in 70% to 80% of patients with RA. Although the test is not totally diagnostic, it has a good diagnostic and prognostic value when the factor is present in high titers (above 1:1,280). In these patients, the disease has a more severe and progressive course. However, the test is also occasionally positive in patients with one of the rheumatoid variants and in approximately 5% of healthy subjects.[30]

The Westergren ESR, although not a highly specific test for RA, is elevated in approximately 90% of patients during active stages of the disease, and the test often is used to follow the course of the disease.[21] The complete and differential blood cell counts frequently show a normal white blood cell count, although leukocytosis or leukocytopenia can occur in patients with RA. An elevated platelet count may accompany the stages of high activity of the disease, while mild anemia is reported in approximately 25% of patients. Most of the latter patients have a normochromic or slightly hypochromic, normocytic anemia. Synovial fluid aspirated from a joint with RA is usually cloudy; the viscosity is reduced and the white cell count is high (greater than 20,000/μL).

Other test results that are less specific for RA include a decreased serum albumin level and the presence of ANA in 15% of RA patients; HLA-Dw5 and HLA-DRw antigens are also both positive in 50% of RA patients.[1,3,20]

Diagnosis

The criteria for diagnosis of generalized RA are based on the presence of several clinical, radiographic, and laboratory findings for at least 6 weeks.[1,3] The diagnosis of RA of the TMJ is frequently less difficult because involvement of the TMJ often occurs in the advanced stages of the disease and, at that point, the diagnosis of RA has already been established. In these instances, the signs and symptoms, along with the positive radiographic findings, form the basis for diagnosing involvement of the TMJ by the disease.[30] However, in the absence of an already established diagnosis, the differential diagnosis of TMJ involvement should include PA, AS, gout, and OA.

Differentiation of RA from the rheumatoid variants is based on factors such as age of the patient, pattern of involvement (symmetry), number and type of joints involved (polyarticular and peripheral joints), presence of rheumatoid nodules, and, to a lesser degree, laboratory findings (positive RF). Differentiation of RA from OA is less difficult and also is based on the clinical and radiographic findings and, to a greater extent, on some of the laboratory tests. The distinguishing general systemic findings of RA and OA are listed in Table 15-2, and the distinguishing TMJ features of the two forms of arthritis are listed on Table 15-3.[31]

Table 15-2 Distinguishing general and systemic features of rheumatoid arthritis and osteoarthritis*

Feature	Rheumatoid arthritis	Osteoarthritis
Sedimentation rate	Usually elevated	Normal
Rheumatoid factor	Present (60% to 80%)	Rarely present
Anemia	Hypochromic, normocytic	None
Synovial fluid	Inflammatory	Noninflammatory
Nodules	20%	None
Morning stiffness	> 30 min	< 30 min
Joint involvement	Symmetric	Symmetric or nonsymmetric
Hand joints commonly involved	Proximal interphalangeal and metacarpophalangeal	Distal interphalangeal
Type of hand swelling	Soft	Hard
Extra-articular findings	May be present	Absent
Radiographic findings	Erosive (symmetric loss of cartilage)	Erosive + exophytic (asymmetric cartilage loss)
Pathogenesis	Synovial reaction	Articular cartilage failure

*From Zide et al.[31]

Table 15-3 Distinguishing local features of rheumatoid arthritis and osteoarthritis of the temporomandibular joint (TMJ)*

Features	Rheumatoid arthritis	Osteoarthritis
Incidence	50%–70% of patients have TMJ symptoms	20%–30% of patients have TMJ symptoms
Symptoms	Deep, dull preauricular pain; high incidence of ear complaints; crepitant joint noises; joint stiffness; symptoms worse in morning	Preauricular and referred pain onset after function; popping, clicking, and crepitation; myogenic pain; symptoms worse in evening
Signs	Edema; tender to palpation; limited function; occlusal changes; profile alteration	Occasionally tender to palpation; myospasm, popping, clicking, crepitation; functional abnormalities due to muscle splinting and disc dysfunction; no occlusal-facial alteration
Radiographic presentation	Cloudy joint space; condyle and glenoid fossa erosion; severe cases show spiking and/or extensive bone loss from lytic enzymes and osteoclastic activity	Hazy joint space; narrowing of joint space; subchondral remodeling and repair most oftens resulting in a broader articulating surface; occasionally incomplete repair leaving osteophytes and erosions that are symptomatic
Pathophysiology	Synovial hyperplasia and inflammation (pannus); bony erosion from lytic enzyme osteoclastic activity	Pressure loading, causing articular breakdown extending into subchondral bone; remodeling and repair most often resulting in a broader articulating surface; occasionally incomplete repair, leaving osteophytes and erosions that are symptomatic
Vertical ramus	Progressive loss of vertical dimension; open bite/retrognathia in advanced cases	Minor regressive remodeling with slight shortening of the condyle

*From Zide et al.[31]

Juvenile Rheumatoid Arthritis

Juvenile rheumatoid arthritis is a chronic inflammatory involvement of the joint lining that has an onset before the age of 16 years. The overall prevalence of JRA is uncertain, but estimates of the number of children affected in the United States range from 30,000 to 250,000.[32] The disease occurs predominantly in girls, with a female-male ratio of 1:2 to 1:3, and it has two peaks of onset, one between the ages of 1 and 3 years and the other between the ages of 8 and 12 years.[1]

The reported TMJ involvement in patients with JRA varies considerably, mostly because of the difference in the methods of examination in different studies. Nonetheless, up to 41% of children with JRA have TMJ involvement, with significant adverse effects on occlusion, oral health, and facial growth.[33–36]

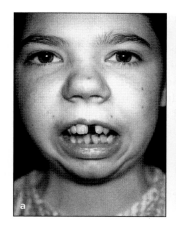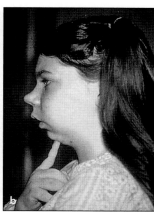

Fig 15-2 Child with juvenile rheumatoid arthritis who developed bilateral ankylosis. *(a)* Frontal view revealing the limited mouth opening. *(b)* Lateral view revealing the severe mandibular retrognathia. (Courtesy of Dr Daniel M. Laskin.)

Clinical findings

Based on the manifestations of the disease during the first 6 months and a number of other factors, JRA is classified into three major subtypes: systemic, polyarticular, and pauciarticular. The last two are often further subdivided into two subtypes.[1,3]

Systemic JRA, called *Still disease*, occurs mostly in boys 5 years of age or younger, can affect any joint, and is usually accompanied by several systemic signs, including high fever, a rheumatoid rash, cardiopulmonary involvement, lymphadenopathy, and hepatosplenomegaly. The major complication of this disease is cardiac failure, but the majority of patients go into remission with minimal or no residual articular complications. Generally, patients in this subtypes are seronegative for both RF and ANA.

Polyarticular onset JRA involves more than four joints and has fewer systemic signs. This subtype can be seropositive for RF and ANA in 50% of patients. The major complication of this subtype is the long-term possibility of deformity and disability from the polyarthritis.[37]

Pauciarticular JRA affects girls more often than boys, involves four or fewer joints, and has fewer systemic signs. This subtype usually affects large joints such as the knee, hip, and sacroiliac, but patients rarely experience severe arthritis. Patients in this group are generally seronegative for RF, but the ANA test is positive in 60% to 80% of patients.[1] The major hazards of this subtype are iridocyclitis and blindness, and the prognosis for articular disability is greater than with the other two forms of JRA.

Although the TMJ can be involved in any of these subtypes, it is mostly affected by the polyarticular subtype. The clinical features of JRA of the TMJ include pain, joint tenderness, crepitation, stiffness, and decreased range of motion.[33] Some patients may even develop fibrous or bony ankylosis.

A characteristic feature associated with advanced JRA of the TMJ is a combination of micrognathia and a Class II skeletal deformity,[38,39] which is frequently referred to as *birdface deformity* (Fig 15-2). This deformity is a result of the impaired growth of the mandible caused by destruction of the condylar growth site. Alterations in the soft tissues adjacent to the TMJ, such as scarring of the capsule and ligaments and the changes in the muscle strength, also can interfere with the normal growth processes of the mandible. The prevalence and severity of such deformity in patients with JRA of the TMJ are influenced by the age of onset of the involvement and by the duration of the disease. The prevalence of this deformity ranges from 0% to 38%.[23,39]

Imaging findings

The early radiographic changes of JRA of the TMJ may not be visible on a conventional radiograph. However, these changes can be detected on MRI, and include cortical bone erosion, disc thinning and perforation, reduction of the joint space, and pannus and effusion in the joint[40,41] (see Fig 10-33). The radiographic changes usually appear late, and the severity of these changes is generally related to the duration of the disease. The radiographic findings in JRA of the TMJ in general resemble those of the adult disease and include erosion of the superior surface of the condyle (leaving a flat, horizontal, or inclined articular surface). The eminence may be eroded and flattened to the same degree as the condyle.

In advanced stages of the disease, these changes may significantly affect growth of the mandible and face. The mandible appears micrognathic, with a downward and backward rotation of the chin and an anterior open bite. This deformity is associated with radiographic evidence of deepening of the antegonial notch.[42–44]

Laboratory findings

Laboratory findings in patients with JRA are not consistent and, when present, the abnormality varies with the mode of onset. RF is positive in 5% to 20% of patients with JRA, mostly with the pauciarticular and polyarticular subtypes, while the ANA test is positive mostly in patients with the pauciarticular subtypes (60% to 80% of these patients). Other laboratory findings, including low-grade anemia, leukocytes, thrombocytopenia, and elevated ESR, may also vary according to the subtype of JRA.

Diagnosis

A diagnosis of JRA of the TMJ is often not difficult to make because involvement of the TMJ usually occurs in the later stages. Because of the presence of fever and generalized arthralgia with the onset of systemic JRA, the differential diagnosis should include bacterial infection, viral polyarthritis, traumatic arthritis, infectious arthritis, and joint involvement with rheumatic fever.

Psoriatic Arthritis

Psoriasis (also see chapter 9) is a dermatologic disease that affects approximately 1% to 2% of the general population. It is characterized by a rash of silvery scales affecting the elbow, scalp, and back. Approximately 5% to 7% of patients with psoriasis develop psoriatic arthritis.[45–47] In 75% of these patients, skin lesions appear before the joint symptoms, whereas arthritis appears first in 10% to 15% of patients; in another 10% to 15% of patients, the symptoms appear simultaneously.[48] PA is an inflammatory, mostly asymmetric, oligoarticular, seronegative arthritis that affects a limited number of joints including those of the hand, knee, and foot.

Reports on the disease incidence relative to sex differ from a predilection for males to equal predilection for males and females.[48,49] The onset of the disease is usually between the ages of 35 and 45 years.

The cause is probably multifactorial, but histocompatibility studies support a propensity for the condition to be associated with several other systemic conditions such as Crohn disease; Reiter, Behçet, and Sjögren syndrome; and aortic incompetence.[3] Heredity and a history of trauma[1,4,48,50] are significant factors in the development of PA.

Despite the prevalence of PA in other joints, fewer than 35 cases of PA of the TMJ have been reported in the English literature.[51–53] However, some authors suggest that involvement of the TMJ with PA is more common and could be as great as 20%.[54] When PA affects the TMJ, the onset of symptoms occurs by the fourth decade of life and is usually associated with a history of trauma.[55,56]

Clinical findings

The arthritic changes of PA are mostly limited to the distal interphalangeal and metacarpophalangeal joints, but occasionally may extend to the proximal interphalangeal joints, producing characteristic sausage-shaped digits. Systemic symptoms of PA include fever, fatigue, myalgia, weight loss, and malaise. Joint symptoms include morning stiffness and pain, swelling, and limitation of motion. Other associated symptoms may include nail dystrophy in the form of pitting and oncolysis in 80% of patients and eye symptoms including conjunctivitis, iritis, and uveitis.[46,57] Mitral valve prolapse occurs with a greater incidence in PA patients than in the general population.[58]

Based on the presence of different clinical features, four distinct patterns of PA are currently recognized: (1) arthritis affecting mostly the distal interphalangeal joints; (2) severe arthritis affecting single or multiple joints, with widespread bone destruction and ankylosis; (3) seronegative polyarthritis that may be difficult to distinguish from seronegative RA; and (4) arthritis that is characterized by the presence of sacroiliitis, spondylitis, and peripheral joint involvement, as well as the presence of HLA-B27 antigen.[1,3]

PA of the TMJ often is unilateral, has a sudden onset, is episodic in nature, and may have a spontaneous remission. Symptoms include pain and tenderness of the joint area and the muscles of mastication, morning stiffness, tiredness in the jaws, joint crepitation, occasional painful swelling of the TMJ capsule, and painful mandibular movements associated with a progressive decrease in the interincisal opening.[51] In severe cases, ankylosis of the TMJ may occur.[52]

Imaging findings

Radiographic changes associated with PA may be seen in as many as 82% of patients with affected TMJs and include erosion, flattening, osteoporosis, loss of joint mobility, and extreme joint space narrowing. Subchondral bone cysts, subluxation, and ankylosis are also observed occasionally.[54,56,59,60] The radiographic changes are nonspecific and cannot be easily distinguished from those of other types of arthritis, particularly RA and AS.

Diagnosis

Because the symptoms of TMJ involvement are generally nonspecific, the diagnosis of PA of the TMJ is difficult and is made mainly on the basis of the systemic presentation of the disease. In general, the diagnosis is based on a triad of *(1)* psoriasis, *(2)* radiographic evidence of erosive poly-arthritis, and *(3)* a negative serologic test for RF. However, even in the presence of a skin rash, the diagnosis of PA cannot be absolutely confirmed. The differential diagnosis of PA should always include entities such as RA, Reiter syndrome, AS, and gout.

Ankylosing Spondylitis

Ankylosing spondylitis (also see chapter 9) is a disease known by many other terms, but two of the most commonly used are *Marie-Strümpell disease* and *seronegative spondylitis*. It is a chronic and usually progressive inflammatory disease that primarily affects the axial skeleton, most commonly the sacroiliac joint and the vertebral column. When the disease spreads to the peripheral joints, the most commonly affected are the hips, shoulders, knees, wrists, hands, and TMJ. The disease has a prevalence of 0.4% to 1.6% among whites, with a strong familial tendency.[1,3] It affects both sexes, with a predilection for men up to 10 times greater that for women, and has an onset between the ages of 20 and 30 years.[3,61]

When affected, the TMJ is usually involved several years after the onset of the systemic disease and frequently during the late stages of spinal and peripheral joint involvement. Although only sporadic case reports of AS of the TMJ have been published, involvement with AS is reported to occur in 4% to 50% of such patients.[62–64]

Clinical findings

The clinical signs and symptoms of AS generally arise from chronic inflammation of the synovial tissues and joint capsule and sites of insertion of ligaments and tendons. The inflammation later progresses to ossification and eventually causes limitation of joint motion. In the spine, this results in low back pain and stiffness that are usually worse in the morning but that can be alleviated by mobility and exercise. In the late stages, fusion of the adjacent vertebrae and fixation of the back in extreme flexion causes decreased spinal mobility, lumbar lordosis, and increased thoracic and lumbar kyphosis with limitation of chest movement. The back pain may be referred to the buttocks and the posterior aspect of the leg. Extra-articular manifestations of AS include iritis or anterior uveitis and cardiac symptoms such as aortic insufficiency and conduction defects.[1,3]

When the TMJ is affected, pain, stiffness, limitation of jaw movements, and, in advanced cases, ankylosis of the joint may occur.[65–68] Often the severity of the TMJ involvement correlates with the severity of the spinal and peripheral involvement, although the presence of TMJ symptoms has been reported in patients with only a slightly affected spine.

Imaging findings

The radiographic features of the disease usually include ossification of ligaments and tendons and sclerotic fusion between the vertebrae. In the late stages of the disease, calcification of the annulus under the paraspinal ligaments gives rise to the characteristic "bamboo spine" appearance. The pelvic radiographs usually show fusion of the sacroiliac joint and sclerotic widening of the margins of the pubic symphysis.[65]

The radiographic features of AS in the TMJ are nonspecific and are observed in 30% of patients. These features usually involve erosive changes in the condyle and fossa, subchondral sclerosis, and osteophyte formation (see Fig 10-29). In the later stages of the disease, narrowing of the joint space and radiographic evidence of restricted anterior translation of the condyle may be detected.[65,67,69]

Laboratory findings

AS characteristically has a hereditary component; the incidence of occurrence of HLA-B27 antigen is higher in patients with AS than in patients with any other disease of the inflammatory arthritis group. An elevated ESR is reported in as many as 70% of patients with AS, although the test is generally nonspecific and only serves as a rough gauge of the disease. Tests for RF are generally negative.[1,3]

Diagnosis

Because of the similarities among RA, PS, and AS, the differential diagnosis should include these entities. However, some features exist that may be helpful in distinguishing AS from the other two conditions. These include involvement of the sacroiliac joint, which, although possible with any of the other types, is only common in AS and is rare in RA. Furthermore, whereas AS may involve peripheral joints, it usually spares the small joints of the hands and feet. Although radiographically apparent erosive changes and narrowing of joint space and osteophyte formation are common in all three diseases, localized or extensive sclerosis is more common in AS, whereas cortical erosion and subcortical bone cyst formation are more common in RA.[70,71]

Reiter Syndrome

Classically, Reiter syndrome (also see chapter 9) is a triad of arthritis, conjunctivitis, and urethritis occurring mostly in men between the ages of 20 and 30 years. More recently, additional frequent features of the disease have been recognized, including mucocutaneous lesions and cardiac and central or peripheral nervous system involvement. The exact cause of the disease is unknown, but the frequent presence of HLA-B27 alloantigen in the patient population has been established. The disease occurs mostly in young men after venereal infection and in both men and women after dysenteric infection.[12]

The arthritis in Reiter syndrome often involves multiple joints (resembling RA), but affects mainly the lower extremities. Involvement of the TMJ is rare, but some authors believe its incidence may be grossly underreported because of the lack of specific clinical or histologic features of the disease.[72]

Clinical findings

The manifestations of the disease include development of urethritis, conjunctivitis, and finally arthritis either sequentially or simultaneously. Fever, fatigue, weight loss, and lymphadenopathy often accompany the arthritis. Both the urethritis and the conjunctivitis can develop and resolve without sequelae, or they can cause long-lasting urologic and ocular complications. Skin lesions, known as *keratoderma blennorrhagica*, may occur on the palms, soles, and glans penis. As many as 80% of patients with Reiter syndrome may show oral lesions in the form of 1- to 10-mm papules on the lips, gingivae, buccal mucosa, and tongue.[55]

When the TMJ is affected, the symptoms are generally acute and asymmetric and include tenderness, erythema, and warmness of the joint.[72]

Imaging and laboratory findings

Radiographically, bony changes in the joints affected by Reiter syndrome are only observed in the late stages and consist of erosion of the condyle and loss of the joint space.[72,73] The laboratory findings are mostly nonspecific and may include an elevated ESR, leukocytosis, mild anemia, and negative tests for RF and ANA. Serologic evidence of recent infection and a HLA-B27 marker may be present.[12]

Diagnosis

The diagnosis of Reiter syndrome is clinical and is based on the triad of symptoms that are present in 70% of patients in the first 10 days. However, only the presence of seronegative, oligoarticular, asymmetric arthritis and urethritis is adequate for diagnosis of the syndrome. The differential diagnosis should include PA and other forms of reactive arthritis, such as those associated with ulcerative colitis and regional enteritis and that occurring after intestinal bypass surgery.

Degenerative (Osteo)Arthritis

Osteoarthritis is a chronic noninflammatory disease that characteristically affects the articular cartilage of synovial joints and is associated with simultaneous remodeling of the underlying subchondral bone and secondary involvement of the synovium. Synonymous terms such as *osteoarthrosis*, *arthrosis*, and *arthritis deformans* are commonly used in Europe, whereas *osteoarthritis*, *degenerative joint disease*, and *degenerative arthritis* are the most commonly used terms in North America. However, many prefer the terms *osteroarthrosis* and *degenerative joint disease* because they reflect the noninflammatory nature of the disease.

OA is the most common form of arthritis affecting the human skeleton and is related to increased mechanical loading, physical stress, and traumatic injury of the joint. Consequently, the joints most often affected are the weight-bearing joints such as the hips, spine, and knees. Hand joints are also commonly affected, especially in women. Systemic, genetic, endocrinologic, metabolic, and/or vascular factors, in combination with local mechanical factors, influence the development and progression of the disease.[74,75]

OA is the most common disease affecting the TMJ. Radiographic evidence of OA of the TMJ occurs in 14% to 44% of symptom-free individuals,[76] and histologic evidence of the disease occurs in 40% to 60% of studied populations.[77,78] However, clinical evidence of the disease occurs in only 8% to 16% of the population.[79,80] OA of the TMJ has a strong predilection for women and affects patients at any age, but is more prevalent beyond the age of 40 years.[22,81] Generally OA is unilateral, although bilateral involvement does occur; in these cases, one side usually shows greater severity.[82]

Clinical findings

Generally OA has a gradual onset and runs a chronic course, with clinical features predominantly in the large weight-bearing joints. When the disease involves the hands, the most frequently affected joints are the distal interphalangeal joints, producing the characteristic enlargement known as *Heberden nodes* (Fig 15-3). When the proximal interphalangeal joints are affected, the nodes are called *Bouchard nodes*.

When the TMJ is affected, the patient usually complains of pain and tenderness in the joint and masticatory muscles. The patient may also complain of jaw muscle fatigue, stiffness and tiredness, difficulty opening the mouth, reduced range of motion, and crepitation during mandibular movements.[83] Osteoarthritis is usually characterized by a lack of morning jaw stiffness; if present, this stiffness lasts no more than 30 minutes.[84] The TMJ symptoms may be present in the absence of similar symptoms in other joints of the body. Because of the bony thickening and marginal osteophyte formation in the mandibular condyle, a palpable swelling may occur over the joint.

Although radiographic changes in the TMJ may be observed bilaterally, only one side may be symptomatic. Other associated symptoms include referred head and neck pain and earache.

OA may affect the TMJ primarily (primary OA) as a result of the normal wear and tear of the joint components that occur with aging. This form of OA usually begins in the fifth decade of life, with slow onset, and runs a course of mild symptoms. The other form of OA of the TMJ is secondary and is usually associated with macrotrauma or chronic microtrauma. This form affects patients 20 to 40 years old and produces more symptoms than the primary form. In these patients, the symptoms may be associated with chronic myofascial pain and dysfunction (MPD) or intra-articular disc derangement.[85,86]

Imaging findings

Radiographic studies of OA of the TMJ reveal an incidence of 40% in patients older than 40 years and 100% in patients older than 80 years. Approximately 50% of the population has radiographic changes, but only 30% of these patients are symptomatic.[87] Because OA affects the articular cartilage first, the early changes may escape radiographic detection or the radiograph may only show a reduced joint space, indicating loss of the articular cartilage and/or perforation of the disc. The most common early radiographic change in the condyle is subchondral bone sclerosis because of thickening of the subchondral bony plate (see Fig 10-11). As the disease progresses, there may

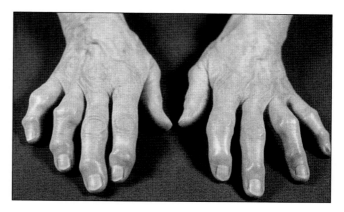

Fig 15-3 Bony enlargement of the proximal interphalangeal joints (Bouchard nodes) and distal interphalangeal joints (Heberden nodes) in a patient with degenerative joint disease of the hands. (©1972–2004 American College of Rheumatology Clinical Slide Collection. Used with permission.)

be flattening and marginal lipping of the condyle and flattening of the articular eminence. In the late stages of the disease the changes are in the form of erosion of the cortical plate, osteophyte formation or both. Occasionally, in the late stages of the disease, subchondral bone breakdown may also occur, causing the formation of a bone "cyst" within the condyle.[85]

MRI of the TMJ with OA may reveal perforation, damage, or displacement of the articular disc, whereas osseous changes are best delineated by computed or linear tomography.[28,88] High resolution ultrasonography may also be a valuable diagnostic aid for the detection of abnormal condylar morphology in OA.[89]

Laboratory findings

In contrast to the results in patients with RA and its variants, the laboratory findings in patients with OA are unremarkable and make no contribution to the diagnosis. The ESD is usually normal or only slightly elevated, and high values may only be present when the disease has an acute inflammatory component. RF is usually absent, and a synovial fluid aspirate shows only a slight elevation of white blood cells (often less than 2000/µL) and fewer than 30% polymorphonuclear cells.[1]

However, studies on synovial fluid analysis for keratan sulfate have shown levels are higher in joints that had arthroscopic evidence of early OA than in normal joints.[90]

The authors suggested that a combination of arthroscopy and synovial fluid analysis is an important diagnostic modality for the early detection of OA. Recent studies using synovial fluid analysis have shown a correlation of pain and disease progression with tumor necrosis factor α, interleukin 1β, stromelysin, and bradykinin[90–93] (see chapter 11).

Diagnosis

The diagnosis of OA is based mostly on clinical findings and radiographic studies and is usually easy to make when the typical features of the disease are present. The most difficulty is encountered in differentiating OA from early MPD and from RA. Therefore, the differential diagnosis of OA of the TMJ should include RA and its variants, MPD, and various forms of intra-articular disc derangement. Features distinguishing OA from MPD include the more localized nature of the pain, the frequent presence of joint tenderness, and the presence of joint crepitation in the former. When both conditions are present concurrently, as is often the case, the history may help determine which is the primary condition.[94] The main distinguishing features between OA and RA are listed in Tables 15-2 and 15-3.[28,31]

Infectious Arthritis

General

Although infectious or septic arthritis of the TMJ is frequently considered a possible complication of such systemic diseases as tuberculosis, syphilis, and gonorrhea, only 22 cases have been reported.[95] Some authors attribute the small number of reported cases to misdiagnosis or underreporting and suggest that misdiagnosed septic arthritis in children may account for a significant percentage of cases of mandibular ankylosis.[96,97]

Infectious arthritis can involve the TMJ by direct extension of local odontogenic infections via the pterygomandibular space, from osteomyelitis of the mandible, or from parotid, ear, or throat infections.[98] Direct infection can also occur as a result of inoculation of organisms into the joint space during traumatic injury or joint surgery.[99]

The other major route of infection of the TMJ is from a systemic disease such as gonorrhea, syphilis, tuberculosis, or actinomycosis.[81] Risk factors for TMJ infection include the presence of RA, diabetes mellitus, intravenous drug abuse,[87,100] burn wounds,[101] sexually transmitted diseases,[102] preexisting joint disease,[103] trauma, and steroid therapy.[1]

Despite the decreased incidence of some of the systemic infectious diseases known to predispose to septic arthritis, an increase in the frequency of septic arthritis can be expected in the future because of the large number of immunocompromised patients with AIDS and the wider use of immunosuppressive agents. This form of septic arthritis may be either bacterial or fungal in origin.[23] Another form of infectious arthritis that can have serious consequences involves infection of a joint prosthesis. Such infection can occur immediately after implant placement or later from hematogenous dissemination of bacteria.[3] However, despite several reports of such infections in the orthopedic literature, only two cases involving the TMJ have been reported.[87,100]

Clinical findings

When the cause of the infectious arthritis is systemic, the joint symptoms may be preceded by a prodromal period of symptoms of the primary disease. The acute presentation of septic arthritis includes signs of malaise, fever, chills, sweating, and regional lymphadenopathy. The affected joint (usually one side) is painful, tender, swollen, warm, and erythematous. Movement of the mandible is usually limited and typically elicits severe pain. Occasionally, malocclusion, deviation of the mandible to the contralateral side, and a posterior open bite will occur secondary to the increased amount of joint fluid.

Fluctuation may be present in the region of the joint if the fluid collection is not drained. If septic arthritis is left untreated, it may progress to complete destruction of the condylar cartilage and bone, causing ankylosis, which in children may cause underdevelopment of the mandible and facial asymmetry later in life.

Imaging findings

Because no bony involvement occurs in the first 7 to 10 days of infectious arthritis, radiographic changes are not demonstrable.[23] However, because of accumulation of intra-articular fluid or pus, a separation of the articular surfaces, in which the mandibular condyle is in a more anteroinferior position, can be seen on either a panoramic radiograph or CT scan of the joint. Later, if the infection is left untreated, bony changes range from destruction of the articular cartilage to total destruction of the joint.

MRI can be used to detect intra-articular pus or accumulation of exudate,[85] although it is not helpful in distinguishing infection from inflammatory, traumatic, or degenerative processes in the joint.[104] A bone scan usually shows an increased uptake in the joint capsule in the presence of sep-

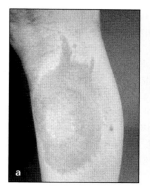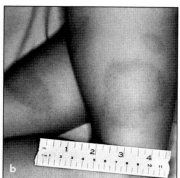

Fig 15-4 *(a and b)* Erythema chronicum migrans, one of the early signs of Lyme disease, begins as a red macule or papule and expands to a larger lesion with red borders and central clearing. (©1972–2004 American College of Rheumatology Clinical Slide Collecton. Used with permission.)

tic arthritis, and it can detect bone changes sooner than other imaging studies.[95]

Laboratory findings

Laboratory tests for septic arthritis in the presence of systemic signs should include a complete blood cell count, a differential cell count, ESR, C-reactive protein determination, and blood culture. Joint fluid should be aspirated for analysis and culture whenever feasible. The aspirated fluid should be examined with a Gram stain, culture, and antibiotic sensitivity testing, a complete blood cell count, and a differential cell count. Glucose and hyaluronic acid levels also should be analyzed; these levels are usually decreased. Typically, the aspirated fluid from an infected joint contains cloudy exudate and sometimes pus. The number of leukocytes is elevated, and the cells are predominantly of the polymorphonuclear type.

Although bacterial growth is obtained in only 62% of cases,[95] when positive it confirms the diagnosis of septic arthritis. The most commonly isolated organism from patients with septic arthritis of the TMJ is *Staphylococcus aureus*,[105,106] although isolation and growth of the other organisms, such as gonococci[102] and viruses,[107] have also been reported.

Diagnosis

The diagnosis of septic arthritis should be considered in all cases of monoarthritis associated with high-grade fever, acute severe pain, and tenderness of the TMJ. The diagnosis is confirmed by identification of the organism in the joint aspirate. In the absence of such a laboratory finding, the clinical presentation, radiographic features, other positive laboratory values, and response to antibiotic therapy should provide a basis for the diagnosis.[108–110] The differential diagnosis should include RA with acute exacerbation, JRA, PA, traumatic arthritis, viral polyarthritis, disseminated malignancy, and gout.

Lyme Disease–Associated Arthritis

Lyme disease (named after Lyme, Connecticut) is a multisystem disorder that involves the skin, joints, nervous system, and heart. It is caused by the spirochete *Borrelia burgdorferi*, and is mostly transmitted by the tick *Ixodes dammini*. Since the first report of the disease in 1977,[111] it has spread rapidly from the five Northeast Atlantic seaboard states, Wisconsin, and Minnesota (where the disease was originally described) to the rest of the United States, Europe, China, and Australia.[112] Although the disease usually affects only one or two large joints, often the knee, the TMJ can also be involved.[113,114]

Clinical findings

The initial presentation of the disease is marked by the appearance of a characteristic skin lesion called erythema chronicum migrans (ECM), a clinical marker for Lyme disease. ECM begins as a red macule or papule at the site of a tick or insect bite. Days to a month later, the lesion expands to an average diameter of 10 cm (range, 8 to 68 cm), with partial clearing of the center of the lesion (Fig 15-4). The outer borders become red and generally flat, while the center is indurated, vesicular, or necrotic. The lesions are usually warm but not painful. They are frequently associated with constitutional symptoms such as fever, malaise, headaches, and regional lymphadenopathy.[116] Generalized lymphadenopathy and splenomegaly are less common findings.

Within a few days to months of the onset of ECM, secondary lesions develop. These lesions are similar in appearance to the ECM but are usually smaller, migrate less, lack the indurated centers, and are not associated with tick bite sites. In some patients, the secondary lesions are associated with a malar rash, conjunctivitis, or, rarely, with a diffuse urticaria.[1,3] Other systemic signs include neurologic involvement, which appears at the same time as the ECM or weeks to months later. They also include meningoencephalitis, vertigo, short-term memory loss, numbness or tingling of the extremities, atypical facial pain, and bilateral facial nerve paralysis. Cardiac abnormalities are less common, can last from a few days to several weeks, and may be recurrent. They include atrioventricular block, myopericarditis, and cardiomegaly.[116]

Musculoskeletal involvement by Lyme disease occurs in approximately 60% of patients and appears from a few weeks to 7 years after the onset of the disease. The arthritis is usually manifested as a migratory polyarthritis or myalgia associated with joint swelling. Months to years later, frank arthritis occurs, characterized by intermittent attacks of painful swelling of one or two large peripheral joints such as the knee. The pain is often episodic and of short duration, followed by periods of complete remission and then recurrence. The affected joints are usually swollen and may be warm but are rarely erythematous. Occasionally, joint involvement is polyarticular and symmetric, including the small joints of the hands and feet.

In approximately 10% of patients with arthritic signs of Lyme disease, the condition evolves into chronic arthritis, causing deformity and disability.[3]

Diagnosis

Because many of the signs and symptoms of Lyme disease are nonspecific and may mimic TMJ involvement from other causes, the diagnosis can be difficult, especially in the early stages. Therefore, these conditions should be included in the differential diagnosis. The diagnosis of Lyme disease can be facilitated by a history of tick bite and skin rash. In the absence of such a history, the diagnosis is more difficult, but the presence of an immunoglobulin M antibody to spirochetes may be a helpful diagnostic test.

B burgdorferi has also been cultured from the skin lesions of ECM[116] and from several body fluids, including the synovial fluid of affected joints.[117] Lyme arthritis that persists after antibiotic treatment is correlated with persistence of the spirochete in the synovial fluid.[118]

Other laboratory findings useful in the diagnosis include an elevated white blood cell count in the synovial fluid (approximately 25,000/µL) that consists mostly of neutrophils, and an elevated serum aspartate aminotransferase.[4]

Metabolic Arthritis

Gout and Pseudogout

Gout (uric acid arthritis) and pseudogout (pyrophosphate arthropathy, chondrocalcinosis articularis, and calcium pyrophosphate dihydrate arthropathy) are the two main types of metabolic arthritis affecting the TMJ.[23,119] They are characterized by inflammation of the joint tissues caused by deposition of microcrystals in the synovium. In gout these crystals are sodium urate and in pseudogout they are calcium pyrophosphate dihydrate.

Gout is characterized by an increase in the serum level of uric acid, generally arising from an inherited anomaly that causes an increase in purine (and uric acid) production and/or a decrease in the excretion of uric acid in the urine. However, it may also be caused by an increase in uric acid production resulting from blood dyscrasias (where cells rich in purine are broken down) or by use of certain medications, such as diuretics.

Pseudogout is regarded by some as an independent disease that often occurs in association with other metabolic diseases, such as hyperparathyroidism and diabetes mellitus.[23]

Gout is uncommon in both men and women younger than 40 years; it mostly affects men older than 40 years. A suggestion of genetic inheritance exists, with a family prevalence that varies from 40% to 60%. The disease is often associated with tophi (urate deposits) in and around the ear and joints of the extremities, renal disease, uric acid nephrolithiasis, and some degree of renal failure. Although the prevalence of gout is 5% among men 65 years and older and 2% among women of the same age,[119] only a few cases of TMJ involvement have been reported.[119,120] The exact prevalence of pseudogout in the TMJ is uncertain, but it frequently affects persons after the age of 40 to 50 years and has an equal sex predilection.[120,121]

Clinical findings

The clinical presentation of a metabolic arthropathy is quite characteristic. The onset is usually sudden and is most often monoarticular, affecting the proximal inter-phalanx of the great toe (Fig 15-5), the ankle, and the wrists and causing pain and swelling in about 50% to 70% of patients. The affected joint is usually erythematous, warm, and extremely tender. In the acute presentation of the disease, the patient may feel ill and feverish.

When the TMJ is involved, the patient's ability to open the mouth wide and masticate is significantly decreased.[119,121,122] Occasionally, the onset and presentation may be less dramatic in the TMJ than in other joints, and the signs and symptoms are less severe. The latter include mild pain, limited mouth opening, and noise in the joint.

Imaging findings

Radiographic changes do not become apparent in the joint until several years after the onset of gout. Although no specific radiographic features exist for gout, the changes in the advanced form of the disease have been described as bony erosion, "punched out" cystic lesions of the bone, bone spurs, and exostoses.

In the case of pseudogout, osseous tophi within the joint and calcification of the disc may be demonstrable in the radiographs (see Fig 10-43). The crystal deposits may have a punctate or linear appearance.[23,121]

Laboratory findings

Typically, the serum uric acid level is elevated in gout. Aspiration of joint fluid reveals an opalescent fluid; monosodium urate crystals are present when the fluid is examined under the polarizing microscope. Acute attacks are generally associated with leukocytosis and an elevated ESR. In pseudogout, the serum uric acid is increased in only 30% of patients.[23]

Diagnosis

The diagnosis of gout can be readily made if the disease presents in its acute form. If the symptoms are mild, determination of the serum uric acid level may be helpful. Because the serum uric acid level may also be increased in numerous other conditions, the diagnosis can only be confirmed by identification of uric acid crystals in the synovial fluid, in the radiograph, or in the surgical specimen. The monosodium urate crystals are needle shaped and have a strongly negative birefringence when examined by compensated polarized light microscopy. In the absence of such findings, a past history of acute synovitis (especially in the great toe), a history of renal colic, and a family history of gout make the diagnosis more likely. The differential diagnosis of gout should include septic arthritis, pseudogout, acute RA, PA, OA, and local trauma.

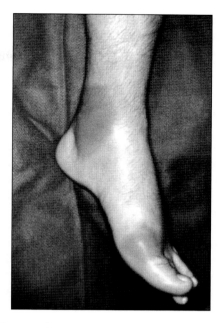

Fig 15-5 Gouty arthritis involving the base of the big toe and the ankle during an acute attack in a patient with gout. (©1972–2004 American College of Rheumatology Clinical Slide Collection. Used with permission.)

Traumatic Arthritis

The term *traumatic arthritis* is generally used to describe the immediate intra-articular response of the joint tissues to single or repetitive episodes of acute trauma.[3] This response is manifested in the form of pathologic and clinical states, the nature of which is generally determined by the magnitude of the trauma sustained by the joint tissues.[123] Minor trauma to the joint tissue may result in compression, or shearing of the retrodiscal tissue and capsule or dislocation of the disc.

Moderate trauma may cause damage to the synovial lining, resulting in subsequent edema and mild serohemorrhagic effusion that can cause hemarthrosis and an inflammatory response in the synovial membrane. This inflammation may eventually result in a hypertrophic synovial response and fibrosis, causing cicatricial contractions and adhesions between the joint components and even fibrous ankylosis. In children, traumatic arthritis can cause growth abnormalities, malocclusion, and facial asymmetry. Severe trauma, short of producing a condylar fracture, can cause damage to the articular surfaces, subchondral bone or both, eventually predisposing to or causing degenerative joint disease.

Clinical Findings

Characteristically, acute traumatic arthritis causes severe jaw pain both at rest and with movement. The joint is tender to palpation, occasionally swollen, and has a decreased range of motion. Effusion in the joint space and edema or hemorrhage in the retrodiscal tissue can cause an increased distance between the articulating components on the traumatized side that results in a posterior open bite. The acute symptoms usually subside within a few days or weeks.[42] In cases of severe trauma, however, the condition may eventually progress to persistent limitation of motion, ganglion formation, intra-articular disc derangement, or degenerative joint disease.

Imaging Findings

The edema and swelling of the intracapsular and capsular structures can cause an increase in their thickness. This can be reflected radiographically as an increased distance between the roof of the glenoid fossa and the condylar surface in the closed-mouth position. Late severe traumatic changes in the joint may be manifested as degenerative joint disease or as bony ankylosis.

Diagnosis

Because no specific features of traumatic arthritis exist, the diagnosis is based primarily on a history of trauma and on the absence of the characteristic features of the other forms of arthritis. A thorough history must be taken and a careful physical examination of the TMJ must be performed after injury to rule out condylar or other mandibular fractures. The use of arthroscopy to evaluate the intra-articular disc and lavage the joint after condylar trauma has been reported, but the long-term benefit of such a procedure is still uncertain.[124,125]

Summary

Arthritis is the most common disease affecting the TMJ. All of the forms that involve other joints in the body also occur in this joint. Therefore, these conditions must be considered in the differential diagnosis whenever a patient presents with chronic TMJ pain and dysfunction.

Acknowledgment

The material in this chapter has been adapted from: Abubaker AO. Differential diagnosis of arthritis of the temporomandibular joint. Oral Maxillofac Surg Clin North Am 1995;7:1–20.

References

1. Katz WA. Diagnosis and Management of Rheumatic Diseases, ed 2. Philadelphia: Lippincott, 1988.
2. Yelin E. Arthritis: The cumulative impact of a common condition. Arthritis Rheum 1992;35:489–497.
3. McCarthy DJ. Differential diagnosis of arthritis; analysis of signs and symptoms. In: McCarthy DJ. Arthritis and Allied Conditions: A Textbook of Rheumatology, ed 9. Philadelphia: Lea & Febiger, 1979:37–50.
4. Kelly W, Harris E, Ruddy S, et al (eds). Textbook of Rheumatology. Philadelphia: Saunders, 1981:1021.
5. Larheim TA, Smith HJ, Asperstraud F. Rheumatic diseases of the temporomandibular joint: MR imaging and tomographic manifestations. Radiology 1990;175:527–531.
6. Gates G. Radionuclide diagnosis. In: Laskin DM, (ed). Oral and Maxillofacial Surgery, vol 1. St Louis: Mosby, 1980: 463–545.
7. Pogrel M. Quantitative assessment of isotope activity in temporomandibular joint regions as a means for assessing unilateral condylar hypertrophy. Oral Surg Oral Med Oral Pathol 1985;60:15–17.
8. Epstein J, Ruprecht A. Bone scintigraphy: An aid in diagnosis and management of facial pain associated with osteoarthrosis. Oral Surg Oral Med Oral Pathol 1982;53:37–42.
9. Melchiorre D, Calderazzi A, Maddali Bongi S, et al. A comparison of ultrasonography and magnetic resonance imaging in the evaluation of temporomandibular joint involvement in rheumatoid arthritis and psoriatic arthritis. Rheumatology (Oxford) 2003;42:673–676.
10. Nordahl S, Alstergren P, Eliasson S, Kopp S. Interleukin-1β in plasma and synovial fluid in relation to radiographic changes in arthritic temporomandibular joints. Eur J Oral Sci 1998;106:559–563.

11. Kubota E, Kubota T, Matsumoto J, Shibata T, Murakami KI. Synovial fluid cytokines and proteinases as markers of temporomandibular joint disease. J Oral Maxillofac Surg 1998; 56:192–198.

12. Wilson JD, Braunwald E, Isselbacher KJ, et al (eds). Harrison's Principles of Internal Medicine, ed 12. New York: McGraw-Hill, 1991.

13. Akerman S, Kopp S, Nilner M, Petersson A, Rohlin M. Relationship between clinical and radiologic findings of the temporomandibular joint in rheumatoid arthritis. Oral Surg Oral Med Oral Pathol 1988;66:639–643.

14. Ogus H. Rheumatoid arthritis of the temporomandibular joint. Br J Oral Surg 1975;12:275–284.

15. Tabeling HG, Dolwick MF. Rheumatoid arthritis: Diagnosis and treatment. Fla Dent J 1985;56:16–18.

16. Koh ET, Yap AU, Koh CK, Chee TS, Chan SP, Boudville IC. Temporomandibular disorders in rheumatoid arthritis. J Rheumatol 1999;26:1918–1922.

17. Ruderman M, Miller LM, Pinals RS. Clinical and serologic observations on 27 patients with Felty's syndrome. Arthritis Rheum 1968;11:377–384.

18. Larheim TA, Floystrand F. Temporomandibular joint abnormalities and bite force in a group of adults with rheumatoid arthritis. J Oral Rehabil 1985;12:477–482.

19. Syrjanen SM. The temporomandibular joint in rheumatoid arthritis. Acta Radiol Diagn (Stockh) 1985;26:235–243.

20. Tegelberg A, Kopp S. Clinical findings in the stomatognathic system of individuals with rheumatoid arthritis and osteoarthrosis. Acta Odontol Scand 1987;45:65–75.

21. Yoshida A, Higuchi Y, Kondo M, Tabata O, Ohishi M. Range of motion of the temporomandibular joint in rheumatoid arthritis: Relationship to the severity of disease. Cranio 1998;16:162–167.

22. Irby W, Zetz R. Osteoarthritis and rheumatoid arthritis affecting the temporomandibular joint. In: Laskin D (ed). The President's Conference on the Examination, Diagnosis and Management of TMJ Disorders. Chicago: American Dental Association, 1982:1–50.

23. Carlsson GE, Kopp S, Oberg T. Arthritis and allied diseases of the TMJ. In: Zarb GA, Carlsson GE (eds). Temporomandibular Joint Function and Dysfunction. St Louis, Mosby, 1979:269–320.

24. Larheim TA, Haanæs HR.. Micrognathia, temporomandibular joint changes and dental occlusion in juvenile rheumatoid arthritis of adolescents and adults. Scand J Dent Res 1981;89:329–338.

25. Fileni A, Amato L, Brizi MG. Radiologic findings related to the TMJ in cases of rheumatoid arthritis. RAYS (Milan) 1968;11:49–51.

26. Voog U, Alstergren P, Eliasson S, Leibur E, Kallikorm R, Kopp S. Progression of radiographic changes in the temporomandibular joints of patients with rheumatoid arthritis in relation to inflammatory markers and mediators in the blood. Acta Odontol Scand 2004;62:7–13.

27. Narvaez JA, Narvaez J, Roca Y, Aguilera C. MR imaging assessment of clinical problems in rheumatoid arthritis. Eur Radiol 2002;12:1819–1828.

28. Gynther GW, Tronje G, Holmlund AB. Radiographic changes in the temporomandibular joint in patients with generalized osteoarthritis and rheumatoid arthritis. Oral Surg Oral Med Oral Pathol Oral Radiol Endod 1996;81: 613–618.

29. Chalmers IM, Blair GS. Rheumatoid arthritis of the temporomandibular joint. A clinical and radiological study using circular tomography. Q J Med 1973;42:369–386.

30. Celiker R, Gokce-Kutsal Y, Eryilmaz M. Temporomandibular joint involvement in rheumatoid arthritis. Relationship with disease activity. Scand J Rheumatol 1995;24:22–25.

31. Zide MF, Carlton DM, Kent JN. Rheumatoid disease and related arthropathies. 1. Systemic findings, medical therapy, and peripheral joint surgery. Oral Surg Oral Med Oral Pathol 1986;61:119–125.

32. Gewanter HL, Roghmann KJ, Baum J. The prevalence of juvenile arthritis. Arthritis Rheum 1983;26:599–603.

33. Larheim TA, Hoeraal HM, Starbrun EA, Haanæs HR. The temporomandibular joint in juvenile rheumatoid arthritis: Radiographic changes related to clinical and laboratory parameters in 100 children. Scand J Rheumatol 1982;11:5–12.

34. Svensson B, Adell R, Kopp S. Temporomandibular disorders in juvenile chronic arthritis patients. A clinical study. Swed Dent J 2000;24:83–92.

35. Harper RP, Brown CM, Triplett MM, Villasenor A, Gatchel RJ. Masticatory function in patients with juvenile rheumatoid arthritis. Pediatr Dent 2000;22:200–206.

36. Ronchezel MV, Hilario MO, Goldenberg J, et al. Temporomandibular joint and mandibular growth alterations in patients with juvenile rheumatoid arthritis J Rheumatol 1995;22:1956–1961.

37. Mericle PM, Wilson VK, Moore TL, et al. Effects of polyarticular and pauciarticular onset juvenile rheumatoid arthritis on facial and mandibular growth. J Rheumatol 1996;23: 159–165.

38. Kjellberg H. Craniofacial growth in juvenile chronic arthritis. Acta Odontol Scand 1998;56:360–365.

39. Hanna VE, Rider SF, Moore TL, et al. Effects of systemic onset juvenile rheumatoid arthritis on facial morphology and temporomandibular joint form and function. J Rheumatol 1996;23:155–158.

40. Taylor B, Babyn P, Blaser S, et al. MR evaluation of the temporomandibular joint in juvenile rheumatoid arthritis. J Comput Assist Tomogr 1993;17:449–454.

41. Kuseler A, Pedersen TK, Herlin T, Gelineck J. Contrast enhanced magnetic resonance imaging as a method to diagnose early inflammatory changes in the temporomandibular joint in children with juvenile chronic arthritis. J Rheumatol 1998;25:1406–1412.

42. Worth HM. Radiology of the temporomandibular joint. In: Zarb GA, Carlson GE (eds). Temporomandibular Joint: Function and Dysfunction. St Louis: Mosby, 1979:321–372.

43. Pearson MH, Ronning O. Lesions of the mandibular condyle in juvenile chronic arthritis. Br J Orthod 1996;23:49–56.

44. Hanna VE, Rider SF, Moore TL, et al. Effects of systemic onset juvenile rheumatoid arthritis on facial morphology and temporomandibular joint form and function. J Rheumatol 1996;23:155–158.

45. Hellgren L. Association between rheumatoid arthritis and psoriasis in total populations. Acta Rheumatol Scand 1969;15:316–326.

46. van Romunde LK, Valkenburg HA, Swart-Bruinsma W, Cats A, Hermans J. Psoriasis and arthritis. 1. A population study. Rheumatol Int 1984;4:55–60.

47. Espinoza LR, Cuellar ML, Silveira LH. Psoriatic arthritis. Curr Opin Rheumatol 1992;4:470–478.

48. Laurent R. Psoriatic arthritis. Clin Rheum Dis 1985;11:61–85.

49. Gladman D, Shuckett R, Russell M, et al. Psoriatic arthritis—Clinical laboratory analysis of 215 patients [abstract]. Ann R Coll Phys Surg Can 1984;17:359.

50. Moll J, Wright V. Psoriatic arthritis. Semin Arthritis Rheum 1973;3:55–78.

51. Koorbusch GE, Zeiter DL, Fotos PG, Doss JB. Psoriatic arthritis of the temporomandibular joint with ankylosis. Oral Surg Oral Med Oral Pathol 1991;17:267–274.

52. Miles DA, Kaugars GA. Psoriatic involvement of the temporomandibular joint: Literature review and report of two cases. Oral Surg Oral Med Oral Pathol 1991;71:770–774 [erratum 1991;72:363].

53. Wilson A, Brown JS, Ord RA. Psoriatic arthropathy of the temporomandibular joint. Oral Surg Oral Med Oral Pathol 1990;70:555–558.

54. Kononen M. Craniomandibular disorders in psoriasis. Community Dent Oral Epidemiol 1987;15:108–112.

55. Blair G. Psoriatic arthritis and the temporomandibular joint. J Dent 1976;4:123–128.

56. Wood N, Stankler L. Psoriatic arthritis of the temporomandibular joint. Br Dent J 1983;154:17–18.

57. Stern R. The epidemiology of joint complaints in patients with psoriasis. J Rheumatol 1985;12:315–320.

58. Pines A, Ejrenfeld M, Fisman E, et al. Mitral valve prolapse in psoriatic arthritis. Arch Intern Med 1986;146:1371–1373.

59. Melchiorre D, Calderazzi A, Maddali Bongi S, et al. A comparison of ultrasonography and magnetic resonance imaging in the evaluation of temporomandibular joint involvement in rheumatoid arthritis and psoriatic arthritis. Rheumatology (Oxford) 2003;42:673–676.

60. Kononen M, Kilpinen E. Comparison of three radiographic methods in screening of temporomandibular joint involvement in patients with psoriatic arthritis. Acta Odontol Scand 1990;48:271–277.

61. Carter ET, McKenna CH, Brian DD, Kurland LT. Epidemiology of ankylosing spondylitis in Rochester, Minnesota, 1935–1973. Arthritis Rheum 1979;22:365–370.

62. Crum RJ, Loiselle RJ. Temporomandibular joint symptoms and ankylosing spondylitis. J Am Dent Assoc 1971;83:630–633.

63. Resnick D. Temporomandibular joint involvement in ankylosing spondylitis: Comparison with rheumatoid arthritis and psoriasis. Radiology 1974;112:587–591.

64. Wenneberg B. Inflammatory involvement of the temporomandibular joint. Diagnostic and therapeutic aspects and a study of individuals with ankylosing spondylitis. Swed Dent J Suppl 1983;20:1–54.

65. Heir GM, Berrett A, Worth DA. Diagnosis and management of TMJ involvement in ankylosing spondylitis. J Craniomandib Pract 1983;1:75–81.

66. Sanders B. Temporomandibular joint ankylosis secondary to Marie-Strümpell disease. J Oral Surg 1975;33:784–786.

67. Wenneberg B, Hollender L, Kopp S. Radiographic changes in the temporomandibular joint in ankylosing spondylitis. Dentomaxillofac Radiol 1983;12:25–30.

68. Ramos-Remus C, Major P, Gomez-Vargas A, et al. Temporomandibular joint osseous morphology in a consecutive sample of ankylosing spondylitis patients. Ann Rheum Dis 1997;56:103–107.

69. Ramos-Remus C, Perez-Rocha O, Ludwig RN, et al. Magnetic resonance changes in the temporomandibular joint in ankylosing spondylitis. J Rheumatol 1997;24:123–127.

70. Ogryzlo MA. Ankylosing spondylitis. In: Hollander JL (ed). Arthritis and Allied Conditions, ed 8. Philadelphia: Lea & Febiger, 1972:399–523.

71. Wenneberg B, Kononen M, Kallenberg A. Radiographic changes in the temporomandibular joint of patients with rheumatoid arthritis, psoriatic arthritis, and ankylosing spondylitis. J Craniomandib Disord 1990;4:35–39.

72. Bomalaski JS, Jiminez SA. Erosive arthritis of the temporomandibular joint of Reiter's syndrome. J Rheumatol 1984;11:400–402.

73. Kononen M, Kovero O, Wenneberg B, Konttinen YT. Radiographic signs in the temporomandibular joint in Reiter's disease. J Orofac Pain 2002;16:143–147.

74. Bole G. Osteoarthritis. In: Cohen A, Bennett J (eds). Rheumatology and Immunology, ed 2. New York: Grune & Stratton, 1986:345–354.

75. Moll J. Osteoarthritis. In: Moll J (ed). Rheumatology in Clinical Practice, ed 2. Boston: Blackwell, 1987.

76. Kellgren JH, Moore R. Generalized osteoarthritis and Heberden's nodes. Br Med J 1952;1(4751):181–187.

77. Macalister AD. A microscopic study of the human temporomandibular joint. N Z Dent J 1954;50:161–172.

78. Dijkgraaf LC, Liem RS, de Bont LG. Synovial membrane involvement in osteoarthritic temporomandibular joints: A light microscopic study. Oral Surg Oral Med Oral Pathol Oral Radiol Endod 1997;83:373–386.

79. Mejersjo C. Therapeutic and prognostic considerations in TMJ osteoarthrosis: A literature review and a long term study in 11 subjects. Cranio 1987;5:6978.

80. Toller P. Temporomandibular arthropathy. Proc R Soc Med 1974;67:153–159.

81. Hansson TL. Pathological aspects of arthritides and derangements. In: Sarnat BG, Laskin DM (eds). The Temporomandibular Joint: A Biological Basis for Clinical Practice, ed 4. Philadelphia: Saunders, 1992:165–182.

82. Gray R. Pain dysfunction syndrome and osteoarthrosis related to unilateral and bilateral TMJ symptoms. J Dent 1986;14:156–159.

83. Rohlin M, Westesson PL, Eriksson L. The correlation of TMJ sounds with joint morphology in fifty-five autopsy specimens. J Oral Maxillofac Surg 1985;43:194–200.

84. Lipstate J, Ball G. Osteoarthritis. In: Ball G, Koopman W (eds). Clinical Rheumatology. Philadelphia: Saunders, 1986:304–314.

85. Laskin DM. Diagnosis of pathology of the temporomandibular joint: Clinical and imaging perspectives. Radiol Clin North Am 1993;31:135–147.

86. Stegenga B. Osteoarthritis of the temporomandibular joint organ and its relationship to disc displacement. J Orofac Pain 2001;15:193–205.

87. Blackwood H. Arthritis of the mandibular joint. Br Dent J 1963;115:317–324.

88. Hansson L, Hansson T, Petersson A. A comparison between clinical and radiologic findings in 259 TMJ patients. J Prosthet Dent 1983;50:89–94.

89. Brandlmaier I, Bertram S, Rudisch A, Bodner G, Emshoff R. Temporomandibular joint osteoarthrosis diagnosed with high resolution ultrasonography versus magnetic resonance imaging: How reliable is high resolution ultrasonography? J Oral Rehabil 2003;30:812–817.

90. Israel HA, Saed-Nejad F, Ratcliffe A. Early diagnosis of osteoarthrosis of the temporomandibular joint: Correlation between arthroscopic diagnosis and keratan sulfate levels in the synovial fluid. J Oral Maxillofac Surg 1991;49:708–711; discussion 712.

91. Nishimura M, Segami N, Kaneyama K, Suzuki T, Miyamaru M. Relationships between pain-related mediators and both synovitis and joint pain in patients with internal derangements and osteoarthritis of the temporomandibular joint. Oral Surg Oral Med Oral Pathol Oral Radiol Endod 2002;94:328–332.

92. Emshoff R, Puffer P, Rudisch A, Gassner R. Temporomandibular joint pain: Relationship to internal derangement type, osteoarthrosis, and synovial fluid mediator level of tumor necrosis factor-alpha. Oral Surg Oral Med Oral Pathol Oral Radiol Endod 2000;90:442–449.

93. Kubota E, Imamura H, Kubota T, Shibata T, Murakami K. Interleukin 1 beta and stromelysin (MMP3) activity of synovial fluid as possible markers of osteoarthritis in the temporomandibular joint. J Oral Maxillofac Surg 1997;55:20–27; discussion 27–28.

94. Laskin DM, Greene CS. Assessment of orofacial pain. In: Turk DC, Melzak R (eds). Handbook of Pain Assessment. New York: Crawford Press, 1992:49–60.

95. Leighty SM, Spach DM, Myall RW, et al. Septic arthritis of the temporomandibular joint: Review of literature and report of two cases in children. Int J Oral Maxillofac Surg 1993;22: 292–297.

96. Irby WB. Etiologic factors in TMJ pain, muscle dysfunction, and mandibular hypomobility. In: Irby WB (ed). Current Advances in Oral Surgery, vol 3. St Louis: Mosby, 1980: 227–252.

97. Topazian RG. Etiology of ankylosis of temporomandibular joint: Analysis of 44 cases. J Oral Anesth Surg Hosp Dent Serv 1964;22:227–233.

98. Thomson HG. Septic arthritis of the temporomandibular joint complicating otitis externa. J Laryngol Otol 1989;103: 319–321.

99. McCain JP, Zabiegalski NA, Levine RL. Joint infection as a complication of temporomandibular joint arthroscopy: A case report. J Oral Maxillofac Surg 1993;51:1389–1392.

100. Haug R, Picard U, Matejczyk MB, Indresano AT. The infected prosthetic total temporomandibular joint replacement: Report of two cases. J Oral Maxillofac Surg 1989;47:1210–1214.

101. Hilbert L, Peters WJ, Tepperman PS. Temporomandibular joint destruction after a burn. Burns Incl Therm Injury 1984;10: 214–216.

102. Chue PWY. Gonococcal arthritis of the temporomandibular joint. Oral Surg Oral Med Oral Pathol 1975;39:572–577.

103. Bounds GA, Hopkins R, Sugar A. Septic arthritis of the temporo-mandibular joint: A problematic diagnosis. Br J Oral Maxillofac Surg 1987;25:61–67.

104. Tang JSH, Gold RH, Bassett LW, Seeger LL. Musculoskeletal infection of the extremities: Evaluation with MR imaging. Radiology 1988;166:205–209.

105. Regev E, Koplewitz BZ, Nitzan DW, Bar-Ziv J. Ankylosis of the temporomandibular joint as a sequela of septic arthritis and neonatal sepsis. Pediatr Infect Dis J 2003;22:99–101.

106. Wang CL, Wang SM, Yang YJ, Tsai CH, Liu CC. Septic arthritis in children: Relationship of causative pathogens, complications, and outcome. J Microbiol Immunol Infect 2003;36: 41–46.

107. Gue TB, Bonner WM Jr. Articular manifestations of infectious hepatitis. J S C Med Assoc 1967;63:279–281.

108. Goldenberg DL, Reed JI. Bacterial arthritis. N Engl J Med 1985;312:764–771.

109. Morrey BF, Bianco AJ Jr, Rhodes KH. Septic arthritis in children. Orthop Clin North Am 1975;6:923–934.

110. Newman JH. Review of septic arthritis throughout the antibiotic era. Ann Rheum Dis 1976;35:198–205.

111. Steere AC, Malawista SE, Syndman DR, et al. Lyme arthritis: An epidemic of oligoarticular arthritis in children and adults in three Connecticut communities. Arthritis Rheum 1977;20:7–17.

112. MacDonald AB. Lyme disease: A neuro-ophthalamologic view. J Clin Neuroophthalmol 1987;7:185–190.

113. Harris RJ. Lyme disease involving the temporomandibular joint. J Oral Maxillofac Surg 1988;46:78–79.

114. Lader E. Lyme disease misdiagnosed as a temporomandibular joint disorder. J Prosthet Dent 1990;63:82–85.

115. Kaplan SA, Buchbinder D. Arthritis. In: Kaplan SA, Assael CA (eds). Temporomandibular Disorders: Diagnosis and Treatment. Philadelphia: Saunders, 1991:165–189.

116. Berger BW, Kaplan MH, Rothenberg IR, Barbour AG. Isolation and characterization of the Lyme disease spirochete from the skin of patients with erythema chronicum migrans. J Am Acad Dermatol 1985;13:444–449.

117. Liebling MR, Nishio MJ, Rodriguez A, Sigal LH, Jin T, Louie JS. The polymerase chain reaction for the detection of *Borrelia burgdorferi* in human body fluids. Arthritis Rheum 1993;36:665–675.

118. Nocton JJ, Dressler F, Rutldege BJ, Rys PN, Persing DH, Steere AC. Detection of *Borrelia burgdorferi* DNA by polymerase chain reaction in synovial fluid from patients with Lyme disease arthritis. N Engl J Med 1994;330:229–234.

119. Gross BD, Williams RB, DiCosimo CJ, Williams SV. Gout and pseudogout of the temporomandibular joint. Oral Med Oral Surg Oral Pathol 1987;63:551–554.

120. De Vos RAI, Brants J, Kusen GJ, Becker AE. Calcium pyrophosphate dihydrate arthropathy of the temporomandibular joint. Oral Surg Oral Med Oral Pathol 1981;51:497–502.

121. Good AE, Upton LG. Acute temporomandibular arthritis in a patient with bruxism and calcium pyrophosphate deposition disease. Arthritis Rheum 1982;25:353–355.

122. Hutton CW, Doherty M, Dieppe PA. Acute pseudogout of the temporomandibular joint: A report of three cases and review of the literature. Br J Rheumatol 1987;26:51–52.

123. Freyberg R. The joints. In: Sodeman W, Sodeman W Jr (eds). Pathologic Physiology: Mechanisms of Disease. Philadelphia: Saunders, 1967:935–959.

124. Goss AN, Bosanquet AG. The arthroscopic appearance of acute temporomandibular joint trauma. J Oral Maxillofac Surg 1990;48:780–783; discussion 784.

125. Nuelle DG, Alpern MC, Ufema JW. Arthroscopic surgery of the temporomandibular joint. Angle Orthod 1986;56:118–142.

Internal Derangements

Daniel M. Laskin

Dentists have long been aware that clicking and popping sounds, as well as locking, can occur in the temporo-mandibular joint (TMJ) as a result of derangement of the intra-articular disc. In fact, in 1887 Annandale[1] wrote, "It is an affliction occurring principally in delicate women, and has been thought to depend upon relaxation of the ligaments of the joint permitting free movement of the bone and possibly a slipping of the intra-articular carti-lage." However, it was not until the technique of arthrog-raphy, first introduced by Nörgaard,[2] was refined[3,4] that the mechanisms underlying these phenomena were finally understood. As a result, the ability to diagnose these conditions has improved considerably and this has led to more successful management.

Classification

An internal derangement of the TMJ can be defined as an abnormal relationship between the mandibular condyle and the intra-articular disc when the teeth are in occlu-sion. In the strictest anatomic interpretation, this implies that the posterior band of the disc is forward of the 12-o'clock position. However, it has been shown that the disc can be in a slightly more anterior position without causing a person to have any symptoms of joint noise, pain, or dysfunction.[5,6]

Internal derangements can be classified into four main categories. The earliest indication of an internal derange-ment has been referred to as an *incoordination phase*. Gen-erally, the patient is unaware of the condition because there is no joint noise or obvious dysfunction. However, when asked to open and close the mouth during an oral examination and questioned about whether the jaw joint moves smoothly, such patients will state that they feel a slight catching sensation. This is the earliest indication that there has been an increase in the frictional properties of the joint.

In the next category, the intra-articular disc has slipped forward and mouth opening is accompanied by a clicking or popping sound. This percussive sound is pro-duced as the condyle passes over the posterior band and returns to a normal relationship with the disc (Fig 16-1). This stage is generally referred to as *anterior disc displace-ment with reduction (ADDwr)*. However, although the con-dition is called *anterior displacement*, anatomically the disc generally lies in an anteromedial position because of the angulation of the condyle and the direction of pull of the lateral pterygoid muscle.

In some patients with ADDwr, a second clicking sound is heard during mouth closure. This has been referred to as a *reciprocal click*, and it occurs as the posterior band of the disc slips forward off the condyle during the closing movement (see Fig 16-1). However, even though such a sound is not heard in every patient, the disc must still slip off the condyle during closure for repetitive clicking on mouth opening to occur. Thus, the presence or absence of a detectable reciprocal click has no clinical significance.

Although clicking sounds in the TMJ are generally pro-duced by anterior disc displacement, occasionally such sounds also can be caused by an irregularity or defect in the surface of the disc or by morphologic changes in the condyle and/or articular eminence.[8] In such instances, these areas act as an impediment to forward movement of the condyle, and the sound is produced as it over-comes this obstruction. These sounds are usually not as pronounced as those caused by anterior disc displace-

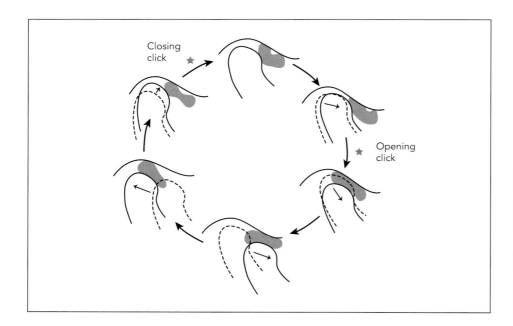

Closing click

Opening click

Fig 16-1 Anterior displacement of the intra-articular disc with reduction on mouth opening. A clicking or popping sound occurs as the disc returns to its normal position in relation to the condyle. During mouth closure, the disc again becomes anteriorly displaced, sometimes accompanied by a second sound (reciprocal click). (Reprinted from McCarty[7p155] with permission.)

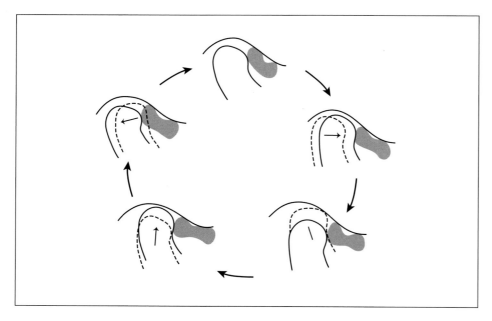

Fig 16-2 Anterior displacement of the intra-articular disc without reduction on attempted mouth opening. The displaced disc acts as a barrier and prevents full translation of the condyle. (Reprinted from McCarty[7p151] with permission.)

ment. Moreover, they also differ because they occur at the same point in the translatory cycle during mouth opening and closing rather than at different points, as occurs when reciprocal clicking is present.

In the third category of internal derangement, the intra-articular disc is located even further forward and the condyle is unable to pass over the posterior band on attempted mouth opening. As a result, there is locking rather than clicking, and the condyle rotates but does not translate (Fig 16-2). This stage is generally referred to as *anterior disc displacement without reduction (ADDwoR)* or *closed lock*.

The fourth category of internal derangement is also characterized by limitation of mouth opening, but is not caused by disc displacement. Rather, the disc is in normal position, but there is adhesion of the disc to the articular eminence so that only condylar rotation can occur (Fig 16-3).

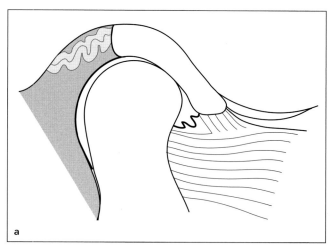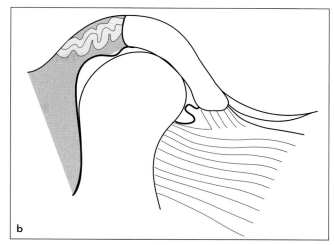

Fig 16-3 Adhesion of the intra-articular disc, resulting in limitation of mouth opening. (Reprinted from Kaplan and Assael[9] with permission.) *(a)* The disc is adherent to the articular eminence in the normal position when the mouth is closed. *(b)* During mouth opening, the disc does not move; this limits condylar translation. Because the condyle can only rotate, mouth opening is limited to 25 to 30 mm.

Clinical Diagnosis

Incoordination

A clinical diagnosis of incoordination is based on the patient's report of a catching sensation or hesitation in the TMJ during mouth opening. It is unaccompanied by joint noise, limitation in mouth opening, or joint tenderness or pain.

Anterior Disc Displacement with Reduction

Patients with ADDwr may be asymptomatic except for the clicking or popping sound, or they may have associated symptoms of joint tenderness on lateral and intrameatal palpation, joint pain that is increased with function, and limitation of mouth opening. When the condition is unilateral, the mandible may deviate to the affected side on mouth opening. In the late stages, the patient may also complain of intermittent locking, which is eliminated by active jiggling or manual manipulation of the jaw. Patients with ADDwr will frequently also have muscle pain, either because of protective splinting of the mandible to limit movement or because of the myofascial pain associated

with chronic parafunction. In the latter instance, the patient may also complain of frequent headache.

Anterior Disc Displacement Without Reduction

The main complaint of patients with ADDwoR is a sudden onset of inability to open the mouth widely, associated with localized pain in the TMJ that increases with attempted mouth opening and chewing. The patient generally also experiences joint tenderness on lateral and intrameatal palpation. In unilateral cases, the mandible will deviate to the affected side with attempted mouth opening. In most instances, there will be a prior history of clicking or popping in the involved joint.

Disc Adhesion to the Articular Eminence

Disc adhesion is also characterized by a sudden onset of restricted mouth opening, but, because the disc is not anatomically displaced, the highly innervated retrodiscal tissue is not compressed; therefore, there is generally no pain unless the patient attempts to open the mouth or chew, which stretches the joint capsule. Because this condition often occurs in persons with chronic tooth-clenching and tooth-grinding habits, it is frequently associated with myofascial pain.

Other Conditions to Consider in Differential Diagnosis

In establishing a diagnosis of internal disc derangement in the TMJ, the clinician must consider a number of other conditions that can cause joints sounds or limited mouth opening. For example, hypertrophy or an osteochondroma of the coronoid process can cause both a limitation in mouth opening and a clicking sound as the enlarged coronoid process passes the zygomatic arch.[10] Irregularities in the surface of the disc can also produce clicking sounds, even though the disc is not displaced.

Intra-articular causes of jaw limitation unrelated to the disc include various forms of arthritis, synovial chondromatosis, and primary and secondary neoplasms involving the TMJ. Extra-articular causes of limited mouth opening, such as myofascial pain, myositis, myositis ossificans, scleroderma, masticatory muscle fibrosis and scarring, hysterical trismus, and depressed fracture of the zygomatic arch, also must be considered in the differential diagnosis. Among the factors that can help distinguish most of these conditions from the limitation in mouth opening produced by an internal derangement are their more gradual onset and the absence of a prior history of clicking and popping.

Imaging Diagnosis

Although in the past arthrography was the most common technique used for imaging the intra-articular disc, the current gold standard is magnetic resonance imaging (MRI). The only current indication for the use of arthrography is to determine or confirm the presence of a perforation in the disc or retrodiscal tissue. Under these circumstances, both the upper and lower joint spaces will fill simultaneously when the first joint space is injected with the radiopaque medium.

With MRI, sequential views starting with the patient's mouth closed and progressing incrementally to the widest possible mouth opening clearly demonstrate the functional relationship between the disc and condyle. Under normal circumstances, the posterior band of the disc is generally located approximately at the 12-o'clock position when the mouth is closed (see Fig 10-1a and 10-1c), although a slightly more anterior position has also been found in normal subjects.[11,12] When the mouth is open, the disc is located between the condyle and the crest of the articular eminence and has a bow-tie configuration (see Fig 10-3c).

In the incoordination stage, the magnetic resonance image is also normal. However, in the patient with clicking or popping in the TMJ, the disc will be anteriorly displaced (forward of the 12-o'clock position) in the closed-mouth sagittal view (see Fig 10-10a). As the patient opens the mouth and a click or pop occurs, the magnetic resonance image will show the disc back in normal relationship with the condyle and it will again have a bow-tie appearance (see Fig 10-10b). In patients with a nonreducing, anteriorly displaced disc (ADDwoR), the disc is located more anteriorly in the closed-mouth position than it is in patients with ADDwr. Moreover, the disc remains anteriorly displaced during attempted mouth opening (see Fig 10-7).

Although disc displacement occurs most frequently in an anteromedial direction, it has been shown that posterior, medial, and lateral displacements also can occur[13] (see Figs 10-8 and 10-9). The last two possibilities are visible only on coronal magnetic resonance image. Because the disc is innervated on its margins, such displacements can account for the presence of pain in the TMJ even though the sagittal magnetic resonance image appears to show that the disc is in normal position.

To avoid the need for an expensive procedure such as MRI, clinicians often make the mistake of trying to determine if the disc is anteriorly displaced based on an evaluation of the width of the joint space in a plain radiograph,[14,15] a panoramic radiograph, or a tomogram. In such circumstances, these clinicians assume that an anteriorly displaced disc will result in a narrowing of the joint space because the condyle is now articulating with the thinner retrodiscal tissue. Even if this were true, and it is not,[16,17] the determination would still be questionable because it is not possible to accurately visualize the joint space on these images. In a plain radiograph, such as a transcranial view, the observer is looking at the widest part of the condyle opposite the narrowest part of the fossa; therefore, even in the normal joint, the intra-articular space appears narrow. In a panoramic radiograph, the inability to compensate for the horizontal and vertical angles of the condyle because of the standardized focal trough generally results in a tangential image that is wider than the actual condyle; this produces an artifactually narrowed joint space.

In a tomogram of the TMJ, each radiographic slice presumably shows that part of the glenoid fossa that is directly opposite any given part of the condyle. However, this is only true if the patient's head is positioned to compensate for the horizontal and vertical condylar angles when the radiograph is made (corrected tomography),[18] so that the radiographic cut is not tangential. Even when this is accomplished, it is unlikely that corrected tomography is sensitive enough to show a difference in the width of the joint space of normal subjects and in patients with anteriorly displaced, nonreducing discs because of the wide variation in both groups.

It has also been proposed that, rather than causing a narrowing of the joint space, anterior disc displacement causes a posterior displacement of the condyle in the glenoid fossa.[14] However, it has been shown that patients with anteriorly displaced, nonreducing discs do not have significantly different condylar positions from normal, asymptomatic subjects.[19]

Because of the possible serious consequences of treating a patient for an internal derangement based on presumptive radiographic evidence, radiographs should never be used as a substitute for magnetic resonance imaging in determining disc position. On the other hand, in patients with a history of persistent clicking or popping in the TMJ, it is generally not necessary to use MRI to establish a diagnosis of ADDwr since the outcome is quite predictable. This is also true when the sudden inability to open the mouth widely is preceded by a history of persistent clicking or popping. However, when locking is present and the prior history is unclear, or when the patient denies ever having clicking in the TMJ, MRI should be performed to distinguish between ADDwoR and disc adhesion.

Summary

If clinicians understand the mechanisms involved in the production of TMJ clicking and locking related to displacement of the intra-articular disc, they can usually make the correct diagnosis on the basis of the history and the clinical findings without the need for imaging. However, when these findings are unclear, proper imaging should be completed before treatment is initiated. This involves the use of MRI. The use of plain radiographs, panoramic radiography, and tomography is not diagnostic for this purpose.

References

1. Annandale T. Displacement of the inter-articular cartilage of the lower jaw, and its treatment by operation. Lancet 1887;1:411.

2. Nörgaard F. Temporomandibular Arthrography [thesis]. Copenhagen: Munksgaard, 1947.

3. Toller PA. Opaque arthrography of the temporomandibular joint. Int J Oral Surg 1974;3:17–28.

4. Wilkes CH. Arthrography of the temporomandibular joint in patients with TMJ pain-dysfunction syndrome. Minn Med 1978;61:645–652.

5. Westesson P-L. Double contrast arthography and internal derangements of the temporomandibular joint. Swed Dent J 1982;(suppl 13):1–57.

6. Katzberg RW. Temporomandibular joint imaging. Radiology 1989;170:297–307.

7. McCarty W. Diagnosis and treatment of internal derangements of the articular disc and mandibular condyle. In: Solberg WK, Clark GT (eds). Temporomandibular Joint Problems: Biologic Diagnosis and Treatment. Chicago: Quintessence, 1980:145–168.

8. Isberg-Holm A, Ivarsson R. The movement pattern of the mandibular condyles in individuals with and without clicking. A clinical cineradiographic study. Dentomaxillofac Radiol 1980;9:58–69.

9. Kaplan AS, Assael LA. Temporomandibular Disorders: Diagnosis and Treatment. Philadelphia: Saunders, 1991:158.

10. Shackelford RT, Brown WH. Osteochondroma of the mandible. Surg Gynecol Obstet 1943;77:51–54.

11. Westesson PL, Eriksson L, Kurita K. Temporomandibular joint: Variation of normal arthrographic anatomy. Oral Surg Oral Med Oral Pathol 1990;69:514–519.

12. Kircos LT, Ortendahl DA, Mark AS, Arakawa M. Magnetic resonance imaging of the TMJ disc in asymptomatic volunteers. J Oral Maxillofac Surg 1987;45:852–854.

13. Leidberg J, Westesson PL, Kurita K. Sideways and rotational displacement of the temporomandibular joint disc: Diagnosis by arthrography and correlation to cryosectional morphology. Oral Surg Oral Med Oral Pathol 1990;69:757–763.

14. Weinberg L. Correlation of temporomandibular dysfunction with radiographic findings. J Prosthet Dent 1972;28:519–539.

15. Farrar WB. Characteristics of the condylar path in internal derangements of the TMJ. J Prosthet Dent 1978;39:319–323.

16. Bean L, Thomas C. Significance of condylar position in patients with temporomandibular disorders. J Am Dent Assoc 1987;114:76–77.

17. Ronquillo H, Guay J, Tallents RH, Katzberg RW, Murphy W. Tomographic analysis of mandibular condyle position as compared to arthrographic findings in the temporomandibular joint. J Craniomandib Disord 1988;2:59–64.

18. Rosenberg HM, Graczyk RJ. Temporomandibular articulation tomography: A corrected anteroposterior and lateral cephalometric technique. Oral Surg Oral Med Oral Pathol 1986;62:198–204.

19. Katzberg RW, Keith DA, Ten Eick WR, Guralnick WC. Internal derangements of the temporomandibular joint: An assessment of condylar position in centric occlusion. J Prosthet Dent 1983;49:250–254.

Masticatory Muscle Pain and Dysfunction

Yoly M. Gonzalez and Norman D. Mohl

There is consensus that pain is the most common feature of most masticatory muscle disorders. However, mandibular dysfunction, such as limited range of motion and chewing difficulties, can also occur. The most common type of masticatory muscle disorder is myofascial pain, but several other muscular disorders, as well as other conditions, have to be considered during the process of differential diagnosis. The muscular disorders include regional problems such as myositis, myospasm, local (nonspecific) myalgia, myofibrotic contracture, and neoplasia[1] as well as the problem of centrally mediated chronic muscle pain (Table 17-1 and Box 17-1). However, these must be differentiated from the primary temporomandibular joint (TMJ) disorders, particularly those that involve pain associated with osteoarthritis, disc displacement, or jaw dysfunction.

In addition, a number of orofacial conditions that are characterized by pain and/or jaw dysfunction also must be considered in the differential diagnosis. Among these are toothache, pericoronitis, maxillary sinusitis, earache, salivary gland pathosis, temporal arteritis, neuralgias, and tension-type headache (see chapter 20). The differential diagnosis of masticatory muscle pain and dysfunction becomes even more complicated when patients have a systemic disorder, such as fibromyalgia, because the clinical features of these disorders have considerable overlap (see chapter 22).

Masticatory Muscle Disorders

Myofascial Pain

Myofascial pain is the most commonly reported type of masticatory muscle disorder as well as the most common type of temporomandibular disorder (TMD).[2,3] It is characterized by a dull regional ache that increases during function. Palpation may reveal localized tender sites in one or more of the masticatory muscles and, in some cases, such palpation can trigger pain in other areas.[1,4] These myofascial symptoms may sometimes be accompanied by tension-type headache, earache, or toothache; an unverifiable sensation of an acute malocclusion; a sensation of muscle stiffness; and a reduced range of motion of the mandible.[1]

These criteria are consistent with the Muscle Diagnosis group of the Axis I section of the Research Diagnostic Criteria for Temporomandibular Disorders (RDC/TMD).[5] The Muscle Diagnosis group of TMDs includes the subgroups myofascial pain with and without limited range of motion, implying that this painful condition may or may not be accompanied by jaw dysfunction. Because the RDC/TMD was developed for research purposes, it was necessary for the diagnostic criteria to be defined in a way that enhances reliability and validity of the diagnostic

Table 17-1	Diagnostic criteria for masticatory muscle disorders	
Disorder	**Definition**	**Diagnostic criteria**
Myofascial pain	Chronic regional muscle pain	Complaint of pain Tenderness on palpation with replication of chief complaint Pain increased by mandibular function or parafunction Affected ROM Possible presence of trigger points
Myospasm	Rare acute condition of involuntary and continuous muscle contraction	Localized pain Limited ROM/dysfunction Electromyography by needle or fine wire for definitive diagnosis
Local myalgia	Acute muscle pain; may be due to protective muscle splinting, postexercise muscle soreness, muscle fatigue, and/or pain from ischemia	Muscle pain and history, after other muscle conditions are ruled out
Myofibrotic contracture	Painless shortening of muscle as a result of fibrosis	Limited ROM/dysfunction Resistance to passive stretch
Neoplasia	Benign or malignant	Presence or absence of pain Structural changes and history Imaging and biopsy for definitive diagnosis
Centrally mediated chronic muscle pain	Chronic generalized muscle pain associated with comorbid conditions	History and biobehavioral assessment Presence of comorbid conditions

outcome and thus reduce the likelihood of false-positive and false-negative diagnoses. As a result, the diagnostic inclusion and exclusion criteria are very specific. For example, the identification of myofascial pain requires the existence of at least three positive palpation sites from among 20 specific locations on several specific muscles.

For purely clinical (nonresearch) purposes, however, these rigid criteria are probably not necessary or even desirable. This means that a patient who has all of the clinical features of myofascial pain but exhibits tenderness in only one or two muscle palpation sites is still a patient and deserves to be cared for accordingly. Despite this limitation, the specifications for clinical examination developed for the RDC/TMD have definite application in the nonresearch clinical environment and are therefore highly recommended.

Myositis

Myositis is a primary inflammation of muscle resulting from infection or trauma. It is characterized by constant acute pain in one or more of the masticatory muscles and is usually accompanied by swelling, redness of the overly-ing skin, and increased temperature over the affected muscle.[1] As a result of the pain and swelling, jaw dysfunction, particularly moderate-to-severe limited range of motion and pain on movement, is a characteristic feature of myositis. Myositis can be differentiated from myofascial pain by the acuteness, quality, and constancy of the reported pain, its associated sequelae, the patient's acute and unambiguous responses to muscle palpation, and a history of recent trauma or infection.

Myospasm

Myospasm, often referred to as a *muscle cramp*, is an acute but rare condition resulting from a sudden, involuntary, and continuous tonic contraction of a muscle or muscles. It is characterized by localized acute pain and severely limited range of motion of the mandible. These characteristics, coupled with their sudden onset at rest, allows the clinician to differentiate myospasm from other masticatory muscle disorders. The term *muscle spasm* has been incorrectly used to describe myofascial pain, but it is now clear that muscles are not in spasm in that condition. Electromyography using needle electrodes can be used to confirm the presence of

Box 17-1	Diagnostic criteria for myofascial pain*

Primary findings
- Patient complaint of pain in one or more masticatory muscles
- Tenderness or pain upon palpation of the masticatory muscles, with replication of the chief complaint
- Tender site pain can be referred to other orofacial areas (trigger points)
- Pain aggravated by mandibular function

Secondary findings
- Restricted ROM
- Maximum assisted opening > maximum unassisted opening > pain-free opening
- ROM increased by use of vapocoolants
- Limited function
- Clinical or behavioral indications of hyperfunction or parafunction
- Acute malocclusion

Possible findings
- TMJ pain
- Joint sounds
- Inflammation
- Restricted ROM unmodified by assisted opening or vapocoolants

myospasm and rule out myofascial pain or other masticatory muscle disorders (see chapter 12).

Local (Nonspecific or Unclassified) Myalgia

Myalgia refers to a general category of acute muscle pain disorders whose etiology and pathology cannot currently be explained and whose clinical features have not been systematically studied or classified. They include conditions such as the protective muscle splinting that accompanies joint inflammation or injury, delayed postexercise muscle soreness, muscle fatigue, and pain from ischemia, among others. Because of the diversity of conditions in this category, their diagnosis can only be based on the objective evaluation of the information gained from a thorough history and clinical examination and after other possible diagnoses are ruled out.[1]

Myofibrotic Contracture

This condition involves a painless shortening of muscle as a result of fibrosis (scarring) in and around the remaining contractile muscle tissue. The disorder often follows an infectious process or trauma-produced myositis, particularly if the patient has experienced a long period of limited range of motion or masticatory function. Although not painful, the myofibrotic contracture results in easily recognizable jaw dysfunction characterized by limited mouth

opening and an unyielding resistance to passive jaw-muscle stretch (hard end-feel).[1]

Neoplasia

As with any tissue or system, the masticatory muscles can also be sites of benign or malignant tumors, some of which can be painful. Depending on the location and size, jaw dysfunction also can occur. In addition to producing structural changes, muscle neoplasms can lead to deviation of the mandible and acute malocclusions. Tumors of the masticatory muscles must be differentiated from adaptive muscle hypertrophy, parotid gland disease, enlarged lymph nodes, or any other regional growth or swelling. However, any muscle disorder suspected of involving a neoplasm requires timely and appropriate imaging and a biopsy for microscopic examination.[1]

Centrally Mediated Chronic Muscle Pain

Masticatory muscle pain, particularly myofascial pain and unclassified myalgia, can sometimes be a regional manifestation of a widespread centrally mediated chronic pain phenomenon such as fibromyalgia (chapter 22). Thus, the diagnostic protocol must include information about other areas or sites in the body that have been consistently painful or tender. In addition, masticatory muscle pain, for whatever reason, can itself become chronic as a result of central mediation. This again emphasizes the importance of gaining information about the duration of the patient's pain complaints.

Any chronic TMD pain situation calls for a thorough psychological diagnostic assessment, such as that promulgated in RDC/TMD Axis II.[5] Such an assessment is necessary to determine if the patient's chronic pain is related to depression, anxiety, somatization, or other psychological, psychosocial, or psychiatric conditions. Failure to recognize these factors will seriously undermine the diagnosis and the effectiveness of subsequent management (see chapter 13 for more detailed information on this subject).

Conditions That Mimic Masticatory Muscle Pain

The literature is replete with case reports in which the signs and symptoms of masticatory muscle pain coexisted with or were initially mistaken for another disorder or disease. Among these conditions are toothache; earache; maxillary sinusitis and carcinoma of the maxillary sinus; trigeminal and other neuralgias; salivary gland pathosis; acromegaly; carcinoma of the nasopharynx; Eagle's syndrome; temporal arteritis; migraine, tension, and other headaches; and angina pectoris.

A complete discussion of these conditions is beyond the scope of this chapter and the reader is referred to other sources, including chapters 20 and 22 in section IIB of this book. However, because so many conditions can be confused with masticatory muscle pain, a thorough and structured diagnostic protocol is required when any patient with orofacial pain is evaluated.

Conditions That Produce Jaw Dysfunction

Jaw dysfunction can be defined as a disturbance, impairment, or abnormality of the function of the mandible. This definition would encompass conditions such as a reduction in the normal mandibular range of motion, a diminished ability to masticate, and a change in the ability to close the mandible into the patient's optimal or normal occlusion (malocclusion).

A primary cause of jaw dysfunction is orofacial pain, particularly when jaw movement increases the pain. Examples of this would be myofascial pain, myositis, and localized myalgia as well as osteoarthritis and arthralgia of the TMJ. Soft or hard tissue swellings in the masticatory system or the contiguous tissues from infection or neoplasia, such as myositis, cellulitis, parotitis, or a condylar

osteochondroma, also interferes with normal jaw function. Fibrosis and scarring, such as occurs in myofibrotic contracture, TMJ ankylosis, and scleroderma, will certainly lead to jaw dysfunction. In addition, acute or developing structural changes, such as nonreducing derangements of the intra-articular disc or hyperplasia of the coronoid process, can interfere with normal jaw function.

The diagnostic problem for the clinician is to obtain sufficient reliable information to determine (differentiate) which disorder, disease, or condition accounts for a patient's particular type of jaw dysfunction. Useful information can be gained from the clinical examination that can differentiate jaw dysfunction resulting from masticatory muscle disorders from dysfunction related to the TMJ. For example, a patient with limited ability to open the mouth, but with a soft end-feel on maximum assisted opening, is more likely to have a masticatory muscle disorder than myofibrotic contracture or a fibrous ankylosis. Furthermore, a patient who has limited ability to open the mouth but who can still move the mandible horizontally (lateral excursion) is more likely to have a masticatory muscle disorder than an intracapsular TMJ disorder, in which both the vertical and horizontal ranges of motion are limited.

The absence of dysfunction does not always rule out the existence of a muscle condition. Some individuals may overcome their dysfunctional limitations by adapting to a new functional status to avoid their symptoms.

Diagnostic Protocol

The gold standard for the differential diagnosis of masticatory muscle pain is the same as that for other TMDs and for most, if not all, other types of orofacial pain. This involves an analytical evaluation of the information gained from the chief complaint, the history of the chief complaint, the dental, medical and psychosocial history, and the clinical examination.

This protocol can be supplemented, when indicated, by imaging of the TMJ or other structures. However, the only image that should be obtained on a routine or screening basis is a panoramic radiograph to detect possible dental, periodontal, or other potential problems that could be the source of the patient's pain. The phrase "common things occur commonly" is appropriate to remember. The decision to obtain other images, particularly of the TMJ, should be deferred until the diagnostic protocol is leading in the direction of a disorder other than masticatory muscle pain.

This diagnostic protocol (in fact, any diagnostic protocol) also must include consideration of alternative diagnoses or alternative hypotheses. Ultimately, this process is intended to reduce uncertainty to the point at which the clinician reaches a reasonable, but never absolute, working diagnosis.[6]

It is also important to remember that a diagnosis of a masticatory muscle condition should not be made until the diagnostic protocol has been completed and a working diagnosis established. Telephone diagnoses, diagnoses suggested by the patients, or presumptive diagnoses made by referring physicians and dentists are never definitive and are therefore never acceptable. The assumption that a patient's orofacial pain complaint is myogenous may lead to self-fulfilling prophesies, which, when coupled with a clinician's preexisting biases, can result in an inaccurate diagnosis and inappropriate treatment.[6]

Chief Complaint and Related History

The chief complaint is the typical reason that patients seek professional help. Although pain, joint sounds, and functional jaw limitation are the most common chief complaints, pain is unquestionably the most prevalent reason. In addition to the chief or primary complaint, patients may describe other symptoms that accompanied the onset of the pain or that accompany the pain episodes. Reports of symptoms such as nausea, photophobia, phonophobia, vertigo, loss of equilibrium, and so on, can provide key information that better enables the clinician to arrive at a reasonable differential diagnosis.

It is best to record the chief complaint in the patient's own words, because this allows the clinician to gain some idea of which system is involved and to create a framework for obtaining more detailed information during the subsequent interview. It also provides some insight into the patient's expectations. A patient could have more than one complaint, requiring that each be addressed according to the patient's reported order of severity. The report of more than one complaint could also suggest that the patient has more than one orofacial pain disorder, therefore requiring more than one diagnosis. Recording the chief complaint in the patient's own words has medicolegal implications, because it establishes a basis upon which progress or lack of progress can be judged.

If the chief complaint is pain, as is highly likely, the clinician should gather all relevant information about the characteristics of that pain. A summary of the pain characteristics that should be recorded during the initial patient interview (ie, location, quality, intensity, onset, pattern, duration, chronicity, modifiers, and associated symptoms), can be found in Box 17-2.

Patients should first be asked to describe and, if possible, identify the location of the pain that they have been experiencing. Asking patients to point to the area or areas where the pain is present helps to identify its location (Fig 17-1). They may point to or touch a specific localized area, or they may respond in a way that suggests that multiple or generalized pain sites are present. In general, patients who specifically localize the facial pain to the preauricular area are most likely identifying an intracapsular TMJ disorder, while those who report diffuse or multiple sites of pain are most likely describing pain of muscle origin. In contrast, patients who are afraid to touch their face because it may bring on a sudden shocklike pain may be suffering from trigeminal neuralgia. Diagrams of the head, face, neck, and upper body are useful tools on which patients can indicate the location or locations of their pain.

There are many descriptors that patients may use to describe the quality of their pain, such as *sharp*, *dull*, *burning*, *electrical*, *aching*, etc. Although these descriptors may help the clinician to differentiate muscular pain from, for example, pain of neuropathic origin, they are not diagnostic per se.

Visual analog scales are very useful instruments that serve to gauge the intensity of the pain or the level of suffering that patients are or have been experiencing. These scales are the best method available to try to quantify an admittedly subjective and very personal sensory experience. Furthermore, when used sequentially, visual analog scales enable the clinician to measure changes in patients' perceived pain intensity (eg, the increase or decrease in pain during the course of intervention). Thus, the use of these instruments is highly recommended.

With regard to onset, pattern, and duration, patients should be asked how long the pain or other symptoms have been present, when and under what conditions their complaints first appeared, and the relative course of the pain since its onset. The initial symptoms may have begun in a gradual or spontaneous way, for no apparent reason, or they may have occurred following some specific event such as a long dental appointment. Questions about the pain pattern provide important information about diurnal, constant, episodic and other pain characteristics over time.

Patients should be asked about so-called modifiers, ie, conditions or situations that exacerbate or diminish the pain. A very effective way to obtain this information is by asking patients what makes their pain better and what makes their pain worse. For example, answers such as, "drinking ice water makes the pain go away," or, "chewing makes the pain worse," are revealing statements that greatly enhance the process of differential diagnosis. Thus, it is important that the clinician obtain as much information as possible about any factors that may mod-

---

Box 17-2 Pain characteristics

Quality
- Patient's description of quality of the pain.
- Pain descriptors can include the terms *sharp, dull, aching, electrical, burning,* etc.

Location
- Patient's description of the location of the pain: A very specific region versus a more generalized area.
- Unilateral versus bilateral pain.
- Pain confined to a particular muscular and/or joint area and/or pain referred to a distant area.

Intensity
- On a scale of 0 to 10, 0 represents no pain and 10 the worst pain that the patient has experienced.

Onset, duration, and pattern
- How long have the pain or other symptoms been present?
- When and under what conditions did the complaints first appear?
- What has been the relative course of the pain since its onset (eg, diurnal, episodic, constant, or fluctuating)?

Modifiers
- What conditions or situations exacerbate or diminish the pain, including self-help methods or past professional treatment?

Chronicity
- Has pain persisted for 3 to 6 months with a record of treatment failures?

Comorbid signs or symptoms
- Does the patient have or experience conditions such as clinical depression, acute anxiety, vomiting, nausea, tearing, visual changes, dizziness, numbness, or generalized pain?

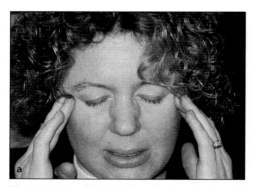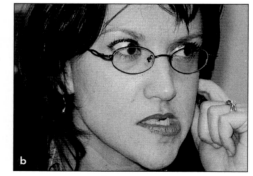

Fig 17-1 *(a and b)* Pain localization by the patient.

ify the course of the pain condition, including self-help methods and past professional interventions.

Information about duration, particularly when past therapeutic attempts have failed, is essential in determining if the condition has become chronic. Chronicity is a very important phenomenon that will have an impact on the differential diagnosis, prognosis, and subsequent management (see Box 17-2; see also chapters 4, 5, and 13 for a discussion of the criteria and implications of chronic pain).

Dental, Medical, and Psychosocial History

In addition to the chief complaint and its history, the information gained from careful questioning of—and listening to—patients regarding their dental, medical, and psychosocial history is pivotal to differentiating masticatory muscle disorders from many other possible orofacial pain conditions (Box 17-3). For example, the medical his-

Box 17-3	Medical history

Systemic conditions
- Past and present illnesses
- History of trauma or surgery to the head, face, or neck
- Operations and hospitalizations
- Current treatments

Current prescription and nonprescription medications
- Prescription or over-the-counter medications being taken for pain associated with the chief complaint or for any other conditions

Review of systems
- Any cardiovascular, dermatologic, gastrointestinal, musculoskeletal, neurologic, otologic, psychiatric, respiratory, or urogenital problems

Dental history
- Recent dental interventions, including dental treatments provided in relation to the chief complaint

Psychosocial history
- Alcohol, tobacco, and recreational drug use
- Changes in patient's life or lifestyle, including family, social, work, financial, and litigation, particularly when associated with onset or duration of the symptoms

tory may help the clinician to determine if the chief complaint is related to a regional phenomenon or is a manifestation of a generalized condition such as fibromyalgia or other systemic disorder.

Information about use of prescription medications, over-the-counter medications, or recreational drugs provides important insight into the medical and/or psychological condition of the individual. In addition, it is important to consider possible drug interactions or side effects, eg, cholesterol-lowering medications that may produce muscle pain.

In taking the dental history, the clinician should obtain information about the type of dental care patients have received or are receiving, if any, and any possible relationship to the current complaints. Questions about the presence or absence of toothache or other intraoral pain, perceived changes in the occlusion, or other oral complaints can provide information about the type and nature of the presumptive disorder.

The psychosocial history is also an integral part of the evaluation, because it can provide very important insights into the differential diagnosis and possible contributing factors. Questions about caffeine, alcohol, tobacco, and recreational drug use, as well as changes in patients' life or lifestyle (eg, in the areas of family, social, work, financial status, or litigation), particularly when associated with the onset or duration of the symptoms, can elicit information about the possible presence of

acute or chronic emotional stress. Stress, which may be present for a variety of intrinsic or extrinsic reasons, can be a major factor underlying oral habits such as bruxism. In addition, stress can affect pain perception, adaptive ability, chronicity, and other factors, so obtaining some information about it is important, particularly when myofascial pain or localized myalgia is among the diagnostic possibilities. Thus, an assessment of these psychosocial factors is a necessary component of the diagnostic protocol. These histories are also vitally important in the assessment of possible comorbid conditions, such as depression, anxiety and somatization (subjects that are thoroughly addressed in chapter 13).

Biobehavioral Assessment

Objective determination of the presence or absence of repetitive or persistent oral behaviors and habits can be difficult, and the same is true for functional limitations of the mandible or other oral structures. Although these behaviors and habits may not have proven diagnostic validity at present, their assessment is important because it provides clinically relevant information about potential causative factors and/or the effects of the disorder on the masticatory system.

In this regard, the Oral Behavior Checklist[7] is a useful instrument for assessing the presence or awareness of oral

Behavior	None of the time	A little of the time	Some of the time	Most of the time	All of the time
Clench or grind teeth when asleep	☐	☐	☐	☐	☐
Sleep in a position that puts pressure on the jaw (eg, on stomach, on the side)	☐	☐	☐	☐	☐
Grind teeth during waking hours	☐	☐	☐	☐	☐
Clench or press teeth together during waking hours	☐	☐	☐	☐	☐
Touch or hold teeth together other than while eating	☐	☐	☐	☐	☐
Hold, tighten, or tense muscles without clenching or bringing teeth together	☐	☐	☐	☐	☐
Hold or jut jaw forward or to the side	☐	☐	☐	☐	☐
Press tongue forcibly against the teeth	☐	☐	☐	☐	☐
Place tongue between the teeth	☐	☐	☐	☐	☐
Bite, chew, or play with tongue, cheeks, or lips	☐	☐	☐	☐	☐
Hold jaw in rigid or tense position to brace or protect the jaw	☐	☐	☐	☐	☐
Bite or hold objects such as hair, pipe, pencil, fingers, fingernails, etc between the teeth	☐	☐	☐	☐	☐
Use chewing gum	☐	☐	☐	☐	☐
Play musical instrument that involves use of the mouth or jaw	☐	☐	☐	☐	☐
Lean with the hand on the jaw, such as cupping or resting the chin in the hand	☐	☐	☐	☐	☐
Chew food on one side only	☐	☐	☐	☐	☐
Eat between meals (food that requires chewing)	☐	☐	☐	☐	☐
Do sustained talking	☐	☐	☐	☐	☐
Sing	☐	☐	☐	☐	☐
Yawn excessively	☐	☐	☐	☐	☐
Hold telephone between the head and shoulder	☐	☐	☐	☐	☐

Fig 17-2 Oral Behaviors Checklist. (Based on Ohrbach et al.[7])

behaviors, because it provides a structured approach to evaluating the functional and parafunctional activities of patients (Fig 17-2). An assessment of functional limitation can be accomplished by using the Jaw Functional Limitation Scale,[8] in which patients are asked to indicate, on a scale of 0 to 10, the level of functional limitation associated with the chief complaint during the last month (Fig 17-3). Although both of these instruments have been developed for research purposes, they do enable the clinician to gather very important information about patients and their problems.

Function	Scale *(circle one)*										
Chewing tough food	0	1	2	3	4	5	6	7	8	9	10
Chewing hard bread	0	1	2	3	4	5	6	7	8	9	10
Chewing chicken (eg, prepared in oven)	0	1	2	3	4	5	6	7	8	9	10
Chewing crackers	0	1	2	3	4	5	6	7	8	9	10
Chewing soft food (eg, macaroni, canned or soft fruits, cooked vegetables, fish)	0	1	2	3	4	5	6	7	8	9	10
Eating soft food requiring no chewing (eg, mashed potatoes, applesauce, pudding, pureed food)	0	1	2	3	4	5	6	7	8	9	10
Opening wide enough to bite a whole apple	0	1	2	3	4	5	6	7	8	9	10
Opening wide enough to bite into a sandwich	0	1	2	3	4	5	6	7	8	9	10
Opening wide enough to talk	0	1	2	3	4	5	6	7	8	9	10
Opening wide enough to drink from a cup	0	1	2	3	4	5	6	7	8	9	10
Swallowing	0	1	2	3	4	5	6	7	8	9	10
Yawning	0	1	2	3	4	5	6	7	8	9	10
Talking	0	1	2	3	4	5	6	7	8	9	10
Singing	0	1	2	3	4	5	6	7	8	9	10
Putting on a happy face	0	1	2	3	4	5	6	7	8	9	10
Putting on an angry face	0	1	2	3	4	5	6	7	8	9	10
Frowning	0	1	2	3	4	5	6	7	8	9	10
Kissing	0	1	2	3	4	5	6	7	8	9	10
Smiling	0	1	2	3	4	5	6	7	8	9	10
Putting on a sad face	0	1	2	3	4	5	6	7	8	9	10
Laughing	0	1	2	3	4	5	6	7	8	9	10

Fig 17-3 Jaw Functional Limitation Scale. (Based on Ohrbach and List.[8]) 0 = no dysfunction, 10 = severe dysfunction.

Clinical Examination

The main objective of the clinical examination is to identify the signs and replicate the symptoms associated with the chief complaint. The examination also serves to identify or rule out conditions that may mimic, but are not necessarily related to, masticatory muscle pain (Box 17-4). The information obtained during the examination should allow the clinician to reduce diagnostic uncertainty by navigating through the diagnostic options in a structured and consistent manner. Toward this end, the examination protocol and techniques recommended in the RDC/TMD are highly recommended.[5]

The clinical evaluation actually begins as soon as the first interaction with the patient commences. During this initial encounter, the clinician should carefully observe such things as body expression and posture, gross and fine motor skills, facial expression and mood, as well as habits that the patient may exhibit while seated in the dental chair (Box 17-5). The face, head, and neck should

Box 17-4	Clinical examination

Facial symmetry
- Evaluation for asymmetry, swelling, inflammation, hypertrophy, and paralysis or paresis.
- Patient awareness and chronicity of the finding are relevant.

Opening pattern
- Evaluation for any deviations during opening, whether corrected or uncorrected, so as to discriminate unilateral from bilateral conditions or to identify self-reducing disc derangements.

Range of motion (ROM)*
- Assessment of vertical ROM includes measurement of pain-free opening, maximum unassisted opening, and maximum assisted opening.
- Average pain-free opening is about 40 ± 3 mm.
- A maximum assisted opening that is greater than the maximum unassisted opening implies that the problem may be muscular and not the result of a mechanical impediment in or around the TMJ.
- Assessment of horizontal ROM includes measurement of lateral and protrusive jaw movements to determine limitations and whether they are unilateral or bilateral.
- Average horizontal ROM is < 7 mm.

Joint palpation
- Detection of joint sounds by palpation with the index and middle fingers in the preauricular region during opening and lateral jaw movements while listening and feeling for sound vibrations.
- Auscultation used to assess mild crepitation or to confirm mild clicks.
- Detection of joint pain by the same palpation technique while asking patient to report presence of tenderness or pain.
- Joint pain can also be detected by applying 1-lb pressure anteriorly in the external auditory meatus with the little finger while the patient's mouth is open and closed and when teeth are in occlusion.

Muscle palpation
- Palpation done unilaterally as patient is asked if any tenderness or pain is the same as or similar to the pain reported as their chief complaint.
- Extraoral sites, assessed using 2 to 4 lb of pressure, include the anterior, middle, and posterior portions of the temporalis muscle; the origin, body, and insertion of the masseter muscle; and the submandibular and posterior mandibular region.
- Intraoral sites, assessed using 1 to 2 lb of pressure, include the lateral pterygoid area and the tendon of the temporalis muscle.

Intraoral examination
- Evaluation for possible odontogenic causes of patient's orofacial pain.
- Examination of oral mucosa, periodontium, and dentition for signs of bruxism or other oral habits, such as wear facets; cheek, nail, or lip biting; lateral tongue scalloping or frictional keratosis from chronic cheek biting; and/or tooth mobility or fremitus, particularly in the absence of attachment loss from periodontal disease.

*All measurements are obtained with a millimeter ruler; the midline is used as a reference point. Reproducibility of these measurements is very consistent.

be evaluated for the presence of asymmetry, developmental abnormalities, trauma, and swelling; this examination should include palpation of lymph nodes, salivary glands, and temporal arteries as well as evaluation of the function of the cranial nerves.

Range of Motion

Observation and recording of the range of motion of the mandible are essential components of the clinical examination. In the vertical plane, pain-free opening of the

Oral habits
- Determination of the presence or absence of repetitive or persistent oral behaviors and habits by observing the patient's communication, interaction, and conduct during the interview.
- Specific instruments, such as the Oral Behaviors Checklist, can be used as a structured assessment of the patient's awareness of parafunctional behaviors.

Functional limitation
- Determination of the presence or absence of functional limitations of the mandible. The Jaw Functional Limitation Scale is an instrument that can provide a structured approach to this assessment.

Comorbid conditions
- Awareness of conditions such as clinical depression, acute anxiety, and somatization during interactions with patients experiencing chronic pain.

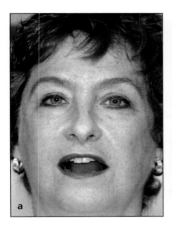 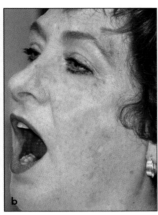 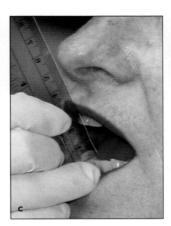 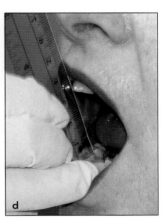

Fig 17-4 (a) Frontal view of pain-free opening. (b) Profile view of maximum unassisted opening. The patient can significantly increase the range of motion, indicating no mechanical interruption of the translation. This may indicate that the condition is muscular. (c) Measuring the interincisal distance of pain-free opening. (d) Measuring the interincisal distance of maximum unassisted opening.

mouth is in the range of 40 ± 3 mm for males and slightly less for females.[9] If the pain-free opening is restricted, it should be compared to maximum unassisted opening and maximum assisted opening, even if pain is present (Fig 17-4). If the interincisal distance during maximum unassisted opening and maximum assisted opening increases several millimeters beyond pain-free opening, it suggests that the patient has a muscle-based limitation, not an intracapsular joint problem.

The pattern of mouth opening and closing can also provide significant clues as to whether the problem is primarily of muscular or intracapsular origin. For example, a corrected unilateral deviation of the mandible on mouth opening, accompanied by a click and return to full midline opening, strongly suggests the presence of a self-reducing disc derangement and not a primary myofascial pain problem.

In the horizontal plane, range of motion is measured by asking patients to move their jaw left, right, and forward as much as possible, even in the presence of pain. Distances and deviations are measured and recorded to assess the significance of any functional limitations (Figs 17-5 and 17-6).

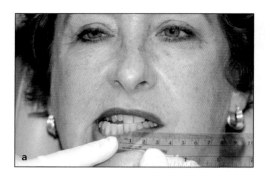

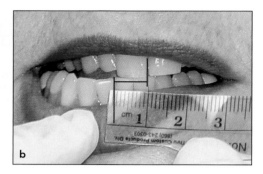

Fig 17-5 *(a and b)* Measuring lateral movement. From the intercuspal position, the patient moves the mandible as far laterally as possible, even if the movement is painful. Measurements are taken from midline to midline.

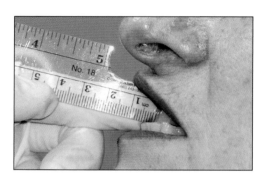

Fig 17-6 Measuring protrusive movement. From the intercuspal position, the patient moves the mandible as far forward as possible, even if the movement is painful. The distance is measured with a ruler.

Joint Sounds

Although joint sounds (especially clicking) are commonly found among patients with either TMJ or masticatory muscle pain, they may also be present without associated pain and therefore they are not pathognomonic for either kind of disorder. Thus, although the presence or absence of joint sounds, whether clicking or crepitation, should be noted and recorded as part of the diagnostic protocol, they have no diagnostic validity in terms of specifically identifying or differentiating one type of pain problem from another (Figs 17-7 and 17-8).

Palpation

Palpation of the masticatory muscles and the TMJ is essential to the diagnosis of any TMD, particularly myofascial pain, myositis, and unclassified myalgias. Because joint soreness on palpation, without significant muscle tenderness, clearly indicates an intracapsular rather than a muscular problem, only muscle palpation techniques are addressed in this chapter.

An accepted method of determining muscle tenderness or pain is to use the fingertips of the middle and index fingers to palpate specific anatomic sites (Figs 17-9 and 17-10). It has been demonstrated that 2 lb of digital pressure on extraoral muscles and 1 lb of digital pressure on intraoral areas,[2,5] held for 3 to 5 seconds, are appropriate procedures for minimizing false-negative and false-positive responses to palpation. The main question is whether patients are able to identify the tenderness or pain from palpation as being the same as or similar to the pain reported as the chief complaint; once patients confirm the replication of the chief complaint, the clinician can be more confident of the diagnosis.

The sites that should be palpated include, but are not necessarily limited to, the anterior, middle, and posterior portions of the temporalis muscle; the origin, body, and insertion of the masseter muscle; the submandibular and posterior mandibular regions; the tendon of temporalis; the lateral pole of the condyle; and, intrameatally, the posterior attachment area. During muscle palpation, attention should be paid to the possible presence of inflammation, hypertrophy, or asymmetry.

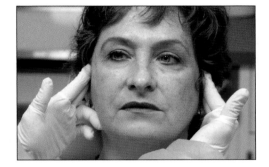

Fig 17-7 Palpation of TMJs for the assessment of joint sounds. The examiner's fingers are placed in the preauricular area and the patient is asked to open and close the mouth.

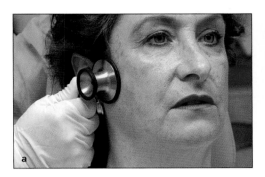

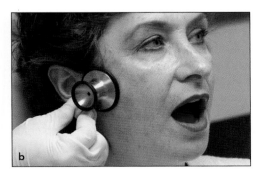

Fig 17-8 Auscultation of the TMJs in the (a) closed-mouth and (b) open-mouth positions. Auscultation becomes very beneficial for the assessment of fine crepitation or to replicate the chief complaint of sounds that are present at the time of the clinical examination and cannot be detected by palpation.

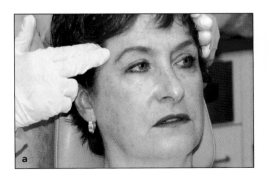

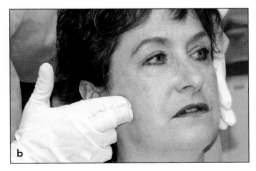

Fig 17-9 Palpation of the masticatory muscles. (a) Extraoral palpation of the anterior temporalis muscle. (b) Extraoral palpation of the masseter muscle.

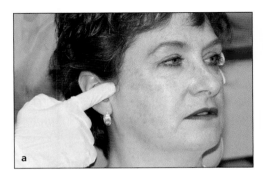

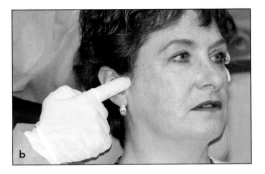

Fig 17-10 (a and b) Palpation of the lateral pole of the condyle. If the condyle is difficult to locate, the patient is asked to protrude the jaw slightly to allow better palpation of the joint and discrimination between it and the deep masseter muscle.

Intraoral Examination

An intraoral examination of presumptive TMD patients should always be conducted to rule out both benign and malignant forms of pathosis that may be causing orofacial pain. Possible dentoalveolar sources of orofacial pain must be identified or ruled out, including deep caries lesions, pulpal hyperemia or pulpitis, cracked teeth, periapical or periodontal abscesses, and pericoronitis. The use of bite-wing, periapical, or panoramic radiographs can be very helpful during this part of the examination. In addition, an examination of the oral mucosa, tongue, and oropharynx is also very important, because one or more of these structures could be the site of a pathologic lesion. Signs of wear facets; cheek, nail, or lip biting; lateral tongue scalloping; frictional keratosis from chronic cheek biting; and tooth mobility or fremitus (particularly in the absence of attachment loss from periodontal disease) strongly suggest the presence of parafunctional oral habits, phenomena that have special relevance to myofascial pain.

Other than identifying any patient-noted acute malocclusion ("my bite feels funny"), which is typically *the result* of a TMD rather than the cause, a specific examination of occlusal relationships is not necessary. Although some authorities continue to argue that such examinations are routinely necessary to establish a diagnosis or to determine an etiology for masticatory muscle pain, the overwhelming evidence from the past 25 years of research shows that neither of these assumptions is correct (see chapters 12 and 27). The presence or absence of occlusal disharmonies cannot be used to substantiate masticatory muscle pain or to differentiate any of these disorders from among other diagnostic possibilities. In addition, it has not been objectively demonstrated that various types of so-called good or poor occlusal relationships have any correlation with the incidence or prevalence of any TMD.

Other Diagnostic Tests

If the results of the history and clinical examination provide a reasonable degree of certainty that the patient is suffering from masticatory muscle pain and not from an intracapsular TMJ disorder, no additional diagnostic testing is routinely required. Other than the use of bitewing, periapical, or panoramic radiographs to look for nonodontogenic pathology or dentoalveolar problems, there is no reason to use additional imaging, including TMJ imaging. Furthermore, the lack of reliability and validity of other diagnostic tests, including electromyography, jaw-tracking devices, sonography, and thermography (see chapter 12) makes them unsuitable for clinical use at ths time. Thus,

the clinical diagnosis of most myogenous TMDs is based primarily on the current gold standard—a thorough history and an appropriate clinical examination.

Conclusion

Despite significant advances during the past 30 years, much more research is needed to elucidate the specific clinical features, the diagnostic criteria, and the pathophysiologic phenomena underlying masticatory muscle disorders. Because of the high prevalence of these problems, the literature is replete with articles on this subject. Unfortunately, many have been based on anecdotal reports of clinical success or on invalidated or unverified clinical evidence.[2] Because myofascial pain is the most commonly reported type of masticatory muscle disorder,[3,10] articles dealing with this type of disorder have been predominant. Fortunately, the clinical research conducted by Laskin and Greene on what they, at the time, called *myofascial pain-dysfunction syndrome* set the standard for soundly designed and unbiased scientific inquiry in this field. The importance of their research accomplishments cannot be overstated, both for the precedent-setting effects and for the valuable data that were produced. For example, these investigations provided important evidence of the role of stress and psychological factors,[11–13] the positive effects of placebo treatments, and the relationship—or lack thereof—of occlusal factors to the etiology of myofascial pain.[14,15] Of particular importance is their evidence that conservative management of myofascial pain is just as effective as, if not more effective than, invasive and irreversible modes of therapy.[16]

Despite these promising early starts, there is still much to learn about masticatory muscle disorders and other types of TMDs. Toward that end, the RDC/TMD was developed and is now being used in many studies and in many locations. However, the RDC/TMD criteria and methods of patient assessment still remain to be scientifically validated. A multicenter study is currently being conducted at three major dental schools (University of Minnesota, University of Washington, and State University of New York at Buffalo),[17] funded by the National Institute of Dental and Craniofacial Research, to determine the reliability and validity of the RDC and other diagnostic tests for TMDs, including masticatory muscle disorders. This ongoing investigation is the first analytical work to test the validity of the diagnostic criteria for some of the conditions discussed in this chapter. Ultimately, the development of a clear and valid diagnostic system will become a milestone for future research in the important but controversy-laden area of temporomandibular disorders.

References

1. Differential diagnosis and management considerations of temporomandibular disorders. In: American Academy of Orofacial Pain, Okeson JP (ed). Orofacial Pain: Guidelines for Assessment, Diagnosis, and Management. Chicago: Quintessence, 1996:113–184.

2. Mohl ND. The anecdotal tradition and the need for evidence-based care for temporomandibular disorders. J Orofac Pain 1999;13:227–231.

3. Schiffman E, Fricton JR, Haley D, et al. The prevalence and treatment needs of subjects with temporomandibular disorders. J Am Dent Assoc 1989;120:295–301.

4. McNeill C, Dubner R. What is pain and how do we classify orofacial pain? In: Lund JP, Lavigne GJ, Dubner R, Sessle BJ (eds). Orofacial Pain: From Basic Science to Clinical Management. Chicago: Quintessence, 2001:3–14.

5. Dworkin SF, LeResche L (eds). Research Diagnostic Criteria for temporomandibular disorders: Review, criteria, examinations and specifications, critique. J Craniomandib Disord 1992;6:302–355.

6. Mohl ND, Ohrbach R. The dilemma of scientific knowledge versus clinical management of temporomandibular disorders. J Prosthet Dent 1992:67:113–120.

7. Ohrbach R, Markiewicz M, McCall WD Jr. Oral Behaviors Checklist: Performance validity of targeted behaviors [abstract 3603]. J Dent Res [serial on CD-ROM]2004;83(special issue A).

8. Ohrbach R, List T. Psychometric properties of the Jaw Functional Limitation Scale [abstract 1023]. J Dent Res 2002;81(special issue A):A-147.

9. Dworkin S, Huggins K, LeResche L, et al. Epidemiology of signs and symptoms in temporomandibular disorders: Clinical signs in cases and controls. J Am Dent Assoc 1990;120:273–281.

10. Lipton JA, Ship JA, Larach-Robinson D. Estimated prevalence and distributions of orofacial pain in the United States. J Am Dent Assoc 1993;124:115–121.

11. Mercuri LG, Olson RO, Laskin DM. The specificity of response to experimental stress in patients with myofascial pain-dysfunction syndrome. J Dent Res 1979;58:1866–1871.

12. Greene CS, Olson RE, Laskin DM. Psychological factors in the etiology, progression, and treatment of MPD syndrome. J Am Dent Assoc 1982;105:443–448.

13. Schwartz RA, Greene CS, Laskin DM. Personality characteristics of patients with myofascial pain-dysfunction (MPD) syndrome unresponsive to conventional therapy. J Dent Res 1979;58:1435–1439.

14. Laskin DM, Greene CS. Influence of the doctor-patient relationship on placebo therapy with myofascial pain-dysfunction (MPD) syndrome. J Am Dent Assoc 1972;85:892–894.

15. Goodman P, Greene CS, Laskin DM. Response of patients with myofascial pain-dysfunction syndrome to mock equilibration. J Am Dent Assoc 1976;92:755–758

16. Greene CS, Laskin DM. Long-term evaluation of conservative treatment for myofascial pain dysfunction syndrome. J Am Dent Assoc 1974;89:1365–1368.

17. Schiffman E. Research Diagnostic Criteria: Reliability and Validity. NIDCR grant DE13331. 2004.

Traumatic Injuries

Dean A. Kolbinson and Frank I. Hohn

Trauma to the temporomandibular joint (TMJ) can occur in many different ways. Major trauma to the joint can be associated with fractures of different components of the mandible, including the symphysis, body, angle, coronoid process, and condylar process; crush injuries; and mandibular dislocation. There can also be minor injuries resulting from either direct or indirect trauma to the TMJ complex, which will produce only soft tissue damage within or around the joint. This chapter discusses the damage caused in the various forms of trauma to the TMJ and the pathophysiology of the tissue changes involved. Management aspects will also be discussed, as will the controversial nature of these topics.

Major Trauma

Fractures of the TMJ Complex

Fractures of the condylar process make up approximately 25% to 50% of all mandibular fractures.[1–3] Accompanying these fractures are both osseous and soft tissue injuries resulting in short-term and, in many cases, long-term dysfunction, deformity, and pain.

Although the primary determinants of the surgical approach to the osseous deformity have always been influenced by the fracture location and the degree of displacement,[4] there historically has been, and continues to be, significant controversy as to the best method of fracture reduction. The primary controversy surrounds the use of a closed reduction versus an open reduction approach and the ensuing degree of posttraumatic deformity and function, depending on the treatment chosen. Even the term *closed reduction*, although still in widespread use, has been challenged in favor of *closed treatment* or *nonsurgical treatment*.[5]

A review of the orthopedic literature echoes a similar controversy to that which oral and maxillofacial surgeons have experienced in the treatment of condylar fractures. In 1961, in *The Closed Treatment of Common Fractures*, Sir John Charnley[6] stated that "perfect anatomical restoration and perfect freedom of joint movement can be obtained simultaneously only by internal fixation." At that time, with the techniques and equipment available, the results of open reduction of fractures were so poor, leading to a high incidence of stiffness, deformity, malunion, and nonunion, that Charnley argued in favor of nonoperative treatment. The frustration and poor results of this era were paralleled in the maxillofacial literature. In 1975, Archer[7] stated, "there is no indication for the open reduction of subcondylar fractures . . . meddlesome surgery in the form of open reduction frequently results in trismus or ankylosis, or sterile or suppurative resorption of the condyle." The miniaturization of rigid fixation systems and the experience gained with arthroscopic intervention for nontraumatic TMJ dysfunction have led to further debate on the indications for, and preferred mechanisms of, open reduction for subcondylar fractures.[8–14]

Zide and Kent[11] originally described the absolute indications for open reduction. Zide[15] later revised these indications. Absolute indications include:

1. Fracture dislocation into the middle cranial fossa or temporal fossa with clinical disability
2. Foreign body in the joint capsule (eg, gunshot wound)
3. Lateral extracapsular displacement of the condyle
4. Inability to open the mouth or bring the mandible into occlusion after 1 week, with radiographic evidence that the fracture segment is in the mechanical path
5. Open fracture in which extensive fibrosis from the injury could occur and that would benefit from rigid fixation and rapid mobilization (eg, gunshot wound)
6. Failure to obtain segment contact with closed reduction because of intervening soft tissue
7. Tympanic plate injury
8. Facial nerve paresis secondary to the initial injury
9. Contraindication to maxillomandibular fixation
10. Open wounds from the initial injury that would provide good access to the fracture site

Relative indications are:

1. Unilateral or bilateral condylar fracture associated with comminuted midfacial fractures
2. Condylar fracture with associated comminuted symphyseal fracture and tooth loss
3. Displaced condylar fracture with clinical evidence of open bite or retrognathia in adults who are developmentally disabled or medically compromised
4. Displaced condylar fracture in an edentulous or a partially edentulous mandible associated with posterior bite collapse
5. Displaced condylar fracture for which treatment was delayed because of concomitant systemic injuries
6. Bilaterally displaced condylar fractures and associated preexisting dental or occlusal abnormalities

For many years, these were the defining principles by which treatment modalities were decided. However, as pointed out by Brandt and Haug,[16] the absolute and relative indications evolved in the years that followed. Zide and Kent,[11] Zide,[15] and Kent et al[17] have contributed to this evolution and transition, perpetuating the controversy. According to the American Association of Oral and Maxillofacial Surgeons, current indications for open reduction include physical evidence of fracture, imaging evidence of fracture, malocclusion, mandibular dysfunction, abnormal relationship of the jaws, presence of foreign bodies, lacerations and/or hemorrhage in the exter-

nal auditory canal, hematotympanum, cerebrospinal fluid otorrhea, effusion, and hemarthrosis.[18]

Despite the controversy regarding the use of open versus closed reduction techniques, the endpoint of successful therapy is universally judged by the following criteria: return to premorbid occlusion, normal mandibular range of motion, pain-free joint function, facial symmetry, and minimal surgical morbidity.[19,20] The role that soft tissue injury plays in the successful outcome after condylar and subcondylar fractures remains largely unexplored.

Associated Soft Tissue Injuries

Historically, the focus of treatment for the traumatized TMJ has centered on the osseous components. Osseous realignment, as determined by radiography, has been the primary determinant of successful treatment outcome. Although the associated soft tissue injuries have long been identified,[21,22] heightened interest in TMJ disorders has fostered emerging ideas about the application of internal derangement treatment procedures to the traumatized joint.[23] The role of the associated periarticular soft tissue injuries and their influence on the outcome of condylar process fractures is now also being considered more carefully. The advent of computerized tomography (CT), magnetic resonance imaging (MRI), and arthroscopic techniques has led to a better understanding of the effect of trauma on the surrounding soft tissues.[22,24–26] In addition, an improved understanding of the biochemical aspects of injury and repair, and their correlation with the TMJ in health and disease, has broadened the biologic basis of treatment.[27] It is not incongruous that soft tissue injury would occur concomitant with osseous injury.

The orthopedic literature describes two common mechanisms of injury resulting in fractures: an indirect force and a direct crushing or axial force. Application of indirect force, the more common of the two mechanisms, produces a bending moment that drives a part of the joint into its opposing articular surface. The surrounding ligamentous and capsular components typically resist this load, thereby causing fracture of the joint surface and resulting in a partial articular fracture. The second, less common mechanism, a direct crushing or axial application of force, causes an explosion of the bone into the soft tissues.[28]

During macrotrauma to the TMJ, it is inevitable that periarticular soft tissue injury as well as injury to the interpositional disc and fibrocartilaginous articular surfaces will occur, regardless of the mechanism of injury. It is relatively easy to determine the amount of energy absorbed by the bone during injury, as evidenced by the presence or absence of a fracture. However, the extent of soft tissue injury is more difficult to qualify and quantify. Studies in the orthopedic literature reveal that hyaline cartilage can fracture prior to bone and that even a single blow can alter the biochemical composition of the fibrocartilaginous matrix.[29,30]

As early as 1961, Pauwels[31] suggested that an equilibrium existed between regeneration and degeneration of articular cartilage, depending on the biochemical environment of the joint. These orthopedic principles of injury are similar in many ways to those in the patient who experiences TMJ trauma. However, some aspects of macrotraumatic soft tissue injury in the TMJ are still poorly understood. Rowe and Killey[32] have discussed the similarity of the TMJ to other joints possessing serous or hemorrhagic effusion. They also suggested that tearing of the lateral pterygoid muscle or the temporomandibular ligament can occur with trauma. It has further been suggested that the intra-articular disc can be displaced following macrotrauma to the TMJ.[33] The most frequently described injuries to the nonosseous structures of the TMJ include hemarthrosis, disc avulsion, and disruption of the lateral capsule.[25,26,34–36] Adhesions and anteriorly displaced discs have also been reported.[37–39]

A bilateral arthroscopic evaluation of 20 patients with mandibular fractures was performed by Goss and Bosanquet.[36] Although 15 patients had fractures of the condylar process (75%), only one joint (out of 40) had a "normal" intra-articular evaluation. The most common injuries included hemarthrosis with shredding of the disc and the articular surface. The most recently injured joints showed more hyperemia of the capsule and hemarthrosis. This was confirmed by Jones and Van Sickels,[26] who also noted more hyperemia of the synovial lining and synovial proliferation but less blood than in those joints examined after a 24-hour delay.

Some experimental histologic evidence of TMJ trauma has been documented in the literature.[40,41] In a rat model, impact trauma was created and the ipsilateral condyle was examined. Proliferative changes, manifested by repair or by a hyperplastic process in the glenoid fossa and mandibular ramus, were observed. These hyperplastic changes seemed to be more intense when the articular disc was torn.

In guinea pigs, indirect trauma via a blow to the symphysis and direct trauma via a blow to both TMJs produced hemorrhage, enlargement of the disc, adhesion of the disc to the condyle, and fracture of the condyle. Degenerative changes in the muscles adjacent to the TMJ were more common in the group subjected to indirect trauma, as were soft tissue changes (ie, fibrosis) adjacent to the TMJ. Direct trauma usually caused injuries in the condyle and the adjacent tissues, such as the disc and glenoid fossa.[41]

It has been suggested that mouth position (open versus closed) may have an influence on the injury sustained by the various structures of the TMJ complex. A closed-mouth position with the teeth in maximum intercuspation dissipates the force of the injury over a larger area, including the dentition and TMJs. However, when trauma occurs while the mouth is open or the mandible is in a relaxed position, more forces are transmitted to the articular structures, muscles, and tendons.[42]

In a study of patients with condylar or subcondylar fractures who underwent MRI preoperatively and after open reduction, the joint capsule and retrodiscal tissues were both noted to be swollen, and some also exhibited tears. All discs were displaced in an anteromedial direction along with the fractured condylar fragment, but no ruptures were recognized. Signal intensity was high in the joint spaces in all cases, and hemarthrosis was recognized in some of these joints during open reduction surgery.[34] Once again, the suggestion that periarticular soft tissue and intra-articular injuries occur concomitant to osseous injury is evident.

Changes in the intra-articular anatomy and their relationship to trauma have also been considered. Merrill[22] arthroscopically evaluated 1,151 joints in 720 patients with internal derangements. Sixty percent of these patients had a history of macrotrauma that was considered an etiologic factor. Although only 10% of the patients had sustained a mandibular fracture, all the patients who were evaluated demonstrated intra-articular abnormalities.[22] Furthermore, the normal asymptomatic population can have variable disc position when examined arthroscopically or with MRIs and approximately 20% have been shown to have marked disc displacement.[43]

The answers to the mysteries of TMJ soft tissue injury and its effect on treatment outcome may once again lie in the orthopedic literature. Hettinga[44] has described the nature of the soft tissue injury in synovial joints. As the force is transmitted to the condyle–glenoid fossa complex, an inflammatory response occurs in the synovial lining. Proliferation of surface cells, increased vascularity, and fibrosis of the subsynovial tissues occur. The endothelium of the blood vessels swells, adventitial cells proliferate, and erythrocytes extravasate. A proliferative synovitis ensues that can lead to the formation of hypertrophied synovial nodules, pigmented villonodular synovitis, and further subsynovial fibrosis.[44]

However, despite this damage, the potential for repair is significant. The synovial tissues enjoy rich vascularity, and their regenerative abilities are excellent. This vascularity and the fact that synovial cells originate from a single undifferentiated mesenchymal cell type contribute to the healing potential. It has been reported that, within weeks of a macrotraumatic injury, the injured synovial tissues cannot be distinguished from normal tissues.[45]

The traumatic (or surgical) disruption of the joint capsule and synovial membrane can lead to an exposure of the articular cartilage. This can alter the composition of the cartilaginous matrix, either by stimulating degradation of the proteoglycans or by suppressing the reparative synthesis of proteoglycans. The decreased concentration of matrix proteoglycans reduces the stiffness of the cartilage and subsequently renders the tissue more susceptible to damage from impact loading.

Restoration of the closed synovial environment results in a repair of this damage. There is controversy as to the acceptable interval between injury and repair of synovial tissue and articular surface, and the influence of this timing on the permanency or reversibility of the damage. It would seem logical that all condylar or subcondylar fractures would induce some degree of soft tissue injury, yet clinical experience, particularly in children, suggests that permanent progressive changes in the articular cartilage are relatively rare following injury.

Long-term Implications

The long-term implications of condylar and subcondylar fractures on the patient's ability to function are frequently debated,[46] regardless of whether the fracture is treated conservatively or via open reduction. In a classic study by Walker,[47] condylar process fractures with dislocation were created in the macaque monkey model, and acceptable results were observed regardless of the degree of displacement or the type of fixation. There was also minimal effect on mandibular growth and symmetry. Neither injury to the intra-articular soft tissues nor nonanatomic repositioning of the fractured segment appeared to have any effect on the development of arthritis, clicking, or the other postfracture sequelae sometimes seen in humans.[47]

A variety of parameters have been evaluated in an effort to gauge treatment outcome, including radiographic evidence of deformity,[48] facial deformity,[48] mandibular deviation on opening,[48] facial symmetry,[49,50] mandibular range of motion,[51,52] masticatory dysfunction,[53] bite force,[54] and occlusal changes.[55] Ellis and Throckmorton[5] performed an excellent review of the functional alterations in the masticatory system after fracture of the condylar process.

The major inadequacy of most studies on mandibular dysfunction after fractures of the condylar process relates to a lack of accurate long-term follow-up. The unreliability of the typical patient pool contributes to this problem. One of the earliest follow-up studies also incorporated one of the longest follow-up periods (19 years).[9] In that review, only 7 of 120 patients (approximately 6%) had "dysfunction" after closed reduction for condylar fractures. Zide and Kent[11] reviewed several studies and concluded that only about 15% of patients with condylar process fractures who underwent closed reduction demonstrated "short-term" problems such as pain, dysfunction, limited opening, or deformity. Sorel[56] reviewed eight studies with a total of 714 patients (865 fractures), all treated with closed reduction or observation only, and reported a complication rate of only 7%.

Despite the plethora of follow-up studies, there is no firm evidence suggesting that open reduction techniques are superior to closed reduction techniques when all quantifiable parameters, including long-term patient function, comfort, joint noise, and mandibular motion, are evaluated. As pointed out by Assael,[46] many of the historically cited articles regarding these measurable parameters have reported findings detected by the clinician rather than those symptoms or deficits reported by the patient. Indeed, the normal, nonpatient population reports pain, deviation, joint noise, and various functional deficits at about the same frequency as do patients who have experienced fracture of the condylar process.[57,58] The logical conclusion is that, unless there are definitive indications for open reduction, as previously discussed, most fractures of the condyloid process in adults can be managed satisfactorily by closed reduction (Figs 18-1a to 18-1d).

Pediatric Trauma

Incidence

Fractures of the mandibular condylar process are particularly common in the pediatric population; from 28% to 62% of mandibular fractures are reported to involve the condyle.[59–68] The mechanism and incidence of injury in the pediatric population vary greatly, depending on the socioeconomic group to which the patient belongs and the country in which he or she lives. The literature is also somewhat misleading about what constitutes a pediatric patient.

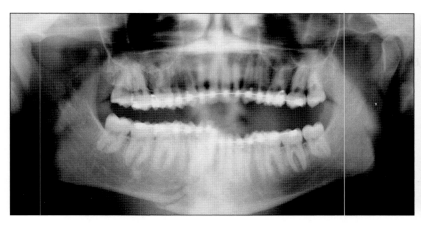

Fig 18-1a Panoramic radiograph of a 22-year-old man with a fractured right parasymphysis and a "minimally" displaced left subcondylar fracture.

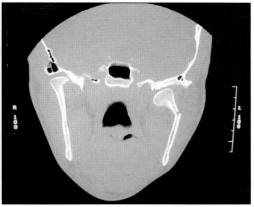

Fig 18-1b CT scan demonstrating the deceptive nature of panoramic radiography. Note the medial displacement of the condylar process.

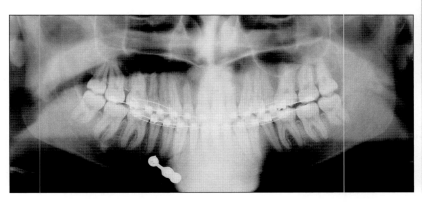

Fig 18-1c Postoperative panoramic radiograph after open reduction of the parasymphysis fracture and nonsurgical, closed reduction of the subcondylar fracture.

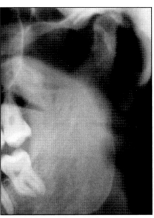

Fig 18-1d Bony union with good alignment of the segment at 8 weeks.

Gassner[69] and Qudah and Bataineh[50] have reported that play accidents represented the major cause of injury in children. Additional studies have implicated sports injuries, motor vehicle accidents (MVAs), and interpersonal violence as the major causes of facial fractures in the pediatric population.[68,70,71] There is a consensus that boys are affected more frequently than girls.[66–68,72–75] There also is some agreement as to the typical pattern of fractures sustained in the pediatric mandible. The condylar neck, condylar head, and angle appear to be the most frequently affected sites, constituting about 80% of mandible fractures.[76,77]

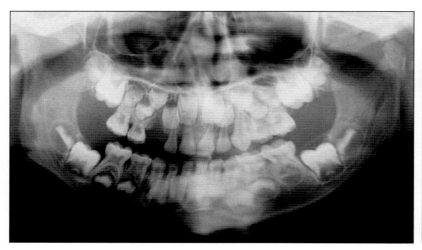

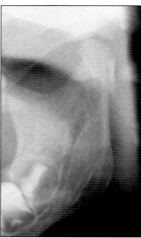

Fig 18-2a Panoramic radiograph of an 8-year-old child who sustained a fall from a bicycle. Note the intracapsular fracture of the left condylar head.

Fig 18-2b Close-up view showing the overlap of the segments.

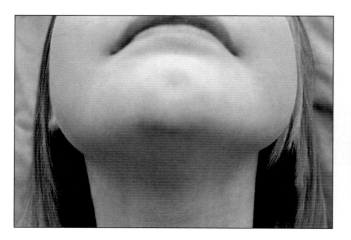

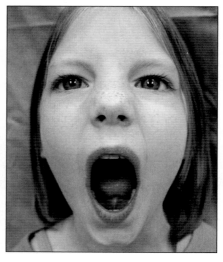

Fig 18-2c Well-healed chin laceration after 1 month.

Fig 18-2d Symmetric range of mandibular movement after 3 weeks on a liquid diet.

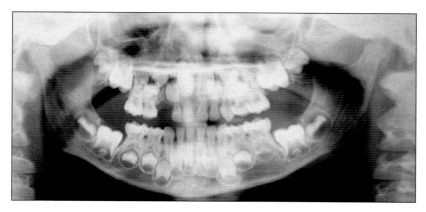

Fig 18-2e Panoramic radiograph 8 weeks postinjury, revealing minimal loss of ramus height on the affected side.

Mechanism of Injury

The mechanism of injury in the pediatric patient is typically a fall, either during play or sports-related activities.[4,75] A blow to the chin creates a propagation of forces posterosuperiorly, driving the condyle into the glenoid fossa and base of the skull. The ensuing injuries can involve bony disruption as well as soft tissue injury, including hemarthrosis[26] and/or capsular tear.[33] Lund[78] suggested that fractures in the condylar region have the greatest potential for causing mandibular growth disturbance. This disturbance can take the form of growth retardation or overgrowth of the mandible.

It has been suggested that the two primary goals of treatment for condylar fractures in this age group should be (1) preservation of function and (2) maintenance of ramus height. Normal growth will typically occur if these two goals are achieved. The preservation of normal mandibular function appears to provide the best chance for normal growth (Figs 18-2a to 18-2e).

Treatment

While the treatment of the condylar and subcondylar fractures in the adult is both historically and currently a hotly debated topic, greater agreement exists regarding the treatment of choice in the pediatric patient. Despite the development of improved endoscopic equipment and techniques, along with the further refinement of rigid fixation devices, closed reduction continues to be the overwhelming treatment of choice for the pediatric patient with a condylar or subcondylar fracture.[10,48,76–84] However, open reduction is indicated in children when a severe unilateral or bilateral loss of ramus height exists. A fracture causing persistent crossbite or chin point deviation also strengthens the argument for an open reduction. The availability of technological advances in rigid internal fixation may also vary from country to country, affecting the mechanism of reduction chosen.

Very little is known about effects of pediatric condylar and subcondylar fractures on TMJ function when that injured child grows to an adult. However, there is general agreement that the likelihood of asymptomatic TMJ function correlates directly with the age of the patient at the time of injury. It is presumed that the favorable adaptive potential of the pediatric patient is responsible for this trend.[85] Lindahl[86] and Lindahl and Hollender[87] have discussed the implications of the patient's age on the ability of the condylar process to adapt and repair after fracture, showing that children 11 years old and younger clearly fare better.

Crush injuries of the condylar head in the pediatric population deserve special attention. This type of injury often creates a concomitant intra-articular hemarthrosis. Although the use of closed reduction in such cases is well agreed on, these intra-articular fractures carry with them a high potential for ankylosis, particularly if the patient is 3 years of age or younger.[81,88] The morphology of the TMJ in the child may contribute to this predisposition. The condylar head tends to be rather broad mediolaterally and have a short condylar neck. There is a large articular surface area, and the bone is well vascularized. Thus a fracture in the area with the attendant hemarthrosis and hypomobility creates a favorable environment for ankylosis. Early mobilization appears to reduce the likelihood of this occurrence.

Thoren and colleagues[82] evaluated the long-term status of dislocated condylar process fractures in children aged 15 years and younger. After a mean follow-up of 8.6 years, the 18 patients evaluated demonstrated minimal signs and symptoms of dysfunction, despite dislocation of the condyle out of the glenoid fossa at the time of fracture. These patients were all treated conservatively with either soft diet and observation or maxillomandibular fixation for 10 to 24 days (mean, 17 days).

Although the signs and symptoms of dysfunction were minimal, the evidence of incomplete repair was more significant. A higher degree of incomplete repair was found in those patients with a history of total fracture and dislocation. The authors concluded that conservative treatment of dislocated condylar process fractures in children remains the treatment of choice despite the high incidence of radiographic aberrations in these patients[82] (Fig 18-3).

Regardless of the nature and location of the mandibular condylar fracture, its management in the pediatric population varies from that in the adult patient. The presence of tooth buds, variable patient cooperation, inherent effects on growth potential, and the enhanced healing potential all influence the management principles. These factors are particularly important when the fracture involves the condylar region. Fractures in this region of the mandible may disrupt the functional matrix, and growth abnormalities can occur. Despite clinical experience that suggests that the majority of pediatric patients with fractures in the condylar region do well, long-term follow-up is always advised. Unilateral and bilateral fractures of the condylar process can create mandibular asymmetry, mandibular retrognathia, and/or apertognathia.

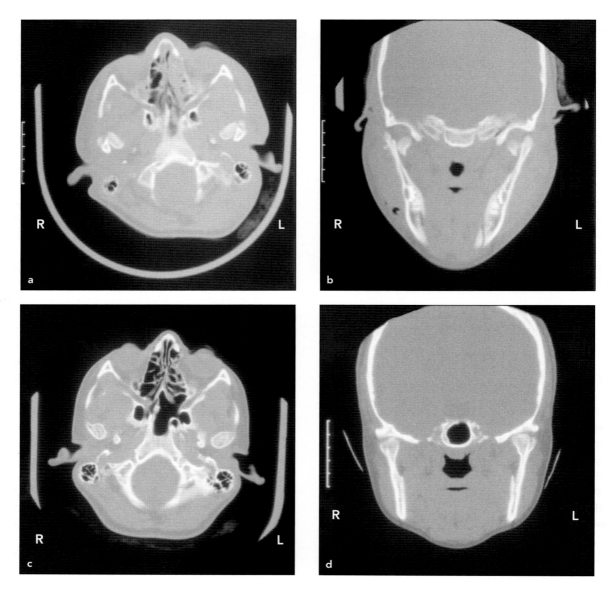

Fig 18-3 *(a)* Axial CT scan of a 14-year-old-child after a motor vehicle accident, revealing bilateral, medially displaced condylar fractures. *(b)* Coronal CT scan of the fractures. *(c)* Axial CT scan 10 months following closed reduction and fixation for 2 weeks. *(d)* Coronal CT scan 10 months following treatment, revealing good alignment of the condylar processes.

Long-term Implications

Fractures of the condylar process (and particularly intra-articular fractures or crush injuries) are of particular concern in the pediatric patient. Disruption of the condylar head can retard growth of the mandible, causing subsequent facial asymmetry.[89] Condylar trauma has been suggested as the cause of 5% to 20% of all clinically signifi-

cant mandibular deficiencies or asymmetries. Growth changes have been reported in 3% to 52% of all patients who experienced pediatric condylar fractures. An alteration of the muscle-bone interaction, resulting in a bowing of the mandibular body on the affected side and a flattening on the unaffected side, has been demonstrated. This results in a deviation of the chin to the fractured side and continued shortening of the ramus.[89]

Proffit and coworkers[90] have reported that facial and occlusal asymmetries are common findings in patients suspected of having sustained a condylar process fracture during childhood. Their suggested initial management of such fractures included a brief period of immobilization followed by a patient-directed regimen of physical therapy and finally close involvement with the orthodontist to monitor jaw growth and symmetry.

In a prospective study of facial growth after condylar trauma, Lund[78] studied 38 patients ranging in age from 4 to 17 years. Fractures occurred bilaterally in 11 of 38 patients (29%) and unilaterally in the other 27 patients (71%). Only two patients had open reductions, while the majority had conservative treatment consisting of observation or maxillomandibular fixation. Surprisingly, results showed that mandibular growth after a condylar fracture was greater on the injured side than on the non-traumatized side. The fractured ramus, made shorter by the trauma, grew more in a relative sense, thereby reducing the height discrepancy. Lund[78] described three types of mandibular growth pattern:

1. Compensatory growth without overgrowth. The fractured side grew more than the normal side but still remained shorter than the unaffected side after the cessation of growth (13 of 27 patients; 48%).
2. Compensatory growth with overgrowth. The fractured side grew more than the normal side (8 of 27 patients; 30%).
3. Dysplastic growth. The fractured side grew less than or equal to the uninjured side, resulting in an increased ramus length discrepancy over time (6 of 27 patients; 22%).

The majority of patients who suffered condylar fractures showed compensatory growth on the injured side and did not develop significant mandibular asymmetry. Historically, it was assumed that decreased mandibular growth on the fractured side creates the mandibular asymmetry. However, this assumption did not take into account the shortening effect that overriding of the fracture segments has on the ramus and mandible.

Lund[78] also described two types of condylar repairing after a condylar process fracture: (1) incomplete repairing, in 37 of 49 condyles (76%), and (2) complete repairing, the so-called functional restitution, in 12 of 49 patients (24%). It appears that incomplete repairing was more likely when fractured condyles were displaced from the glenoid fossa. Younger patients had a much better chance for complete repairing, which is consistent with the findings reported by Thoren and colleagues.[82]

Motor Vehicle Accidents, Whiplash, and TMDs

Temporomandibular disorders (TMDs) generally have a multifactorial etiology (see chapter 14). The role of direct mandibular trauma as one of the etiologic factors is well established, but the role of indirect trauma (eg, whiplash injuries) remains somewhat controversial; some investigators question its significance,[91] while others believe in its importance.[92] In the case of MVAs, it is widely recognized that they may produce cervical whiplash injuries, but the question of whether, or how frequently, cervical whiplash causes TMDs remains extremely controversial.

Whiplash has been defined as an acceleration-deceleration phenomenon of energy transfer to the neck that results from rear-end or side-impact motor vehicle collisions but that can also occur during diving or other mishaps.[93] The collision impact is thought to result in bony and soft tissue injuries to various tissues in the cervical spine (whiplash injury), which in turn leads to a variety of clinical manifestations termed whiplash-associated disorders (WADs). According to an extensive report from the Quebec task force on whiplash-associated disorders, the symptom complex predominantly includes neck and head pain but can also include TMJ pain and other TMDs as well as multiple other presentations.[93] However, other reviews of WADs have questioned the existence of a causative link between whiplash and TMDs.[94]

Whiplash injuries result in acute symptoms,[93] but there is some dispute as to whether they lead to chronic injuries or symptoms. Onset of symptoms several hours after impact tends to be characteristic of whiplash injuries. Most patients reportedly feel little or no pain for the first few minutes after the injury, but symptoms gradually intensify over the next few days. It has been postulated that the delay in onset of symptoms may be due to the time required for traumatic edema and hemorrhage to occur in the injured soft tissues. After several hours, limitation of neck motion, cervical tightness, muscle spasm and/or swelling, and tenderness of both anterior and posterior cervical structures may become apparent.[95]

WADs are usually self-limited, and most patients recover in the first few months.[93,94] As a possible explanation for patients who do not recover early, a biopsychosocial model has been proposed that states that symptom expectation, amplification, and attribution (possibly related to cultural factors) contribute to whiplash victims' reports of chronic pain. The possibility that physical and psychological causes may coexist, but are not necessarily the result of chronic injury, is part of this model.[96] This opinion is based in part on the findings in some low-velocity, rear-end car and bumper-car crash test studies in which no symptoms were reported, as well as findings that approximately 20% of subjects exposed to placebo, low-velocity rear-end collisions reported WAD symptoms.[97] It also draws on studies from Lithuania, Greece, and Germany, where acute whiplash injuries occur but the reporting of chronic symptoms is rare.[98]

Conversely, the concept of a biopsychosocial model as a framework for understanding chronic WADs has been criticized, because some investigators believe that the psychological and social components are overemphasized.[99] Alternatively, a biomechanical framework for understanding WADs has been proposed that states that prevertebral and postvertebral muscles may be torn in whiplash injuries and that some zygapophyseal joints and intervertebral discs are damaged. In addition, the sympathetic trunk, brain, inner ear, and esophagus may possibly be damaged, although much less commonly.[94] A number of studies have claimed that patients with chronic symptoms of whiplash have variations of generalized central hyperexcitability and muscular hyperalgesia, generalized or central hypersensitivity, spinal cord hyperexcitability, or deficits in the motor system that explain their prolonged symptoms. Annular tears of the cervical discs have been detected by discography in a group of patients with neck pain, although these tears went undetected by MRI.

It has also been shown that approximately one third of people exposed to controlled low-speed, rear-end automobile collisions experience symptoms of WADs, especially cervical symptoms and headaches.[100] A group of patients who experienced cervical whiplash and presented with TMJ symptoms, but who had sustained no direct trauma to the face, head, or mandible, underwent MRI of the TMJs. TMJ abnormalities were detected in 95% of these 87 patients, although none had any TMJ complaints prior to the MVA.[101] Furthermore, some studies have reported complaints such as neck pain and headache in more than half of patients up to several years after the original motor vehicle accident.[102]

The natural history of TMDs following MVAs has not been well documented. Scientific articles primarily concerned with other aspects of post-MVA TMDs have reported the onset of symptoms in the majority of their subjects to be within 1 week of the MVA.[103–105] However, onset of TMD symptoms has been reported to occur in a small proportion of subjects from more than 3 months[103] to 18 months[105] to 56 months after the MVA.[104] It is difficult to explain such prolonged delays in the development of symptoms, but it has been speculated that the delay in reporting TMDs is due to the patient's preoccupation

with other problems associated with concomitant injuries (eg, severe pain or fractures).[106] The duration of TMD symptoms has been reported to range from less than 1 month post-MVA[91] to at least 5 years after the MVA.[107]

Biomechanics of Whiplash Injuries

As part of the investigation into whether whiplash is strongly associated with the onset of TMD signs and symptoms, the biomechanics of whiplash injury should be considered. Unfortunately, there are also contradictory opinions in the literature about this issue.

Some propose that hyperextension of the neck during a rear-end impact causes mouth opening that could result in TMJ injuries, including internal disc derangement.[108,109] Weinberg and Lapointe[109] have postulated that during forward acceleration of the person's body after a rear-end impact, the unsupported head accelerates less quickly, resulting in the hyperextension phase of the whiplash mechanism (Figs 18-4a and 18-4b). According to this concept, the mandible moves posteriorly less quickly than the cranium, causing the mouth to open rapidly and resulting in downward and forward displacement of the disc-condyle complex relative to the cranial base. They further speculated that this is accompanied by an initial injury in the form of stretching, tearing, and loosening of the TMJ posterior attachment, medial and lateral disc attachments, and synovial tissues. In the deceleration phase, as the vehicle comes to a sudden stop, the head is propelled forward, causing hyperflexion of the cervical spine and then subsequent mouth closure, resulting in additional crushing, stretching, tearing, or perforation of the previously injured posterior attachment tissues (Figs 18-4c and 18-4d).

Subsequent spasm of the masticatory muscles is proposed to produce further disc displacement and perpetuate the TMJ symptoms. In particular, according to Weinberg and Lapointe,[109] spasm of the superior head of the lateral pterygoid muscle accentuates stretching or tearing of the posterior attachment tissues, inevitably leading to progressive worsening of the disc displacement and the attendant symptoms of pain and persistent locking.

Other investigators, however, have shown in experimental settings that only minor degrees of cervical extension and flexion and submaximal mouth opening occur in rear-end collisions at or below the 10 to 15 km/h range. No cervical hyperextension was observed, and only compressive forces at the TMJ were found; these forces were well within physiologic limits.[110,111]

Howard and coworkers,[111] for instance, used human subjects in rear-end test collisions of motor vehicles in

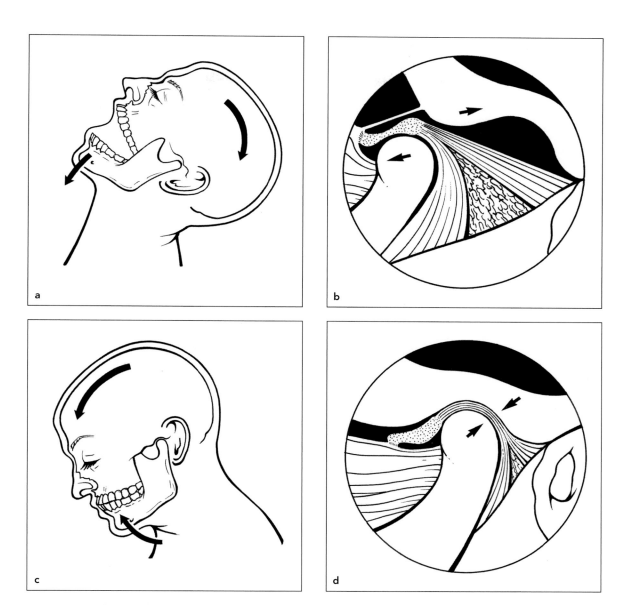

Fig 18-4 Weinberg and Lapointe's proposed mechanism[109] concerning whiplash and the TMJ. *(a and b)* Hyperextension phase. After a rear-end impact, cervical hyperextension occurs and the mouth opens rapidly. This results in injury of the TMJ, including stretching, tearing, and loosening of attachment tissues. *(c and d)* Hyperflexion phase. As the vehicle comes to a stop, cervical hyperflexion and mouth closure occur, resulting in additional crushing, stretching, tearing, or perforation of previously injured attachment tissues.

which the impact velocity changes ranged from approximately 4 to 11 km/h (Fig 18-5). Under these conditions, neck hyperflexion and hyperextension were not noted in any subject. However, the whiplash maneuver was reported to produce a combination of both rotational and translational motions of the head, neck, and mandible; rotational acceleration of the head was found to precede significant translational acceleration.

In the early extension phase, the center of rotation of the head was located in the high forehead region (see Figs 18-5a and 18-5b). It then migrated in a dorsocaudal direction until the angular motion slowed and translational motion increased. Significant vertical translation of the head did not occur, although there was a small rise due to straightening of the kyphotic thoracic curve during the extension phase. Involuntary reflex action of the cervical

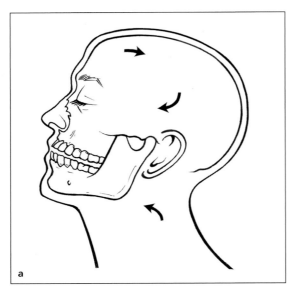

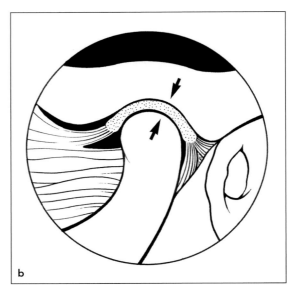

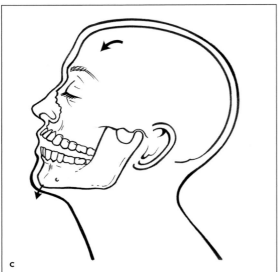

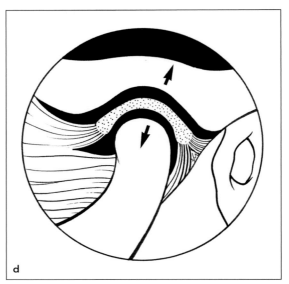

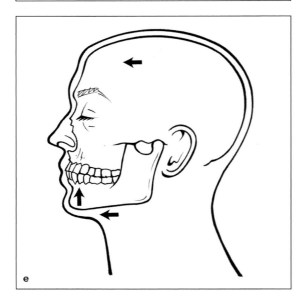

Fig 18-5 Howard and coworkers' proposed mechanism[111] concerning whiplash and the mandible. *(a and b)* Extension phase. No cervical hyperextension occurs. The center of rotation of the head is initially in the high forehead region. There is only forward motion of the TMJ; only a small rise of the head occurs because of straightening of the kyphotic thoracic curve. Resultant mechanical forces at the TMJ are compressive and are only fractions of physiologic forces. *(c and d)* Flexion phase. No cervical hyperflexion occurs. The head is returned to a near-normal position. Trivial tensile forces develop in the TMJ as the head decelerates; there is no stretching of the TMJ ligament. Mouth opening is in the 1.5-cm range. *(e)* Translational acceleration is only forward. Mandibular acceleration is initially horizontal, but later rotates upward. Overall, transient forces imposed on the TMJ and other craniomandibular structures do not represent significant mechanisms of injury in low-velocity–collision whiplash maneuvers.

muscles occurred very early in the extension phase, thereby stabilizing the head posture, and no significant forward flexion of the cervical spine occurred in the latter phases of the whiplash. The head was restored to a near-normal position, with minimal forward flexion overshoot, because of the stabilizing effects of the cervical muscles (see Figs 18-5c and 18-5d).

The translational acceleration could only be forward because it must move in the direction of the applied force; there was no backward motion of the head. The rotational component also produced only forward motion of the TMJ during the extension phase if the center of rotation of the head and neck remained above the TMJ, as it did in their test crashes. Resultant mechanical forces at the TMJ during the extension phase were consequently compressive.

Based on these findings, the authors concluded that there was no basis for TMJ ligament stretch because there was no distraction (see Fig 18-5e). In addition, the compressive forces were only fractions of the typical compressive forces imposed physiologically at the TMJ. Trivial tensile forces developed in the TMJ as the head decelerated. The maximum opening torque that developed in the TMJ during the extension phase was reportedly below that experienced under normal physiologic conditions. Actual mouth opening with respect to the cranium was found to be in the 1.5-cm range. Howard and coauthors[111] suggested that rapid extension of the masseter and temporalis muscle bellies produced a reflexive response that arrested mouth opening.

Prevalence of TMDs After Whiplash

There are conflicting studies in the dental literature concerning the prevalence of TMDs in postwhiplash patients. For example, it has been reported that individuals with a chronic WAD were found to have a higher prevalence of TMD signs and symptoms than were matched general dental practice patients.[112] However, in another study, in which patients were evaluated in the emergency room, it was concluded that the incidence of TMJ pain and clicking following whiplash injury was low, both initially and 1 year later.[91]

In a study by Kasch et al,[113] patients with acute whiplash injury after an MVA involving a rear-end collision were compared to a matched group of patients with an ankle injury. Patients were evaluated within the first month and again 6 months postinjury. The authors concluded that whiplash injury was not a major risk factor for the development of TMD problems, because TMD pain was rare in their subjects after either whiplash or ankle injury.

In addition, it has been reported that Lithuanian accident victims do not report chronic TMD symptoms despite having acute whiplash injuries, which is unlike whiplash claimants in many Western societies.[114] Therefore, the use of a biopsychosocial model to understand the occurrence of TMD symptoms after whiplash may be required in those societies where such factors influence the course and outcome of various other conditions.[114]

Differences in Posttrauma and Nontrauma TMD Patients

If one concedes that chronic TMD symptoms do exist in some postwhiplash victims, are these patients different from TMD patients who do not report previous head and neck trauma? One study found that posttraumatic TMD patients had more facial and head pain, neck pain frequency, masticatory and neck muscle tenderness, and TMJ tenderness than nontrauma TMD patients.[92] However, a different study concluded that patients with neck symptoms after rear-end traffic collisions did not show any significantly greater incidence of disc displacement, joint effusion, or other injury to the TMJ than a control group when studied by MRI.[115]

Furthermore, posttraumatic TMD patients have been described as not responding as well to treatment and requiring more treatments than a nontrauma TMD patient group.[116,117] Kolbinson and coworkers[116] compared treatment regimens and outcomes in TMD patients with MVA-related trauma to those in patients whose TMD was not trauma related. As a whole, posttraumatic TMD patients tended to receive more types of treatment, have more medications prescribed, have more oral medicine clinic visits over a longer period of time, and have a poorer treatment outcome than did the nontrauma group.[116]

On the other hand, other investigators have found that treatment outcomes did not differ significantly between TMD patients with or without a history of trauma.[118] For instance, de Boever and Keersmaekers[119] compared two groups of TMD patients, one without a history of trauma to the head and neck and one with such a history that was linked to the onset of symptoms. The trauma group had more pronounced symptoms initially, but both groups (98 in the trauma group and 302 in the nontrauma group) had responded equally well to conservative treatment when evaluated with the Helkimo dysfunction index after 1 year.

Effects of Litigation

Miller[120,121] proposed in 1961 that postaccident patients fail to respond to therapy until the compensation issue is settled, after which nearly all the cases recover completely without treatment. A study published almost 40 years later also found that the elimination of compensation for pain and suffering was associated with a decreased incidence and improved prognosis of whiplash injury.[122] This more recent study also claimed that under both tort and no-fault systems, the involvement of a lawyer was a strong predictor of a delayed claim closure. In some studies, whiplash injury subjects in litigation have been found to have more pain than nonlitigants, but there are mixed reports as to whether these two groups differ in their psychological status. It has been reported that litigation status does not predict employment status in chronic pain patients who sustain a whiplash injury after a MVA.[123] This suggested that secondary gain does not figure prominently in influencing the functionality of these patients. A study comparing litigating and nonlitigating TMD patients found that litigants have more reported pain sites, more severe neck and face pain, and greater sleep disturbance and level of somatization; receive more and longer treatments; and have poorer treatment outcomes.[124] However, several studies have shown that patients frequently continue to experience chronic whiplash-related symptoms even following litigation.[125] In addition, the majority of previously treated patients with a TMD after MVAs continue to have problems with jaw, head, and neck pain and jaw dysfunction, regardless of their litigation status.[126]

Psychological Aspects of Postwhiplash Subjects

Patients with whiplash injury have been reported to have psychological distress.[127] This seems to be worse in persons with persistent moderate to severe symptoms. It has been postulated that psychological symptoms in posttraumatic whiplash patients are not the cause, but rather the consequence, of somatic symptoms.[128] It has also been reported that TMD patients with a history of MVA trauma have more psychological symptoms than do TMD patients without a history of trauma.[117]

Prognostic Factors

Many articles have been written with the intent of identifying prognostic factors in relation to WADs. A systematic review[129] determined that there was strong evidence that high initial pain intensity was a negative prognostic factor for functional recovery of patients with a whiplash injury. Restricted range of cervical motion and a large number of complaints also had some limited prognostic value for functional recovery. However, this review did not find sufficient evidence supporting a number of factors that have often been mentioned to be of prognostic value concerning outcome, including being older, being female, having an angular deformity of the neck, and receipt of compensation.[129] There are conflicting findings in the literature concerning other potential prognostic factors for recovery including, but not limited to, awareness of impending impact, position of the head at impact, various parameters related to head restraint factors, and premorbid personality traits.

Not much has been written about prognostic indicators in the TMD literature. One study[103] reported that speeds of 40 mph or higher at impact appeared to be associated with significantly more headache days and greater overall pain intensity. Also, an impact other than from the side was more likely to result in a facial injury such as bruising. People in accidents in which there was excessive vehicular damage, such as when the vehicle was "totaled," showed more potential for restricted mouth opening (less than 30 mm). In addition, looking right or left at the time of impact may be associated with significantly greater overall pain and significantly greater masticatory muscle tenderness.[103]

A different study[104] concluded that minimal vehicular damage, lack of headrest use, being in the driver position, and settlement of an insurance claim may be characteristic of patients whose post-MVA TMDs have a poorer prognosis. However, in general, it was not found that patients who reported some type of direct head, facial, or dental injury during their MVAs presented themselves for treatment differently from, or had different treatment needs or outcomes from, patients with no history of these types of direct injuries.

Relationships Between Neck Problems and TMD Symptoms

It has been noted that all patients with post-MVA TMDs report the onset of some type of complaint to have occurred the day of or the day after the MVA.[104] However, only 50% of these patients reported that their TMD symptoms were noticed either immediately or within 1 day of the accident, while 76% identify the beginning of their TMD complaints to be in the first week post-MVA. The first post-MVA complaint was reported to be "TMJ symptoms" in only 12% of patients. Furthermore, the TMJ symptoms were identified by the patients themselves, rather than by the health care providers, in more than 80% of the study patients.[104]

These findings potentially have a number of explanations. One possibility might be related to a situation in which both TMD symptoms and painful neck injuries are present. It is well known that cervical and craniofacial pain can present concurrently, and it has been suggested that this is the result of strong connectivity between trigeminal and cervical motor and sensory responses.[130] It has also been shown that jaw muscle pain can be linked to increases in neck electromyographic activity when the head and jaw are at rest.[131] It has been suggested that trauma to the neck region leading to a WAD can derange integrated jaw and neck behavior, underlining the functional coupling between the mandibular and head-neck motor systems during jaw function. It was hypothesized that pain may be an explanatory factor for this disturbed jaw function in the WAD group.[132]

Additionally, it has been shown that there is a functional connection between the masticatory and cervical motor systems. For example, the sternocleidomastoid muscle has been found to be activated at or below 30% of its maximum capacity in subjects who had normal jaw function and were clenching maximally.[133] Furthermore, patients with WADs report jaw fatigue and pain more often and earlier than do patients with TMDs and healthy control subjects, suggesting an association between neck injury and reduced functional capacity of the jaw motor system.[134]

Air Bag Injuries

Although much of the MVA-related facial trauma literature deals with direct facial impact and whiplash, a more recent consideration is the use of air bags in motor vehicles. When used properly as a supplement to the three-point lap-shoulder belt restraint, air bags afford significant reduction in facial, head, and thoracic injuries as well as a significant reduction in fatalities. However, numerous air bag–related injuries have been reported.[135] These range from facial lacerations and abrasions to eye, extremity, and abdominal injuries. In addition, TMJ injuries from air bag deployment, including effusions and internal derangements as well as subcondylar fractures and nondisplaced zygomatic fractures, have also been reported.[135]

Fatal injuries have also occurred in "out-of-position" drivers, particularly those who are of small stature and require seat adjustments to far-forward positions in close proximity to the air bag assembly.

Intubation Injuries

Trauma to the TMJ can occur during orotracheal intubation. Anterior dislocation of the mandible has been noted, and disc displacement without reduction associated with limited opening has also been reported in a small number of patients. These conditions were noted after emergence from anesthesia in patients who reportedly had no prior history of TMDs.[136] TMJ dislocation has also been noted following endoscopy.

Summary

Because of its prominent location, the mandible is a frequent site of trauma, resulting in a high incidence of injury to one or both TMJ. These injuries involve not only the bony components of the joint but also the associated soft tissues. Whereas it is generally agreed that most fractures of the condyloid process in children can be managed by closed reduction, there is considerable debate over whether this is also true in the adult. Although there have been no good randomized clinical trials comparing treatment by open and closed reduction, most of the case series studies that have been done indicate that, outside of a few specific indications for open reduction, most of these fractures can also be successfully managed conservatively.

The topic of TMDs that result from MVAs or other trauma in which there are no fractures or other direct mandibular area injuries continues to be fraught with controversy. The polarization of arguments on this topic is extreme. Opinions range from the belief that posttraumatic TMD signs and/or symptoms should be treated as minor, transient occurrences that respond readily to conservative treatment protocols to an opposite viewpoint in which such patients are expected to have more severe symptoms and to require more intensive treatment, often with a guarded prognosis.

Much of the science supporting both sides of the argument falls far short of the gold standard of randomized, controlled, prospective studies. Therefore, considerably more research is required to better resolve the multitude of unanswered questions in this area. However, in the meantime, it should be recognized that many patients will continue to present to dental practitioners with signs and symptoms of TMDs following an MVA, and these patients will require the best diagnostic and therapeutic efforts available. Although cervical whiplash is a common injury associated with rear-end or side-impact MVAs, there is considerable controversy regarding the frequency with which soft tissue WADs occur in the TMJ, as well as the mechanism by which they develop. Whereas there is general agreement that some patients with whiplash injuries can also have soft tissue injuries in the TMJ, most studies have shown that this is not a common occurrence. Moreover, the reasons why some of these minor injuries result in chronic pain and dysfunction are not well understood, but there are indications that psychosocial and cultural factors may play a large role in these cases. Clearly, there are still many unanswered questions regarding the pathogenesis, pathophysiology, and treatment of soft tissue as well as bony injuries of the TMJ.

References

1. Bradley P. Injuries of the condylar and coronoid process. In: Rowe NL, Williams JLL (eds). Maxillofacial Injuries. New York: Churchill Livingstone, 1985:337–362.
2. Olson RA, Fonseca RJ, Zeitler DL, Osbon DB. Fractures of the mandible: A review of 580 cases. J Oral Maxillofac Surg 1982;40:23–28.
3. Ellis E 3rd, Moos K, el-Attar A. Ten years of mandible fractures: An analysis of 2137 cases. Oral Surg Oral Med Oral Pathol 1985;59:120–129.
4. Villarreal PM, Monje F, Junquera LM, Mateo J, Morillo AJ, Gonzalez C. Mandibular condyle fractures: Determinants of treatment and outcome. J Oral Maxillofax Surg 2004;62:155–163.
5. Ellis E 3rd, Throckmorton GS. Treatment of mandibular condylar process fractures: Biological considerations. J Oral Maxillofac Surg 2005;63:115–134.
6. Charnley J. The Closed Treatment of Common Fractures. Edinburgh: Livingstone, 1961.
7. Archer HW. Oral and Maxillofacial Surgery. Philadelphia: Saunders, 1975:1157.
8. Zemsky JL. New conservative treatment versus surgical operation for displaced fractures of the neck of the mandibular condyle. Dent Cosmos 1926;68:43–49.
9. Chalmers J. Lyons club: Fractures involving the mandibular condyle: A post-treatment survey of 120 cases. J Oral Surg 1947;5:45–73.
10. MacLennan DW. Considerations of 180 cases of typical fractures of the mandibular condyle process. Br J Plast Surg 1952;5:122–128.
11. Zide MF, Kent JN. Indications for open reduction of mandibular condyle fractures. J Oral Maxillofac Surg 1983;41:89–98.
12. Konstantinovic VS, Dimitrijevic B. Surgical versus conservation treatment of unilateral condylar process fractures: Clinical and radiographic evaluation of 80 patients. J Oral Maxillofac Surg 1992;50:349–352; discussion 352–353.
13. Baker HW, Moos KF. Current consensus on the management of fractures of the mandibular condyle. Int J Oral Maxillofac Surg 1998;27:258–266.
14. Ellis E 3rd. Condylar process fractures of the mandible. Facial Plast Surg 2000;16:193–205.
15. Zide MF. Open reduction of mandibular condyle fractures. Indications and technique. Clin Plast Surg 1989;16:69–76.
16. Brandt MT, Haug RH. Open versus closed reduction of adult mandibular condyle fractures: A review of the literature regarding the evolution of current thoughts on management. J Oral Maxillofac Surg 2003;61:1324–1332.
17. Kent NJ, Neary JP, Silva C, Zide MF. Open reduction of fractured mandibular condyle fractures. Oral Maxillofac Clin North Am 1990;2:69–102.
18. Haug RH, Dodson TB, Morgan JP. Trauma Surgery—Parameters and Pathways: Clinical Practice Guidelines for Oral And Maxillofacial Surgery. Rosemont, IL: American Association of Oral and Maxillofacial Surgeons, 2001:TRA/15.
19. Bos RRM, Ward RP, de Bont LGM. Mandibular condyle fractures: A consensus [editorial]. Br J Oral Maxillofac Surg 1999;37:87.
20. Hayward JR, Scott RF. Fractures of the mandibular condyle. J Oral Maxillofac Surg 1993;51:57–61.
21. Norman JE. Posttraumatic disorders of the jaw joint. Ann R Coll Surg Engl 1982;64:27–36.
22. Merrill RG. The arthroscopic appearance of acute temporomandibular joint trauma [discussion]. J Oral Maxillofac Surg 1990;48:784.
23. Van Sickels JE, Parks WJ. Temporomandibular joint region injuries. In: Fonseca RJ (ed). Oral and Maxillofacial Surgery, vol 3. Philadelphia: Saunders, 2000:136–148.
24. Choi BH, Huh JH, Yoo, JH. Computed tomographic findings of the fractured mandibular condyle after open reduction. Int J Oral Maxillofac Surg 2003;32:469–473.
25. Sullivan SM, Banghart PR, Anderson Q. Magnetic resonance imaging assessment of acute soft tissue injuries to the temporomandibular joint. J Oral Maxillofac Surg 1995;53:763–766.
26. Jones JK, Van Sickels JE. A preliminary report of arthroscopic findings following acute condylar trauma. J Oral Maxillofac Surg 1991;49:55–60.
27. Milam SB, Schmitz JP. Molecular biology of temporomandibular joint disorders: Proposed mechanism of disease. J Oral Maxillofac Surg 1995;53:1448–1454.
28. Stover MD, Kellam JF. Articular fractures: Principles. In: Rüedi TP, Murphy WM (eds). AO Principles of Fracture Management. Stuttgart: Thieme, 2000:105–120.
29. Borrelli J, Torzilli PA, Grigiene R, et al. Effect of impact load on articular cartilage: Development of an intra-articular fracture model. J Orthrop Trauma 1997;11:319–326.
30. Mankin HJ. The response of articular cartilage in mechanical injury. J Bone Joint Surg Am 1986;64:460–466.
31. Pauwels F. Neue richtlinien fur die operative behandlung der coxarthrose. Verh Dtsch Orthrop Ges 1961;48:322–366.
32. Rowe NL, Killey HC. Fractures of the Facial Skeleton, ed 2. Baltimore: Williams & Wilkins, 1970:137–172.

33. Raustia AM, Pyhtinen J, Oikarinen KS, Altonen M. Conventional radiographic and computed tomographic findings in cases of fracture of the mandibular condylar process. J Oral Maxillofac Surg 1990;48:1258–1262.

34. Zarb GA, Fenton AH, MacKay HF. Maxillofacial prosthesis and orofacial trauma. Dent Clin North Am 1982;26:613–630.

35. Takaku S, Yoshida M, Sano T, Toyoda T. Magnetic resonance images in patients with acute traumatic injury of the temporomandibular joint: A preliminary report. J Craniomaxillofac Surg 1996;24:173–177.

36. Goss A, Bosanquet AG. The arthroscopic appearance of acute temporomandibular joint trauma. J Oral Maxillofac Surg 1990;48:780–783.

37. Chuong R, Piper MA. Open reduction of condylar fractures of the mandible in conjunction with repair of discal injury: A preliminary report. J Oral Maxillofac Surg 1988;46:257–263.

38. Murakami KI. Diagnostic arthroscopy. In: Sanders B, Murakami KI, Clark GT (eds). Diagnostic and Surgical Arthroscopy of the Temporomandibular Joint. Philadelphia: Saunders, 1989:73–94.

39. Sanders B, Buoncristiani RD. Surgical arthroscopy. In: Sanders B, Murakami KI, Clark GT (eds). Diagnostic and Surgical Arthroscopy of the Temporomandibular Joint. Philadelphia: Saunders, 1989:95–114.

40. Luz JG, Jaeger RG, de Araujo VC, de Rezende JR. The effect of indirect trauma on the rat temporomandibular joint. Int J Oral Maxillofac Surg 1991;20:48–52.

41. Yucel E, Borkan U, Mollaoglu N, Erkmen E, Gunhan O. Histological evaluation of changes in the temporomandibular joint after direct and indirect trauma: An experimental study. Dent Traumatol 2002;18:212–216.

42. Feinerman DM. Soft tissue temporomandibular joint trauma. Oral Maxillofac Surg Clin North Am 1998;10:619–625.

43. Hatala MP, Westesson P-L, Tallents RH, Katzberg RWl. TMJ disc displacement in symptomatic volunteers detected by MR imaging [abstract100]. J Dent Res 1991;70:278–625.

44. Hettinga D. II. Normal joint structures and their reaction to injury. J Orthop Sports Med 1979;1:83–88.

45. Hettinga D. III. Normal joint structures and their reaction to injury. J Orthop Sports Med 1980;1:178–185.

46. Assael LA. Open versus closed reduction of adult mandibular condyle fractures: An alternative interpretation of the evidence. J Oral Maxillofac Surg 2003;61:1333–1339.

47. Walker RV. Traumatic mandibular condyle fracture dislocation: Effect of growth in the *Macaca* monkey. Am J Surg 1960;100:850–863.

48. MacLennan WD, Simpson W. Treatment of fractured mandibular condylar process in children. Br J Plast Surg 1965;18:423–427.

49. Ellis E 3rd, Throckmorton G. Facial symmetry after closed and open treatment of fractures of the mandibular condylar process. J Oral Maxillofac Surg 2000;58:719–728; discussion 729–730.

50. Qudah MA, Bataineh AB. A retrospective study of selected oral and maxillofacial fractures in a group of Jordanian children. Oral Surg Oral Med Oral Pathol Oral Radiol Endod 2002; 94:310–314.

51. Blevins C, Gores R. Fractures of the mandibular condyloid process: Results of conservative treatment with 140 patients. J Oral Surg 1961;19:393–407.

52. Palmieri C, Ellis E 3rd, Throckmorton G. Mandibular motion after closed and open treatment of unilateral condylar process fractures. J Oral Maxillofac Surg 1999;57:764–775; discussion 775–776.

53. Throckmorton G, Ellis E 3rd, Hayasaki H. Masticatory motion after surgical or nonsurgical treatment for unilateral fractures of the condylar process. J Oral Maxillofac Surg 2004;62:127–138.

54. Ellis E 3rd, Throckmorton GS. Bite forces after open or closed treatment of mandibular condylar process fractures. J Oral Maxillofac Surg 2001;59:389–395.

55. Ellis E 3rd, Simon P, Throckmorton GS. Occlusal results after open or closed treatment of fractures of the mandibular condylar process. J Oral Maxillofac Surg 2000;58:260–268.

56. Sorel B. Open versus closed reduction of mandible fractures. Oral Maxillofac Surg Clin North Am 1998;10:541–565.

57. Burakoff R. Epidemiology. In: Kaplan A, Assael L (eds). Temporomandibular Disorders, Diagnosis and Treatment. Philadelphia: Saunders, 1991:95–103.

58. Pullinger AG, Seligman DA, Solberg WK. Temporomandibular disorders. Part I: Functional status, dentomorphologic features, and sex differences in a nonpatient population. J Prosthet Dent 1988;59:228–235 [erratum 1988;60:132].

59. Morgan WC. Pediatric mandibular fractures. Oral Surg Oral Med Oral Pathol 1975;40:320–326.

60. Fortunato MA, Fielding AF, Guernsey LH. Facial bone fractures in children. Oral Surg Oral Med Oral Pathol 1982;53:225–230.

61. Ramba J. Fractures of facial bones in children. Int J Oral Surg 1985;14:472–478.

62. Amaratunga NA. A study of condylar fractures in Sri Lankan patients with special reference to the recent views on treatment, healing and sequelae. Br J Oral Maxillofac Surg 1987;25:391–397.

63. Andersson L, Hultin M, Kjellman O, Nordenram A, Ramstrom G. Jaw fractures in the county of Stockholm (1970–1980). Jaw fractures in children and adolescents. Swed Dent J 1989;13:201–207.

64. Stylogianni L, Arsenopoulos A, Patrikiou A. Fractures of the facial skeleton in children. Br J Oral Maxillofac Surg 1991;29:9–11.

65. Guven O. Fractures of the maxillofacial region in children. J Craniomaxillofac Surg 1992;20:244–247.

66. Thoren H, Iizuka T, Hallikainen D, Lindqvist C. Different patterns of mandibular fractures in children. An analysis of 220 fractures in 157 patients. J Craniomaxillofac Surg 1992;20:292–296.

67. Posnick JF, Wells M, Pron GE. Pediatric facial fractures: Evolving patterns of treatment. J Oral Maxillofac Surg 1993;51:836–844; discussion 844–845.

68. Infante Cossio P, Espin Galvez F, Gutierrez Perez JL, Garcia-Perla A, Hernandez Guisado JM. Mandibular fractures in children. A retrospective study of 99 fractures in 59 patients. Int J Oral Maxillofac Surg 1994;23:329–331.

69. Gassner R. Pediatric craniomaxillofacial trauma: Review of 3385 cases with 6060 injuries in 10 years. Presented at the Oral Abstract Session, American Association of Oral and Maxillofacial Surgeons Annual Meeting, Chicago, Oct 2002.

70. Haug RH, Foss J. Maxillofacial injuries in the pediatric patient. Oral Surg Oral Med Oral Pathol Oral Radiol Endod 2000;90:126–134.

71. Bamjee Y, Lownie JF, Cleaton-Jones PE, Lownie MA. Maxillofacial injuries in a group of South Africans under 18 years of age. Br J Oral Maxillofac Surg 1996;34:298–302.

72. Hayrinen-Immonen R, Sane J, Perkki K, Malmstrom M. A six-year follow-up study of sports-related injuries in children and adolescents. Endod Dent Traumatol 1990;6:208–212.

73. Tanaka N, Uchide N, Suzuki K, et al. Maxillofacial fractures in children. J Craniomaxillofac Surg 1993; 21:289–293.

74. Lustmann J, Milhem I. Mandibular fractures in infants: Review of the literature and report of seven cases. J Oral Maxillofac Surg 1994;52:240–245.

75. Iida S, Matsuya T. Pediatric maxillofacial fractures: Their aetiological characters and fracture patterns. J Craniomaxillofac Surg 2002;30:237–241.

76. Schultz RC, Meilman J. Facial fractures in children. In: Goldwyn RM (ed). Long-term Results in Plastic and Reconstructive Surgery. Boston: Little, Brown, 1980:458–480.

77. Kaban LB, Mulliken JB, Murray JE. Facial fractures in children: An analysis of 122 fractures in 109 patients. Plastic Reconstr Surg 1997;59:15–20.

78. Lund K. Mandibular growth and remodeling processes after condylar fracture: A longitudinal roentgencephalometric study. Acta Odontol Scand Suppl 1974;32(64):3–117.

79. Leake DJ, Doykos J, Habal MB, et al. Long-term follow-up of fractures of the mandibular condyle in children. Plast Reconstr Surg 1971;47:127–131.

80. MacGregor AB, Fordyce GL. The treatment of fracture of the neck of the mandibular condyle. Br Dent J 1957;102:351–357.

81. Dodson TB. Mandibular fractures in children. Oral Maxillofac Surg Knowledge Update 1995;1(pt 2):95–107.

82. Thoren H, Hallikainen D, Iizuka T, Lindqvist C. Condylar process fractures in children: A follow-up study of fractures with total dislocation of the condyle from the glenoid fossa. J Oral Maxillofac Surg 2001;59:768–773.

83. Guven O, Keskin A. Remodelling following condylar fractures in children. J Craniomaxillofac Surg 2001;29:232–237.

84. Dahlstrom L, Kahnberg KE, Lindahl L. 15 years follow-up on condylar fractures. Int J Oral Maxillofac Surg 1989;18:18–23.

85. Norholt SE, Krishnan V, Sindet-Pedersen S, Jensen I. Pediatric condylar fractures: A long term follow-up study of 55 patients. J Oral Maxillofac Surg 1993;51:1302–1310.

86. Lindahl L. Condylar fractures of the mandible. 1. Classification and relation to age, occlusion, and concomitant injuries of teeth and teeth supporting structures and fractures of the mandibular body. Int J Oral Surg 1977;6:12–21.

87. Lindahl L, Hollender L. Condylar fracture of the mandible. 2. A radiographic study of remodeling processes in the temporomandibular joint. Int J Oral Surg 1977;6:153–165.

88. Kaban LB. Facial trauma. 2. Dentoalveolar injuries and mandibular fractures. In: Kaban LB (ed). Pediatric Oral and Maxillofacial Surgery. Philadelphia: Saunders, 1990:233–260.

89. Sorel B. Management of condylar fractures. Oral Maxillofac Surg Knowledge Update 2001;3:47–62.

90. Proffit WR, Vig KW, Turvey TA. Early fracture of the mandibular condyles: Frequently an unsuspected cause of growth disturbances. Am J Orthod 1980;78:1–24.

91. Heise AP, Laskin DM, Gervin AS. Incidence of temporomandibular joint symptoms following whiplash injury. J Oral Maxillofac Surg 1992;50:825–828.

92. Kolbinson DA, Epstein JB, Senthilselvan A, Burgess JA. A comparison of TMD patients with or without prior motor vehicle accident involvement: Initial signs, symptoms and diagnostic characteristics. J Orofac Pain 1997;11:206–214.

93. Spitzer WO, Skovron ML, Salmi LR, et al. Scientific monograph of the Quebec task force on whiplash-associated disorders: Redefining 'whiplash' and its management. Spine 1995;20(suppl 8):1–73.

94. Barnsley L, Lord S, Bogduk N. Whiplash injury. Pain 1994;58:283–307.

95. Teasell RW. The clinical picture of whiplash injuries: An overview. In: Teasell RW, Shapiro AP (eds). Spine: State of the Art Reviews, vol 7. Cervical Flexion-Extension/Whiplash Injuries. Philadelphia: Hanley and Belfus, 1993:373–389.

96. Ferrari R, Schrader H. The late whiplash syndrome: A biopsychosocial approach. J Neurol Neurosurg Psychiatr 2001;70:722–726.

97. Castro WHM, Meyer SJ, Becke MER, et al. No stress—No whiplash? Prevalence of "whiplash" symptoms following exposure to a placebo rear-end collision. Int J Legal Med 2001;114:316–322.

98. Ferrari R, Russell AS. Epidemiology of whiplash: An international dilemma. Ann Rheum Dis 1999;58:1–5.

99. Freeman MD, Croft AC, Rossignol AM, Weaver DS, Reiser M. A review and methodologic critique of the literature refuting whiplash syndrome. Spine 1999;24:86–98.

100. Brault JR, Wheeler JB, Siegmund GP, Brault EJ. Clinical response of human subjects to rear-end automobile collisions. Arch Phys Med Rehabil 1998;79: 72–80.

101. Garcia R Jr, Arrington JA. The relationship between cervical whiplash and temporomandibular joint injuries: An MRI study. Cranio 1996;14:233–239.

102. Bunketorp L, Nordholm L, Carlsson J. A descriptive analysis of disorders in patients 17 years following motor vehicle accidents. Eur Spine J 2002;11:227–234.

103. Burgess JA, Kolbinson DA, Lee PT, Epstein JB. Motor vehicle accidents and TMDs: Assessing the relationship. J Am Dent Assoc 1996;127:1767–1772.

104. Kolbinson DA, Epstein JB, Senthilselvan A, Burgess JA. Effect of impact and injury characteristics on post–motor vehicle accident temporomandibular disorders. Oral Surg Oral Med Oral Pathol Oral Radiol Endod 1998;85:665–673.

105. Probert TCS, Wiesenfeld D, Reade PC. Temporomandibular pain dysfunction disorder resulting from road traffic accidents—An Australian study. Int J Oral Maxillofac Surg 1994;23:338–341.

106. Brooke RI, Lapointe HJ. Temporomandibular joint disorders following whiplash. In: Teasell RW, Shapiro AP (eds). Spine: State of the Art Reviews, vol 7. Cervical Flexion-Extension/Whiplash Injuries. Philadelphia: Hanley and Belfus, 1993:443–454.

107. Romanelli GG, Mock D, Tenenbaum HC. Characteristics and response to treatment of posttraumatic temporomandibular disorder: A retrospective study. Clin J Pain 1992;8:6–17.

108. Huang SC. Dynamics modeling of human temporomandibular joint during whiplash. Biomed Mater Eng 1999;9:233–241.

109. Weinberg S, Lapointe H. Cervical extension-flexion injury (whiplash) and internal derangement of the temporomandibular joint. J Oral Maxillofac Surg 1987;45:653–656.

110. Castro WHM, Schilgen M, Meyer S, Weber M, Peuker C, Wörtler K. Do "whiplash injuries" occur in low-speed rear impacts? Eur Spine J 1997;6:366–375.

111. Howard RP, Bowles AP, Guzman HM, Krenrich SW. Head, neck and mandible dynamics generated by 'whiplash.' Accid Anal Prev 1998;30:525–534.

112. Klobas L, Tegelberg A, Axelsson S. Symptoms and signs of temporomandibular disorders in individuals with chronic whiplash-associated disorders. Swed Dent J 2004;28:29–36.

113. Kasch H, Hjorth T, Svensson P, Nyhuus L, Jensen TS. Temporomandibular disorders after whiplash injury: A controlled, prospective study. J Orofac Pain 2002;16:118–128.

114. Ferrari R, Schrader H, Obelieniene D. Prevalence of temporomandibular disorders associated with whiplash injury in Lithuania. Oral Surg Oral Med Oral Pathol Oral Radiol Endod 1999;87:653–657.

115. Bergman H, Andersson F, Isberg A. Incidence of temporomandibular joint changes after whiplash trauma: A prospective study using MR imaging. AJR Am J Roentgenol 1998;171:1237–1243.

116. Kolbinson DA, Epstein JB, Senthilselvan A, Burgess JA. A comparison of TMD patients with or without prior motor vehicle accident involvement: Treatment and outcomes. J Orofac Pain 1997;11:337–345.

117. Krogstad BS, Jokstad A, Dahl BL, Soboleva U. Somatic complaints, psychologic distress, and treatment outcome in two groups of TMD patients, one previously subjected to whiplash injury. J Orofac Pain 1998;12:136–144.

118. Steed PA, Wexler GB. Temporomandibular disorders—Traumatic etiology vs. nontraumatic etiology: A clinical and methodological inquiry into symptomatology and treatment outcomes. Cranio 2001;19:188–194.

119. de Boever JA, Keersmaekers K. Trauma in patients with temporomandibular disorders: Frequency and treatment outcome. J Oral Rehabil 1996;23:91–96.

120. Miller H. Accident neurosis. Br Med J 1961;1(5230):919–925.

121. Miller H. Accident neurosis. Br Med J 1961;1(5231):992–998.

122. Cassidy JD, Carroll LJ, Côté P, Lemstra M, Berglund A, Nygren A. Effect of eliminating compensation for pain and suffering on the outcome of insurance claims for whiplash injury. N Engl J Med 2000;342:1179–1186.

123. Swartzman LC, Teasell RW, Shapiro AP, McDermid AJ. The effect of litigation status on adjustment to whiplash injury. Spine 1996;21:53–58.

124. Burgess JA, Dworkin SF. Litigation and post-traumatic TMD: How patients report treatment outcome. J Am Dent Assoc 1993;124:105–110.

125. Kolbinson DA, Epstein JB, Burgess JA. Temporomandibular disorders, headaches, and neck pain following motor vehicle accidents and the effect of litigation: Review of the literature. J Orofac Pain 1996;10:101–125.

126. Kolbinson DA, Epstein JB, Burgess JA, Senthilselvan A. Temporomandibular disorders, headaches, and neck pain after motor vehicle accidents: A pilot investigation of persistence and litigation effects. J Prosthet Dent 1997;77:46–53.

127. Sterling M, Kenardy J, Jull G, Vicenzino B. The development of psychological changes following whiplash injury. Pain 2003;106:481–489.

128. Radanov BP, Begré S, Sturzenegger M, Augustiny KF. Course of psychological variables in whiplash injury—A 2-year follow-up with age, gender and education pair-matched patients. Pain 1996;64:429–434.

129. Scholten-Peeters GGM, Verhagen AP, Bekkering GE, et al. Prognostic factors of whiplash-associated disorders: A systematic review of prospective cohort studies. Pain 2003;104:303–322.

130. Browne PA, Clark GT, Kuboki T, Adachi NY. Concurrent cervical and craniofacial pain: A review of empiric and basic science evidence. Oral Surg Oral Med Oral Pathol Oral Radiol Endod 1998;86:633–640.

131. Svensson P, Wang K, Sessle BJ, Arendt-Nielsen L. Associations between pain and neuromuscular activity in the human jaw and neck muscles. Pain 2004;109:225–232.

132. Häggman-Henrikson B, Zafar H, Eriksson P-O. Disturbed jaw behavior in whiplash-associated disorders during rhythmic jaw movements. J Dent Res 2002;81:747–751.

133. Clark GT, Browne PA, Nakano M, Yang Q. Co-activation of sternocleidomastoid muscles during maximum clenching. J Dent Res 1993;72:1499–1502.

134. Häggman-Henrikson B, Österlund C, Eriksson P-O. Endurance during chewing in whiplash-associated disorders and TMD. J Dent Res 2004;83:946–950.

135. Boyd BC. Automobile supplemental restraint system–induced injuries. Oral Surg Oral Med Oral Pathol Oral Radiol Endod 2002;94:143–148.

136. Gould DB, Banes CH. Iatrogenic disruptions of right temporomandibular joints during orotracheal intubation causing permanent closed lock of the jaw. Anesth Analg 1995;81:191–194.

Maxillofacial Movement Disorders

Leon A. Assael

Because most temporomandibular disorders (TMDs) involve a disturbance in mandibular function as well as pain, it is essential to understand those unrelated movement disorders that must be considered in the differential diagnosis. Movement disorders are defined clinical sign and symptom patterns (syndromes) in which normal functional movements are altered. Movement may be too fast or too slow; too frequent or too infrequent; too powerful or too weak; too rigid or too flaccid; overly deliberate or spastic. Although these abnormal movements can frequently be mitigated through the volitional effort of the affected individual or the peripherally directed therapeutic efforts of clinicians, often only pharmacologic treatment directed at the central nervous system (CNS) or neurosurgery can influence the underlying impetus of many of these conditions.

Movement disorders are capable of affecting all voluntary muscles. They are generally the result of CNS neurologic disease. Thus, most movement disorders are not confined to the head and neck region.

Most maxillofacial movement disorders are expressions of pathologic conditions in the basal ganglia (previously referred to as the *extrapyramidal system* when the thalamus is included) and/or their connections. The five basal ganglia (the caudate, putamen, globus pallidus, subthalamic, and substantia nigra) are gray matter nuclear groups located deep in the cerebral hemispheres. They communicate with the cerebral cortex and outflow tracts via the thalamus through loop connections with the cerebral cortex. The basal ganglia have only minimal direct connections with the motor spinal and cranial nerves.

A principal role of the basal ganglia is to process motor commands from the cerebral cortex that modulate, learn, form, and execute complex motor activities. Failure of one or more activities of the basal ganglia produces movement disorders. Functional problems in the basal ganglia may be the result of anatomic derangements, neurodegenerative diseases, or deficits in neurotransmitter function. Less frequently, diseases of the cerebellum are associated with movement disorders, producing impairment of coordination.

The unknown cause of some movement disorders has led clinicians to consider that these may be psychophysiologic, noxious habit, or neurotic disorders. Temporary improvement through the use of psychotropic drugs serves only to limit the cerebral cortex's initiation of motor activity but does nothing to eradicate the underlying disorder. Many functional derangements of the masticatory system, including myofascial pain and dysfunction, mandibular subluxation, internal derangements of the temporomandibular joint (TMJ), and bruxism are *not* recognized movement disorders with proven basal ganglia association. Yet the continuous and recalcitrant nature of these diseases is compelling in terms of identifying a basal ganglia etiology for some cases. As more is learned about the neuropathology of these disorders, fewer are considered to be psychological or peripheral in origin.

The most visible and affecting nature of the recognized maxillofacial movement disorders can be in the head and neck. Maxillofacial movement disorders are initially often misdiagnosed. When there is no preexisting confirmed global diagnosis, maxillofacial movement disorders may be mistakenly treated as a local peripheral disease such as myofascial pain and dysfunction, a malocclusion, or a TMD. Patients may undergo months or years of useless treatment before a correct diagnosis directs a path toward appropriate therapy. Treatment directed at the affected structures, such as the teeth, jaw, or neck, is unlikely to offer more than brief symptomatic relief for patients with centrally generated movement disorders. Thus, it is essen-

Hypokinesia

- Decreased degree or amplitude of muscle activity.
- Frequency of movement not necessarily altered.
- Not necessarily associated with hypotonia (decreased resting strength) of muscles.
- Facioscapulohumoral muscular dystrophy is a good example of a hypokinesia-hypotonia syndrome affecting the maxillofacial region.

Bradykinesia

- Slowing of movements that may reach a normal range of motion and strength.
- Catatonia, obsessional slowness, and clinical depression are symptom complexes that may produce bradykinesia.

Akinesia

- Loss of movement of a voluntary muscle.
- Etiologic site may include all tracts from the cerebral cortex to the peripheral nerve.
- Parkinson disease is a classic cause of akinesia.

Hypotonia

- Reduction in tone of the skeletal muscles.

Hyperkinesia

- Excessive movement of muscles.
- Often rhythmic in nature with deeper amplitude of function.
- May be continuous or vary with activity, alertness, sleep cycle, or emotional state.
- Hemifacial spasms and tics are examples of the expression of this condition in the head and neck.

Tics

- Brief, rapid involuntary movements that are stereotypical, repetitive, and rhythmic.
- Often involve the face and may be psychogenic or neurogenic in origin.

Dystonia

- Sustained abnormal posture and disruption of ongoing movement that results from alterations in muscle tone.
- In the maxillofacial region, involuntary co-contraction of the laryngeal muscles may result in a strained or hoarse voice.

Myoclonus

- Very brief involuntary contraction of a muscle or group of muscles.
- May occur normally, as with hiccups, or accompany certain metabolic derangements (eg, uremia), degenerative diseases of the central nervous system, or closed head trauma.

Chorea

- Brief, rapid, purposeless movement that appears to be well coordinated but is performed involuntarily.
- Frequently involves the face.

Fig 19-1 Categories of involuntary movement disorders.

tial to include movement disorders in the differential diagnosis and assessment of all patients presenting with pain-producing functional derangements of the maxillofacial region.

Movement disorders are among the most frequent conditions affecting the contemporary patient population. The onset of a movement disorder may occur at any time during growth, adulthood, or aging. Parkinson disease alone affects about 187 out of 100,000 people, which means that the average dentist serving 2,000 patients will have about 4 with Parkinson disease.[1] Moreover, the presence of an essential tremor is more than twice as frequent as Parkinson disease. Furthermore pharmacologically induced movement disorders (typically caused by psychotropic drugs or illegal and designer drugs) are a growing problem among dental patients.

Categories

The classification of involuntary movement disorders (dyskinesias) is usually based on the predominant clinical findings. In general, they can be categorized as either hypokinesias or hyperkinesias, as shown in Fig 19-1.

Diagnosis

For the purposes of the practicing clinician who primarily treats disorders affecting the maxillofacial region, some of the most pertinent movement disorders are presented, with an emphasis on their manifestations in the head and neck.

Hypokinesias

Parkinson disease and parkinsonian syndromes

Parkinson disease is the prototypical bradykinesia syndrome that causes a progressive movement disorder. Its frequency and importance as a pathophysiologic process is such that all movement disorders can be classified into parkinsonian or nonparkinsonian type.

Parkinson disease is a diagnosis of exclusion once the other conditions that produce parkinsonian signs and symptoms have been ruled out.[2] Parkinson disease and other syndromes producing parkinsonism may be initially indistinguishable. So many conditions produce secondary parkinsonism that only a thorough history, clinical exam-

ination, computerized tomography (CT) and magnetic resonance imaging (MRI) evaluations, and laboratory assessment can begin to exclude other causes. Most substantially, a strong clinical response to levodopa in patients for whom other causes have been eliminated is a good indication of Parkinson disease.

The clinical signs of Parkinson disease and parkinsonian syndromes (secondary parkinsonism) include the following key findings that are immediately evident in the maxillofacial complex:

Rest tremor
A shaking or nodding movement of the head and/or trembling of the lips and facial muscles may be apparent. A tremulous voice is often noted. A common finding is arrhythmic tremor of the thumb and fingers ("pill-rolling tremor").

Bradykinesia
The patient may exhibit a slow response to verbal commands and subsequent slow movement of the jaw (indicated by slow mastication), facial muscles (indicated by delayed response in muscles of facial expression in communication), and neck (indicated by slow turning of the head in response to request).

Rigidity
In severe Parkinson disease, rigidity may so restrict jaw, head, and neck movement that the patient remains immobile and is unable to be positioned for treatment in the dental operatory. In milder forms of progressive parkinsonism, loss of relaxed natural positioning of the jaw is expressed through a decrease in interincisal opening and clenching. If the jaw is placed in a static position, as with a mouth prop, the parkinsonian dental patient often maintains that position for a long period after the prop is removed.

Altered posture
The patient becomes stooped, with the head postured forward and downward and the arms held close to the body. The altered head position may not be adjustable because of rigidity, and the head returns to its abnormal position with the first movement after adjustment.

Drooling
Patients with moderate Parkinson disease will often carry a handkerchief to manage copious saliva production. They also may complain of a pasty or viscous feeling in the mouth. The drooling may result from excessive saliva production, an inability to provide muscle control of oral fluids, or both.

Table 19-1	Parkinsonian motor symptoms	
Symptom	**Locations**	**Findings**
Tremor	Face, tongue, jaw, extremities	Rest tremor Action tremor
Rigidity	Shoulder, calf, thigh, neck, face	Painful, hard muscles
Bradykinesia	Face, hand, legs	Micrographia (tiny writing) Slow gait Facial masking Hypophonia (quiet voice) Drooling
Tachykinesia	Extremities	Festination (faster, shorter gait) Other fast, repetitive upper and lower extremity movements
Dystonia	Hands and feet	Early morning spasm and stiffness
"Freezing"	Whole body	During walking (midstride), writing, speech (midsentence) Start hesitation at boundaries
Postural instability	Whole body	Falling forward or backward Inability to right oneself

Parkinsonian facial appearance

Patients with Parkinson disease will stare; in more severe cases, the patient's face becomes masklike, with a flaccid appearance in which the lips are apart, the mouth is open, and the eyebrows are raised. The stooped posture with the eyes lifted may give the patient a quizzical look. They also may exhibit vigorous closure of the eyes (blepharospasm).

Dental aspects

Deteriorating oral hygiene is expected with this and other progressive movement disorders, because the affected individual is less able to initiate and control the fine motor movements.

Parkinsonian motor symptoms also extend to a host of inconsistently observed general findings, presented in Table 19-1.[3]

Other parkinsonian conditions

Parkinson disease is but one of many conditions that may produce parkinsonian symptoms. If a patient presents with one or more of these findings, the clinician should observe for other signs, to assess if a parkinsonian clinical complex is emerging. Diagnosis of the various parkinsonian syndromes may rely on detection of an underlying cause. A remarkable list of potential precipitating factors for this disorder of the basal ganglia must be considered. Furthermore, some of the features of parkinsonian activity can be considered normal through different stages of life.

Secondary parkinsonian syndrome is known to be a clinical finding in some of the following major etiologic categories.

Drug induced

Some or all of these symptoms may be produced by some illegal "designer" drugs, as well as heroin; dopamine depleters, such as reserpine; dopamine receptor blockers; promethazine; lithium; neuroleptic major tranquilizers; alcohol; and calcium channel blockers, such as diltiazem. Idiosyncratic reactions to a large variety of drugs capable of causing modulation in neurotransmitter activity also have produced secondary parkinsonian syndrome.

Trauma

Chronic repeated head trauma, as occurs in boxer's encephalopathy, may produce secondary parkinsonian syndrome. A cerebrovascular event, hypoxia, or acute injury to the basal ganglia may be the precipitating cause.

Infection

HIV infection, fungal infection, viral encephalitis, and Creutzfeldt-Jakob disease are among the infectious diseases that may cause parkinsonian syndrome.

Neoplasia

Parkinsonian syndrome may be the first manifestation of a neoplasm of the basal ganglia or other CNS structure that is causing pressure on the basal ganglia.

Metabolic

Glycogen storage diseases, hypocalcemia, and enzyme deficits of CNS metabolism can produce parkinsonian symptoms.

Toxins

Sniffing carbon monoxide, methanol, gasoline, and glue, among other toxic substances, is known to produce symptoms.

Because of the progressive, debilitating, and often life-threatening nature of the diagnoses underlying parkinsonian symptoms, all patients with any of these symptoms should undergo a complete neurologic assessment. CT and MRI may reveal some of the underlying causes, but the images are often normal. Functional imaging with positron emission tomographic scanning using fluorodopa can reveal a decrease in uptake in the effected portions of the basal ganglia. If no other underlying cause is evident, a diagnosis of Parkinson disease is usually confirmed by a good clinical response to levodopa.[4]

Muscular dystrophy

Muscular dystrophies are progressive disorders resulting in weakness, atrophy, and loss of function as muscle is replaced by connective tissue and fat. Of the 250,000 cases in the United States, most occur in children. The most common form severely affects the lower extremities and trunk before affecting the head and neck. Patients with Duchenne muscular dystrophy may have atonal muscles of facial expression, jaw weakness, malocclusion, and difficulty in maintaining normal head posture.

Dental malocclusions associated with muscular dystrophy are characterized by mandibular deficiency, open bite, and a high, arched palate.[5] Measurable weakening of the muscles of mastication, tongue, buccinator, and muscles of facial expression also may result in a crossbite and drifting of the teeth. The skeletofacial deformity, as well as the disease, may be progressive during the course of growth and development.[6]

Facioscapulohumeral muscular dystrophy is a milder form of progressive muscular weakness that primarily affects the head, neck, and shoulders. While it affects 1 in 20,000 individuals, it remains an obscure entity that may remain undiagnosed. It usually begins between 7 and 20 years of age, and there is no gender predilection. Because of the slow, progressive nature of this condition, diagnosis is often delayed or never made in mild cases.[7]

Clinical findings in patients with facioscapulohumeral muscular dystrophy include progressive weakness, hypotonality, and atrophy of the muscles of facial expression, supporting muscles of the neck, and muscles of mastication. Patients sometimes present with facial or myofascial pain symptoms. Weakness and atrophy of the supporting muscles of the scapula, resulting in eventual winglike projection of the scapula and inability to raise the arms, and variable weakness of the pelvic girdle (hip and thigh) muscles may also occur. Unlike patients with other forms of muscular dystrophy, patients with facioscapulohumeral muscular dystrophy do not develop respiratory failure. The condition does not progress beyond moderate severity, and it often improves with aging. Patients generally have a normal lifespan.

Myotonic dystrophy

Myotonic dystrophy is an adult form of muscular dystrophy in which the muscles are both weak and have sustained contraction after motor effort. It is genetic in origin. The first muscles to be affected may be in the face and neck. Early diagnosis is important not only because of the progressive nature of this disease but also because of the associated cardiac conduction defects and lens cataracts that result.

The muscles of mastication are frequently seriously affected in myotonic dystrophy. Not only are they weak, but fatty degeneration, wasting, malocclusion, and TMJ modeling and remodeling are also noted.[8] Spasms in muscles of mastication that mimic myofascial pain and dysfunction may be the presenting symptom in patients with myotonic dystrophy.

Peripheral nerve injury

Peripheral nerve injury may initiate a centrally mediated movement disorder because the usual afferent input is no longer processed in the basal ganglia. Sensory nerve injury such as neurotmesis of the lingual nerve is known to produce altered articulation in speech.[9] Alteration of appropriate afferent feedback mechanisms may subtly alter functional movements. Peripheral motor nerve injury involving cranial nerves may be the result of trauma, tumor, or infection. Generalized hypokinesia may be obvious, but partial motor nerve injury may produce incomplete recruitment of muscle activity, resulting in spasm and ineffective function.

Hyperkinesias

Tremor is the rhythmic synchronous movement of opposing muscle groups in a nonfunctional continuous fashion. Tremors may be *resting tremors*, in which the patient exhibits continuous movement, or *acting tremors*, in which an activity induces the tremor. An *intention tremor* is one is which the tremor increases during an intended action. Resting tremors are associated with Parkinson disease, but acting tremors are more diverse in origin. Tremors may also be physiologic, because of fatigue, anxiety, or stress, and they may be caused by drugs such as caffeine.

An *essential tremor* is a rhythmic movement of the head, spine, extremities, or voice in response to intended function (intentional tremor or kinetic tremor) or in response to attempts to maintain position against gravity (postural tremor) Manifestations in the head and neck can result in rhythmic movement of the cervical spine, tremulous voice, rhythmic movement of the jaw, or trembling lips. Essential tremor increases with age, affecting as many as 10% of elderly patients.[10]

Tardive dyskinesia

Tardive dyskinesia is an involuntary, continuous movement involving the head, neck, trunk, and extremities resulting from the use of neuroleptic medications that block dopamine receptors in patients with psychosis. Classically identified with use of chlorpromazine hydrochloride (Thorazine, GlaxoSmithKline), the incidence of tardive dyskinesia has been reduced in recent years through control of dosing as well as prophylactic administration of anticholinergic drugs or antihistamines. Although withdrawal of the causative drug can eliminate the symptoms, this is not always the case.

A common form of tardive dyskinesia is orobuccolingual tardive dyskinesia. This classically produces lip and tongue smacking, lip pursing, tongue-in-cheek movements, severe tooth impressions in the tongue, and chewing motions. In the most severe form, the patient's head is thrown backward and the mouth may be thrust open while the tongue protrudes continuously.

A milder form of spontaneous oral dyskinesia has been noted in elderly nursing home patients not currently taking psychotropic drugs.[10] These patients often have ill-fitting dentures as well as dentoalveolar pain. They also often suffer from senile dementia.

Oculogyric crisis is a severe form of dyskinesia caused by dopamine receptor–blocking agents or occurring after encephalitis. The affected patient deviates the eyes (usually upward), thrusts the neck backward, forces the jaw open and protrudes the tongue. Increasing doses of the blocking agents may increase the frequency of attacks.[11]

Dystonia

In dystonia, tonic contractions or spasms cause deformity in body position. In contrast to myoclonic movements, dystonic muscle contractions are sustained, unidirectional, and formed in a clear pattern. When dystonias appear in adults, they are often mistakenly believed to be due to cervical trauma or emotional stress. Dystonias are centrally mediated and thus differ from peripherally mediated muscle spasms and cramps that are caused by overwork and hypoxia.

Dystonias involve the same muscle groups with each occurrence. In action dystonia, a specific motor activity, such as writing, may precipitate the spasm. Maxillofacial movement disorders that are dystonias include cranial cervical dystonia, blepharospasm, and torticollis (cervical dystonia). The twisting deformity of the upper body produced in torticollis is a classic dystonia.

A characteristic of dystonia is that the afflicted person often learns to induce afferent sensory triggers to relieve the spasm. Termed *gestes antagoniste*, they may include finger pressure on the side of the face for torticollis or an object wedged between the teeth for oromandibular dystonia.[12]

Dystonias may have an onset at any time during life. Many dystonias have a genetic origin; they are most frequently seen in individuals of Eastern European Jewish origin and in Mennonites. Although young individuals generally have symptoms in the extremities, adult-onset dystonia more often affects the head and neck.

Craniocervical dystonia

This condition may produce sustained contraction of the neck and jaw muscles, resulting in alteration of head posture. Such alterations have been associated with dental malocclusion and TMDs.[13]

Oromandibular dystonia (Meige syndrome; Brueghel syndrome)

This disorder produces involuntary contraction of the muscles of mastication, the suprahyoid muscles, and/or the intrinsic tongue muscles. The patient exhibits ocular blinking, tooth grinding, and grimacing. These involuntary contractions may be rigid and painful. Oromandibular dystonia has been associated with impaired movement-related cortical potentials, indicating that this disorder has a cerebral cortex component.[14]

Blepharospasm

This is a dystonia that can occur in isolation or as part of a complete hemifacial spasm. This startling disorder causes rigid contraction of the muscles innervated by cranial nerve VII. It is not due to a basal ganglion defect but rather is more often a result of multiple sclerosis, a tumor, or a vascular malformation in the cranial base.

Hemifacial spasm

This is a unilateral condition that involves chronic twitching of the face, caused by spasm of muscles innervated by cranial nerve VII and occasionally by those innervated by cranial nerve V. Simple hemifacial spasms variably occur after injury of the seventh cranial nerve or while Bell palsy is resolving. In Meige syndrome, the muscles of the eyes and neck are also affected.

Torticollis

Torticollis is a cervical dystonia that can be congenital or acquired. It occurs in about 1% of births and is associated with firmness of the sternocleidomastoid muscle. It usually resolves spontaneously. Plagiocephaly of the frontal bone and facial asymmetry with facial scoliosis may be associated with torticollis.[15] Whereas the head and neck relationship in congenital muscular torticollis is easily apparent, the true extent of anteroposterior growth restriction and frontal asymmetry becomes progressively apparent during growth.[16]

Torticollis is also a symptom that can be the result of trauma to the neck or CNS diseases. Turning of the neck that frequently cannot be controlled during normal activities such as driving can be noted in the adult forms. Adult cervical dystonias can often be controlled with a geste antagoniste.

Choreas

Choreas are involuntary muscle movements that flow from one body part to another. These movements are rapid, startling, and unpredictable. Facial choreic movements occur in patients with Huntington disease. Choreic movements in the face can be puzzling to the observer, who may misinterpret the condition as involving the emotional state of the individual suffering from the chorea. The sequential series of movements can include smiling, frowning, lip smacking, squeezing the eyes shut and raising the eyebrows, and other sequences of rolling facial movement.

Huntington disease

This disease is an autosomal-dominant genetic disorder. The onset can be at any age, but it often does not become apparent until the fifth decade of life. In addition to the involuntary facial muscle movements, other maxillofacial symptoms may include dysphagia, dystonia, noisy clicking of the palate, and dysarthric speech. Severe psychiatric symptoms of depression, withdrawal, and paranoia may accompany the disease at the time of primary diagnosis.

Other causes

Choreas may also be caused by HIV and AIDS, hypernatremia, hypomagnesemia, rheumatic fever, and infectious mononucleosis as well as by lightning injury.

Tics

Tics are abnormal functional movements that have the appearance of noxious habits to the casual observer. Typical tics affecting the maxillofacial region include lip smacking, blinking, squinting, throat clearing, and nose twitching. The etiology of tics is not completely understood but both the basal ganglia and the limbic structures may be involved in their pathogenesis.

Tourette syndrome

An inherited condition, Tourette syndrome develops in childhood and involves a sequence of rapid tics (involuntary vocalizations, movements, and activities) that are repetitive but not rhythmic. These events may occur infrequently or several times a day and are startling to both observers and the patient. The tics occur in bouts and may be induced by social interaction. Oral manifestations of Tourette syndrome include a high incidence of dental caries, injuries to the oral mucosa, and buccolingual choreaform movements.[17]

Myoclonic disorders

Myoclonus is a sudden shocklike muscle contraction measurable in milliseconds. The contractions may be single or repeated randomly. The myoclonic jerk may be generalized or it may affect a single group of muscles. A myoclonic jerk is an event seen in motor epilepsies. However, myoclonus is not necessarily the manifestation of disease. Hiccups and sleep jerks are physiologic myoclonic events. While myoclonic movements most often affect the extremities, there are also head and neck manifestations.

Palatal myoclonus

This condition causes spasmodic rhythmic movement of the soft palate musculature and parapharyngeal muscles, often producing an audible clicking.[18] It may be associated with an eye movement disorder, in which case it is called *oculopalatal myoclonus*. It may result from brainstem trauma, tumor, stroke, multiple sclerosis, or other diseases that produce brainstem pathosis.

Summary

The signs and symptoms of maxillofacial movement disorders are diverse and often mimic other conditions. A thorough review of the signs and symptoms exhibited, the use of clinical databases, and, most important, consultation with a neurologist are indicated when a movement disorder is suspected.

References

1. Schoenberg BS, Anderson DW, Haerer AF. Prevalence of Parkinson's disease in the population of Copiah County, Mississippi. Neurology 1985;35:841–845.

2. Jankovic J, Rajput AH, McDermott MP, Perl DP. The evolution of diagnosis in early Parkinson disease. Arch Neurol 2000;57:369–372.

3. Parkinsonism. In: Fahn S, Greene PE, Ford B, Bressman SB (eds). Handbook of Movement Disorders. Philadelphia: Current Medicine, 1998:11–48.

4. Jankovic J, Rajput AH, McDermott MP, Perl DP. The evolution of diagnosis in early Parkinson disease. Arch Neurol 2000;57:369–372.

5. Guler AU, Ceylan G, Ozkoc O, Aydiin M, Cengiz N. Prosthetic treatment of a patient with facioscapulohumeral muscular dystrophy: A clinical report. J Prosthet Dent 2003; 90:321–324.

6. Matsumoto S, Morinushi T, Ogura T. Time dependent changes of variables associated with malocclusion in patients with Duchenne muscular dystrophy. J Clin Pediatr Dent 2002; 27:53–61.

7. Facioscapulohumeral Muscular Dystrophy Society [website]. Available at: http://www.fshsociety.org/fsh/fshd.html. Accessed November 16, 2004.

8. Zanoteli E, Yamashita HK, Suzuki H, Oliveira AS, Gabbai A. Temporomandibular joint and masticatory muscle involvement in myotonic dystrophy: A study by magnetic resonance imaging. Oral Surg Oral Med Oral Pathol Oral Radiol Endod 2002;94:262–271.

9. Niemi M, Laaksonen JP, Vahatalo K, Tuomainen J, Aaltonen O, Happonen RP. Effects of transitory lingual nerve impairment on speech: An acoustic study of vowel sounds. J Oral Maxillofac Surg 2002;60:647–652; discussion 653.

10. Louis ED, Marder K, Cote L, et al. Prevalence of a history of shaking in persons 65 years of age or older: Diagnostic and functional correlates. Mov Disord 1996;11:63–69.

11. Movement disorders induced by dopamine receptor blocking agents. In: Fahn S, Greene PE, Ford B, Bressman SB (eds). Handbook of Movement Disorders. Philadelphia: Current Medicine, 1998:127–134.

12. Muller J, Wissel J, Masuhr F, Ebersbach G, Wenning GK, Poewe W. Clinical characteristics of the geste antagoniste in cervical dystonia. J Neurol 2001;248:478–482.

13. Kondo E, Aoba T. Case report of malocclusion with abnormal head posture and TMJ symptoms. Am J Orthod Dentofac Orthop 1999;116:481–493.

14. Yoshida K, Kaji R, Kohara N, Murase N, Ikeda A, Shibasaki H. Movement related cortical potentials before jaw excursions in oromandibular dystonia. Mov Disord 2003;18: 94–100.

15. Putnam G, Postlethwaite K, Chate R, Ilnakovan V. Facial scoliosis—A diagnostic dilemma. Int J Oral Maxillofac Surg 1993;22:324–327.

16. Ferguson J. Cephalometric interpretation and assessment of facial asymmetry secondary to congenital torticollis. Int J Oral Maxillofac Surg 1993;22:7–10.

17. Friedlander AH, Cummings JL. Dental treatment of patients with Gilles de la Tourette's syndrome. Oral Surg Oral Med Oral Pathol 1992;73:299–303.

18. Deuschl G, Mischke G, Schenck E, Schulte-Monting J, Lucking CH. Symptomatic and essential rhythmic palatal myoclonus. Brain 1990;113:1645–1672.

Differential Diagnosis of Orofacial Pain

Robert L. Merrill

It is appropriate that current texts on temporomandibular disorders (TMDs) include a discussion of the scope and differential diagnosis of orofacial pain in order to place such disorders in the broader context of pain syndromes that occur in the head. These pain syndromes are often confused with TMDs by both dentists and physicians, and this issue has been a major impetus for expanding the field of orofacial pain disorders within the dental profession to include conditions heretofore considered to be exclusively a part of medicine.

To date, there is no generally accepted and standardized classification system for orofacial pain, making the task of performing a differential diagnosis difficult. The most recent effort to categorize and classify all of the known craniofacial pain conditions was published by the International Headache Society (IHS) in 2004.[1] The IHS included TMDs and neuropathic pain in its system of diagnostic criteria for headache disorders, cranial neuralgias, and facial pain. The classification system grouped headache or head pain in a hierarchically constructed system using operational diagnostic criteria for all headache disorders, including the neuropathies and TMDs.

The IHS sought to use definitions rather than descriptions and endeavored to avoid the use of descriptive modifiers such as *often*, *commonly*, or *frequently*. Addition-

ally, the IHS recognized that each condition had to have one set of criteria but that any one patient could have more than one form of head pain. Although the ideal classification would be characterized by both high specificity and high sensitivity, the IHS acknowledged that a usable system would have to be a compromise between these standards.

The purposes of this chapter are to review the process of forming a differential diagnosis for orofacial pain, to discuss the various conditions that can cause persistent pain, and to suggest an examination process to help clinicians form an accurate diagnosis more consistently. It is hoped that this information will help dentists avoid needlessly altering occlusal relationships, sacrificing teeth, or performing unnecessary temporomandibular joint (TMJ) surgery when treating patients with orofacial pain.

Figure 20-1 shows a general scheme for the conditions seen in the orofacial, cranial, and cervical areas. The scheme goes far beyond what was originally envisioned as TMJ or nonodontogenic orofacial pain. However, all of these possibilities have to be considered, because most of the listed disorders can manifest as pain in the TMJ or orofacial region and can be confused with odontogenic or TMJ pain. Therefore, clinicians must be aware of the conditions in the taxonomic scheme and know their distinguishing characteristics, in order to make an appropriate

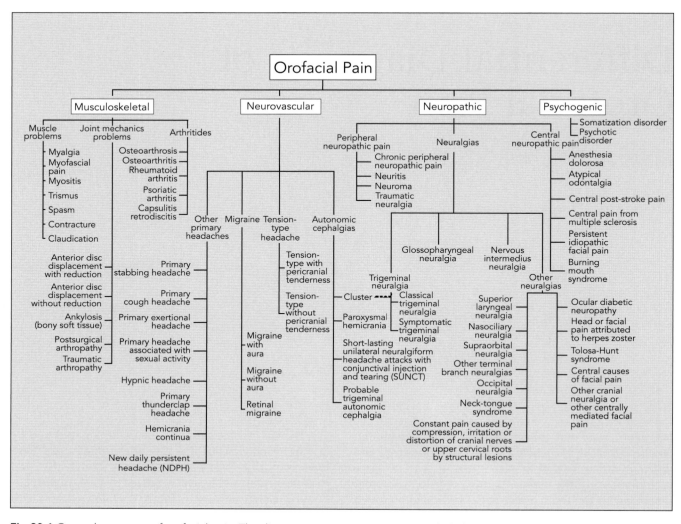

Fig 20-1 General taxonomy of orofacial pain. The diagram separates pain into musculoskeletal, neuropathic, neurovascular, and psychogenic disorders.

differential diagnosis of the pain presented by each patient.

Orofacial pain can be caused by extracranial disorders, such as infections or lesions, intracranial lesions (eg, tumors), or vascular compression of sensory fibers from the facial region. These potential sources of pain must also be considered in the differential diagnosis, and the clinician must rule in or rule out each source by obtaining a thorough history of the pain and doing a careful clinical examination. Figure 20-2 shows a flow chart or step-by-step analytic thought process that can serve as a guide to the clinician during patient evaluation.

The clinician should obtain a detailed history of the presenting problem, with a focused inquiry about the

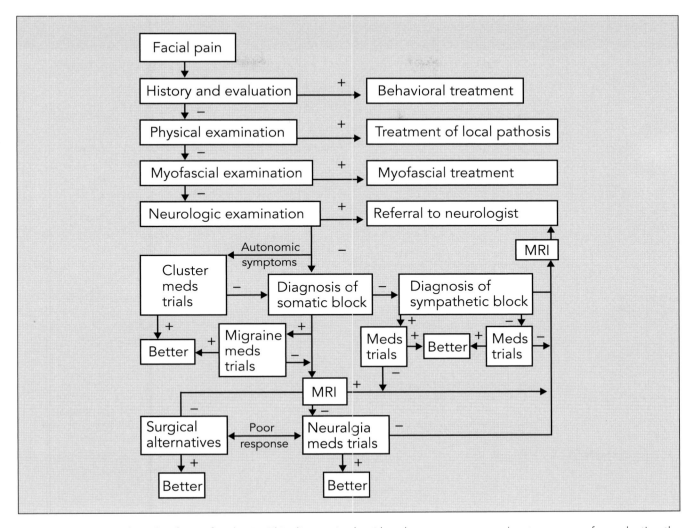

Fig 20-2 Diagnostic algorithm for orofacial pain. This diagnostic algorithm demonstrates a step-by-step process for evaluating the complex pain problems found in the orofacial region.[2] (MRI) Magnetic resonance imaging; (meds) medicines.

description and temporal pattern of the pain, the exacerbating and alleviating factors, and associated symptoms. As the thought process is pursued through this algorithm, pain and organ systems that should be ruled in or out are considered and added to or excluded from the differential diagnosis. Additionally, Fig 20-2 suggests diagnostic procedures that should be performed and specialist referrals that should be made for those conditions that fail to be diagnosed during the evaluation process.[2] Table 20-1 shows the sources of pain that should be considered during the evaluation process; example disorders are included for each of the potential causes of orofacial pain.

Table 20-1	Sources of pain in the orofacial region		
System	**Pain pattern**	**Pain description**	**Example disorders**
Extracranial	Becomes continuous	Variable, but usually aching or throbbing	Dental pain Acute sinusitis Mucogingival lesions Oropharyngeal tumors
Intracranial	Continuous	Aching, throbbing, sharp, or lancinating	Acoustic neuroma Aneurysms Tumors
Neurovascular	Episodic or intermittent	Aching, throbbing, may have episodes of sharp or boring pain	Facial migraine Migraine Cluster headache Paroxysmal hemicrania
Musculoskeletal	Continuous and variable with exacerbations with function or provocation	Aching	Myalgia Myofascial pain Arthritides
Peripheral neuropathic pain	Continuous, variable; exacerbated by static mechanical stimulation; variable response to local analgesic blocking, but generally blockable	Deep aching	Peripheral trigeminal neuropathy Neuritis Neuroma
Central neuropathic pain	Continuous, may or may not be variable; exacerbated by dynamic light touch; not responsive to local analgesic blocking	Aching, burning	Chronic centralized trigeminal neuropathy (atypical odontalgia) Complex regional pain syndromes I and II
Psychogenic pain	Variable	Variable	Somatization disorders Psychotic disorders

Extracranial and Intracranial Sources of Pain

Because of the rich innervation of the head and neck area, there are many potential problems that can impact sensory nerves, resulting in pain. The clinician always must consider the possibility that persistent pain in the orofacial region is caused by a tumor or central lesion. Dentists are aware that some maxillary toothaches may be caused by acute sinusitis, but they may not consider the fact that peripheral lesions such as nasopharyngeal or oropharyngeal tumors also cause orofacial pain. As the verbal history of the pain complaint is developed, the clinician should ask questions that would rule in or rule out potential extracranial or intracranial lesions.

Central Nervous System Lesions

Pain resulting from central lesions is usually described as increasing in intensity with time, and often the patient will describe pain accompaniments such as numbness, tingling, or weakness.

Acoustic neuroma

Acoustic neuroma is the most common brain tumor that causes pain in the orofacial region. Commonly, the pain is similar to and often mistaken for trigeminal neuralgia until magnetic resonance imaging (MRI) of the posterior fossa is performed. The orofacial and dental symptoms of acoustic neuroma are episodic aching or a sharp, electric-like toothache or jaw ache. The patient may only complain of toothache and be unaware of other symptoms. Often, but not always, acoustic neuroma will be associated with decreased hearing or hypoacusis on the side of the pain because it involves the eighth cranial nerve. Acoustic neuromas are slow growing, and the patient may tolerate the episodic pain for significant periods. These patients are vulnerable to having inappropriate dental procedures performed to treat a misdiagnosed problem.

Aneurysms and blood vessel dissection

Aneurysms and dissection of intracranial blood vessels coursing through the cavernous sinus area may also impinge on trigeminal nerve branches V1 and V2, resulting in pain in the upper face and headache. Headaches that develop rapidly to maximum intensity within minutes are termed *thunderclap* headaches, and they may be a premonitory sign of an aneurysm or blood vessel dissection. These headaches may also be associated with double vision caused by oculomotor or trochlear nerve paresis, because these nerves also pass through the cavernous sinus and may be impacted by pressure from the aneurysm, dissection, or rupture of a blood vessel. Additionally, parasympathetic fibers in the oculomotor nerve can be affected by the increased pressure, decreasing the ipsilateral pupillary response to bright light.

Multiple sclerosis

Commonly, multiple sclerosis is associated with numbness, tingling, and pain in the orofacial region. The pain and tingling may present as trigeminal neuralgia when the central demyelinating lesions involve the trigeminal tract and root.

Peripheral Lesions

Dental disease is one of the most common causes of orofacial pain. Disorders involving tissues in and around the face, such as sialadenitis, salivary gland blockage, sinusitis, sinus polyps, mucogingival lesions, and oral and nasopharyngeal cancers, can also be associated with orofacial pain and should be investigated and ruled out during the evaluation stage.

Dental disease

Although dental pain is most often due to obvious caries or periodontal disease, one of the most perplexing problems in dentistry is the diagnosis of pain in a tooth that does not show obvious pathosis on intraoral examination or in the radiographs. When the tooth shows an obvious crack or periapical radiolucency, the diagnosis is more certain. However, cases have been reported in which no disease could be found during clinical examination or on the radiograph, but the tooth was treated or eventually extracted and the pain was resolved, indicating that the initial pain problem was indeed odontogenic. On the other hand, often dental treatment is undertaken, despite the lack of a definitive diagnosis, in the hope that the symptoms will be alleviated, but the pain continues even after the tooth is extracted.

The term *cracked tooth syndrome* was first used by Cameron[3] in 1964. It has been defined as an incomplete fracture of a vital tooth involving the dentin and possibly the dental pulp. The fracture most often is vertical, involving both the crown and root of the tooth.[3–6] A review of the literature on cracked tooth syndrome shows a focus on examination for a crack, with no mention of other conditions that can cause tooth pain, eg, neurovascular, neuropathic, or musculoskeletal conditions.[3,7–10]

Clinicians must be aware that the reports of cracked teeth given in the literature are, for the most part, descriptions of teeth successfully treated or extracted to discover the crack.[5–7,11–15] Little is said about those situations in which the teeth were unsuccessfully treated and eventually extracted, and no cracks were found. This omission is, in part, because of a general lack of awareness and understanding in the dental community of the different pain conditions that may imitate a toothache and may be mistaken for a cracked tooth. The clinician must evaluate the tooth in question carefully and consider all factors and disorders that can imitate a toothache while performing a thorough dental evaluation of the tooth through intraoral and radiographic examinations.[2,15,16]

Symptoms of a cracked tooth range from vague discomfort or mild pain during mastication to severe, stabbing, lancinating pain.[7,10,12] The most commonly reported symptoms are pain associated with chewing, sensitivity to hot or cold stimuli or chemical changes,[7] and pain following release of chewing pressure. However, frequently the patient reports no increase in symptoms with any provocation.[10]

Incomplete fractures of posterior teeth rarely occur in people younger than 40 years. The mandibular molars and maxillary premolars are the most commonly involved teeth, and many are noncarious and unrestored.[5–7,10,15,17]

Salivary gland disorders

Pain from sialadenitis or salivary gland blockage may be confused with toothache, a TMD, or trigeminal neuralgia. Salivary gland pain is often described as aching with accompanying sharp, stabbing pain when the patient eats. The affected glands are usually swollen and painful to the touch. When the blocked parotid gland is stimulated by food, the reflex parasympathetic sudomotor stimulation causes sharp pain as the sudomotor muscles contract, attempting to expel glandular fluid. The patient should be carefully questioned about the actual incident inciting the pain, to determine if it is the act of chewing the causes the pain or simply the placement of food in the mouth. The latter type of pain must be differentiated from a TMD, which is aggravated by chewing. Parotid pain also should be assessed by palpation and manipulation of the inflamed tissue.

Nasopharyngeal and oropharyngeal lesions

As peripheral tumors develop, the patient will usually become aware of swelling and alteration of sensation. Pain ensues from pressure and traction on the sensory fibers in the affected area, becoming continuous, although brief episodes of sharp or shooting pain may be associated with the nerve irritation. Additionally, motor nerves that traverse the area affected by the tumor may be irritated, resulting in paresis of the associated muscles. These symptoms should be evaluated carefully during the clinical examination and, if any doubt or question persists, the patient should be referred to an ear, nose, and throat specialist for further evaluation.

Sinus disorders

Acute sinusitis typically causes pain in the teeth whose roots are in close proximity to the floor of the maxillary sinus. The association between nasal congestion or discharge and tooth pain is easily determined. Pain that occurs when pressure is applied to the maxillary sinus and sinus radiographs will usually confirm the diagnosis.

Although chronic sinusitis is often blamed for facial pain, it is generally not a painful disorder. There may or may not be clear, nonpurulent nasal discharge, and finger pressure applied to the sinus areas is not painful. However, sinus polyps, often associated with clear discharge and/or bleeding, may be painful when chronically irritated. Such patients should be evaluated by an ear, nose, and throat specialist after other potential causes of pain in the sinus region are ruled out.

Nonpurulent sinus congestion associated with chronic sinusitis may be a rebound phenomenon from the overuse of antihistamines. Discontinuation of the medication allows the sinuses to clear.

Pain from migraine headaches may have a facial component that is easily confused with sinusitis, and the patient's pain may even respond to antihistamines. These patients often chronically use antihistamines to treat the pain, which is actually caused by the neurovascular inflammation of migraine.

Acute otitis media

TMD symptoms may be easily confused with acute otitis externa or otitis media. Acute otitis media is usually due to bacterial or viral infection that accompanies a viral upper respiratory tract infection and is often associated with fever. The ear feels full, and there is decreased hearing on the affected side. Because the infection also may affect the vestibular system, the patient may experience loss of balance. Examination of the tympanic membrane reveals opacity and bulging, and the membrane appears yellow or inflamed. The swelling or bulging is best viewed with a pneumatic otoscope. If the results of the ear examination are normal, the symptoms may be caused by pain referred from the TMJ, the masticatory muscles, or teeth.

Chronic otitis media

Acute otitis media can become chronic if the inflammatory response is not resolved. The associated pain may be mistaken for a TMJ disorder, and, as with acute otitis media, it may also be referred to the ipsilateral teeth.[18]

Musculoskeletal Pain

A detailed discussion of the differential diagnosis of musculoskeletal pain can be found in chapter 17. Craniocervical musculoskeletal disorders are the most prevalent of all conditions falling within the rubric of orofacial pain. Therefore, the astute clinician must carefully distinguish between musculoskeletal pain and the other orofacial pain conditions described in the present chapter.

Table 20-2	Comparison of neurovascular headaches				
Headache disorder	Location	Provoking/ aggravating factors	Temporal pattern	Pain quality	Associated symptoms
Facial migraine/ migraine	Cranium or maxilla involving posterior teeth	None or migraine triggers; pain aggravated with physical effort	Intermittent, lasting 2 to 72 hours	Throbbing and aching	Nausea, photophobia, and/or phonophobia
Jabs and jolts syndrome	Temples; parietal and occipital	None	Episodic, lasting seconds	Sharp jabs (not electrical)	With or without migraine
Cluster headache	Strictly unilateral, typically behind eye but may be in maxilla or TMJ	None or cluster triggers such as smoking, alcohol, high altitude	Episodic, lasting 20 minutes to 1 hour; bouts occurring 1 to 15 times per day	Sharp, stabbing	Rhinorrhea, nasal stuffiness, red sclera, drooping or swollen eyelid
Paroxysmal hemicrania	Strictly unilateral, typically behind eye but may be in maxilla or TMJ	None	Intermittent, lasting minutes; bouts occurring 15 to 40 times per day	Sharp, stabbing	Rhinorrhea, nasal stuffiness, red sclera, drooping or swollen eyelid

Neurovascular Pain

The second edition of *The International Classification of Headache Disorders* (ICHD-II)[1] is the definitive and most widely accepted document for the classification of such conditions. The system lists 14 categories of headache. The first four categories represent the primary headache disorders, while the remaining 10 categories contain secondary headache conditions, including headache from sources such as neuropathic pain and disorders of the teeth, jaws, and cervical structures. All headache symptoms or complaints should be evaluated and included in the differential diagnosis, because these problems, if ignored, may limit the successful management of the patient's condition. However, the astute clinician also may note a decrease in certain headache symptoms, particularly migraine and tension-type headache disorders,

as successful treatment of a primary musculoskeletal pain progresses.

The primary headache disorders to be included in a differential diagnosis of orofacial pain include migraine headache, tension-type headache, and the autonomic cephalgias, such as cluster headache (Table 20-2). Although these headache disorders are most often present in the V1 distribution of the trigeminal nerve, they may cause pain in the face and be confused with a TMD or odontogenic pain.[19-21]

In his classic book, *Headache*, Raskin[22] describes facial migraine or chronic carotidynia as a neurovascular headache disorder that has its primary symptoms in the face and more specifically in the maxillary molar and premolar and maxillary sinus regions. The patient typically complains of a toothache; however, during the clinician's careful exploration of the problem, such patients also will report nausea and sensitivity to light as well as toothache.[22]

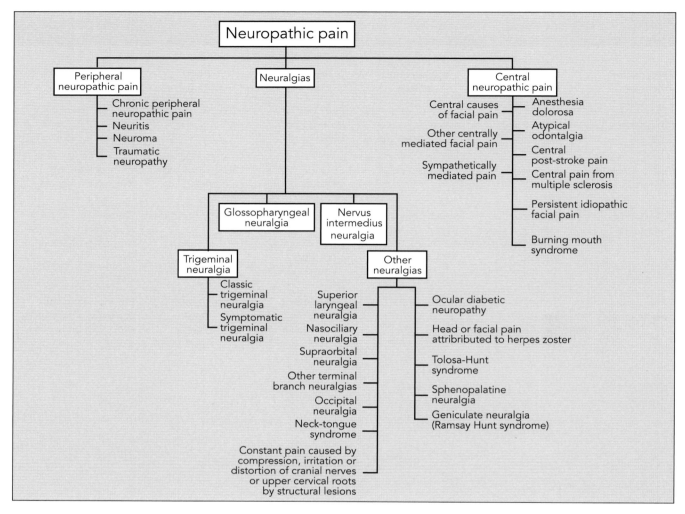

Fig 20-3 Taxonomy of neuropathic pain.

Neuropathic Pain

The trigeminal nerve richly innervates the orofacial region, and its nerve endings are typically traumatized by most dental procedures. Considering the number of dental procedures performed on a daily basis, it is amazing that traumatically induced neuropathic pain is not more common. Figure 20-3 shows the general categories of neuropathic pain and divides those categories into more specific disorders. There is still much disagreement as to the specific neuropathic disorders that occur in the orofacial region, so the information in this classification system undoubtedly will become obsolete as newer information is developed through research.

The spectrum of neuropathic pain conditions is diagrammed in Fig 20-4. This diagram displays peripheral and central neuropathic pain conditions as suggested by the IASP and IHS classification systems. The neuralgias that are characterized by lancinating pain are also included in this diagram. Neuralgias have characteristics that suggest either a peripheral problem, a centralized problem, or a combination of both. One of the initial tasks of the clinician is to determine which category of pain accounts for the patient's complaint. If the pain is thought to be neuropathic, then the clinician must ascertain whether the pain is responsive to local and/or topical anesthetics. A positive response would be indicative of a peripheral neuropathy. If the response is negative, although the patient shows indications of anesthesia in the area, it would be indicative of a non-neuropathic problem or a centralized neuropathic pain condition. Table 20-3 reviews the diagnostic criteria for various neuropathic pain conditions.

Fig 20-4 Spectrum of neuropathic pain.

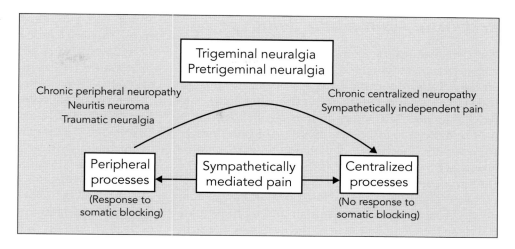

Table 20-3	Diagnostic criteria for neuropathic pain	
Pain generator location	**Types**	**Signs and symptoms**
Peripheral > central	C-fiber sensitization Neuroma Traumatic neuralgia Chronic peripheral Trigeminal neuropathy	Continuous variable aching pain History of trauma to area No obvious local cause Pain aggravated by local stimuli (hyperalgesia and allodynia) Normal radiograph Positive response to somatic block Response to thermography not defined Sympathetic block does not define this disorder
Both central and peripheral	Atypical odontalgia (partially blockable) Complex regional pain syndrome II or III (CRPS II or III)	Continuous, variable diurnal aching pain History of trauma to area Pain present longer than 4 months Pain aggravated by local stimuli (hyperalgesia and allodynia) No obvious local cause Normal radiograph Equivocal response to somatic block Positive response to sympathetic block (> 60%) not a defining characteristic
Central > peripheral	Atypical odontalgia (nonblockable) Sympathetically independent pain (SIP)	Continuous, variable diurnal aching pain History of trauma to area Pain present longer than 4 months Pain aggravated by local stimuli (hyperalgesia and allodynia) No obvious local cause Normal radiograph Negative response to somatic block Negative response to sympathetic block, although not a defining characteristic

Peripheral Neuropathic Pain

Peripheral neuropathic orofacial pain is characterized by a moderately intense aching and/or burning sensation in an area of previous nerve trauma, whether extraoral or intraoral. Chronic peripheral neuropathic pain can develop from a trivial injury; in the oral environment, it may be difficult to associate a causal event with the subsequent pain. Procedures as simple as a dental prophylaxis have been associated with the development of chronic neuropathic pain. Because nerve injury is so prevalent during dental procedures, it raises the question of why persistent posttreatment jaw and tooth pain are not more common. Fortunately, the healing response in the vast majority of patients resolves most types of neuronal activation, so the pain or discomfort is eliminated as the healing process is completed.

Nevertheless, persistent or chronic pain does occur in some patients even after mild peripheral nerve activation. The challenge for the clinician is to render an appropriate diagnosis and treatment plan for such pain. The clinician must obtain a careful history of the initiating event and the progression of the pain. Additionally, he or she should develop careful descriptions of the quality of the pain, the temporal pattern, aggravating and alleviating factors, and associated symptoms. The physical evaluation should include a cranial nerve examination and careful neurosensory testing of the site of pain.

One of the best distinguishing characteristics of peripheral neuropathies is their response to topical or local anesthetic blocking, which should eliminate such pain. On the other hand, pain from a central neuropathy will not be affected by a peripheral block, because the pain-generating mechanism is located within the central nervous system and is not the result of peripheral neuronal activity.

Peripheral sensitization and irritable nociceptors

In 1989, Cline et al,[23] in evaluating a chronic neuropathic pain that was responsive to local anesthetic blocking and lacked sympathetic involvement, proposed that C fibers were sensitized and continued to produce action potentials even though the injury from the traumatic event had long since healed. The pain was described as chronic, spontaneous burning with a painful response to normally nonpainful tactile stimuli.

Subsequently, Fields et al[24] proposed a similar mechanism for ongoing pain associated with postherpetic neuralgia, and implicated "irritable" nociceptors. The characteristics of this condition would be chronic but blockable

aching and burning pain subsequent to a traumatic event. This mechanism undoubtedly accounts for some of the persistent painful conditions found in the oral environment (see chapters 4 and 5 for a discussion of the neurophysiology of the trigeminal system).

Fields et al[24] suggested that a sensory examination of a field of irritable nociceptors would find *static mechanical hyperalgesia*. The use of this term is confusing, because the International Association for the Study of Pain (IASP) classification[25] defines *hyperalgesia* as an increased response to a stimulus that is normally painful, but the stimulus used by Fields and colleagues[24] in the examination was finger pressure to the affected area. This pressure normally would not be painful, so the term *hyperalgesia* is inaccurate. A better term would be *allodynia*, which is defined as a painful response to a normally nonpainful stimulus. Therefore, the response to a static, normally nonpainful force applied to the affected area would be described as *static mechanical allodynia*.[26]

Use of this term also suggests the probable mechanism for the ongoing pain, ie, sensitized C fibers. These nociceptors would be responsive to topical and/or local anesthetic application, reducing or eliminating the pain. The features distinguishing peripheral neuropathy from central neuropathy, therefore, are the chronic activation and lowered threshold to stimulation of the C-fiber nociceptors and a positive response to anesthetics.

Researchers in the pain field have opined that a mechanistic approach to the diagnosis and treatment of chronic pain can lead to better treatment outcomes; however, it is generally recognized that the scientific community is far from understanding all of the mechanisms involved in chronic pain and that knowledge about the subject is somewhat superficial at the present time. Those conditions that normally respond to topical or local anesthetics because C fibers are sensitized (the "irritable nociceptors" described by Fields et al[24]) are chronic peripheral trigeminal neuropathy, neuritis, neuroma, and traumatic neuralgia (see Fig 20-3). Painful neuropathies not responding to local anesthetic blocking will be discussed under the classification of central neuropathic pain.

Neuritis

Neuritis is defined by the IASP as "inflammation of a nerve or nerves (not to be used unless inflammation is thought to be present)."[25] Observable evidence of inflammation should be present if this term is used. Local inflammation of a nerve should respond to topical and local anesthetics and should be characterized by aching and burning pain. This form of neuropathy does not include conditions caused by neuropraxis, neurotmesis, or deafferentation.

Optic neuritis

The ICHD-II classification committee has included optic neuritis in its classification system of chronic head pain. Optic neuritis is characterized by pain behind one or both eyes accompanied by impairment of central vision caused by demyelination of the optic nerve. The pain usually precedes the development of visual symptoms by less than 4 weeks. The conditions may be a manifestation of multiple sclerosis.[1]

Pain associated with optic neuritis is characteristically noted in the involved eye and could be mistaken for headache. Both migraine and optic neuritis may be associated with blurred vision and increased pain in the eye when the eyes are moved. These conditions can be differentiated by the apparent progressive nature of the neuritis. The optic nerve inflammation causes progressive visual loss and loss of color information because the inflammation inhibits signal transmission from the retina to the brain. Half of the axons in the optic nerve carry signals from the fovea, so the major change in vision is a loss of acuity and color in the central vision. Because optic nerve conduction is reduced by the inflammation, the pupillary light reflex is also affected (efferent pupillary defect). The persistent symptoms of optic neuritis are in contrast to the intraictal changes of vision that occur with migraine. Additionally, migraine is not associated with an efferent pupillary defect.

Diagnostic criteria

1. Dull pain is present behind one or both eyes; the pain is worsened by eye movement and fulfills criteria 3 and 4.
2. A central or paracentral scotoma is present, causing visual impairment.
3. Onset of pain and onset of visual impairment are separated by less than 4 weeks.
4. Pain resolves within 4 weeks.
5. A compressive lesion has been ruled out.

Optic neuritis is usually associated with an afferent pupillary defect in the affected eye and is detected by testing the pupillary reflex. When the optic nerve is inflamed, light shined in the affected eye does not cause normal pupillary constriction in either eye, because the message is not carried along the optic nerve fibers that course to the pretectal area of the rostral midbrain and stimulate the reflex pupillary constriction. Light shined in the normal eye will cause the reflex pupillary constriction in both eyes. Additionally, visual acuity and color perception are decreased.

Optic neuritis may be confused with other headache disorders as well as certain TMDs because the pain may be experienced as deep, aching periorbital and brow pain.

Neuroma

The orofacial region is susceptible to nerve damage and the possibility of neuroma formation. When a peripheral nerve axon is injured, the damaged terminal produces sprouts that grow peripherally toward the structure it innervated. If the sheath is also damaged and the sprout cannot enter, it continues to grow outside the sheath, producing a gnarled mass of nerve fibers called a *neuroma*.

The neuroma is sensitive to stimulation and develops spontaneous discharge activity within a week. It is most sensitive within the first 2 weeks of development but pain may continue at lesser levels for longer periods. Both animal studies and anecdotal reports suggest that ectopic discharge occurs not only at the site of the neuroma but also at sites proximal to it.

A neuroma can be identified by a painful response to tapping (Tinel sign) over the neuroma site. Additionally, static mechanical allodynia may be present over the area.[27–30]

Traumatic neuropathy

The IASP defines *neuropathy* as "a disturbance of function or pathological change in a nerve."[25] Trauma to a sensory nerve can lead to dysfunction of the affected nerve, characterized primarily by spontaneous pain. The term *traumatic neuropathy* has been used to describe sensory nerve dysfunction when the inciting incident can be clearly identified. However, the term is generic in reference to clinical manifestations and does not indicate whether peripheral or central processes drive the pain.

Symptoms of traumatic neuropathy are similar to the symptoms of peripheral neuropathy, but the traumatic incident is clear. Often areas in the damaged tissue will display peripheral pain (blockable, with indications of static mechanical allodynia), central pain (not blockable, with indications of dynamic mechanical allodynia), dysesthesia, and anesthesia similar to that occurring in postherpetic neuralgia.

Neuralgias

Trigeminal neuralgia

Classic trigeminal neuralgia and pretrigeminal neuralgia (trigeminal neuralgia variant)

No description of pretrigeminal neuralgia has been included in the present IASP or the IHS classification systems because there is disagreement about the actual nature of the condition.[1,25] Some critics contend that the condition does not exists or that it is merely a variant of classic trigeminal neuralgia.

Pretrigeminal and trigeminal neuralgia have both peripheral and central mechanisms. The clinical presentation of trigeminal neuralgia has been described as a "sudden, usually unilateral, severe brief stabbing recurrent pain in the distribution of one or more branches of the Vth cranial nerve."[25] If the individual is young, the presence of a tumor or multiple sclerosis must be ruled out. The posterior fossa or cerebellopontile angle is the area most affected by a tumor. If the neuralgia is caused by a demonstrable lesion it is considered a symptomatic trigeminal neuralgia; if no lesion is identifiable, the neuralgia is regarded as idiopathic.

Pretrigeminal neuralgia, a variant presentation of trigeminal neuralgia without sharp, shooting pain, has been mentioned infrequently in the literature, and it is only relatively recently that the condition has been suggested to be a pretrigeminal disorder developmentally.[2,31–34] Symonds[34] described a subgroup of facial neuralgias that had an atypical presentation, not fitting the accepted categories of that time. The patients were often thought to have psychogenic pain until the condition changed to the more characteristic symptoms of trigeminal neuralgia.

The site of pretrigeminal neuralgia pain most commonly involves the maxilla or mandible (V2 or V3), an area of the alveolar process (usually in the molar region), or the base of the tongue. Several case studies describe the presenting complaint, often in the area of a tooth, as a dull, continuous toothache that may have been present for days to years. The pain is not lancinating and paroxysmal, and the aching quality mimics the familiar toothache. The temporal pattern of pretrigeminal neuralgia is similar to that of trigeminal neuralgia; long periods of remission between attacks are common.

Inappropriate dental or TMJ therapies are often undertaken before the pain complaint is carefully differentiated. Patients who are finally diagnosed with pretrigeminal neuralgia often demonstrate a prior history of multiple dental procedures performed to alleviate what was assumed to be tooth pain. These treatments may involve multiple endodontic procedures, apical surgery, extractions, bite appliances, and dental reconstructive procedures.

Imaging by computed tomography (CT) or MRI should be considered in the assessment of any neuropathic pain, such as trigeminal neuralgia and pretrigeminal neuralgia, that is not associated with trauma. The age group most commonly associated with trigeminal neuralgia or pretrigeminal neuralgia is 50 to 70 years, and the prevalence is 3 to 5 per 100,000 per year.

Symptomatic trigeminal neuralgia

Trigeminal and pretrigeminal neuralgias must be differentiated from neuralgia secondary to a tumor or an aberrant blood vessel that is pressing on the trigeminal root. Central or cerebellopontile angle tumors are most often accompanied by cranial nerve deficits. Trigeminal neuralgia may be mistaken for glossopharyngeal neuralgia when the active area of the mandibular division is near the pharynx.

The paroxysmal pain of trigeminal neuralgia can also be confused with idiopathic stabbing headache (jabs and jolts syndrome) and with short-lasting, unilateral neuralgiform pain with conjunctival injection and tearing (SUNCT). Idiopathic stabbing headache is marked by paroxysms of cephalic pain in multiple sites, with varying frequency and often occurring in bouts. SUNCT is marked by short-lasting unilateral paroxysmal pain, usually in the ocular region, that is accompanied by autonomic phenomena such as conjunctival injection, lacrimation, and rhinorrhea.[35–39] Table 20-4 provides a comparative listing of the diagnostic features and management of the facial neuralgias.

Glossopharyngeal neuralgia

Glossopharyngeal neuralgia, like trigeminal neuralgia, is subclassified as symptomatic or classic.[1] Glossopharyngeal neuralgia is an uncommon disorder of the ninth cranial nerve with a prevalence of 0.5 persons per 100,000 per year. It has been reported that it is more common in people older than 50 years (57%), but 43% of cases occur in persons between 18 and 50 years of age.[1]

The clinical picture of glossopharyngeal neuralgia is different from that of trigeminal neuralgia. Pain is reported to radiate from the oropharyngeal area upward and backward toward the ear. It is rare for the pain to begin in the ear and radiate downward. Swallowing, stimulation of the back of the throat, coughing, talking, or rapid movement of the head are the most common triggers. Mechanical stimulation of the external auditory canal, lateral cervical region, and preauricular and postauricular skin can trigger the pain during bouts of activity.

The pain characteristically begins suddenly, rapidly reaching maximum intensity, lasts several seconds, then ends abruptly. A background pain, described as continuous, dull, and aching, is often located in the oropharynx. The painful paroxysms occur five to 30 times per day and will frequently awaken the patient from sleep. Coughing occurs in 10% of patients, and there may be an attendant hoarseness that lasts for several minutes after an episode of severe pain.

Table 20-4	Comparison of neuralgiform disorders and treatment		
Neuralgia	**Features**	**Differential**	**Treatment**
Trigeminal neuralgia	Sharp, electric-like episodic pain	V3> V2 > V1 distribution Blockable with local anesthetic	Antiseizure medications Neurolytic procedures if unresponsive
Pretrigeminal neuralgia	Episodic dull, aching pain	V3 > V2 > V1 distribution Blockable with local anesthetic	Antiseizure medications Neurolytic procedures if unresponsive
Glossopharyngeal neuralgia	Episodic pain in pharyngeal area with swallowing or speaking; radiates to ear	Blockable with topical anesthetic at back of throat	Antiseizure medications Neurolytic procedures if unresponsive
Geniculate neuralgia	Lancinating pain deep in auditory canal; may have hemifacial spasm	Preceded by herpes zoster over concha and mastoid	Antiseizure medications
Nervus intermedius neuralgia	Paroxysmal pain deep in ear and over ipsilateral face and neck	Similar to geniculate neuralgia but no preceding herpes zoster; if tearing and nasal stuffiness, rule out cluster headache	Antiseizure medications Neurolytic procedures if unresponsive
Superior laryngeal neuralgia	Lancinating pain with talking, coughing, yawning, or turning of head	Blockade of superior laryngeal nerve is diagnostic	Antiseizure medications Neurolytic procedures if unresponsive
SUNCT*	Unilateral, short-lasting pain in ocular area with lacrimation and rhinorrhea	Rule out trigeminal neuralgia of first division; rule out cluster; fails to respond to medication trials	May respond to carbamazepine but generally unresponsive to management with medications
Occipital neuralgia	Deep and aching suboccipital area pain with occasional stabbing jolts, radiating to the vertex	Rule out cervical myofascial pain by palpation of splenius capitis and semispinalis capitis muscles	Local anesthetic blockade and physical therapy
Superior laryngeal neuralgia	Brief paroxysmal pain in the throat, submandibular region, and/or under the ear; paroxysms triggered by swallowing, straining the voice, or turning of head; trigger point present on the lateral aspect of the throat overlying the hypothyroid membrane	Blocking the superior laryngeal nerve	Condition relieved by local anesthetic block and cured by section of the superior laryngeal nerve
Nasociliary neuralgia	Stabbing pain lasting seconds to hours in one side of the nose; pain radiates upward to the medial frontal region; precipitated by touching the lateral aspect of the ipsilateral nostril	Positive response to topical anesthetic block of the affected nostril	Section of the nasociliary nerve or application of cocaine to the nostril on the affected side

*SUNCT = Short-lasting unilateral neuralgiform headache pain with conjunctival injection and tearing.

The pain can persist for weeks to months and then remit spontaneously; however, as with trigeminal neuralgia, the periods of remission tend to become shorter with time. It is typical for a patient to have two or three bouts of pain per year. Topical and local anesthetic applied to the back of the throat can be useful in diagnosing glossopharyngeal neuralgia.

It has been reported that syncope or seizures may be associated with attacks of pain in 2% of patients with glossopharyngeal neuralgia.[40] Because of the proximity of cranial nerves IX and X, activity in cranial nerve IX can cause bradycardia or asystole. It is assumed that this is not attributable to carotid sinus hypersensitivity, because sinus stimulation by massage does not cause syncope in these individuals.[40] The presence of a vasovagal reaction characterizes those reflex cardiovascular syncopes in which the glossopharyngeal nerve constitutes the main afferent nerve pathway.

Glossopharyngeal neuralgia must be differentiated from carotid sinus syndrome, which is also marked by asystole. If the syncopal episodes consistently follow the neuralgia episodes, it is more likely that the vasomotor activity is a result of the neuralgia and not caused by other vasomotor phenomena.

A number of causes for glossopharyngeal neuralgia have been mentioned in the literature. These range from oropharyngeal squamous cell carcinoma to compression at the root entry zone of cranial nerves IX and X. Olds and colleagues[41] have described the phenomenon of contact between the ninth cranial nerve and the inferior posterior cerebellar artery.

Nervus intermedius neuralgia

Nervus intermedius neuralgia is very rare and, as with sphenopalatine neuralgia, there is controversy over whether it actually exists.[42-49] In the most recent IHS classification,[1] it is differentiated from geniculate neuralgia, which is preceded by herpes zoster eruptions and hemifacial spasms (Ramsay Hunt syndrome).

The nervus intermedius, which is a component of the seventh cranial nerve, contains sensory afferents whose cell bodies are located in the geniculate ganglion in the roof of the temporal bone. Axons from this nerve supply part of the external auditory canal and tympanic membrane, the skin in the angle between the ear and mastoid process, the tonsillar region, and some other deep structures of the head and neck.

Nervus intermedius neuralgia is marked by recurrent paroxysmal stabbing and shooting pain felt deep in the ear and over the ipsilateral face and neck. This condition must be differentiated from glossopharyngeal neuralgia, geniculate neuralgia, and trigeminal neuralgia.

Afferent sensory facial nerve fibers are known to pass not only through the nervus intermedius but also through the main motor trunk of the facial nerve. Touching the posterior wall of the external ear canal may trigger the pain. Other reported symptoms during the attack include vertigo, tinnitus, nasal discharge, salivation, and a bitter taste. Compression of the eighth cranial nerve has also been associated with this neuralgia. Because of the overlap of these symptoms with those of cluster headache, this condition should be part of the differential diagnosis of nervus intermedius neuralgia and should be ruled out in the workup. Nervus intermedius neuralgia must also be differentiated from the "ice pick" pain of migraine, which can manifest as a repetitive lancinating pain deep to the ear.[48]

Lacrimation, salivation, or attendant taste phenomena may accompany the pain. The condition has been reported to be associated with herpes zoster. Some have suggested that nervus intermedius neuralgia may be an otalgic variant of glossopharyngeal neuralgia.[40]

Superior laryngeal neuralgia (vagus nerve neuralgia)

Superior laryngeal neuralgia was first described at the turn of the century. It is a rare disorder and, although it has been distinguished from glossopharyngeal neuralgia, it is sometimes difficult to differentiate between the two.[50,51] As a result, some consider these two conditions to be one disorder, termed *vagoglossopharyngeal neuralgia*.[52] In the absence of accompanying disease in the organs adjacent to the nerve, idiopathic superior laryngeal neuralgia is the most likely condition to produce pain around the thyroid cartilage and pyriform sinus.

Superior laryngeal neuralgia occurs equally between the sexes. It is marked by paroxysmal unilateral submandibular pain that can radiate to the ear, eye, or shoulder. The stabbing pain lasts for seconds to minutes and is provoked by activity that causes movements of the cricothyroid apparatus, such as talking, swallowing, coughing, yawning, and turning of the head. Local anesthetic blockade of the superior laryngeal nerve is considered to be diagnostic.

Because of overlap of symptoms with glossopharyngeal neuralgia and carotidynia, these conditions must be included in the differential diagnosis. Carotidynia is marked by tenderness of the carotid artery ipsilateral to the pain.

Treatment of superior laryngeal neuralgia includes use of antiseizure medication, as well as neurosurgical approaches. Neurectomy has been reported to bring relief in those patients unresponsive to medications.

Nasociliary neuralgia

Nasociliary neuralgia (Charlin syndrome) is characterized by sharp, lancinating pain in the distribution of the nasociliary nerve and the ciliary ganglion.[53-57] Touching the outer aspect of the ipsilateral nostril provokes a lancinating pain that radiates to the medial frontal region of the face.

Peripheral and terminal branch neuralgias

A number of neuralgias have more peripheral characteristics and usually do not reflect central problems; nevertheless, the clinician should always assess the patient carefully to rule out central or secondary causes for these problems. The peripheral and terminal branch neuralgias are usually caused by nerve injury or entrapment, giving rise to neuralgiform pain of the affected distribution.

Central Neuropathic Pain

Central neuropathic pain is characterized by pain that does not respond to topical or local anesthetic blockade. In addition to the lack of response to anesthetic blocking, there is dynamic mechanical allodynia or pain when a nonpainful moving stimulus, such as a wisp of cotton, is brushed across the area of pain. This response is thought to be mediated by central neuroplastic changes involving activation of N-methyl-D-aspartate receptors and central neurophysiologic changes in A beta–fiber activity (see chapter 5). There is also an exaggerated pain response to pinprick in the area subserved by the damaged nociceptors. This response is termed *hyperalgesia*.

Complex regional pain syndrome

The term *complex regional pain syndrome (CRPS)* was introduced to describe those painful syndromes that were formerly termed *reflex sympathetic dystrophy* or *causalgia*. In part, this was done because not all cases of reflex sympathetic dystrophy were sympathetically mediated, nor were dystrophic changes always present. In additional, sympathetic involvement was also noted in a number of other pain syndromes.[58,59]

The key symptoms of CRPS in the orofacial region are pain, abnormal regulation of blood flow, edema of the skin with trophic changes, and limited movement of the mandible. Symptoms may occur in areas that were not traumatized or closely related to the injured site. Sympathetic involvement (sympathetically mediated pain [SMP]) is usually, but not always, a part of this syndrome. Blockade of the appropriate sympathetic paravertebral ganglion usually results in pain relief that outlasts the duration of the anesthesia, while physiologic activation of the sympathetic neurons or application of norepinephrine will increase the pain.

There are two main divisions of CRPS disorders: CRPS I and CRPS II. CRPS I is more common than CRPS II and may develop after minor nerve damage without any nerve lesion, whereas CRPS II is usually associated with obvious nerve lesions. CRPS I is more commonly localized in the deep somatic tissue and associated with sympathetic changes, but historically both have been associated with sympathetic mediation. However, the mechanism of sympathetic involvement may differ between the two syndromes. Jänig[60] has indicated that, of the two syndromes, CRPS II is most frequently associated with SMP and that CRPS II can be more justifiably labeled a neuropathy than CRPS I.

CRPS I

CRPS I occurs after a traumatic event and is not limited to the distribution of just one nerve. Additionally, the symptoms produced by the trauma are disproportional to the severity of the initiating event. As the syndrome develops, additional changes are noted, such as alteration of blood flow, edema, alteration of sudomotor activity in the skin, allodynia, and hyperalgesia. The reaction is usually evident in extremities but has been reported to occur in the mouth and particularly in patients with TMJs that have undergone multiple surgeries.[61–6]

Symptoms of CRPS I usually occur within a month of the initiating trauma. The pain is described as continuous, aching, and burning. The intensity of the pain is variable but is increased with movement or stress.

Diagnostic criteria[64]
1. An initiating noxious event or a cause of immobilization is present.
2. There is continued pain, allodynia, or hyperalgesia in which the pain is disproportionate to any inciting event.
3. There is evidence at some time of edema, changes in skin blood flow, or abnormal sudomotor activity in the region of pain.
4. Diagnosis of CRPS I is excluded by the existence of conditions that would otherwise account for the degree of pain and dysfunction.

Associated signs and symptoms
1. Soft tissue atrophy.
2. Loss of joint mobility.
3. Impaired motor function, including weakness, tremor, and dystonia.
4. Sympathetically maintained pain may be present.

CRPS II

CRPS II is associated with burning pain (the old term was *causalgia*). This condition is usually associated with a known nerve injury in an extremity. The pain is spontaneous and is exacerbated by light touch, stress, temperature changes, or movement of the involved limb. Visual and auditory stimuli, as well as emotional disturbances, may also exacerbate the pain.[65] SMP may be present.

Diagnostic criteria
1. There is continued pain, allodynia, or hyperalgesia after demonstrated peripheral nerve injury.
2. There is evidence at some time of edema, changes in skin blood flow, or abnormal sudomotor activity in the region of the pain.
3. Diagnosis of CRPS II is excluded by the existence of conditions that would otherwise account for the degree of pain and dysfunction.

Sympathethically mediated pain

Sympathetically mediated pain may be associated with a number of pain conditions and is not in itself a sufficient criterion for the diagnosis of CRPS. SMP is pain that is maintained by sympathetic efferent activation of adrenergic receptors thought to be on nociceptors. The diagnosis of SMP is confirmed when a sympathetic block of the appropriate paravertebral autonomic ganglion provides pain relief. The blockade does not imply a mechanism for the pain but simply demonstrates a clinical observation that sympathetic nervous system blocks may relieve the pain in some pain conditions.[65] SMP is considered to be an associated symptom and not a disorder itself.[58]

Anesthesia dolorosa

Anesthesia dolorosa is a central condition characterized by persistent pain and dysesthesia in an area of nerve deafferentation. The area will also be anesthetic.

Diagnostic criteria[1]
1. Persistent pain and dysesthesia are present in the area of distribution of one or more divisions of the trigeminal or occipital nerves.
2. Sensation to pinprick is diminished.

Central poststroke pain

The ICHD II describes central poststroke pain as "unilateral pain and dysesthesia associated with impaired sensation involving part or the whole of the face, not explicable by a lesion of the trigeminal nerve." It is attributed to a lesion of the quintothalamic (trigeminothalamic) pathway, thalamus, or thalamocortical projection. Symptoms may also involve the trunk and/or limbs of the affected or contralateral side. Pain resulting from a thalamic lesion may occur in isolation in half of the face but is frequently associated with crossed hemidysesthesia. The pain is usually persistent.[1]

Diagnostic criteria
1. Pain and dysesthesia are present in one half of the face, associated with loss of sensation to pinprick, temperature, and/or touch, and the condition fulfills criteria 3 and 4.
2. One or both of the following is true: There is a history of sudden onset, suggesting a vascular lesion (stroke), or CT or MRI demonstrates a vascular lesion in an appropriate site.
3. Pain and dysesthesia develop within 6 months after stroke.
4. The symptoms are not explicable by a lesion of the trigeminal nerve.

Central pain from multiple sclerosis

Facial pain attributed to multiple sclerosis is described as either unilateral or bilateral and may be associated with dysesthesia. The pain is due to demyelination of central connections of the trigeminal nerve. The pain remits and relapses spontaneously and may mimic trigeminal neuralgia, which is why clinicians should be concerned when young individuals present with trigeminal neuralgia–like pain.

Diagnostic criteria[1]
1. Pain with or without dysesthesia is present in one or both sides of the face.
2. There is evidence that the patient has multiple sclerosis.
3. Pain and dysesthesia develop in close temporal relation to, and with MRI demonstration of, a demyelinating lesion in the pons or quintothalamic (trigeminothalamic) pathway.
4. Other causes have been ruled out.

Persistent idiopathic facial pain

The category of persistent idiopathic facial pain reclassifies disparate and poorly understood conditions previously classified as *atypical facial pain*. Historically, the persistent nonodontogenic tooth pain disorders had been placed under this nonspecific rubric by physicians and dentists. As research continues to reevaluate and assess these conditions in terms of known pathophysiologic processes, new insights have been gained; these disorders have been removed from the former junk heap of "atypical facial pain" and reclassified as a form of neuropathic pain. Atypical odontalgia and burning mouth syndrome are subcategories of persistent idiopathic facial pain.

Atypical odontalgia (chronic central trigeminal neuropathy)

The IASP's classification of chronic pain[65] includes atypical odontalgia but, based on some early articles, implies that it is a result of emotional problems.[66,67] However, recent articles have suggested that this condition is neuropathic and that a significant number of these cases are sympathetically maintained.[61,62,67] There is usually a history of trauma to the area but no current obvious local cause for the pain (CRPS I).

There may be two major subgroups in the category of traumatic trigeminal neuralgia or atypical odontalgia: *(1)* traumatic trigeminal neuralgia without SMP (ie, sympathetically independent pain) and *(2)* traumatic trigeminal neuralgia with SMP. Orofacial pain syndromes generally mirror pain syndromes in other areas of the body and have similar underlying mechanisms. In Graff-Radford and Solberg's study of atypical odontalgia,[61,62] a majority of the patients responded to sympathetic block and would be considered to have sympathetically maintained pain as part of the neuropathy. The unresponsive patients may have had sympathetically independent traumatic trigeminal neuropathy, but this was not discussed. The term *phantom tooth pain* is still being used to describe a similarly poorly defined population of patients. However, this diagnosis also carries an unfortunate psychological burden and should not be used.

Atypical odontalgia is characterized by a continuous nonodontogenic toothache or alveolar pain that is described as aching and burning. The pain tends to be persistent over a 24-hour period but varies in intensity. There may or may not be an identifiable causative event, and there is no observable lesion.

Diagnostic criteria
1. There is a 3-month history of unresolving pain in a tooth or tooth site.
2. Pain is continuous but variable.
3. There is no demonstrable lesion.
4. Pain is not blockable with local anesthetic.
5. There may be gingival dysesthesia, hyperalgesia, or allodynia.

Burning mouth syndrome

Burning mouth syndrome is a puzzling chronic pain disorder for which there is no known cause; the pathophysiology is unclear. The pain is usually bilateral and there is no known inciting event associated with its onset. Intraoral examination usually reveals nothing of significance. Occasionally, systemic disorders and bacterial infections have been associated with burning intraoral pain, and these conditions should be ruled out when the diagnosis is made. The pain is often confined to the tongue (glossodynia) and patients may complain of associated symptoms such as dry mouth, altered taste, or tingling sensations. It has been reported in the literature that most cases of burning mouth occur in perimenopausal and postmenopausal women.[1]

Diagnostic criteria
1. Pain in the mouth is present daily and persists for most of the day.
2. Oral mucosa is of normal appearance.
3. Local and systemic diseases have been excluded.

Psychogenic Pain

Psychogenic pain is not discussed in this chapter. It is a diagnosis that is made only by using the criteria in the psychiatric manual *Diagnostic and Statistical Manual for Mental Disorders*.

Conclusion

This chapter has discussed the differential diagnosis of orofacial pain using the perspective of the IHS classification system for headache and facial pain, but with a relevant focus on those pain conditions that can be experienced in the orofacial environment. This classification scheme and its suggested differential diagnostic protocol go far beyond what is currently understood scientifically and clinically, even by most orofacial pain specialists. However, it is necessary that the vision of clinicians be expanded to limit the possibility of misdiagnosing and mistreating both acute and chronic orofacial pain. The field of orofacial pain is slowly expanding its purview, and more university-based orofacial pain programs are including the expansion in their curricula.

References

1. Olesen J (ed). The International Classification of Headache Disorders, ed 2. Cephalalgia 2004;24(suppl 1):1–150.
2. Merrill RL, Graff-Radford SB. Trigeminal neuralgia: How to rule out the wrong treatment. J Am Dent Assoc 1992;123: 63–68.
3. Cameron C. Cracked tooth syndrome. J Am Dent Assoc 1964;68:405–11.
4. Rosen H. Cracked tooth syndrome. J Prosthet Dent 1982; 47:36–43.
5. Ehrmann EH, Tyas MJ. Cracked tooth syndrome. Aust Dent J 1990;35:390–391.
6. Ehrmann EH, Tyas MJ. Cracked tooth syndrome: Diagnosis, treatment and correlation between symptoms and post-extraction findings. Aust Dent J 1990;35:105–112.
7. Cameron C. The cracked tooth syndrome: Additional findings. J Am Dent Assoc 1976;93:971–975.
8. Gher M, Dunlap RM, Anderson M, Kuhl L. Clinical survey of fractured teeth. J Am Dent Assoc 1987;114:174–177.
9. Hawks M, Mullaney TP. A false diagnosis of a cracked tooth; report of case. J Am Dent Assoc 1987;114:478–479.
10. Stanley H. The cracked tooth syndrome. Am Acad Gold Foil Oper 1968;11:36–47.
11. Baer P, Savoia V, Andors L, Gwinnett J. The cracked tooth syndrome. N Y State Dent J 1978;44:144–145.
12. Silvestri A Jr. The undiagnosed split-root syndrome. J Am Dent Assoc 1976;92:930–935.
13. Goose D. Cracked tooth syndrome. Br Dent J 1981;150: 224–225.
14. Reuben HL, Nathanson D. Initial misdiagnosis of the cracked tooth syndrome—A case report. Quintessence Int 1978; 9(10):15–18.
15. Geurtsen W. The cracked-tooth syndrome: Clinical features and case reports. Int J Periodontics Restorative Dent 1992; 12:395–405.
16. Snyder D. The cracked-tooth syndrome and fractured posterior cusp. Oral Surg Oral Med Oral Pathol 1976;41:698–704.
17. Hiatt W. Incomplete crown-root fracture and pulpal-periodontal disease. J Periodontol 1973;44:369–379.
18. Smirnova MG, Birchall JP, Pearson JP. The immunoregulatory and allergy-associated cytokines in the aetiology of the otitis media with effusion. Mediators Inflamm 2004;13:75–88.
19. Delcanho RE, Graff-Radford SB. Chronic paroxysmal hemicrania presenting as toothache. J Orofac Pain 1993;7: 300–306.
20. Moncada E, Graff-Radford SB. Cough headache presenting as a toothache. Headache 1993;33:240–243.
21. Graff-Radford SB. Headache problems that can present as toothache. Dent Clin North Am 1991;55:155–170.
22. Raskin NH. Headache, ed 2. New York: Churchill Livingstone, 1988:333–373.
23. Cline MA, Ochoa J, Torebjork HI. Chronic hyperalgesia and skin warming caused by sensitized C nociceptors. Brain 1989;112:621–647.
24. Fields HL, Rowbotham M, Baron R. Postherpetic neuralgia: Irritable nociceptors and deafferentation. Neurobiol Dis 1998;5:209–227.
25. Classification of chronic pain. Descriptions of chronic pain syndromes and definitions of pain terms. Prepared by the International Association for the Study of Pain, Subcommittee on Taxonomy. Pain Suppl 1986; 3:S1–S226.
26. Dworkin RH, Backonja M, Rowbotham MC, et al. Advances in neuropathic pain: Diagnosis, mechanisms, and treatment recommendations. Arch Neurol 2003;60:1524–1534.
27. Bennett GJ. Chronic pain due to peripheral nerve damage: An overview. In: Fields HL, Liebeskind JC (eds). Pharmacological Approaches to the Treatment of Chronic Pain: New Concepts and Critical Issues. Progress in Pain Research and Management, vol 1. Seattle: IASP Press, 1994:51–59.
28. Devor M, Govrin-Lippmann R, Raber P. Corticosteroids suppress ectopic neural discharge origination in experimental neuromas. Pain 1985;22:127–137.
29. Burchiel KJ. Carbamazepine inhibits spontaneous activity in experimental neuromas. Exp Neurol 1988;102:249–253.
30. Yaari Y, Devor M. Phenytoin suppresses spontaneous ectopic discharge in rat sciatic nerve neuromas. Neurosci Lett 1985; 58:117–122.
31. Fromm GH, Sessle BJ. Introduction and historical review. In: Fromm G, Sessle BJ (eds). Trigeminal Neuralgia, Current Concepts Regarding Pathogenesis and Treatment. Boston: Butterworth-Heinemann, 1991:1–26.
32. Fromm GH, Graff-Radford SB, Terrence CF, Sweet WH. Pre-trigeminal neuralgia. Neurology 1990;40:1493–1495.
33. Mitchell RG. Pre-trigeminal neuralgia. Br Dent J 1980;149: 167–170.
34. Symonds SC. Facial pain. Ann R Coll Surg Engl 1949;4: 206–212.
35. Pareja J, Joubert J, Sjaastad O. SUNCT syndrome. Atypical temporal patterns. Headache 1996;36:108–110.
36. Zhao J, Sjaastad O. SUNCT syndrome. 8. Pupillary reaction and corneal sensitivity. Funct Neurol 1993;8:409–414.
37. Pareja JA, Sjaastad O. SUNCT syndrome. A clinical review. Headache 1997;37:195–202.
38. Sjaastad O, Kruszewski P. Trigeminal neuralgia and "SUNCT" syndrome: Similarities and differences in the clinical pictures. An overview. Funct Neurol 1992;7:103–107.
39. Sjaastad O, Zhao JM, Kruszewski P, Stovner LJ. Short-lasting unilateral neuralgiform headache attacks with conjunctival injection, tearing, etc. (SUNCT). 3. Another Norwegian case. Headache 1991;31:175–177.
40. Bruyn GW. Glossopharyngeal neuralgia. Cephalalgia 1983; 3:143–157.
41. Olds MJ, Woods CI, Winfield JA. Microvascular decompression in glossopharyngeal neuralgia. Am J Otol 1995;16: 326–330.

42. Rupa V, Weider DJ, Glasner S, Saunders RL. Geniculate ganglion: Anatomic study with surgical implications. Am J Otol 1992;13:470–473.

43. Dubuisson D. Nerve root damage and arachnoiditis. In: Wall PD, Melzack R (eds). Textbook of Pain, ed 2. New York: Churchill Livingstone, 1989:544–565.

44. Bruyn GW. Nervus intermedius neuralgia (Hunt). Cephalalgia 1984;4(1):71–8.

45. Yentur EA, Yegul I. Nervus intermedius neuralgia: An uncommon pain syndrome with an uncommon etiology. J Pain Symptom Manage 2000;19:407–408.

46. Yeh H, Tew JMJ. Tic convulsif, the combination of geniculate neuralgia and hemifacial spasm relieved by vascular decompression. Neurology 1984;34:682–683.

47. Ouaknine GE, Robert F, Molina-Negro P, Hardy J. Geniculate neuralgia and audio-vestibular disturbances due to compression of the intermediate and eighth nerves by the postero-inferior cerebellar artery. Surg Neurol 1980;13:147–150.

48. Raskin NH, Schwartz RK. Icepick-like pain. Neurology 1980; 30:203–205.

49. Pulec JL. Geniculate neuralgia: Diagnosis and surgical management. Laryngoscope 1976;86:955–964.

50. Bagatzounis A, Geyer G. Lateral pharyngeal diverticulum as a cause of superior laryngeal nerve neuralgia [in German]. Laryngorhinootologie 1994;73:219–221.

51. Bruyn GW. Superior laryngeal neuralgia. Cephalalgia 1983; 3:235–240.

52. Zaal MJ, Volker-Dieben HJ, D'Amaro J. Prognostic value of Hutchinson's sign in acute herpes zoster ophthalmicus. Graefes Arch Clin Exp Ophthalmol 2003;241:187–191.

53. Rothova Z, Boguszakova J, Roth J. Charlin's syndrome—Nasociliary nerve neuralgia [in Czech]. Cesk Oftalmol 1992; 48:354–358.

54. Izakson KA. Neuralgia of the nasociliary nerve—Charlin's syndrome [in Russian]. Med Sestra 1986;45(11):55–56.

55. Mashak VK. Neuralgia of the nasociliary nerve in a patient with chronic sphenoiditis [in Russian]. Vestn Otorinolaringol 1986;(5):81–82.

56. Lambert WC, Okorodudu AO, Schwartz RA. Cutaneous nasociliary neuralgia. Acta Derm Venereol 1985;65:257–258.

57. Mironenko IT. Syndrome of the nasociliary nerve [in Russian]. Zh Ushn Nos Gorl Bolezn 1973;33(2):88–89.

58. Boas RA. Complex regional pain syndromes: Symptoms, signs, and differential diagnosis. In: Jänig W, Stanton-Hicks M (eds). Reflex Sympathetic Dystrophy: A Reappraisal. Progress in Pain Research and Management, vol 6. Seattle: IASP Press, 1996:79–92.

59. Stanton-Hicks M, Jänig W, Hassenbusch S, Haddox JD, Boas R, Wilson P. Reflex sympathetic dystrophy: Changing concepts and taxonomy. Pain 1995;63:127–133.

60. Jänig W. CRPS-I and CRPS-II: A strategic view. In: Harden RN, Baron R, Jänig W (eds). Complex Regional Pain Syndrome. Seattle: IASP Press, 2001:3–15.

61. Graff-Radford SB, Solberg WK. Atypical odontalgia. J Craniomandib Disord 1992;6:260–265.

62. Graff-Radford SB, Solberg WK. Atypical odontalgia. CDA J 1986;14(12):27–32.

63. Vickers ER, Cousins MJ, Walker S, Chisholm K. Analysis of 50 patients with atypical odontalgia. A preliminary report on pharmacological procedures for diagnosis and treatment. Oral Surg Oral Med Oral Pathol Oral Radiol Endod 1998;85:24–32.

64. Stanos SP Jr, Harden RN, Wagner-Raphael L, Saltz SL. A prospective clinical model for investigating the development of CRPS. In: Harden RN, Baron R, Janig W (eds). Complex Regional Pain Syndrome. Seattle: IASP Press, 2001: 151–164.

65. Merskey H, Bogduk N (eds). Classification of Chronic Pain: Descriptions of Chronic Pain Syndromes and Definitions of Pain Terms, ed 2. Seattle: IASP Press, 1994:53–56.

66. Paulson GW. Atypical facial pain. Oral Surg Oral Med Oral Pathol 1977;43:338–341.

67. Brooke RI. Atypical odontalgia. A report of 22 cases. Oral Surg Oral Med Oral Pathol 1980;49:196–199.

Benign and Malignant Tumors

Diane Stern

Tumors of the temporomandibular joint (TMJ) occur infrequently. They may arise from the articulating bones (glenoid fossa of the temporal bone and mandibular condyle), the disc, the synovial membrane, and the articular capsule. Those that arise from the articulating bones (the majority develop from the mandibular condyle) for the most part resemble those that arise in other parts of the jaw. However, the synovium is unique to joints and therefore emphasis will be placed on tumors arising from this area. As in most other sites, benign proliferations are considerably more common than malignancies, and, as in other bones, the most frequently occurring malignancy is metastatic carcinoma.

Diagnosis of neoplasms in the TMJ can be difficult because of their infrequent occurrence as well as the fact that the symptoms often mimic those of regional masticatory muscle pain, which is a far more common temporomandibular disorder. Consequently, correct diagnosis is often delayed. Too often patients receive treatment for such myofascial pain, sometimes over several years, before ultimate failure leads to the true diagnosis. The adage that a "diagnosis not thought of is a diagnosis not made" is all too true in the field of TMJ pathoses.

Radiographic interpretation may also be challenging, and computerized tomography (CT) and magnetic resonance imaging (MRI) techniques are often indispensable to obtaining the correct diagnosis.

Once a tumor mass attains sufficient size, it may invade through the glenoid fossa posteriorly and present as a lesion of the external auditory canal or middle ear. It may also extend into the middle cranial fossa through the roof of the glenoid fossa. Growing laterally, it may mimic a parotid neoplasm, creating a preauricular swelling. Anteromedially it can extend into the infratemporal and pterygopalatine fossae and produce symptoms of cranial nerve involvement. Pathologic fracture with sudden onset of pain may also occur. The signs and symptoms pertaining to these situations are all indicative of advanced disease. Earlier findings are more consistent with an internal derangement: limited mouth opening, jaw deviation, and clicking or popping joint sounds.

The entities discussed in this chapter include those arising in the synovium and an assortment of other lesions that have been reported in the literature as occurring in the TMJ. The benign conditions that will be considered do not all represent neoplasms (also see chapter 35). Some are cystic lesions but are important in differential diagnosis; others may be reactive or hyperplastic proliferations, in which the distinction from a benign neoplasm is often unclear.

Benign Tumors, Cysts, and Cystlike Lesions

Synovial Chondromatosis

This uncommon entity has generally been considered to represent a non-neoplastic, metaplastic process. However, certain characteristics suggest the possibility that it may be neoplastic. The evidence of monoclonal chromosomal changes has given this theory strong support.[1] In addition, not only may synovial chondromatosis (SC) recur,

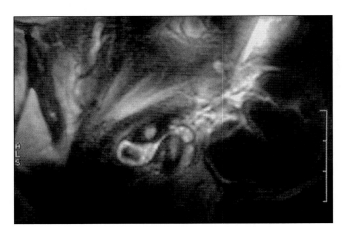

Fig 21-1 T2-weighted MRI (sagittal view) of the TMJ, showing synovial osteochondromatosis in which the cartilage nodules are located within the joint space. The central voids represent ossification. (From Marx and Stern.[4] Reprinted with permission.)

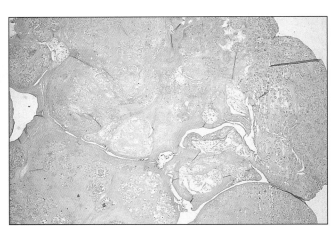

Fig 21-2 Synovial chondromatosis. Cartilaginous masses have proliferated into the joint space and are covered by synovium but have not yet broken free. This represents the first stage of synovial chondromatosis. (Hematoxylin-eosin stain.)

but also the cartilaginous component may exhibit atypia. Synovial chondrosarcoma has also developed within pre-existing SC.[2] In some cases, SC reaches considerable size and behaves in a destructive fashion.[3] SC may develop as a primary lesion or may arise secondary to trauma or another disease process such as osteoarthritis. The aggressive neoplastic features appear to be associated with the primary disease. Thus, it is possible that the primary type is neoplastic and the secondary form is metaplastic.

SC usually affects the joints of the knee, hip, elbow, and ankle; approximately 70% of cases occur in the knee. It is rare in the TMJ; slightly fewer than 100 cases have been reported in the literature. In at least one reported case, the lesion developed from the disc. In the TMJ, SC occurs more frequently in females than in males and usually in the fourth through sixth decades. At other sites, there is a male preponderance and presentation generally occurs two decades earlier.

Pain is the most frequently cited symptom, followed by swelling, clicking, mandibular deviation, and limited mouth opening. CT scans and MRI can be very helpful diagnostically (Fig 21-1), although the presence of loose bodies in the joint space is not pathognomonic, because they may also be seen with intracapsular fractures and the osteoarthroses.

Initially, the lesion develops within the synovium as a proliferation of undifferentiated cells. Then fibroblast-like cells form a chondroid matrix from which cartilaginous nodules develop. This early phase has been called *Stage 1.*

Subsequently the nodules begin to lose their attachment and extrude into the joint cavity (Fig 21-2). The synovial fluid helps to maintain their nutrition and growth. Stage 2 is the transitional phase, in which there is synovial involvement and detached nodules are found in the joint space. The cartilaginous foci within the synovium and joint space may calcify or even ossify, at which time the term *osteochondromatosis* is appropriate. This process commences at the periphery of the nodule and progresses inward. Eventually the nodules may coalesce to form an irregular mass. Stage 3 is advanced disease in which there is no longer synovial involvement and all the nodules have detached (Figs 21-3a and 21-3b). Although the nodules or masses are typically confined to the joint space, in some cases they may erode the underlying bone or joint capsule and invade the periarticular tissues.

Cellular atypia is not unusual in SC, where large cells and binucleated cells may be observed (Fig 21-4). However, this does not indicate aggressive behavior. The most important consideration in the differential diagnosis is chondrosarcoma.

Pigmented Villonodular Synovitis

This term is applied to a group of fibrohistiocytic lesions that involve joints, tendon sheaths, bursae, and adjacent fascial and ligamentous tissues. They are believed to represent a reactive inflammatory process. However, the fact that

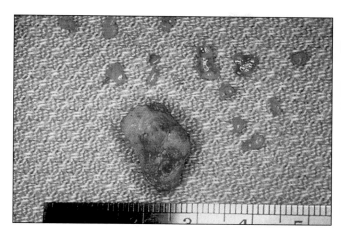

Fig 21-3a Discrete masses of cartilage that have been removed from the joint space, together with the condyle. This represents the third stage of synovial chondromatosis. (Courtesy of Dr Sheldon Mintz.)

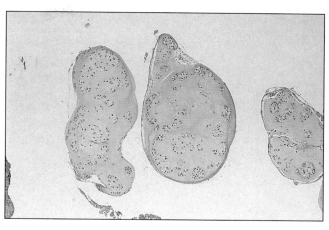

Fig 21-3b Section through the free nodules of cartilage. (Hematoxylin-eosin stain.)

there may be bone destruction and a significant rate of recurrence suggests a locally aggressive neoplastic process. Clonal chromosomal aberrations[5] and aneuploidy have been found in some cases, particularly in those lesions that are extra-articular, but other studies have shown no evidence of clonality.[6]

Essentially, these are destructive lesions that produce villous and nodular protrusions of the articular and extra-articular synovial membranes. They have been divided into intra-articular (diffuse and localized) and extra-articular (diffuse and nodular) forms. However, the nomenclature and classification involving these lesions have not been consistent.

They are relatively rare lesions, constituting fewer than 5% of all primary soft tissue tumors, and occur over a wide age range, with a peak in the third and fourth decades. Most are located intra-articularly. Eighty percent of cases involve the knee (including both diffuse and local types). The nodular extra-articular form (also called *pigmented villonodular tenosynovitis* or *giant cell tumor of tendon sheath*) is seen predominantly in the finger, carpal, and metacarpal joints.

These lesions are very rare in the TMJ. The majority are extra-articular, although this cannot always be confirmed. Although only about 22 cases have been reported in the literature, approximately a third of them have extended into the temporal bone and middle cranial fossa.[7]

Among the presenting symptoms, preauricular swelling is the most frequent. Hearing loss and tinnitus arising from

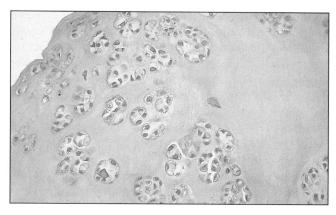

Fig 21-4 Synovial chondromatosis showing cytologic atypia. This does not indicate malignant change, but may make it difficult to distinguish the lesion from synovial chondrosarcoma. (Hematoxylin-eosin stain.)

compression of the auditory canal, as well as pain, trismus, and clicking, may also be present. Some cases have occurred in conjunction with SC.

The lesions have typically been described grossly as red to yellow-orange to brown masses that adhere to the external capsular surface. They may also involve the surrounding soft tissue and bone. The borders are ill defined and blend into the adjacent tissues.

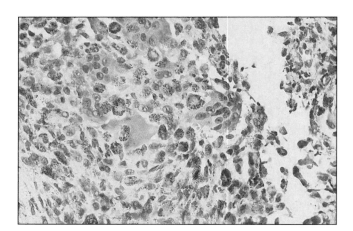

Fig 21-5 Inflammatory cells, multinucleated giant cells, and hemosiderin, typical components of pigmented villonodular synovitis. (Hematoxylin-eosin stain.)

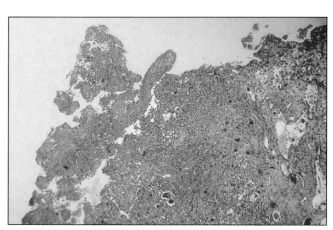

Fig 21-6 Low-power view of pigmented villonodular synovitis revealing some villous projections, ulceration of the synovium, proliferation of multinucleated giant cells, fibrous tissue, and inflammatory cells. (Hematoxylin-eosin stain.)

Histologically, the lesions consist of fibroblasts, mononuclear histiocytic cells, and irregularly interspersed multinucleated giant cells. Scattered and clustered foamy histiocytes are present, giving the lesion its yellow color, and there is abundant hemosiderin, responsible for the brown color. The hemosiderin may be found in the synovial cells and macrophages or lying free in the proliferative connective tissue, associated with multinucleated giant cells (Fig 21-5). The irregular villi are covered by thickened synovium or may be denuded (Fig 21-6). The histiocytes and giant cells are of monocyte-macrophage origin.

The histologic components of the different fibrohistiocytic lesions under this rubric are similar; the distinction is in the clinical presentation and behavior. Localized lesions are well circumscribed and may be partially encapsulated, while the diffuse lesions exhibit infiltrative and destructive growth. Thus the overall prognosis is more favorable for localized disease. This issue has not been addressed directly in the reported TMJ cases, but it is clear that many of these cases did behave in an aggressive fashion.

Osteochondroma (Osteocartilaginous Exostosis)

The osteochondroma constitutes about 35% of all benign bone tumors. It is a hamartomatous proliferation that arises from endochondral bone and is thus usually found in the long bones, most frequently the distal metaphysis of the femur and proximal metaphysis of the tibia. Patients are usually younger than 20 years and there is a 2:1 male predilection, but tumors of the condyle occur over a much wider age range and have a 2:1 female predilection.

Seventy-five percent are solitary lesions, and 25% are multiple lesions. Multiple osteochondromatosis is an autosomal-dominant hereditary disorder. In these cases, about 11% undergo sarcomatous change, in contrast to 1% of the solitary lesions. However, no cases of sarcomatous change have been reported in the condyle.

Osteochondromas occur infrequently in the mandibular condyle. They form an exophytic mass emanating from the cortex that may cause limited mouth opening, jaw deviation, and unilateral open bite. The radiographic appearance of an osteochondroma of the condyle is pathognomonic. A tapering radiopaque mass extends from the anteromedial aspect of the condyle along the tendon of the lateral pterygoid (Fig 21-7).

Histologically, the bony mass is covered by a cap of fibrocartilage and hyaline cartilage of varying thickness and cellularity, which is surrounded by the fibrous tissue of the perichondrium. In the deepest aspect of the cartilage, where it interfaces with bone, endochondral ossification occurs (Fig 21-8).

Spontaneous regression of an osteochondroma has occurred in rare instances.[8] This is most likely due to cessation of growth of the cartilage cap and subsequent resorption and incorporation of the lesion into the cortex through appositional growth. Cessation of growth also may be the consequence of a pathologic fracture. It is also possible that involution of the cartilage cap may result in the lesion resembling an osteoma.

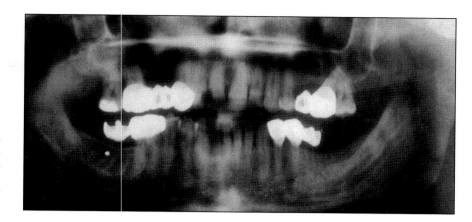

Fig 21-7 Panoramic radiograph presenting a pathognomonic picture of an osteochondroma projecting anteromedially from the condyle along the lateral pterygoid tendon. (From Marx and Stern.[4] Reprinted with permission.)

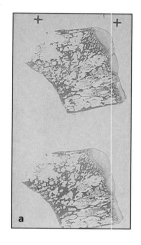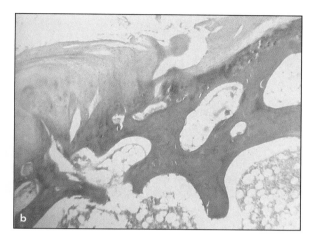

Fig 21-8 (a) Osteochondroma, which has formed a cap of cartilage on the surface of the condyle. (Hematoxylin-eosin stain.) (b) Pale-staining cap of hyaline cartilage. Endochondral ossification is present at the bony interface. (Hematoxylin-eosin stain.)

Chondroblastoma

These tumors develop in the medullary cavity of a bone and are thought to arise from the cartilage of the growth plates. Thus, most of the cases occur prior to skeletal maturity; the vast majority occur in patients aged 10 to 20 years.

Chondroblastomas usually involve the epiphysis of the distal femur and proximal tibia. These sites are followed in frequency by the proximal humerus and proximal femur. When the tumors develop in more unusual locations, the patients are usually older. Thus, the mean age of patients with tumors of a long bone is 16 years, while the mean age in patients with flat and short tubular bone involvement is 28 years.[9] In the condyle the reported age range has been from 27 to 41 years,[10] and there is a 2:1 male predilection.

Pain is the dominant symptom in the extremities, but swelling or limited motion is prevalent with condylar tumors. Radiographically, they produce a well-defined radiolucency with a sclerotic margin. Flocculent radiopacities may be seen within the lesion.

Chondroblastomas of the skull and facial bones are very uncommon, but it is interesting to note that among the 30 cases reported from the Mayo Clinic, three arose in the condyle. Twenty-one patients had tumors in the temporal bone and two of these also extended into the TMJ.[11]

The chondroblastoma is a benign tumor of immature cartilage cells with foci of cartilage matrix formation. The proliferating cell is believed to be a chondroblast. The cells are round to oval, with central or eccentric round to oval nuclei that may have a longitudinal cleft. These cells may be densely packed, and scattered multinucleated giant cells are usually prominent (Figs 21-9a and 21-9b). Interspersed areas show cartilage differentiation and an immature cartilaginous matrix, which appears as an amorphous pinkish tissue. The proportion of these two types of tissue is quite variable. Calcifications tend to form a fine, "chicken wire" pattern around the chondroblastic cells, although a coarser pattern may be present (Fig 21-10). Aneurysmal bone cysts develop in about 20% of cases.

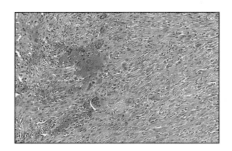

Fig 21-9a Chondroblastoma. Numerous multinucleated giant cells, in a background of chondroblastic cells, are visible. (Hematoxylin-eosin stain.)

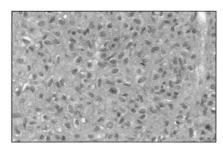

Fig 21-9b Sheet of chondroblasts. (Hematoxylin-eosin stain.)

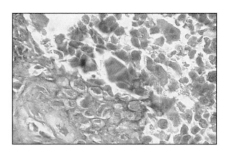

Fig 21-10 Fine, "chicken wire" calcification that surrounds individual cells, visible in the lower left quadrant. (Hematoxylin-eosin stain.)

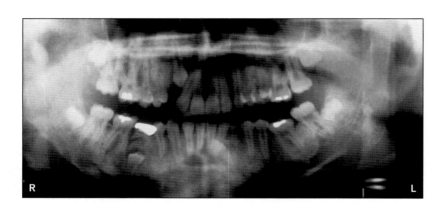

Fig 21-11 Panoramic radiograph of a 14-year-old boy with Gardner syndrome. An osteoma of the right condyle is present. In addition, other stigmata of the syndrome are present, including multiple endosteal osteomas, impacted teeth, and fibromatosis involving the left mandible. (Courtesy of Dr Stanley Stewart.)

Osteoma

Osteomas occur in several clinicopathologic guises, and frequent sites of involvement include the cranium, mandible, facial bones, orbit, and paranasal sinuses. In the condyle, osteomas usually appear as spherical or lobular enlargements. They may even have a pedicle. They generally consist of dense lamellar cortical bone that is well circumscribed, but a cancellous form also has been described. Although usually occurring as single, isolated lesions, osteomas may also arise in the condyle as part of Gardner syndrome (Fig 21-11).

Osteoid Osteoma

These tumors are very uncommon in the jaws. One case has been reported in which the inferolateral aspect of the mandibular condyle was involved.[12] The patient was a 21-year-old woman who experienced trismus and spontaneous pain that, in the classic presentation of this tumor, occurred essentially at night. The radiographic appearance was also classic, in that it appeared as a subcortical nodule, 0.8 cm in diameter, with a sclerotic border.

Osteoid osteomas consist of active osteoblasts that deposit abundant osteoid to form a small nidus within normal bone. The lesion generally does not exceed 1.0 cm in diameter (Fig 21-12).

In general, osteoid osteomas are found in the 10- to 25-year age group, and there is a 3:1 male predilection. About half the cases involve the lower extremity. They have a limited growth potential and may undergo spontaneous regression.

Benign Osteoblastoma

Osteoblastomas do not occur frequently in the jaws. In this region, the most common site is the body of the mandible, but several cases involving the TMJ have been reported.[13]

Most osteoblastomas arise in the vertebrae and long bones, with a 2:1 male to female ratio. The average age of patients is 17 years, and the age range is from the first through eighth decades. The sex and age distributions of TMJ lesions are similar to those in other locations.

They are typically well-circumscribed, solitary lesions that expand within the medullary cavity and exceed 1 cm

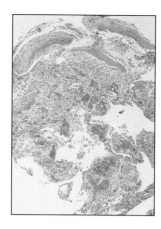

Fig 21-12 Osteoid osteoma. There is a central focus of osteoblastic activity with deposition of osteoid; peripheral bone is normal. (Hematoxylin-eosin stain.)

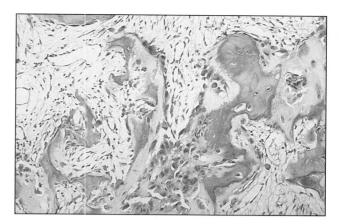

Fig 21-13 Osteoblastoma in which numerous plump osteoblasts are layered along seams of osteoid. The fibrous stroma contains a prominent vascular component. (Hematoxylin-eosin stain.)

in diameter. They often produce a tender swelling. When osteoblastomas occur in the TMJ, there is often a history of trauma and, as in other locations, a tender swelling is the frequent presentation. In some cases, there is not only an expanding deformity of the condyle but also a secondary deformity of the glenoid fossa.

These neoplasms, as in the osteoid osteoma, consist of active osteoblasts that lay down abundant osteoid. The osteoblasts are concentrated along the osteoid seams. The fibrous stroma is very vascular with numerous dilated capillaries (Fig 21-13). Because of the vascularity of the lesion, angiography and scintigraphy are diagnostically useful.

Nonossifying Fibroma (Fibrous Cortical Defect)

This is a common benign lesion that is generally noted as an incidental radiographic finding in the metaphyses of long bones in skeletally immature patients. It appears to be a self-limiting process that is related to incomplete ossification. It is found almost exclusively in children and adolescents. The lesion frequently resolves spontaneously. The lower extremity is the site of predilection; the distal femoral metaphysis is the most frequent site, followed by the proximal tibial metaphysis.

Occasionally these lesions are multifocal and symmetric. Multiple lesions have been associated with neurofibromatosis and are also found in Jaffe-Campanacci syndrome.

Nonossifying fibromas are typically asymptomatic, but when large, they may cause some expansion and even a

pathologic fracture. When found in its typical location, the radiographic appearance is pathognomonic. It appears as an eccentric cortical-based radiolucency with scalloped sclerotic margins. The overlying cortex may be considerably thinned and slightly expanded.

Involvement of the TMJ is extremely rare. Several cases have been reported in the neck of the condyloid process.[14–16] These lesions have not caused joint dysfunction and are typically asymptomatic. The jaw lesions appear to favor females, whereas in the long bones more males are affected.

Histologically, the lesion consists of a cellular fibroblastic stroma with a storiform pattern. Some multinucleated giant cells and foci of foamy histiocytes are present, and hemosiderin is visible in the stromal cells. Some mononuclear inflammatory cells are usually present.

Cystic change, hemorrhage, and necrosis may occur and secondary aneurysmal bone cysts have developed. The nonossifying fibroma tends to stabilize at puberty and heals by peripheral sclerosis or solid opacification.

Central Giant Cell Granuloma

Central giant cell granuloma represent fewer than 7% of all benign jaw tumors; of these, 70% occur in the mandible. The body of the mandible is the area of predilection. There is a female preponderance, and the majority of patients are younger than 30 years. The condyle is an unusual location, although several cases have been reported.[17]

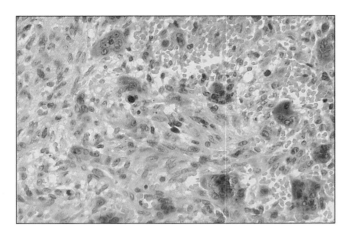

Fig 21-14 Fibrous stroma with numerous multinucleated giant cells, extravasated blood, and some hemosiderin, characteristic of the central giant cell tumor. (Hematoxylin-eosin stain.)

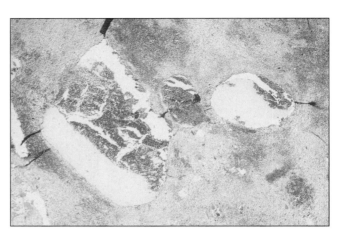

Fig 21-15 Central giant cell tumor in which dilated, blood-filled spaces that lack an endothelial lining are present. Because of this characteristic, such lesions are sometimes called *aneurysmal bone cysts*. (Hematoxylin-eosin stain.)

In the condyle, both unilocular and multilocular lesions have been described. Some have been asymptomatic, without functional impairment, even in the presence of preauricular swelling.

Histologically, these tumors consist of randomly scattered multinucleated giant cells within a cellular fibrous stroma that also contains extravasated blood (Fig 21-14). The giant cells are osteoclastic cells, so these lesions represent an osteoclastoma.

A more aggressive giant cell lesion, referred to as a *giant cell tumor*, has been described in the jaws and facial bones but not in the mandibular condyle.

Aneurysmal Bone Cyst

Several cases of aneurysmal bone cyst have been reported in the TMJ.[18] These lesions are not actually cysts but rather tumors in which there are widely dilated, blood-filled spaces that are not lined by endothelium. Frequently these tumors occur as a secondary phenomenon within a preexisting pathologic process, most often a giant cell tumor (Fig 21-15), but also with other conditions such as osteoblastoma, chondroblastoma, and nonossifying fibroma. There is a near equal distribution between the sexes, and the majority arise in individuals younger than 20 years. In 32 cases in the mandible reported by Trent and Byl,[19] only 2% occurred in the condyle.

The histories concerning the cases in the condyle have varied from rapidly expanding, destructive lesions to incidental findings. The majority of patients had experienced previous trauma.

Hemangioma

Intraosseous hemangioma

Only five cases of intraosseous hemangioma in the TMJ have been reported.[20] Hemangiomas of bone are found most frequently in the vertebrae and are uncommon in the jaws, where their usual location is in the body of the mandible. These lesions have a 2:1 female-to-male ratio and there is a predilection for the second decade.

Among the patients with a lesion involving the TMJ, one was asymptomatic. The others presented with joint pain, aggravated by movement of the mandible, as well as tenderness over the joint and restricted mouth opening.

Synovial hemangioma

Synovial hemangiomas are rare lesions, occurring predominantly in the knee joint. They are most unusual in other sites. There is a predilection for female children and young adults.

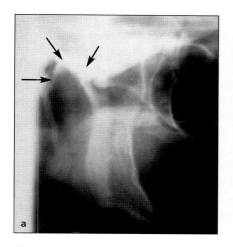
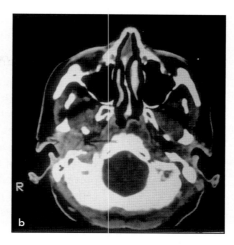

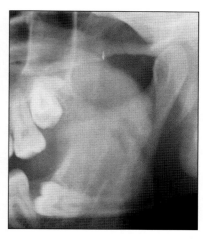

Fig 21-16 Synovial hemangioma. (Courtesy of Dr Sheldon Mintz.) *(a)* In the panoramic radiograph, a radiolucency *(arrows)* is visible posterior to the condyle, which is displaced anteriorly. *(b)* CT scan of the same patient.

Fig 21-17 Pseudocyst of the mandibular condyle, presenting as a well-defined radiolucency with a sclerotic rim in the anterior aspect of the condyle. (Courtesy of Dr Timothy Collins.)

The findings are typically recurrent, long-standing pain, decreased range of motion, and a spongy, compressible mass over the joint. They may be localized and well circumscribed or diffuse and infiltrative. These hemangiomas are of the cavernous type, with large, dilated, blood-filled vessels that are separated by an edematous, myxoid, or focally hyalinized matrix. Inflammatory cells may also be present. The synovium may develop villous projections, with hemosiderin deposition in the synovial cells.

These lesions may be juxta-articular, intra-articular, or mixed. The intra-articular type is the most frequent, and the tumor is lined by a synovial membrane. The mixed type originates from the synovium and lies both juxta-articularly and intra-articularly, while the juxta-articular type is located adjacent to the joint without actual involvement of the synovial membrane.

Radiographs usually reveal nonspecific radiolucencies or opacities. However, the presence of phleboliths is a helpful diagnostic feature.

TMJ involvement has been reported.[21] The case was that of a 43-year-old woman who had been treated for 3 years for masticatory myalgia associated with localized intermittent preauricular pain, restricted motion, and deviation on opening. However, there was no muscle tenderness and no preauricular mass, although there was a painful preauricular depression. Aspiration was not productive. A CT scan showed a soft tissue mass in the posterior portion of the joint. Grossly it was confluent with the synovial membrane (Fig 21-16).

Pseudocysts

Pseudocysts of the mandibular condyle are asymptomatic radiolucencies with corticated margins. They are seen in the anterior aspect of the condyle (Fig 21-17) and are the result of cupping of the pterygoid fovea; the margins are formed by the dense medial and lateral condylar ridges.

The image is the result of a radiographic distortion when the central x-ray beam does not pass through the condyle at right angles but rather passes obliquely in the horizontal plane and superiorly in the vertical plane. Consequently, the medial ridge is projected posteriorly and superiorly, and the lateral ridge is projected anteriorly and inferiorly. These "lesions" are thus not pathologic processes.

In a Veterans Affairs population of 507 patients aged 22 to 96 years, 9 (1.8%) such cases were found.[22] In a population of 1193 patients aged 18 years and younger, 18 (1.5%) such cases were found.[23]

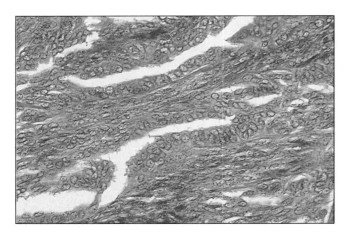

Fig 21-18 Synovial sarcoma showing the typical biphasic pattern. Clefts are lined by epithelial-like cells, beneath which spindle cells are found. (Hematoxylin-eosin stain.)

Idiopathic Bone Cavity (Traumatic Bone Cyst, Hemorrhagic Bone Cyst, Simple Bone Cyst)

Idiopathic bone cavities in the jaw usually are located in the body or symphysis. Approximately 10 cases have been reported in the TMJ.[24] These are essentially asymptomatic lesions. When associated symptoms have occurred, they have usually been caused by a pathologic fracture.

The diagnostic criteria for an idiopathic bone cavity include the presence of a single lesion, the absence of an epithelial lining, and the absence of infection. The lumen should be empty save for some fluid or gas. The wall is bony, although a scant amount of fibrous tissue may be present. Many of these cavities appear to undergo spontaneous regression. Similar lesions may be observed in association with other entities, such as florid osseous dysplasia and other fibro-osseous processes.

Ganglion and Synovial Cysts

The literature does not always clearly distinguish these two lesions. While the synovial cyst is a true cyst with an epithelial lining, the ganglion cyst is not. Ganglion cysts arise in a joint capsule as a consequence of myxoid degeneration of the connective tissue, possibly secondary to a deficiency in the vascular supply. They are not connected to the joint cavity. There is a female predilection with an age range of 30 to 50 years. These lesions are very rare in the TMJ area; only about 10 cases have been reported.[25]

They present as a preauricular swelling and there may also be joint dysfunction, pain, and tenderness. Bone scans will reveal an increased uptake of technetium 99. Histologically, these lesions are lined by fibrous tissue and contain a gelatinous material.

Synovial cysts are also uncommon in the TMJ. Five cases have been reported, two of which were associated with a history of trauma.[26] These lesions also present as a preauricular swelling. They are lined by flat or cuboidal cells, which are of synovial origin, and the lumen contains a gelatinous material. These cysts may be the consequence of herniation of the synovium or possibly the result of displacement of tissue during embryogenesis. Following trauma, increased intracapsular pressure may cause degeneration of the adjacent connective tissue.

Malignant Neoplasms

Synovial Sarcoma

These tumors represent about 5% to 10% of all soft tissue sarcomas. They are the fourth most frequently occurring soft tissue sarcoma, following malignant fibrous histiocytoma, liposarcoma, and rhabdomyosarcoma. They arise near tendons and tendon sheaths and next to joint capsules. They do not arise from mature synovial cells but rather from pluripotential mesenchyme.

Joint involvement per se is very uncommon, occurring in less than 5% of cases. Usually they occur in para-articular areas of the extremities, particularly around the knee, but approximately 9% occur in the head and neck, where the paravertebral structures give rise to most of the tumors, which then present in the pharynx, larynx, or esophagus. The tumors are generally rather slow growing. Up to 50% show calcifications radiographically, a helpful finding diagnostically.

Most cases occur in patients in the 15- to 40-year age range. The four patients with lesions in the TMJ ranged from 22 to 57 years in age.[26] At this site they have tended to present as a preauricular mass, which was painless in some instances.

Histologically, two types of synovial sarcoma may occur: biphasic and monophasic. Both types have occurred in the TMJ. The biphasic tumor consists of plump, uniform spindle cells that resemble a fibrosarcoma but lack a herringbone pattern and cuboidal to columnar epithelial-like cells that line spaces or clefts and form nests. There also may be a pseudoglandular pattern (Fig 21-18). Both the

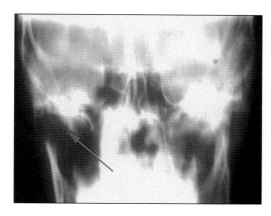

Fig 21-19 Osteosarcoma of the TMJ (*arrow*), presenting as an expansile destructive mass. (Courtesy of Dr Louis Mercuri.)

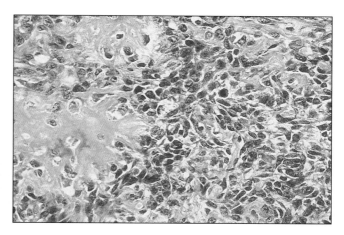

Fig 21-20 Osteosarcoma. The osteoid (pale pink stain) is formed directly from a malignant stroma. (Hematoxylin-eosin stain.)

spindle and epithelial-type cells stain positively for cytokeratin and epithelial membrane antigen. Mitoses are infrequent, and calcifications may be present.

The monophasic form is usually of the fibrous type, and most of the spindle cells exhibit the same immunohistochemistry as the biphasic form. A monophasic epithelial form also exists but is very rare. Synovial sarcomas are associated with the chromosomal translocation t (X:18)(p11.2;q11.2).

About half the cases of synovial sarcoma will have local recurrences, even after wide surgical excision and a neck dissection. Most recur within the first 2 years, but recurrence may also take place many years later. Although the lung is the most frequent metastatic site, synovial sarcoma is one sarcoma that may metastasize to the lymph nodes (20% of cases).

Osteosarcoma

Osteosarcomas represent about 30% of all primary bone malignancies, and 6% to 13% involve the craniofacial bones. The maxilla and mandible are involved in almost equal frequency. It is unusual for these tumors to originate in the TMJ.[27] The age of patients with such tumors has ranged from 17 to 69 years.

Patients generally complain of pain, often mild; limited mouth opening; and altered occlusion. Radiographically, the lesions show extensive destruction (Fig 21-19).

These tumors arise from pluripotential mesenchymal stem cells and may thus show considerable histologic diversity. This includes chondroid and fibrous differentiation. The diagnosis rests on the identification of osteoid formed directly from a malignant stroma (Fig 21-20).

Lung metastases may occur early in the course of the disease.

Chondrosarcoma

The majority of reported sarcomas arising in the TMJ have been chondrosarcomas. However, because this amounts to some 14 cases, this is still a very rare occurrence.[28] The age and sex of the patients were not known in three cases. Among the others, the age ranged from 17 to 75 years; four cases arose in the patient's fifth decade. Six patients were female and three were male.

Swelling was a consistent finding and, in most instances, pain or discomfort was also noted. Limited mouth opening and diminished hearing have also been described. Overall, chondrosarcomas constitute about 25% of primary bone sarcomas, with only 1% to 3% arising in the facial bones and jaws.

These tumors develop from mesenchymal stem cells, which show partial chondroblastic differentiation. They are typically slow-growing tumors, and the majority are low grade. They tend to show a lobular growth pattern with hypercellularity. The cells are often pleomorphic and may be binucleated. Malignant cartilage is formed but, in distinction to the osteosarcoma, no osteoid is formed directly from the malignant stroma.

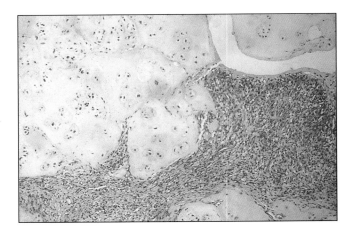

Fig 21-21a Synovial chondrosarcoma with a lobular arrangement of cartilaginous tissue. The cellular area represents the more poorly differentiated cells. (Hematoxylin-eosin stain.)

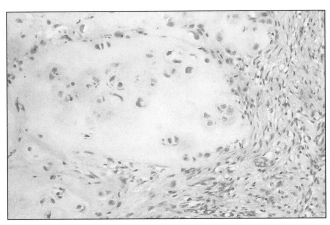

Fig 21-21b Same synovial chondrosarcoma showing cellular pleomorphism. (Hematoxylin-eosin stain.)

High-grade tumors may metastasize to regional lymph nodes. Low-grade tumors have an excellent prognosis, but recurrences can develop, often after many years.

Synovial chondrosarcoma

These tumors may arise as a primary malignancy of the synovium or secondarily in a preexisting synovial chondromatosis. They are rare occurrences, and only 21 cases have been reported in the literature. The knee, hip, and ankle are the sites of predilection. The age range of the patients is 30 to 70 years, and two thirds occur in the fifth to seventh decades. There is a female preponderance. The tumors form a soft tissue mass associated with pain and joint dysfunction.

Only six cases occurring in the TMJ have been reported.[29–33] Because there are very close similarities in the clinical, radiologic, and histologic aspects between synovial chondromatosis and synovial chondrosarcoma, the diagnosis may be difficult. Local recurrence and invasion of bone and surrounding soft tissue are clinical features that are also shared by these two entities. Radiographically, in addition to the presence of a soft tissue mass, clumps of calcification may be seen within the lesion, and there may be marginal erosion of the articular bone. As in synovial chondromatosis, nodules may be seen grossly, lying free within the joint space and/or the soft tissues.

The histology may also be ambiguous because cytologic atypia is common in synovial chondromatosis (Figs 21-21a and 21-21b). The following histologic criteria are suggested to recognize malignancy:

1. Qualitative differences in the cartilage in different parts of the tumor, in which a clustering pattern is juxtaposed with abundant matrix and tumor cells arranged in sheets
2. Myxoid changes in the matrix
3. Hypercellularity, with crowding and spindling of the nuclei at the periphery
4. Necrosis
5. Permeation of trabecular bone, with "filling up" of marrow spaces rather than a pushing margin[2]

In the series reported by Bertoni et al,[2] the nine patients available for follow-up, in whom the tumors occurred in the lower extremity (knee, hip, and ankle), all developed recurrences following local excision with "lesional margins." In spite of aggressive follow-up surgery, five patients developed metastases.

Langerhans Cell Histiocytosis

Approximately 13 cases of Langerhans cell histiocytosis have been reported in the condyle.[34] The majority were solitary lesions. One patient was found to have additional bone lesions at presentation, and another developed an additional lesion in the bone within 6 months. Four patients were female and nine were male. Three cases

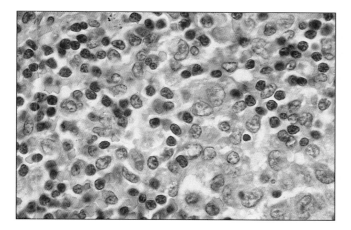

Fig 21-22a Langerhans cell histiocytosis revealing pale-staining histiocytic cells and smaller, darker-staining eosinophils. (Hematoxylin-eosin stain.)

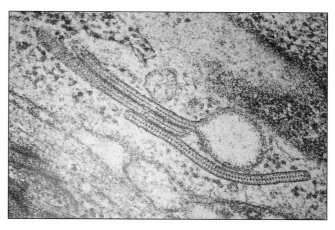

Fig 21-22b Electron photomicrograph showing the zipperlike intracytoplasmic Birbeck granules that characterize the histiocytic cell as a Langerhans cell.

occurred in the patients' first decade, three in the third, four in the fourth, and three in the fifth.

All patients had pain in the area of the TMJ. Most had preauricular swelling, and limited mouth opening was also frequently reported. At least four patients developed pathologic fractures. In all cases, a lytic lesion could be identified radiographically within the condyle.

Histologically these tumors consist of sheets of histiocytes with focal collections of eosinophils (Fig 21-22a). Some plasma cells and lymphocytes may also be present. The proliferating histiocytic cells can be identified as Langerhans cells by staining for S100 protein and more definitively by immunostaining for CD1a antigen, as well as by ultrastructural examination and identification of cytoplasmic Birbeck granules (Fig 21-22b).

Although there is still some controversy concerning the nature of these lesions, the finding that these are clonal proliferations suggests that they are indeed neoplasms.

Multiple Myeloma

Multiple myeloma represents about 43% of malignant tumors of bone. Most cases arise in individuals older than 60 years, and there is a slight male preponderance.

There appear to be seven cases of multiple myeloma reported in the literature in which there was a condylar lesion.[35] These patients ranged from 41 to 70 years in age, which is typical for this disease. Two patients had patho-

logic fractures. The most frequent finding was pain, usually associated with trismus. One patient had a tender preauricular swelling. In some patients, additional bone lesions were found at time of presentation, but in others no additional bone lesions were identified.

Multiple myeloma is a plasma cell dyscrasia in which sheets of proliferating plasma cells form bone tumors. Radiographically, the lesions are typically well-defined radiolucencies that lack a sclerotic rim.

Metastatic Carcinoma

Metastatic carcinoma is the most frequently occurring malignancy of bone. However, the jaws are an uncommon site for metastases, and the condyle is an even less frequent location. In a review of 390 cases of metastatic tumors to the jaws, Hirshberg et al[36] reported that 81% occurred in the mandible but only 11 cases (3.5%) involved the condyle. They also noted that overall there was a female preponderance, probably accounting for the fact that the breast was the most prevalent primary tumor site. Other reported primary sites with metastases to the condyle have included lung, prostate, liver, pancreas uterus, rectum, and skin of the toe. One particularly unusual report involved a testicular teratoma with metastases to both condyles.[37]

The most prevalent presentation of metastases to the condyle was TMJ dysfunction, but a pathologic fracture

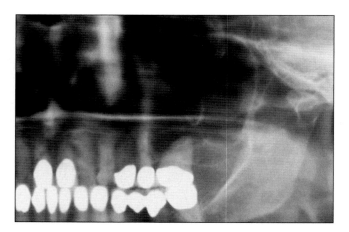

Fig 21-23 Radiograph of breast carcinoma metastatic to the condyle, associated with a pathologic fracture. (Courtesy of Dr Sheldon Mintz.)

may also be found (Fig 21-23). Although in many cases the patient may have a known primary lesion, in some series the condylar metastasis was the first sign of a neoplasm in as many as half of the patients. Unfortunately, patients with these metastases have a very poor prognosis and treatment is generally palliative.

Hypotheses regarding the reason for the paucity of metastases to the condyle include the scant amount of red marrow, the separate blood supply from the circular penetrating branches of the maxillary and superficial temporal arteries, the slow circulation, and limiting osseous plate, which shuts off the condylar marrow cavity from the spongiosa of the rest of the mandible.

Other Tumors

Many other tumors have been described as occurring within the condyle. Most of these have been single cases. They have included nodular fasciitis,[38] neurofibroma,[39] malignant schwannoma,[40] leiomyosarcoma,[41] malignant fibrous histiocytoma,[42] fibrosarcoma,[43] and Ewing sarcoma,[44] (see chapter 35).

Conclusion

In the study of temporomandibular disorders, much emphasis has been placed on the commonly occurring conditions such as masticatory myalgia and internal derangements. Practitioners must approach such patients with an open mind, because many other conditions can produce similar signs and symptoms. These include neoplasms. Although most neoplasms of the TMJ are benign, features that may suggest the possibility of malignancy include swelling; parasthesia; paresis; trismus; and occlusal changes. In addition, there may be auditory changes, including tinnitus and vertigo secondary to eighth nerve involvement and decreased auditory acuity secondary to eustachian tube involvement. When occlusal changes are of sudden onset, the immediate cause may be a pathologic fracture. The development of symptoms of myofascial pain and jaw dysfunction later in life (ie, beyond the typical 20- to 40-year age range for patients with masticatory myalgia) or failure of the initial treatment for this condition, should make clinicians suspicious of more serious problems.

The use of good radiographs and other imaging studies is of paramount importance in developing a correct diagnosis. Although the diagnosis is frequently suggested by the clinical and imaging information, in most cases the final diagnosis will only be made by microscopic tissue examination. However, histologic analysis alone is not sufficient. Only by assessing the clinical, radiographic, and histologic information together can the clinician achieve an accurate diagnosis.

References

1. Sciot R, Dal Cin P, Bellemans J, Samson I. Synovial chondromatosis: Clonal chromosome changes provide further evidence for a neoplastic disorder. Virchows Arch 1998;433:189–191.
2. Bertoni F, Unni K, Beabout JW, Sim FH. Chondrosarcoma of the synovium. Cancer 1991;67:155–162.
3. Karlis V, Glickman RS, Zaslow M. Synovial chondromatosis of the temporomandibular joint with intracranial extension. Oral Surg Oral Med Oral Pathol Oral Radiol Endod 1998;86:664–666.
4. Marx RE, Stern D. Oral and Maxillofacial Pathology: A Rationale for Diagnosis and Treatment. Chicago: Quintessence, 2003.
5. Sciot R, Rosai J, Dal Cin P, et al. Analysis of 35 cases of localized and diffuse tenosynovial giant cell tumor: A report from the Chromosomes and Morphology (CHAMP) Study Group. Mod Pathol 1999;12:576–579.
6. Vogrincic GS, O'Connell JX, Gilks CB. Giant cell tumor of tendon sheath is a polyclonal cellular proliferation. Hum Pathol 1997;28:815–819.
7. Chow LTC, Kumta SM, King WWK. Extra-articular pigmented villonodular synovitis of the temporomandibular joint. J Laryngol Otol 1998;112:182–185.

8. Copeland RL, Meehan PL, Morrissy RT. Spontaneous regression of osteochondroma. Two case reports. J Bone Joint Surg 1985;67:971–973.

9. Bloem JL, Mulder JD. Chondroblastoma: A clinical and radiologic study of 104 cases. Skeletal Radiol 1985;14:1–9.

10. Kondoh T, Hamada Y, Kamei K, Seto K. Chondroblastoma of the mandibular condyle: Report of a case. J Oral Maxillofac Surg 2002;60:198–203.

11. Bertoni F, Unni KK, Beabout JW, Harner S, Dahlin DC. Chondroblastoma of the skull and facial bones. Am J Clin Pathol 1987;88:1–9.

12. Tochihara S, Sato T, Yamamoto H, Asada K, Ishibashi K. Osteoid osteoma in mandibular condyle. Int J Oral Maxillofac Surg 2001;30:455–457.

13. Weinberg S, Katsikeris N, Pharaoh M. Osteoblastoma of the mandibular condyle: Review of the literature and report of a case. J Oral Maxillofac Surg 1987;45:350–355.

14. Makek M. Non-ossifying fibroma of the mandible. A common lesion with unusual location. Arch Orthop Trauma Surg 1980;96:225–227.

15. Aldred MJ, Breckon JJW, Holland CS. Non-osteogenic fibroma of the mandibular condyle. Br J Oral Maxillofac Surg 1989;27:412–416.

16. Hudson JW, Livesay KW, McCoy JM. Condylar lesion. J Oral Maxillofac Surg 2003;61:824–826.

17. Abu-El-Naaj I, Ardekian L, Liberman R, Peled M. Central giant cell granuloma of the mandibular condyle: A rare presentation. J Oral Maxillofac Surg 2002;60:939–941.

18. Motamedi MHK. Destructive aneurysmal bone cyst of the mandibular condyle: Report of a case and review of the literature. J Oral Maxillofac Surg 2002;60:1357–1361.

19. Trent C, Byl FM. Aneurysmal bone cyst of the mandible. Ann Otol Rhinol Laryngol 1993;102:917–924.

20. Whear NM. Condylar haemangioma—A case report and review of the literature. Br J Oral Maxillofac Surg 1991;29:44–47.

21. Atkinson T J, Wolf S, Anavi Y, Wesley R. Synovial hemangioma of the temporomandibular joint; report of a case and review of the literature. J Oral Maxillofac Surg 1988;46:804–808.

22. Friedlander AH, Monson ML, Friedlander MD, Esquerra AC. Pseudocysts of the mandibular condyle. J Oral Maxillofac Surg 1992;50:821–824.

23. Collins TE, Laskin DM, Farrington FH, Shetty NS, Mourino A. Pseudocysts of the mandibular condyle in children. J Am Dent Assoc 1997;128:747–750.

24. Tanaka H, Westesson PL, Emmings FG, Marashi AH. Simple bone cyst of the mandibular condyle: Report of a case. J Oral Maxillofac Surg 1996;54:1454–1458.

25. Chang YM, Chan CP, Kung Wu SF, Hao SP, Chang LC. Ganglion cyst and synovial cyst of the temporomandibular joint; two case reports. Int J Oral Maxillofac Surg 1997;26:179–181.

26. Warner BF, Luna MA, Newland JR. Temporomandibular joint neoplasms and pseudotumors. Adv Anat Pathol 2000;7:365–368.

27. Zorzan G, Tullio A, Bertolini F, Sesenna E. Osteosarcoma of the mandibular condyle: Case report. J Oral Maxillofac Surg 2001;59:574–577.

28. Sesenna E, Tullio A, Ferrari S. Chondrosarcoma of the temporomandibular joint; a case report and review of the literature. J Oral Maxillofac Surg 1997;55:1348–1352.

29. Merrill RG, Yih WY, Shamloo J. Synovial chondrosarcoma of the temporomandibular joint; a case report. J Oral Maxillofac Surg 1997;55:1312–1316.

30. Ichikawa T, Miyauchi M, Nikai H, Yoshiga K. Synovial chondrosarcoma arising in the temporomandibular joint. J Oral Maxillofac Surg 1998;56:890–894.

31. Allias-Montmayeur F, Durroux R, Dodart L, Combelles R. Tumours and pseudotumorous lesions of the temporomandibular joint: A diagnostic challenge. J Laryngol Otol 1997;111:776–781.

32. Stadelmann WK, Cruse CW, Messina J. Synovial cell sarcoma of the temporomandibular joint. Ann Plast Surg 1995;35:664–668.

33. Delbalso M, Pyatt RS, Busch RF, Hirokawa R, Fink CS. Synovial cell sarcoma of the temporomandibular joint. Computed tomographic findings. Arch Otolaryngol 1982;108:520–522.

34. Wong GB, Pharaoh MJ, Weinberg S, Brown DH. Eosinophilic granuloma of the mandibular condyle: Report of three cases and review of the literature. J Oral Maxillofac Surg 1997;55:870–878.

35. Gonzalez J, Elizondo J, Trull JM, De Torres I. Plasma-cell tumours of the condyle. Br J Oral Maxillofac Surg 1991;29:274–276.

36. Hirshberg A, Leibovich P, Buchner A. Metastatic tumors to the jawbones: Analysis of 390 cases. J Oral Pathol Med 1994;23:337–341.

37. Porter SR, Chaudhry Z, Griffiths MJ, Scully C, Kabala J, Whipp E. Bilateral metastatic spread of testicular teratoma to mandibular condyles. Eur J Cancer B Oral Oncol 1996;32B:359–361.

38. Van Royen C, Wackens G, Goossens A. Nodular fasciitis in a temporomandibular joint. Int J Oral Maxillofac Surg 1993;22:168–170.

39. Pasturel A, Bellavoir A, Cantaloube D, Dandrau JP, Perichaud P, Payement G. Temporomandibular joint dysfunction and neurofibromatosis: Apropos of a case [in French]. Rev Stomatol Chir Maxillofac 1989;90:17–19.

40. Bavitz JB, Chewning LC. Malignant disease as temporomandibular joint dysfunction: Review of the literature and report of a case. J Am Dent Assoc 1990;120:163–166.

41. Farole A, Manalo AE, Iranpour B. Lesion of the temporomandibular joint. J Oral Maxillofac Surg 1992;50:510–514.

42. Yoshimura Y, Kawano T, Takada K, et al. Malignant fibrous histiocytoma of the temporomandibular joint: Report of a case. Int J Oral Surg 1978;7:573–579.

43. Gobetti JP, Turp JC. Fibrosarcoma misdiagnosed as a temporomandibular disorder: A cautionary tale. Oral Surg Oral Med Oral Pathol Oral Radiol Endod 1998;85:404–409.

44. Talesh KT, Motamedi MHK, Jeihounian M. Ewing's sarcoma of the mandibular condyle: Report of a case. J Oral Maxillofac Surg 2003;61:1216–1219.

Fibromyalgia

Octavia Plesh and Stuart A. Gansky

The relationship between fibromyalgia (FM) and chronic temporomandibular disorders (TMDs) is a matter of current interest for both clinicians and researchers. FM, a chronic widespread body pain syndrome, often coexists with the regional musculoskeletal pain characteristic of many types of TMD. Both FM and chronic musculoskeletal TMDs are unexplained clinical conditions, sharing other common symptoms beyond chronic pain, such as fatigue, disability out of proportion to physical manifestations, inconsistent demonstration of laboratory abnormalities, and an association with stress and psychosocial factors.

The diagnosis assigned to patients with these types of illness has been suggested to depend more on the patient's chief complaint and the clinician's specialty than on the actual illness.[1,2] Considerable progress has been made in understanding the epidemiologic aspects of these two conditions, and recently, unified hypotheses have emerged regarding possible common pathophysiologic mechanisms. However, many questions regarding the nature of the two conditions, their natural history, and the relationship between them remain unanswered. This chapter presents the current scientific perspectives about FM and its relationship with musculoskeletal TMD pain and delineates the needs for future research.

Definition

Fibromyalgia, as defined by the American College of Rheumatology (ACR), is a disorder characterized by at least 3 months of widespread pain and tenderness in at least 11 of 18 musculoskeletal sites.[3] The points are nine paired regions of the body, and tenderness is defined as pain on palpation with 4 kg of pressure.

Widespread pain is considered to be present if a subject reports axial skeleton pain, pain in the left and right sides of the body, and pain above and below the waist. Although generalized tenderness is associated with widespread pain, a high percentage of people presenting 11 of 18 tender points report only regional pain or nonaxial pain.[4] The number of tender points was found to correlate more with the level of distress, such as depression, fatigue, and sleep problems, and less with the degree of widespread pain.[5,6] Increased tenderness (more than 11 of 18 points) was reported to be roughly 10 times more common in women than in men.[7,8]

Although considered a defining criterion for FM, widespread tenderness is currently believed to represent a marker of pain severity and distress rather than a symptom of a muscular disorder. As a result, FM is currently regarded as being at the end of a continuum or spectrum of conditions that are chiefly characterized by chronic widespread pain (CWP).[8–12] The requirement that a specific number of tender points be identified, as specified by the original ACR criteria, skews the identified FM population toward being hyperalgesic and female, capturing only about 20% of cases of chronic widespread pain.[11,13]

Investigators in this field currently believe that FM is a subset of CWP, sharing common symptoms including fatigue, sleep disturbances, chronic headaches, and psychological distress. The construct of FM as a distinct rheumatologic disorder has been questioned; as a result, it has been suggested that perhaps subsets of CWP, based on the degree of hyperalgesia and tenderness and the contribution of psychological and cognitive factors to the symptom expression, should be considered for clinical and research studies and clinical management goals.[13,14] However, since the ACR criteria were published in 1990, most studies have been conducted on FM, and therefore much less is known about people with CWP and fewer than 11 tender points. This change in the conceptualization of FM has led to different hypotheses to explain its pathophysiology, which will be discussed later in the chapter.

Epidemiology

Fibromyalgia is considered to affect about 2% to 3% of the North American population,[1,7,15] and 80% of those affected are women.[1] Among the US population, a midwestern study (in Wichita, Kansas) reported the prevalence of FM in women to rise steadily with age from less than 1% in 18- to 30-year-olds to 8% to 9% in 55 to 64-year-olds.[1,7] The peak prevalence in men, although lower (0.5%), appears to increase with age as well.[1,7]

Chronic widespread pain without at least 11 of 18 tender points has been reported to affect about 12% to 14% of the general population, and regional chronic pain (RCP) has been reported to affect about 20% to 25% of the population, depending on whether the pain was episodic, recurrent, or persistent and on the number of body sites involved.[7,10,16] The prevalence of CWP in women is only 1.5 times greater than that in men.[5] Thus, CWP without the requirement of at least 11 of 18 tender points for a diagnosis of FM affects more men than does CWP with the requirement of 11 or more tender points.

Only about 20% to 22% of patients with widespread pain fulfill the 11 or more tender points criterion for FM.[5] In clinical populations, especially US rheumatology clinics, the prevalence of FM is much higher (12% to 20%), being one of the three most commonly diagnosed conditions.[1] Furthermore, the natural history of FM has been described as persistent without undergoing a transition to other clinical disorders.[6,9]

Socioeconomic factors seem to play an important role in the epidemiology of FM. The prevalence of FM was reported to increase among those with lower family income, lower educational level, and increased divorce rates.[6] Studies from non-US and US populations also show that FM has familial aggregation, which is a tendency for disorders, traits, or characteristics to present as clusters within families rather than as random distributions in the population.[17-19] The detection of familial aggregation is usually the first step in suggesting that a genetic mechanism may play an etiologic role in the development of a disorder, either as a main effect or part of an interaction with environmental factors. Pain conditions other than FM are also reported to aggregate in families[20,21] through a variety of mechanisms, including hereditary and psychosocial factors, described as the roles of family functioning and pain "modeling."

Although chronic pains are considered to run in families, some types of chronic pain have been reported not to run in families.[21] Raphael et al,[21] in a comparison of randomly selected first-degree relatives of index probands with the myofascial type of TMD and first-degree relatives of acquaintance control probands, found no difference in the myofascial type of TMD pain. This study raised the question of whether regional pain conditions, such as myofascial pain, differ from widespread pain.

Ongoing studies among a twin registry population are investigating the genetic and environmental contributions to chronic fatigue syndrome (CFS) and FM.[22,23] This paradigm is being used to test a more complex model of genetic predisposing factors versus environmental factors.

Much of the information on FM comes from clinical population studies conducted primarily in rheumatology specialty clinics. FM among care-seeking and non–care-seeking individuals in the community differs from FM among clinic patients in many characteristics, such as degree of pain, psychological distress, and other symptoms.[3,24] Most North American general population studies have been conducted on relatively homogenous populations, such as in Kansas,[1] in Pima Indians,[25] in Ontario, Canada, and in Canadian Amish.[26] Results from these studies demonstrate that FM is more common in whites (Kansas and Ontario populations: 2% to 3%; Amish community: 7%) and nonexistent in Pima Indians. However, less is known about community-dwelling adults of different racial and ethnic backgrounds.

In a recent study (Gansky and Plesh, unpublished data, 2005) of 1,334 young women aged 22 to 25 years, approximately half of whom were African American and half of whom were whites from two urban locations (California and Ohio), the researchers found that the prevalences of regional chronic pain (11%), chronic widespread pain (5.4%), and FM (2.4%) were within the ranges of those reported previously (Fig 22-1). Tenderness to palpation was unexpectedly far more common than widespread pain; among the 553 women examined for tenderness according to the ACR criteria, 33% had at least 11 of 18 tender points. Thus, tenderness (11 of 18 points or more) extended beyond that of CWP, including women with nonaxial and localized self-reported body pain. Among African Americans, 27.0% had 11 or more tender points, 8.5% had RCP, 6.4% had CWP, and 2.8% had FM, while among whites, 39.0% had 11 or more tender points, 13.0% had RCP, 4.3% had CWP, and 2.0% had FM. The prevalences of tenderness and RCP were significantly greater in whites (see Fig 22-1), while the prevalence of CWP was significantly greater in African Americans. TMDs are also more common in women. Unlike FM, however, TMDs are more prevalent at younger ages, with a peak around the reproductive age

(12%), decreasing thereafter.[27] As with RCP, TMDs of mostly myofascial origin have been reported to show racial differences.[28] Thus, white women of young age demonstrate a significantly greater prevalence of chronic regional body pain than do African American women, who demonstrate a significantly greater prevalence of chronic widespread body pain.

Clinical Features

FM is considered a disorder of chronic pain and the most common form of nonarticular rheumatism. The impact of FM on the everyday life is considerable.[3,9,29] Pain and tenderness are the main symptoms distinguishing FM from other unexplained syndromes. The pain resulting from the application of 4 kg pressure at the 18 specified points has been used to distinguish people with FM from control subjects.[3] However, FM patients often display more generalized tenderness, beyond the specified points, extending throughout the entire body.[29–31]

In addition to pain and tenderness, which alone form the criteria for FM, additional symptoms have been reported to be common. They include sleep disturbances, fatigue, memory difficulties, morning stiffness, irritable bowel syndrome (IBS), psychological disturbances, and other somatic symptoms of chronic pain and nonpain that were recognized but not included in the ACR criteria.[3] The number of these symptoms and their severity increase were considered to predict worse outcomes.[3,32] In general, the results of routine laboratory tests are normal, and no diagnostic tests exist for FM or CWP.

Comorbid Conditions

FM often coexists with other musculoskeletal and nonmusculoskeletal syndromes. They include systemic conditions, such as CFS and multiple chemical sensitivity (MCS), and regional or organ-related conditions, such as myofascial-type TMD, IBS, chronic tension-type headaches, chronic pelvic pain, chronic low back pain, and interstitial cystitis.[33–35] The most extensively investigated conditions for comorbidity are CFS, FM, IBS, TMDs, and tension-type headaches.

A recent literature review of studies investigating the overlap of these unexplained clinical conditions reveals that, despite methodologic limitations such as unclear case definition and case-control selection and recruitment, there is substantial evidence of coexistence among these

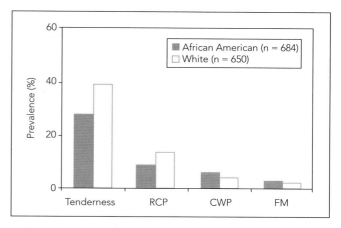

Fig 22-1 Prevalence of body pain (tenderness, spread, and fibromyalgia) in a community cohort of young (23- to 25-year-old) African American and white women from California and Ohio. Tenderness represents at least 11 of 18 positive tender points from the American College of Rheumatology (ACR) examination of a subset of subjects (African American women, n = 291; white women, n = 262). (RCP) Regional chronic pain (axial pain not in all four quadrants); (CWP) chronic widespread pain (axial pain above and below the waist, left and right sides); (FM) fibromyalgia, defined by ACR as tenderness plus CWP.

syndromes or shared common symptoms.[34] These studies show that a high percentage (70%) of FM patients also meet the criteria for CFS and 35% to 70% of patients with CFS meet the FM criteria, while 75% of FM patients meet the Research Diagnostic Criteria for TMDs (RDC/TMD) and 18% of patients with mostly myofascial TMDs meet the FM criteria.[34] Moreover, 32% to 80% of FM patients, 58% to 92% of CFS patients, and 64% of TMD patients meet the criteria for IBS.[33] In addition, 55% of patients with FM present symptoms of MCS, 30% of patients with MCS meet the criteria for CFS, and 10% to 80% of patients with FM present with headaches. Other recent studies have shown similarly high rates of TMDs (68.6%) and other types of orofacial pain in FM patients.[36]

Therefore, coexistence of FM with other unexplained clinical conditions has been documented. However, there is a lack of studies exploring the possible mechanisms responsible for the overlap. Several hypotheses have been proposed. One hypothesis is that these conditions may share similar pathophysiology and that the diagnosis received depends on the patient's present complaint and healthcare provider.[2] Another hypothesis considers FM and the comorbid conditions as consequences of psychiatric distress and the amplification of body sensations.[2,37,38] This hypothesis is based on observations that psychiatric problems are common among patients with these conditions, and stress (psychological and/or physical), although lower, is present even in care-seeking and non–care-seeking individuals in the community.[16,39] However, other studies have shown that not all patients have psychiatric problems and that few psychiatric patients have these syndromes.[32]

Currently, the most accepted hypothesis to explain the comorbidity among these unexplained conditions involves the central nervous system. One of the most common findings among patients with FM, CFS, IBS, TMDs, and chronic headaches is a reduction in pain threshold and tolerance.[35,36] Because this occurs in systemic conditions such as FM and CFS and in localized, organ-specific conditions such as IBS and TMDs, it has been postulated that alteration in pain perception is mediated by central mechanisms.[13,34]

Stress is also reported to be associated with these conditions,[34,40,41] and many clinicians and patients share the view that stress pays an important role in the initiation and perpetuation of most of these conditions. Disruption and dysregulation at different levels involved in pain processing and in the stress systems have been considered.[13,40–44] Psychological distress, such as depression and somatization, is also greater in these unexplained conditions (see chapter 13).[45–47]

A biopsychosocial model has been recently proposed[49] in which genetic predisposing factors, along with physical, environmental, and psychosocial initiating and consequential factors are considered to contribute to altering the functional relationship among the hypothalamic-pituitary-adrenal (HPA) axis, autonomic nervous system (ANS), and pain processing at the central and peripheral levels.[13,41] Ongoing twin studies conducted in subjects with CFS or FM are investigating the role and contribution of genetic and environmental factors.[22,23] Future longitudinal studies are needed to explore the contribution and interplay among these factors in determining the pathophysiology of these overlapping, unexplained syndromes and symptoms.

Pathophysiology

The etiology of FM remains poorly understood, with disparate abnormal findings and no definitive biologic marker. Although some patients implicate acute trauma or infections as triggers for FM, most patients report the insidious onset of symptoms without a clear etiology. Earlier theories on FM focused on peripheral tissue sites, such as abnormalities in muscle metabolism and function, sleep changes, infections, hormonal status, and psychosocial stressors. However, none of these factors alone can explain the pathophysiology of FM. A more complex biopsychosocial model that was recently proposed considers an interplay among genetic, predisposing, and environmental factors to trigger and maintain the symptom expression and persistence.[13,34,43] Several factors that have been reported to be associated with FM are reviewed in the next sections.

Hypothalamic-Pituitary-Adrenal Axis Function

Diverse environmental stressors (eg, psychological or physical trauma) have been considered as triggers for the development of CWP and FM.[34] Stressful events and other forms of stress, such as noise and light,[49] also have been reported to exacerbate symptoms of FM. Daily stress is considered to negatively impact clinical severity.[3,40,50] The heightened sensitivity to stress in FM is also shared with the other unexplained overlapping syndromes, such as CFS, IBS, and TMDs, as previously mentioned.[40,41,51]

Earlier studies of HPA axis dysfunction in FM have demonstrated reduced 24-hour urinary free cortisol excretion, increased plasma cortisol levels with loss of diurnal fluctuation, and exaggerated corticotropin levels. Blunted cortisol response to exogenous corticotropin-releasing hormone indicates a decrease in adrenal responsiveness.[40,52] A study comparing the response of serum cortisol levels in an FM group after exercise and a non-FM sedentary group showed a significant drop in the FM group.[53] Subjects exposed to different stressors in a strictly monitored setting demonstrated elevated salivary and plasma cortisol throughout the day but normal urinary cortisol levels.[54]

However, other studies have failed to show any differences in the functioning of the HPA axis of FM subjects and control subjects. A study of monozygotic and dizygotic twins incorporated a provocation test with corticotropin-releasing hormone, physical stress, and psychological stress.[55] Biochemical responses in monozygotic twins were highly correlated under all three conditions, but the correlations were weaker in dizygotic twins. The conclusion was that HPA response has a strong genetic determinant.[55]

A recent review of the literature on the HPA axis in patients with FM and CFS articulated inconsistencies regarding the relationship between neuroendocrine factors, viewed as disturbances in the HPA axis, and the presence and degree of symptoms of both FM and CFS.[56] The relationship between FM and stress is complex, and the degree to which stress can initiate, maintain, or exacerbate the symptoms of FM remains to be determined.

Autonomic Nervous System

The ANS and, in particular, the sympathetic nervous system are important components of the human stress response. Pain and emotional stress enhance the adrenomedullary response.[57] Common experimental methods to assess the ANS in FM patients include tilt table testing and heart rate variability measures.[58,59] A recent review of the evidence regarding the role of the sympathetic nervous system in FM[56] showed that 60% of such patients demonstrated abnormal ANS responses. Furthermore, abnormal ANS responses have been documented in other comorbid conditions, such as CFS, IBS, and migraine headache. Several studies have suggested that both sympathetic and parasympathetic dysregulation occur in IBS.[57] However, these studies show that, similar to the HPA axis dysregulation response, the ANS response is abnormal only in a subset of patients.

Sleep Disturbances

One primary symptom of FM is disturbed, unrefreshing sleep.[3] Poor sleep was reported to be associated with increased pain, in general.[60] Sleep deprivation also is associated with increased pain in FM patients, and it can induce FM-like symptoms in normal subjects.[49]

Early polysomnographic findings in individuals with FM reported non–rapid eye movement sleep anomalies characterized by an intrusion of the alpha frequency electroencephalogram during non–rapid eye movement sleep.[61,62] Miniarousals, fragmented sleep, and frequent sleep stage changes characterize these sleep perturbations. However, these findings are not specific to persons with FM, being common in healthy as well as depressed individuals.[63,64]

More recently, Moldofsky[65] reviewed the role of sleep in FM and related syndromes such as CFS and IBS, showing that there is a reciprocal relationship between sleep and pain; not only do sleep problems contribute to increases in pain and other symptoms, but increased pain and other symptoms will also disturb sleep.[65] However, the exact role that sleep plays in the pain mechanisms of FM requires clarification.

Exercise Capacity

The exercise capacity of patients with FM is usually compromised. Their fitness level is reported to be significantly lower than that of age- and sex-matched controls.[66] Also, in highly aerobically fit individuals, sleep deprivation–induced FM-like symptoms are almost nonexistent.[64] However, abnormal muscle metabolism has been inconsistently demonstrated in patients with FM.[67,68] Furthermore, one of the most consistent reports regarding treatment of FM involves the benefit of aerobic exercises.[69] However, the role of exercise capacity as a predisposing or consequential factor in individuals with CWP and FM remains to be established.

Pain Processing

Widespread pain and general tenderness extending beyond the specified points are the main features of FM, and sensitization to thermal, chemical, and mechanical stimuli is also present in FM patients.[42] Because psychological distress can influence the pain response, an increased response to different stimuli could be biased, especially in FM patients, who are frequently in distress. However, even when stimuli were presented in a random paradigm, thus reducing the role of hypervigilance or other psychological factors that could enhance pain, the increased sensitivity persisted.[43]

The presence of other centrally associated phenomena such as sleep disturbances and a blunted HPA stress response, and the diffuse nature of the pain in FM patients, suggest a central mechanism.[43] A deficiency in endogenous pain modulation was considered to be part of the central mechanism contributing to FM pain.[70] Brain imaging studies have demonstrated reduced blood flow in the thalamus and caudate nucleus in patients experiencing FM and other pain states.[71] Also, functional imaging studies of the brain using magnetic resonance imaging demonstrated that the amount of pressure stimulus required to activate brain regions involved in pain processing was much lower in FM subjects than in controls.[43] Previous neuropeptide studies showed increased levels of pronociceptive peptides and decreased levels of antinociceptive peptides in FM patients. The concentration of substance P was reported to be three times higher in the cerebrospinal fluid of FM subjects than in that of controls.[72,73] Patients with other chronic pain syndromes also demonstrate elevated levels of substance P. Levels of serum serotonin and its precursor, L-tryptophan, may also be lower in individuals with FM.[74] All these findings support the central mechanism hypothesis for FM.

However, other studies have shown that FM patients under conditions of experimental mechanical and thermal skin stimulation produced a "wind-up" phenomenon, which in animal studies has been demonstrated to induce hyperalgesia and allodynia.[42,75] Moreover, evidence from clinical studies showing that local anesthetic injections at tender points or sympathetic block also result in clinical improvement supports the idea that peripheral mechanisms are at work.[76,77] Therefore, both central and peripheral mechanisms are considered to be involved in FM pain,[78] but their exact contributions and interplay remain to be established.

Psychiatric and Psychosocial Factors

Major depression, panic disorders, and somatization are reported to be associated with FM. Frequent diagnoses include somatization and lifetime panic disorders. Almost two thirds of patients with FM have been reported to have a lifetime history of major depression,[79] and more than 20% report a current psychiatric problem. Hudson and Pope[80] proposed that FM is part of an affective spectrum of disorders with a common pathophysiology. However, Yunus[81] reported that psychological factors are not necessary for development of FM, and only 30% to 35% of FM patients have significant psychological problems.

Whether FM and depression share a common pathophysiology remains to be determined. However, psychological distress may reinforce pain and thus mediate the relationship between pain and healthcare-seeking behavior, because patients attending FM clinics demonstrate a higher rate of psychiatric disorders than do care-seeking and non–care-seeking community-dwelling individuals with FM.[31] Also, women with FM who reported a history of sexual abuse had significantly more symptoms than did women with FM who reported no history of sexual abuse, but the prevalence of sexual abuse did not differ significantly between women with FM and controls without FM.[82] Other psychosocial factors, such as having a lower socioeconomic status, being an immigrant, living in a socially compromised housing area, and lacking community support, were reported to be associated with persistence of FM.[83]

Thus, many factors influence or interact with FM, but none of them alone can explain the pathophysiology of FM. Most parameters were investigated individually and are difficult to integrate with other findings. One main issue has been to integrate these findings into a model and test their association with FM. The multifactorial approach, proposed recently as a biopsychosocial model,[48] incorporates the biologic (HPA axis, ANS, and central nervous system) with the environmental and psychosocial factors and integrates their roles as predisposing to, causative of, concurrent with, or a consequence of FM.[13] Longitudinal studies are needed to test such a model.

Fibromyalgia and TMDs

Both FM and the chronic pain associated with certain TMDs have traditionally been regarded as chronic musculoskeletal pain conditions. While the conceptual basis for both has been shifting in recent years, the comorbidity between them is evident. Although the craniofacial region is not included in the ACR's criteria for FM, there is no reason to expect that the diffuse, generalized pain of FM could not extend to the craniofacial region. Earlier reports have demonstrated that FM patients present with symptoms associated with certain TMDs, such as jaw muscle and temporomandibular joint pain, and that some TMD patients report more generalized pain extending beyond the craniofacial region.[1,7,8] A literature review of studies investigating the overlap between FM and TMDs reveals that, despite methodologic limitations such as unclear case definition (especially of TMDs) and use of mostly clinic samples of homogenous ethnicity, there is substantial evidence of coexistence between the two conditions (Table 22-1).

One study using standardized criteria for both conditions and a clear patient definition demonstrated a difference in overlap between the two conditions based on where the sample was recruited (TMD versus FM clinic).[84] When each condition was assessed according to defined criteria, a high percentage (75%) of FM patients fulfilled the RDC criteria for most types of TMDs.[84] Conversely, a much lower percentage (18%) of patients from the TMD clinic fulfilled the ACR criteria for FM. Only a low percentage (20%) of the 45 FM patients satisfying the criteria for TMDs were currently seeking treatment for their problem (Plesh, unpublished data, 2005).

A comparison between the FM and TMD patients revealed significant differences in general clinical severity scores and pain scores, but no difference in anxiety scores (Table 22-2).[84] This was not surprising, because the FM patients were significantly older than the TMD patients, and FM morbidity increases with age. However, the severity of the TMDs, based on the clinical findings from RDC/TMD Axis I,[46] was not significantly different between TMD patients with and without FM. Patients reported that the general symptoms related to FM constituted more important health issues than those related specifically to the TMD. Perhaps this explains why most FM patients with a TMD do not seek TMD treatment.

The differences in treatment-seeking behavior between FM patients with TMD symptoms and TMD patients without FM must be investigated further to determine why only

Table 22-1	Overlap of fibromyalgia (FM) and TMD symptoms and other somatic complaints*			
Study	**Patient group**	**Eligibility criteria**	**Study methods**	**Major findings**
Hedenberg-Magnusson et al[86]	FM (n = 191)	Clinical diagnosis of FM	Questionnaires	94% of FM patients report TMD symptoms.
Dao et al[87]	FM (n = 29) TMD (n = 19)	ACR RDC/TMD	Questionnaires	69% with FM reported current facial pain. 79.3% reported facial pain in last 6 months. 42% to 68% with MFP reported upper back, lower back, and neck pain. Pain more continuous in FM and more episodic in TMD.
Plesh et al[85]	FM (n = 60) TMD (n = 39)	ACR RDC/TMD	Questionnaires Physical examination	75% with FM met RDC/TMD criteria. 18.4% with TMD met ACR criteria for FM. FM group had greater severity and global distress than TMD group.
Turp et al[88]	Facial pain (n = 278)	Clinical cases with facial pain	Body pain mapping	18.5% reported pain restricted to facial region. About 17% reported pain extending to neck region. 65% reported pain extending to other body segments.
Raphael et al[89]	MFP of temporo-mandibular region (n = 162)	Clinical cases with MFP	Questionnaires Physical examination	23.5% with MFP reported widespread pain like FM. MFP group with widespread pain had more disability and higher severity than MFP group without widespread pain.
Rhodus et al[37]	FM (n = 67)	ACR	Questionnaires Physical examination	67.6% with FM had clinical TMD symptoms and other oral symptoms.
Aaron et al[34]	FM (n = 22) TMD (n = 25)	ACR RDC/TMD	Questionnaires Physical examination	24% with TMD were previously diagnosed with FM. 9% with FM were previously diagnosed with TMD.

*ACR = American College of Rheumatology; RDC/TMD = Research Diagnostic Criteria for Temporomandibular Disorders; MFP = myofascial pain.

a small percentage of FM patients who satisfy the RDC criteria for a TMD seek treatment for the TMD-related symptoms. Other differences between TMD patients who satisfy the criteria for FM (and perhaps other comorbid conditions such as CFS or IBS) and TMD patients without any comorbid conditions also need to be clarified further. Moreover, based on the new data, the TMD classification itself probably needs to be revised. The treatment outcomes for TMD patients with FM and other comorbid conditions may differ greatly from those without any of these syndromes. Very few evidence-based studies differentiating these patient types exist, and more thorough exploration is necessary.

Most studies of comorbidity have been conducted on clinical populations that are known to have a high severity of symptoms. Very little is known about the comorbidity of FM and TMD in community-wide cases of different ethnic origin. A recent study (Gansky and Plesh, unpublished data, 2005) conducted on a community-dwelling population of young women, about half of whom were African Americans and half of whom were white, showed that the percentage of people fulfilling the RDC/TMD criteria increased from 11% in those without widespread body pain to 32% in those reporting widespread pain. However, the pattern for the two races was

Table 22-2	Comparison of patients with fibromyalgia (FM) and patients with a TMD*		
Variable†	**FM (n = 60), mean (SD)**	**TMD (n = 39), mean (SD)**	**P value**
Age (y)	50.5 (9.9)	44.4 (13.2)	.012
AIMS anxiety scores (0–9.9)	4.9 (1.5)	4.3 (1.4)	.076
AIMS depression	3.9 (1.4)	3.2 (1.0)	.003
HAQ disability (0–3)	1.1 (0.6)	0.3 (0.5)	< .001
Fatigue (VAS: 0–3)	2.2 (0.8)	1.5 (0.8)	.001
GI symptoms (VAS: 0–3)	1.7 (0.9)	0.7 (1.0)	< .001
Sleep disturbance (VAS: 0–3)	2.0 (1.0)	1.1 (1.0)	< .001
Pain (VAS: 0–3)	1.8 (0.8)	1.0 (0.9)	< .001
Pain diagram scores (0–20)	12.2 (5.5)	4.6 (4.0)	< .001
Dolorimetry score (0–4 kg)	2.3 (1.0)	2.9 (0.7)	.003
Tender point count (0–18)	11.4 (5.1)	6.3 (0.7)	< .001
Control point count (0–3)	2.5 (1.9)	1.2 (1.0)	< .001

*Based on Plesh et al.[85]

†AIMS = Arthritis Impact Measurement Scale; HAQ = Health Assessment Questionnaire; VAS = visual analog scale.

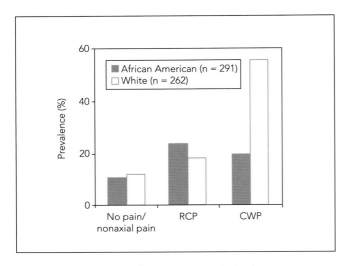

Fig 22-2 Percentage of women in each body pain category meeting Research Diagnostic Criteria for Temporomandibular Disorders (RDC/TMD). Logistic regression predicting RDC/TMD status from body pain, race, and their interaction, adjusting for subjective MacArthur socioeconomic status, showed a statistically significant interaction between body pain and race (P = .015), indicating that the relationship between body pain and TMDs differs for the two races. (RCP) Regional chronic pain; (CWP) chronic widespread pain.

very different, as indicated by a statistically significant interaction between body pain and race (Fig 22-2). For whites, the percentage of subjects with a TMD increased from 12% of those reporting no or nonaxial body pain to 55% of those reporting widespread pain. African Americans demonstrated very little change in the percentage with TMDs, ranging from 11% of those reporting no or nonaxial body pain to only 19% of those reporting widespread pain. Similar to previous reports about a white clinic sample,[84] this study of a community population showed that 17% of all TMD patients had FM and 61% of white FM patients had a TMD. However, among African Americans, only 32% of FM patients had a TMD, suggesting that the overlap between patients with a TMD and FM differs in African Americans and whites.

Based on these latest reports, daunting questions regarding the relationship between TMDs and FM still remain unanswered. The links that Wolfe[1] suggested included the idea that a decreased generalized pain threshold in fibromyalgia patients results in facial pain. The concept proposed was that FM, the underlying problem, leads to a TMD, a resulting manifestation. The previously discussed more recent data show that many young women have a TMD but no FM, while a much lower percentage of young African American women with FM present with a TMD. These racial data regarding prevalences do not support the idea that FM and TMDs share similar pathophysiologic mechanisms. Thus, some processes other than, or perhaps in addition to, decreased pain threshold seem to be responsible for the coexistence of FM and certain TMDs.

The recently proposed biopsychosocial model[48] considers biologic hereditary factors such as stress pathways (HPA axis and ANS) to be predisposing factors, while physical and psychosocial factors and associated symptoms such as pain processing and sleep activity are regarded as triggering, maintaining, or aggravating factors. Future studies should investigate this biopsychosocial model in depth to test its plausibility.

References

1. Wolfe F. Fibromyalgia. In: Sessle BJ, Bryant PS, Dionne RA (eds). Temporomandibular Disorders and Related Conditions. IASP Press, 1995:31–46.

2. Wessely S, Nimnuan C, Sharpe M. Functional somatic syndrome: One or many. Lancet 1999;354:936–939.

3. Wolfe F, Smythe HA, Yunus MB, et al. The American College of Rheumatology 1990 Criteria for Classification of Fibromyalgia: Report of multicenter criteria committee. Arthritis Rheum 1990;33:160–172.

4. Schochat T, Raspe H. Elements of fibromyalgia in an open population. Rheumatology 2003;42:829–835.

5. Croft P, Rigby AS, Boswell R, Schollum J, Silman A. The prevalence of chronic widespread pain in general population. J Rheumatol 1993;20:710–713.

6. Wolfe F. The relation between tender points and fibromyalgia symptom variables: Evidence that fibromyalgia is not a discrete disorder in the clinic. Ann Rheum Dis 1997;56:268–271.

7. Wolfe F, Roses K, Anderson J, Russell IJ, Hebert L. The prevalence and characteristics of fibromyalgia in the general population. Arthritis Rheum 1995;38:19–28.

8. Wolfe F, Ross K, Anderson J, Russell IJ. Aspects of fibromyalgia in the general population: Sex, pain threshold and fibromyalgia symptoms. J Rheumatol 1995;22:151–156.

9. Wolfe F, Anderson J, Harkness D, et al. Health status and disease severity in fibromyalgia: Results of a six center longitudinal study. Arthritis Rheum 1997;40:1571–1579.

10. Croft P, Schollum J, Silman A. Population study of tender points count and pain as evidence of fibromyalgia. BMJ 1994;309:696–699.

11. Croft P, Burt J, Schollum J, Macfarlane G, Silman A. More pain, more tender points: Is fibromyalgia just one end of a continuous spectrum? Ann Rheum Dis 1996;55:482–485.

12. Croft P. Testing for tenderness: What's the point? J Rheumatol 2000;27:2531–2533.

13. Clauw D, Crofford LJ. Chronic widespread pain and fibromyalgia: What we know and what we need to know. Best Pract Res Clin Rheumatol 2003;17:685–701.

14. Giesecke T, Williams DA, Harris RE, et al. Subgrouping of fibromyalgia patients on the bases of pressure-pain thresholds and psychological factors. Arthritis Rheum 2003;48:2916–2922.

15. White KP, Speechley M, Harth M, Ostbye T. The London fibromyalgia epidemiology study: The prevalence of fibromyalgia syndrome in London, Ontario. J Rheumatol 1999;26:1570–1576.

16. White KP, Nielson WR, Harth M, Ostbye T, Speechley M. Chronic widespread musculoskeletal pain with or without fibromyalgia: Psychological distress in a representative community adult sample. J Rheumatol 2002;29:588–594.

17. Pellegrino MJ, Waylonis GW, Sommer A. Familial occurrence of fibromyalgia. Arch Phys Med Rehabil 1989;70:61–63.

18. Stormorken H, Brosstad F. Fibromyalgia: Family clustering and sensory urgency with early onset indicate genetic predisposition and thus a "true" disease. Scand J Rheumatol 1992;21:207–209.

19. Buskila D, Neumann L. Fibromyalgia syndrome (FM) and nonarticular tenderness in relatives of patients with FM. J Rheumatol 1997;24:941–944.

20. Kashikar-Zuck S, Graham TB, Huenefeld MD, Powers SW. A review of biobehavioral research in juvenile primary fibromyalgia syndrome. Arthritis Care Res 2000;13:388–397.

21. Raphael KG, Marbach JJ, Gallagher RM, Dohrenwend BP. Myofascial TMD does not run in families. Pain 1999;80:15–22.

22. Buchwald D, Herrell R, Ashton S, et al. A twin study of chronic fatigue. Psychosom Med 2001;63:936–943.

23. Mahurin RK, Claypoole KH, Goldberg JH, Arguelles L, Ashton S, Buchwald D. Cognitive processing in monozygotic twins discordant for chronic fatigue syndrome. Neuropsychology 2004;18:232–239.

24. Macfarlane GJ, Morris S, Hunt IM, et al. Chronic widespread pain in the community: The influence of psychological symptoms and healthcare seeking behavior. J Rheumatol 1999;26:413–419.

25. Jacobsson LT, Nagi DK, Pillemer SR, et al. Low prevalences of chronic widespread pain and shoulder disorders among the Pima Indians. J Rheumatol 1996;23:907–909.

26. White KP, Thompson J. Fibromyalgia syndrome in an Amish community: A controlled study to determine disease and symptom severity. J Rheumatol 2003;30:1835–1840.

27. Drangsholt M, LeResche L. Temporomandibular disorder pain. In: Crombie IK, Croft PR, Linton SJ, LeResche L, Von Korff M (eds). Epidemiology of Pain. Seattle: IASP Press, 1999:203–233.

28. Plesh O, Sinisi SE, Crawford PB, Gansky SA. Diagnoses based on the Research Diagnostic Criteria for Temporomandibular Disorders in a biracial population of young women. J Orofac Pain 2005;19:65–75.

29. Henriksson C, Buckhardt C. Impact of fibromyalgia in everyday life: A study of women in USA and Sweden. Disabil Rehabil 1994;18:241–248.

30. Granges G, Littlejohn G. Pressure pain threshold in pain-free subjects, in patients with chronic regional pain syndromes and in subjects with fibromyalgia syndrome. Arthritis Rheum 1993;36:642–646.

31. Aaron LA, Bradley LA, Alarcon GS, et al. Psychiatric diagnoses in patients with fibromyalgia are related to health care–seeking behavior rather than illness. Arthritis Rheum 1996;39:436–445.

32. McBeth J, Macfarlane GJ, Hunt IM, Silman AJ. Risk factors for persistent chronic widespread pain: A community based study. Rheumatology 2001;40:95–101.

33. Aaron LA, Burke MM, Buchwald D. Overlapping conditions among patients with chronic fatigue syndrome, fibromyalgia, and temporomandibular disorders. Arch Intern Med 2000;160:221–227.

34. Aaron LA, Buchwald D. A review of the evidence for overlap among unexplained clinical conditions. Ann Intern Med 2001;134:868–881.

35. Aaron LA, Buchwald D. Chronic diffuse musculoskeletal pain, fibromyalgia and co-morbid unexplained clinical conditions. Best Pract Res Clin Rheumatol 2003;17:563–574.

36. Rhodus NL, Fricton J, Carlson P, Messner R. Oral symptoms associated with fibromyalgia syndrome. J Rheumatol 2003;30:1841–1845.

37. Bohr TW. Fibromyalgia syndrome and myofascial pain syndrome: Do they exist? Neurol Clin 1995;13:365–384.

38. Barsky A, Borus JF. Functional somatic syndromes. Ann Intern Med 1999;130;910–921.

39. Benjamin S, Morris S, McBeth J. The association between chronic widespread pain and mental disorder. A population-based study. Arthritis Rheum 2000;43:561–567.

40. Crofford LJ, Engleberg NC, Demitrack MA. Neurohormonal perturbations in fibromyalgia. Baillieres Clin Rheum 1996;10:365–378.

41. Clauw DJ, Chrousos GP. Chronic pain and fatigue syndromes: Overlapping clinical and neuroendocrine features and potential pathogenic mechanisms. Neuroimmunomodulation 1997;4:134–153.

42. Price DD, Staud R, Robinson ME, Mauderli AP, Cannon R, Vierck CJ. Enhanced temporal summation of second pain and its central modulation in fibromyalgia patients. Pain 2002;99:49–59.

43. Gracely RH, Grant MA, Giesecke T. Evoked pain measures in fibromyalgia. Best Pract Res Clin Rheumatol 2003;17:593–609.

44. Gracely RH, Geisser ME, Giesecke T, et al. Pain catastrophizing and neural response to pain among persons with fibromyalgia. Brain 2004;127:835–843.

45. Thompson WG, Longstreth GF, Drossman DA, Heaton KW, Irvine EJ, Muller-Lissner SA. Functional bowel disorders and functional abdominal pain. Gut 1999;54(suppl 2):II43–II47.

46. Dworkin SF, LeResche L. Research Diagnostic Criteria for Temporomandibular Disorders: Review criteria, examinations and specifications, critique. J Craniomandib Disord 1992;6:301–355.

47. Loeser JD, Melzack R. Pain: An overview. Lancet 1999;353:1607–1609.

48. Ferrari R. The biopsychosocial model: A tool for rheumatologists. Baillieres Clin Rheumatol 2000;14:787–795.

49. Waylonis GW, Heck W. Fibromyalgia syndrome. New associations. Am J Phys Med Rehabil 1992;71:343–348.

50. Uveges JM, Parker JC, Smarr KL, et al. Psychological symptoms in primary fibromyalgia syndrome: Relationship to pain, life stress, and sleep disturbance. Arthritis Rheum 1990;33:1279–1283.

51. Adler GK, Kinsley BT, Hurwitz S, Mossey CJ, Goldenberg DL. Reduced hypothalamic-pituitary and sympathoadrenal responses to hypoglycemia in women with fibromyalgia syndrome. Am J Med 1999;106:534–543.

52. Griep EN, Boersma JW, de Kloet ER. Altered reactivity of hypothalamic-pituitary-adrenal axis in the primary fibromyalgia syndrome. J Rheumatol 1993;20:469–474.

53. van Denderen JC, Boersma JW, Zeinstra P, Hollander AP, van Neerbos BR. Psychological effects of exhaustive physical exercise in primary fibromyalgia syndrome (PFS): Is PFS a disorder of neuroendocrine reactivity? Scand J Rheumatol 1992;21:35–37.

54. Kosek E, Ekholm J, Hansson P. Sensory dysfunction in fibromyalgia patients with implications for pathogenic mechanism. Pain 1996;68:375–383.

55. Hellhammer DH, Wade S. Endocrine correlates of stress vulnerability. Psychother Psychosom 1993;60:8–17.

56. Parker AJ, Wessely S, Cleare AJ. The neuroendocrinology of chronic fatigue syndrome and fibromyalgia. Psychol Med 2001;31:1331–1345.

57. Petzke F, Clauw DJ. Sympathetic nervous system function in fibromyalgia. Curr Rheumatol Rep 2000;2:116–122.

58. Martinez-Lavin M, Hermosillo AG, Mendoza C, et al. Orthostatic sympathetic derangement in subjects with fibromyalgia. J Rheumatol 1997;24:714–718.

59. Bou-Holaigah I, Calkins H, Flynn JA, et al. Provocation of hypotension and pain during upright tilt table testing in adults with fibromyalgia. Clin Exp Rheumatol 1997;15:239–246.

60. Affleck G, Urrows S, Tennen H, Higgins P, Abeles M. Sequential daily relationship of sleep, pain intensity, and attention to pain among women with fibromyalgia. Pain 1996;68:363–368.

61. Moldofsky H, Scarisbrick P, England R, Smythe H. Musculoskeletal symptoms and non-REM sleep disturbance in patients with "fibrositis syndrome" and healthy subjects. Psychosom Med 1975;37:341–351.

62. Shaver JL, Lentz M, Landis CA, Heitkemper MM, Buchwald DS, Woods NF. Sleep physiology and stress arousal in women with fibromyalgia. Res Nurs Health 1997;20:47–57.

63. Moldofsky H, Scarisbrick P. Induction of neurasthenic musculoskeletal pain syndrome by selective sleep stage deprivation. Psychosom Med 1976:38:35–44.

64. Manu P, Lane TJ, Matthews DA, Castriotta RJ, Watson RK, Abeles M. Alpha-delta sleep in patients with a chief complaint of chronic fatigue. Am Med J 1994;87:465–470.

65. Moldofsky H. Sleep and pain. Sleep Med Rev 2001;5:385–396.

66. Bennett RM, Clark SR, Goldberg L, et al. Aerobic fitness in the fibromyalgia syndrome. A controlled study of respiratory gas exchange and Xenon 133 clearance from exercising muscles. Arthritis Rheum 1989;32:454–460.

67. Lund N, Bengtsson A, Thorborg P. Muscle tissue oxygen pressure in primary fibromyalgia. Scand J Rheumatol 1986;15:165–173.

68. Bengtsson A, Henricksson KG, Larsson J. Reduced high-energy phosphate levels in the painful muscles of patients with primary fibromyalgia. Arthritis Rheum 1986;29:817–821.

69. Jones KD, Clark SR. Individualizing the exercise prescription for persons with fibromyalgia. Rheum Dis Clin North Am 2002;28:419–436.

70. Lautenbacher S, Rollman GB. Possible deficiencies in pain modulation in fibromyalgia. Clin J Pain 1997;13:189–196.

71. Mountz JM, Bradley LA, Modell JC, et al. Fibromyalgia in women. Abnormalities of regional cerebral blood flow in the thalamus and the caudate nucleus are associated with low pain threshold levels. Arthritis Rheum 1995;38:926–938.

72. Russell IJ, Orr MD, Littman B, et al. Elevated cerebrospinal fluid levels of substance P in patients with fibromyalgia syndrome. Arthritis Rheum 1994;37:1593–1601.

73. Russell IJ, Vaeroy H, Javors M, Nyberg F. Cerebrospinal fluid biogenic amine metabolites in fibromyalgia/fibrositis syndrome and rheumatoid arthritis. Arthritis Rheum 1992;35:550–556.

74. Yunus MB, Dailey JW, Aldag JC, Masi AT, Jobe PC. Plasma tryptophan and other amino acids in primary fibromyalgia: A controlled study. J Rheumatol 1992;19:90–94.

75. Staud R, Vierck CJ, Cannon RL. Abnormal sensitization and temporal summation of second pain (wind-up) in patients with fibromyalgia syndrome. Pain 2001;91:165–175.

76. Bennett RM, Clark SR, Campbell SM, Burckhardt CS. Low levels of somatomedin C in patients with the fibromyalgia syndrome. A possible link between sleep and muscle pain. Arthritis Rheum 1992;35:1113–1116.

77. Bengtsson A, Bengtsson M. Regional sympathetic blockade in primary fibromyalgia. Pain 1988;33:161–167.

78. Yunus MB. Towards a model of pathophysiology of fibromyalgia: Aberrant central pain mechanisms with peripheral modulation. J Rheumatol 1992;19:846–850.

79. Hudson JI, Goldenberg DL, Pope HG Jr, Keck PE Jr, Schlesinger L. Comorbidity of fibromyalgia with medical and psychiatric disorder. Am J Med 1992;92:363–367.

80. Hudson JI, Pope HG Jr. Affective spectrum disorders: Does antidepressant response identify a family of disorders with a common pathophysiology? Am J Psychiatry 1989;147:552–564.

81. Yunus MB. Psychological aspects of fibromyalgia syndrome: A component of the dysfunctional spectrum syndrome. Baillieres Clin Rheumatol 1994;8:811–837.

82. Taylor ML, Trotter DR, Csuka ME. The prevalence of sexual abuse in women with fibromyalgia. Arthritis Rheum 1995;38:229–234.

83. Bergman S, Herrstrom P, Lennart TH, Jacobsson T, Pettersson F. Chronic widespread pain: A three year followup of pain distribution and risk factors. J Rheumatol 2002;29:818–825.

84. Plesh O, Wolfe F, Lane N. The relationship between fibromyalgia and temporomandibular disorders: Prevalence and symptom severity. J Rheumatol 1996;23:1948–1952.

85. Hedenberg-Magnusson B, Ernberg M, Kopp S. Presence of orofacial pain and temporomandibular disorders in fibromyalgia. Swed Dent J 1999;23:185–192.

86. Dao TT, Reynolds WJ, Tenenbaum HC. Comorbidity between myofascial pain of the masticatory muscles and fibromyalgia. J Orofac Pain 1997;11:232–241.

87. Turp JC, Kowalski CJ, O'Leary N, Stohler CS. Pain maps from facial pain patients indicate a broad pain geography. J Dent Res 1998;77:1465–1472.

88. Raphael KG, Marbach JJ, Klausner J. Myofascial face pain. Clinical characteristics of those with regional vs. widespread pain. J Am Dent Assoc 2000;131:854–858.

Pharmacologic Approaches

Raymond A. Dionne

Drug classes for the treatment of pain associated with temporomandibular disorders (TMDs) range from short-term treatment with nonsteroidal anti-inflammatory drugs (NSAIDs) and muscle relaxants for pain of muscular and/or joint origin to chronic administration of antidepressants and anticonvulsants for less well-characterized pain. A recent systematic review[1] of clinical trials that studied treatments for several types of chronic orofacial pain could only identify 11 trials that met minimal criteria for scientific quality; most therapeutic modalities used for this purpose fell into the category of an unvalidated clinical treatment. Yet patients presenting with acute or chronic TMD pain expect treatment for their pain, often with medications that carry significant risk with chronic administration (eg, NSAIDs). In the absence of an evidentiary basis from studies in patients with chronic TMD pain, therapeutic recommendations are often extrapolated from other indications.

Pharmacologic intervention in the management of chronic TMD pain is usually considered adjunctive on the assumption that more definitive treatments will eventually correct the underlying pathophysiologic process. It is now recognized, however, that many so-called definitive dental and surgical therapies for TMDs have not withstood scientific scrutiny for adequate efficacy and safety; this fact has led to the use of medications as the primary intervention for many of these disorders. The multiplicity of pain pathways and the involvement of many well-characterized inflammatory mediators, such as cyclooxygenase 2 (COX-2), bradykinin, and substance P, at the site of injury in the periphery and neuro-transmitters in the nucleus caudalis provide logical targets for pharmacologic interventions (Fig 23-1). Long-term palliative treatment of intractable pain through pharmacologic management may be the only option for some individuals when pain is poorly controlled following failed surgical interventions. This chapter reviews the use of analgesic medications for TMDs where adequate evidence supports their efficacy and safety for this indication. The discussion also includes other drug classes that may be considered because of their documented effectiveness for related chronic pain conditions.

Clinical Evaluation of Drugs

Lack of consensus on the treatment of TMDs is often fostered by a lack of appreciation for the differences between clinical observations, which may form the basis for therapeutic interventions, and the need to verify the safety and effectiveness of treatments in studies that control for factors that can mimic clinical success. Although these considerations apply to all areas of therapy, the management of chronic orofacial pain has a history of therapeutic misadventures, charismatic-based treatment philosophies, and a lack of scientific documentation for most clinical practices. The potential for significant morbidity with drug classes used for TMDs mandates that their effectiveness be documented and outweigh safety concerns, especially when these medications will be administered chronically.

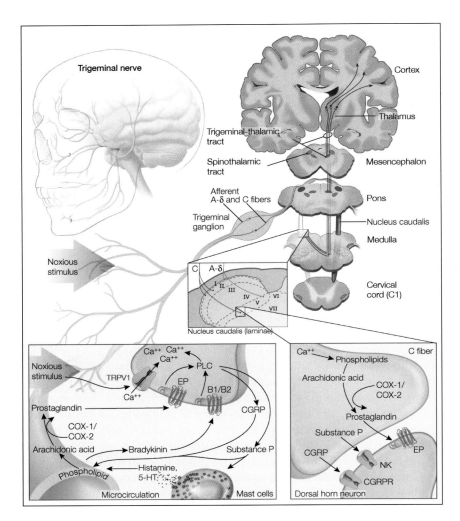

Fig 23-1 Trigeminal pain pathways originate at peripheral nerve endings located throughout the maxilla and mandible and travel along the branches of the trigeminal nerve to the trigeminal ganglion and the nucleus caudalis, which is the trigeminal equivalent of the dorsal horn in the spinal cord. Nociceptive information is then transmitted along two major pathways to the thalamus and eventually results in pain perception at the cortical level. Some of the major inflammatory mediators in the periphery and neurotransmitters that transmit and modulate nociceptive impulses in the nucleus caudalis are illustrated in the insets. (TRPV1) Transient receptor potential Subtype 1; (EP) E-prostanoid; (PLC) phospholipase C; (CGRP) calcitonin gene–related peptide; (COX) cyclooxygenase; (5-HT) 5-hydroxytryptamine; (NK) neurokinin; (CGRPR) calcitonin gene–related peptide receptor.

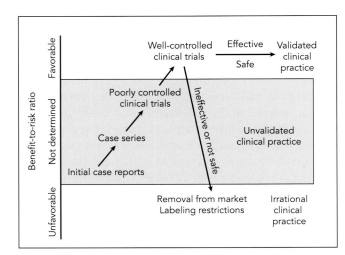

Fig 23-2 Natural history of putative therapies for chronic orofacial pain. Results of novel treatments first identified in case reports and case series are usually very favorable or else they would not have been published, but they represent the lowest form of evidence. Clinical trials that are poorly controlled also do not provide sufficient evidence to consider a novel treatment as validated for use in clinical practice. Well-controlled clinical trials may provide evidence of efficacy and safety to consider the treatment as a validated clinical practice or may demonstrate that it is ineffective or unsafe, resulting in removal from the marketplace or labeling restrictions. Treatments that do not meet criteria for a validated clinical practice remain in the category of unvalidated or irrational clinical practices (shaded area).

The natural history of therapeutic interventions for the management of pain is illustrated in Fig 23-2. Novel treatments first described on the basis of initial case reports, case series, or poorly controlled clinical trials usually appear to have therapeutic benefit, or the results would not be publicized. Following evaluation of a putative therapy in well-controlled clinical trials, however, a number of alternative interpretations are possible. If several trials indicate that the treatment is effective and has minimum toxicity, it is then considered to be a validated therapy. An example of this outcome is the use of nonsteroidal anti-inflammatory drugs for the control of acute pain. If the treatment is found not to be effective, or toxicity becomes evident, the drug is withdrawn from the market, as recently occurred with rofecoxib (Vioxx, Merck) and valdecoxib (Bextra, Pfizer), or labeling restrictions are imposed, as was done for ketorolac (Toradol, Roche).

Most nonpharmacologic therapies that are used for chronic TMD pain do not fall under the jurisdiction of the US Food and Drug Administration (FDA) as either drugs or devices and therefore are not subjected to rigorous examination before being used in humans. Other review processes, such as the US Pharmacopeial Convention, use expert panels to review non–FDA-approved uses for marketed drugs but do not address devices or clinical practices. As a consequence, most drugs, devices, and therapeutic strategies that are used for managing acute and/or chronic TMD pain fall into the category of unvalidated clinical practices. This does not imply that these treatment modalities do not have some therapeutic value. Rather, they have not been subjected to well-controlled trials to determine if the modality is a validated clinical practice whose efficacy exceeds the potential for toxicity or, possibly, if their use represents an irrational clinical practice that should not be continued. The hazard of using a seemingly effective therapy in humans without appropriate validation of safety is illustrated by the current plight of patients who received Proplast-Teflon TMJ disc implants (Vitek) for the surgical treatment of TMDs[2] (see chapter 31).

Another factor that may affect the evaluation of treatment outcome to drug therapy for TMDs is the fluctuating nature of musculoskeletal pain, which may undergo remissions or exacerbations independent of treatment.[3] The high psychological comorbidity described in this population may also influence the onset of symptoms, reporting of pain intensity or its affective component, and treatment response (see chapters 13 and 26).[4] Many patients eventually improve even if an initial course of therapy is not successful or if they receive no treatment at all. Such responses may explain the high rates of success reported in case series and loosely controlled studies for many of the therapeutic modalities used for TMDs.

In general, claims of efficacy based on initial clinical observations are often superseded by equivocal findings of efficacy or belated recognition of adverse effects and toxicity with long-term administration. The principles of pain management for TMDs rest on the same principles that apply to the use of all drugs: demonstrated efficacy for the indication, an acceptable incidence of adverse reactions for the condition being treated, and safety when used in large numbers of patients for prolonged periods of time.

Anti-inflammatory Drugs

Nonsteroidal Anti-inflammatory Drugs

NSAIDs comprise a heterogenous group of drugs with diverse structures, similar therapeutic effects, good oral efficacy, and similar side effects. They are better tolerated by ambulatory patients than opioid drugs, have fewer sedative side effects, and are not likely to produce dependence or result in tolerance. Conversely, the hazards of long-term administration of NSAIDs have been belatedly recognized as involving renal disease and serious toxicity to the gastrointestinal tract, as well as increasing the risks of adverse cardiovascular events.

A comprehensive review of the primary literature reveals modest scientific support for the assertion that the daily use of NSAIDs offers benefit for patients with chronic TMD pain.[1] Standard texts and summaries of expert opinion often provide recommendations or extrapolate from chronic inflammatory conditions such as arthritis. Yet the results of two placebo-controlled studies suggest that NSAIDs are ineffective for the treatment of chronic TMD pain. The analgesic effects of ibuprofen (2,400 mg daily for 4 weeks) could not be separated from placebo in a group of patients with chronic myogenous pain.[5] A similar comparison of piroxicam (20 mg daily for 12 days) to placebo for the treatment of temporomandibular pain also failed to demonstrate any therapeutic advantage for the NSAID.[6]

A recent publication, however, provides stronger evidence for the efficacy of NSAIDs for the treatment of arthrogenous TMJ pain. The administration of naproxen (500 mg twice daily) resulted in a significant reduction in pain over 6 weeks in comparison to both placebo and celecoxib[7]; the mean pain score at the end of the study was approximately one quarter that at the start of the study (Fig 23-3a). Significantly greater improvement in the range of mandibular motion was also observed in the naproxen group than in the placebo and celecoxib groups (Fig 23-3b). The incidence and severity of adverse events were similar in the placebo and NSAID groups, indicating

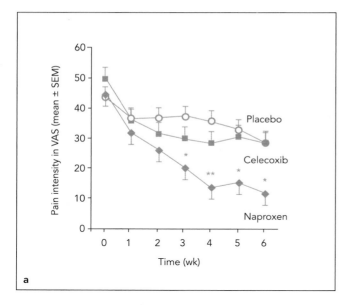

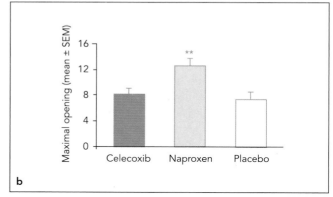

Fig 23-3 Comparison of the effectiveness of naproxen to celecoxib and placebo for providing analgesia and improving range of motion in patients with chronic orofacial pain. *(a)* Use of naproxen resulted in a significantly greater reduction in pain than both celecoxib and placebo. *(b)* Use of naproxen resulted in significantly greater increase in maximal opening than celecoxib and placebo. (VAS) Visual analog scale; (SEM) standard error of the mean. *$P < .05$. **$P < .01$. (Data from Ta and Dionne.[7])

that the drugs are well tolerated at this dose over the 6-week duration of the study. The dual cyclooxygenase 1 (COX-1) and COX-2 inhibition by naproxen was demonstrated to be more effective for the treatment of painful temporomandibular joints (TMJs) than only the selective COX-2 inhibitor, suggesting that inhibition of both COX isoenzymes is needed to achieve effective analgesia for this type of pain.[7]

Both clinical and animal studies suggest that tolerance to NSAIDs can develop with repeated administration. The mean reduction in the intensity of chronic lower back pain following an initial dose of 1,200 mg of ibuprofen was 23%.[8] After 2 weeks' ingestion of 2,400 mg per day of ibuprofen or placebo, the mean reduction in pain intensity after the last dose was fourfold lower in the drug group. Moreover, the initial low level of response suggests that lower back pain is not particularly sensitive to ibuprofen and may also explain, in part, the poor response observed

for treatment of chronic musculoskeletal pain in the orofacial area. The development of tolerance over 2 weeks would suggest a similar process with TMD pain that could make the analgesic response negligible by the end of 4 weeks.

Tolerance to the NSAIDs with repeated administration has been demonstrated in animals. Following 3 days of diflunisal, the same dose resulted in similar blood levels but less clinical effect.[9] This suggests a functional change in the pharmacologic response rather than enhanced pharmacokinetic disposition, because the same amount of drug elicited less analgesia.

There is a growing body of evidence on the potential serious toxic effects of NSAIDs when taken chronically at high doses.[10] A short trial of an NSAID may be considered for patients whose pain complaint has an inflammatory component. However, a lack of therapeutic effect after a 7- to 10-day trial, or the development of any gastrointestinal symptoms, should prompt discontinuation of the drug.

Selective COX-2 Inhibitors

At standard therapeutic doses, conventional NSAIDs exert their analgesic and anti-inflammatory effects through COX-2 inhibition, yet at the same time they also block COX-1. This latter action in turn leads to diminished production of the prostaglandins that regulate homeostatic functions. As a consequence, these agents induce substantial platelet effects, along with the potential for renal and gastrointestinal toxicity, which may interfere with clinical usage.

The discovery and characterization of the COX-2 isoform led to the hypothesis that selective inhibition of COX-2 would provide the potent anti-inflammatory and analgesic effects of an NSAID without influencing COX-1 and its important physiologic functions. Based on this hypothesis, and discouraged by the significant morbidity associated with NSAIDs, there have been substantial efforts to develop specific inhibitors of the COX-2 isoform. A number of studies have suggested that the original paradigm regarding the roles of COX-1 and COX-2 was overly simplistic. Findings from animal studies have demonstrated constitutive expression of COX-2 in the kidney, brain, ovary, uterus, cartilage, and bone.[11–14] There is also evidence that, in some circumstances, COX-1 can be induced by stressful stimuli such as radiation injury to the intestine, and that it may play a protective role in this circumstance.[15] This emerging information strongly suggests that both COX-1 and COX-2 have more complex physiologic and pathophysiologic roles than originally thought.

Originally, three COX-2 inhibitors were commercially available on the market. They were highly selective for COX-2 suppression at the doses administered clinically and had minimal effects on COX-1 activity. Celecoxib (Celebrex, Searle), a sulfonamide, was the first of the COX-2–specific inhibitors approved by the FDA for the treatment of rheumatoid arthritis (RA) and osteoarthritis (OA). Rofecoxib (Vioxx, Merck) was subsequently approved for indications including treatment of OA, RA in adults, and primary dysmenorrhea but was withdrawn from the market in 2004 because of an increased incidence of cardiovascular events in patients who took it chronically. Valdecoxib (Bextra, Pfizer) was later introduced for similar indications but then withdrawn from the market for the same reason in 2005.

Celecoxib has been extensively evaluated for efficacy in patients with OA and RA of the knees and hips, which should be comparable to the response in patients with OA and RA of the TMJ. Dosage ranges of 100 to 400 mg a day for OA and 200 to 800 mg a day for RA, established in phase II trials, have demonstrated efficacy in phase III trials. Celecoxib administered at these dosages has been shown to have similar efficacy as 1,000 mg a day of naproxen or 150 mg a day of diclofenac for the management of the symptoms of OA and RA. In a 12-week trial involving a large sample of patients with OA of the knee, significant pain relief and improvement in physical function were achieved with celecoxib (100 or 200 mg twice daily) and naproxen (500 mg twice daily).[16]

Despite these promising observations for RA and OA, 100 mg of celecoxib administered twice daily failed to result in greater relief of TMD pain or improvement in function than a placebo in a study with demonstrated bioassay sensitivity (see Fig 23-3).[7] Retrospective analysis of treatment responders, defined as 50% reduction from starting pain, showed a marginally nonsignificant trend for a celecoxib response in approximately two thirds of patients, in comparison to one third in the placebo-treated patients.

Although this observation has to be prospectively replicated, in the interim celecoxib may be considered for the treatment of chronic TMD pain as an alternative that might be effective in some patients and is likely to be better tolerated than classic NSAIDs. Upper gastrointestinal complications, in the presence of a confirmed upper gastrointestinal mucosal lesion, occur eightfold less frequently in patients receiving celecoxib than in those receiving standard NSAIDs.[17] The incidence of endoscopically demonstrable ulceration is consistently low with celecoxib and comparable to rates reported with placebo.

Corticosteroids

Corticosteroids have been injected directly into the TMJ and applied topically in an attempt to reduce the pain and dysfunction associated with TMDs (see chapter 30). Very few controlled studies of intra-articular injection have been reported, and results have varied from demonstration of efficacy, to no difference in comparison to placebo, to deleterious effects in the absence of any therapeutic benefit.

The iontophoretic administration of steroids has also been recommended by some clinicians, based on clinical observations. It is hypothesized that iontophoresis, the application of an electrical current to ionized drug solutions, will result in higher drug levels at the site of injury or pain, in this case the TMJ. One study compared iontophoresis with dexamethasone in a lidocaine vehicle to a saline placebo for TMJ pain.[18] Patients met diagnostic criteria for painful TMJ disc displacement with reduction, disc displacement without reduction, or OA. Three drug administration sessions took place over 5 days, and there were 7- and 14-day follow-ups.

Both groups of subjects (active drug and placebo) showed improvement over the course of therapy and continued to report less pain and improved range of motion at

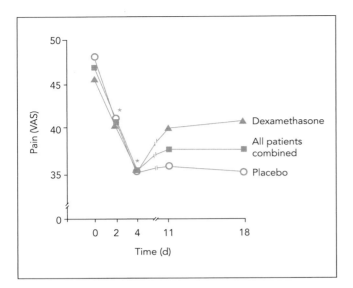

Fig 23-4 Clinical evaluation of a steroid applied by iontophoresis to the TMJ. Both the dexamethasone-treated and placebo-treated patients showed a significant decrease in pain over the first 4 days of treatment that was maintained up to 2 weeks following the last drug treatment. These data illustrate the regression in symptoms that is often observed, independent of any genuine therapeutic effect. (VAS) Visual analog scale. *$P <$ .05. (Data from Reid et al.[13])

the 7- and 14-day follow-ups.[18] These data illustrate the dichotomy that often exists between clinical observations and the results of a controlled clinical trial. If the pain and dysfunction reported before treatment and at the follow-up appointments are compared (Fig 23-4), it would appear logical to conclude that the improvement was the result of the treatment being evaluated, in this case the iontophoretic application of a steroid to the TMJ. Evaluation of the active drug in the presence of a placebo-controlled clinical trial, however, leads to the opposite conclusion, that the drug has no detectable therapeutic effect. Alternative explanations for the results include cyclic fluctuations in symptoms over time and patient expectations of improvement from receiving medications applied by a novel method in a therapeutic environment.

Benzodiazepines

Drugs of the benzodiazepine class are frequently administered to patients with chronic pain, often for prolonged periods, despite long-standing concern about the potential for their abuse and the development of dependence, as well as the possibility that they may initiate or exacerbate depression in patients with chronic pain. Although the efficacy of benzodiazepines for the treatment of chronic pain is not generally recognized, several studies have demonstrated their therapeutic effects for musculoskeletal pain. A study evaluating diazepam, ibuprofen, and the combination of both in patients with chronic orofacial pain of myogenic origin showed a significantly greater decrease in pain in the diazepam and diazepam plus ibuprofen groups than in the placebo group, indicating that the pain relief was attributable to the diazepam.[5] The effects of clonazepam in patients with chronic myofascial pain in the orofacial region were also shown to be superior to those of placebo in a double-blind, 30-day trial.[19] No instances of dependence or withdrawal symptoms were noted on discontinuation of the drug in either of these studies.

A larger study of patients with fibromyalgia receiving alprazolam, ibuprofen, or a combination of both reported decreases in patients' rating of disease severity and tenderness on palpation after 6 weeks in the group receiving the drug combination.[20] The dose of alprazolam (0.5 to 3.0 mg per day) was well tolerated while patients completed 24 weeks of drug administration; it was reported that many patients tapered their daily dosage, contrary to a pattern of drug abuse. The data from these three studies[5,19,20] are supportive of benzodiazepine-mediated relief of symptoms in patients with chronic orofacial pain of myogenic origin.

A nonsystematic review of the long-term use of benzodiazepines for chronic pain also concluded that they are effective for some musculoskeletal symptoms.[21] However, the authors suggested that the antidepressant effects attributable to triazolo-benzodiazepines, such as alprazolam, may be artifactual because of overlap in the diagnostic criteria used for depression and anxiety disorders and the sedative effects on rating scales used to assess depression. Conversely, they concluded that high doses of benzodiazepines produce reversible side effects that are mistakenly interpreted as depression.

The scientific literature does not provide either unequivocal support for the use of benzodiazepines on the basis of their efficacy or universal condemnation of their use because of potential toxicity. Patients whose pain appears to be of musculoskeletal origin may benefit from a 2- to 4-week course of a benzodiazepine. The drugs should not be prescribed in large amounts that would permit dose escalation without professional supervision.

A lack of treatment response or the onset of sedative side effects or depressive symptoms should be an indication to reduce the dose or discontinue the drug. If difficulties in sleep onset or duration are the primary complaint, consideration should be given to the use of a hypnotic benzodiazepine to minimize drug effects during the day. Patients who present with depressive symptoms should be further evaluated by a psychiatrist to rule out depression or other mood disorders. Antidepressant therapy, if indicated, should be pursued in this manner rather than through the prescription of a benzodiazepine with putative antidepressant properties.

Therapy with a benzodiazepine should not be extended beyond a few weeks. Patients for whom a therapeutic course of a benzodiazepine and conservative therapy do not produce a therapeutic response should be reevaluated rather than mismanaged with long-term benzodiazepine treatment.

Muscle Relaxants

Drugs that are thought to reduce skeletal muscle tone are often administered to patients with certain TMD subtypes to help alleviate the increased muscle activity. Muscle relaxants are thought to decrease muscle tone without impairment in motor function by acting centrally to depress polysynaptic reflexes. Drugs with sedative properties also depress polysynaptic reflexes, making it difficult to differentiate between drugs that may be centrally acting muscle relaxants and nonspecific sedatives that also produce muscle relaxation. Benzodiazepines (eg, diazepam) are used in myofascial pain patients partly on the basis of putative muscle relaxant properties, but they only decrease muscle tone at doses that produce unacceptable levels of central nervous system depression.

A critical review of carisoprodol and related propanediols concluded that they are better than placebo for the treatment of acute musculoskeletal disorders but less effective for chronic conditions.[22] A possible exception to this generalization is cyclobenzaprine, which has been demonstrated to be effective in patients with some chronic musculoskeletal disorders. Cyclobenzaprine is superior to placebo for treating pain in the cervical and lumbar regions that is associated with skeletal muscle spasms, and it reduces electromyographic signs of muscle spasm.[23] Although it has not been directly assessed for TMD-related myofascial pain, these findings are suggestive of efficacy for muscle relaxation in the orofacial region.

There appears to be a discrepancy between common clinical use of skeletal muscle relaxants and the results of controlled clinical trials comparing their efficacy to that of a placebo. It is also not clear whether they are specific for muscle relaxation or whether they produce central nervous system depression, thereby reducing muscle tone. Little evidence exists for their efficacy in alleviating TMD pain of myogenic origin, nor has it been demonstrated that they provide an additive effect to exercises or bite appliance therapy aimed at muscle relaxation. Given this modest scientific support, use of muscle relaxants to decrease muscle tone in TMD patients should probably be limited to a brief trial in conjunction with physical therapy.

Opioids

Administration of opioids for nonmalignant pain is controversial but may be considered for patients with certain orofacial pain conditions, especially if other, more conservative options have failed or more surgery is likely to result in iatrogenic injury. Both open-label and double-blind studies have demonstrated that orally administered opioids such as codeine and morphine produce significant analgesia and no signs of respiratory depression but have a greater incidence of adverse events than either a placebo or an NSAID. Although patients with head and neck pain were included in these studies, no direct evaluation was made of long-term administration of opioids for patients with TMD pain.

Most concern over the chronic use of opioids relates to the potential for "addiction," the maladaptive behaviors associated with illicit drug seeking. This term implies the development of physical dependence and tolerance requiring continued opioid use with increasing doses. Physical dependence or the development of tolerance in a therapeutic context do not necessarily equate with addictive behavior, because drug seeking is not necessary if the drug is medically available. Similarly, cycles of intoxication and withdrawal should not occur with sustained-release formulations.

Given the serious adverse effects associated with chronic use of NSAIDs, and the absence of effective therapies for certain chronic orofacial pain conditions, the use of opioids should be considered when more conservative measures have failed. Sustained-release formulations should minimize cyclic fluctuations in pain associated with standard-release formulations with a short duration of action. The chronic use of opioids for patients with TMD pain requires careful patient selection to rule out drug-seeking behavior or other personality disorders, careful monitoring to individualize the dose and minimize side effects and dose escalation, and careful attention to regulatory procedures. The clinical pharmacology of opioids, recommended doses, and therapeutic recommendations to minimize abuse and the development of tolerance are extensively reviewed in standard texts and are beyond the scope of this chapter.

Antidepressants

Antidepressant drugs have been used for more than 30 years for the management of pain arising from a wide variety of conditions, including orofacial pain. Three independent reviews of controlled studies of the use of antidepressants for pain management have indicated that their analgesic effects are largely independent of their antidepressant activity.[24–26] The analgesic effects can be differentiated from placebo, are found at doses lower than those usually effective in depression, and can occur in patients who are not depressed. Studies in patients with nondental chronic pain, primarily diabetic and postherpetic neuropathy, have indicated that drugs that inhibit reuptake of both serotonin and norepinephrine, such as amitriptyline, are more efficacious than drugs that are selective for either neurotransmitter.[27]

Evidence that antidepressants produce analgesia independent of the alleviation of depression comes from studies in which low doses of amitriptyline were administered to patients with chronic pain. A low dose of amitriptyline (mean dose of 24 mg) was as effective for chronic orofacial pain as a higher dose (mean of 129 mg) that was in the range of the usual (75- to 150-mg) daily antidepressant dose.[28] A daily dose of 25 mg of amitriptyline for 3 weeks was also demonstrated to be superior to placebo in a variety of patients with chronic nonmalignant pain.[29]

A dose-response comparison of 25, 50, and 75 mg of amitriptyline showed increased analgesia with increasing doses and improved sleep with the 75-mg dose but a significantly higher incidence of adverse effects at the 75-mg dose.[30] Another study also reported analgesia and improved sleep with 75 mg of amitriptyline daily over 6 weeks.[31] If antidepressants produced therapeutic effects solely through alleviation of depression, the doses used in these studies would have to be similar to those used to treat depression.

The biomedical literature clearly supports the clinical use of antidepressants for treatment of neuropathic pain as well as for chronic nonmalignant pain when other treatments have failed or if depression accompanies the pain. Tricyclic antidepressants with both serotonergic and noradrenergic effects (eg, amitriptyline or doxepin) appear to be most effective. Lower dosages (25 to 75 mg) should be used initially for nondepressed patients. Antidepressant doses should be reserved for patients who are depressed, best prescribed in consultation with a clinician experienced in the diagnosis and treatment of psychiatric illness. Sedative antidepressants may be useful when patients have sleeping problems and may help to reduce the dose of other hypnotic drugs.

The dose of antidepressant will usually be limited by anticholinergic side effects (dry mouth, constipation, blurred vision, and urinary retention) and should be adjusted in response to individual variation in analgesic response and side effects. Cardiovascular effects can occur, ranging from postural hypotension to serious ventricular arrhythmias, especially in patients with preexisting heart disease; medical consultation or parallel management is advisable in at-risk patients.

Drugs for Neuropathic Orofacial Pain

A wide spectrum of drugs is used for the treatment of neuropathic disorders. Anticonvulsant medications have been reported to provide effective treatments for many orofacial pain disorders such as trigeminal neuralgia and related pain disorders (eg, migraine headache). Additionally, the use of N-methyl-D-aspartate (NMDA) receptor antagonists may provide a new line of therapy for orofacial pain. Although most of these drug classes are used in the treatment of other neuropathic disorders, their use in the treatment of orofacial pain has not been systematically evaluated nor is there any evidence for their use in the treatment of early-onset TMD pain. However, as TMD pain persists, central nervous system changes may occur (eg, central plasticity), making use of these medications a therapeutic option.

Gabapentin represents a new-generation drug that was originally developed as an antiepileptic agent; however, it has been studied as an analgesic for chronic conditions as well. Although structurally similar to the inhibitory neurotransmitter γ-aminobutyric acid, the mechanism of action for pain inhibition is still unknown. The use of gabapentin for a wide variety of disorders, including epilepsy, movement disorders, migraine prophylaxis, and chronic pain, suggests a nonspecific mechanism. Benefits of gabapentin include low toxicity and a favorable side-effect profile, and it is well tolerated compared to other anticonvulsants, such as carbamazepine. These attributes make it a suitable candidate for management of chronic pain disorders such as trigeminal neuralgia.

Numerous placebo-controlled, double-blind studies have demonstrated the effectiveness of gabapentin for reducing pain and improving the quality of life for patients suffering from postherpetic neuralgia and diabetic neuropathies.[32,33] Only a limited number of studies have evaluated the use of gabapentin for the treatment of orofacial neuropathic pain.[34–36] None of these studies, however, can be considered prospective, double-blind, or placebo-controlled, leaving its true therapeutic value uncertain. Gabapentin may be considered as a single treatment agent for patients suffering from neuropathic pain that has been refractory to other medications or who cannot tolerate its untoward effects.

A large body of animal data and more limited results of clinical trials suggest that drugs that block the effects of excitatory amino acids at the NMDA receptor interfere with the development and maintenance of central hyperalgesia. In a double-blind, placebo-controlled crossover study comparing the effects of dextromethorphan in patients with either postherpetic neuralgia or diabetic neuropathy, dextromethorphan significantly reduced pain in the diabetic neuropathy group but not the postherpetic neuralgia group, as compared to placebo.[37–40]

While a number of studies have demonstrated the effectiveness of NMDA receptor antagonists in the reduction and treatment of chronic pain, their use is primarily limited because of the intolerability of the side effects associated with these drugs. These include sedation, dizziness, dissociative effects, nausea, and visual disturbances. NMDA receptor antagonists may be useful when combined with opioids, because there appears to be a synergistic effect in reducing pain and a decrease in the development of tolerance to the opioid. This strategy may have particular usefulness in patients whose TMJ surgery failed and whose only treatment options are sometimes limited to use of high doses of opioids.

Despite the scientific literature supporting the use of anticonvulsant drugs for the treatment of pain, most studies do not provide well-controlled clinical data to support the use of anticonvulsant medications for the treatment of TMD pain, because the pathophysiolgic basis for these disorders is primarily arthritic and muscular in origin. However, it is increasingly recognized that secondary central changes occur as these conditions become chronic. There is evidence of central activation and changes occurring following a focal TMJ injury that may contribute to the long-lasting symptoms reported by this group of patients. In this instance, such pain sufferers may experience a spreading, lancinating, or burning quality to their pain that may relate to development of a neuropathic component. With this transition, these patients may not be merely classified as TMD patients; rather, they fall in a broader realm of patients with chronic orofacial pain. In patients who develop these secondary changes, appropriate incorporation of an anticonvulsant or NMDA antagonist may be beneficial, as previously outlined.

Therapeutic Recommendations

Review of the drug classes most commonly used for TMDs and other types of chronic orofacial pain does not reveal a wealth of data on which to base therapy. Given the potential for serious toxicity that can accompany long-term administration of drugs that are safe enough to be marketed without a prescription (ie, the NSAIDs), the use of some drug classes may involve risk to the patient with minimal therapeutic benefit. A need exists for well-controlled studies of drugs for TMDs and related orofacial pain in the relevant patient populations. These studies should ensure that the medications are used for a duration of administration that approximates their clinical use, with appropriate indices of therapeutic efficacy and toxicity, and with appropriate patient groups that control for cyclic fluctuations in symptoms. In the interim, clinicians should consider the use of many drug classes for TMD pain as unvalidated clinical practices and limit treatment to short trials subject to some evidence of clinical efficacy and careful attention to potential adverse events.

The decision to use traditional NSAIDs or one of the newer selective COX-2 inhibitors is first predicated on whether any NSAID is appropriate therapy. In a patient with a high risk for gastropathy, a COX-2–selective NSAID may provide a useful alternative to combination therapy with a gastric-protective drug and a nonselective NSAID. When treating inflammation associated with a TMD, the nonselective NSAIDs and selective COX-2 inhibitors should be considered based on their proven efficacy in the oral surgery model and for both RA and OA. A short trial of celecoxib may be considered for patients with TMJ synovitis, capsulitis, or an acute flare of TMJ osteoarthritis. Whether a nonselective NSAID or a COX-2–selective inhibitor is prescribed, close monitoring is important to ensure patient safety. Although cardiovascular risks have been reported to be associated with the use of COX-2–selective inhibitors, this occurred with long-term use, and it has not been shown that short-term use causes similar problems.

Pain that is primarily of musculoskeletal origin is best managed by physical medicine procedures (see chapter 24), possibly along with a short trial of a muscle relaxant or benzodiazepine. As with many other chronic pain conditions, low doses (10 to 75 mg a day) of tricyclic antidepressants may be considered for individuals with persistent musculoskeletal pain. This is particularly helpful for those individuals who are mildly depressed or have sleep disturbances.

The use of antidepressant and anticonvulsant medications has been reported to provide effective treatments for many orofacial pain disorders, including various neuropathies (diabetic and trigeminal), muscle disorders (myofascial pain and fibromyalgia), and related pain disorders (eg, migraine headache). Additionally, the use of NMDA receptor antagonists may provide a new line of pharmacotherapy or adjuvant therapy for patients with chronic TMD pain. Although most of these drug classes are routinely used in the treatment of neuropathic disorders, their use in the treatment of TMD pain has not been systematically evaluated, nor is there any evidence for their use in the treatment of early-onset TMD pain.

The decision to treat patients with complex neuropathic pain depends on the clinician's knowledge, training, experience, and comfort with diagnosing and managing these patients; alternatively, the patient could be referred to a dentist with advanced training in orofacial pain management or a neurologist. In either case, it is important to recognize signs and symptoms that require immediate evaluation and referral. These may include presentation of new, unusual, systemic, and unresolving or worsening symptoms. Additionally, the clinician must consider that many of the medications (for example, carbamazepine) require careful management and monitoring through the course of treatment. The choice of medications is based on presenting symptoms, the patient's history, the presence of certain systemic conditions, and general logistical considerations. These are merely guidelines, because each patient's treatment response may vary and the clinical presentation of TMD pain must be assessed individually.

For patients in whom other therapeutic modalities have failed or for whom a specific treatment is not readily apparent, such as patients with failed TMJ implants or multiple surgeries, a trial with an opioid should be considered. Although concerns about the patient's potential development of tolerance and dependence must be considered, opioids may represent a more favorable therapeutic choice than further surgery that increases the risk of iatrogenic injury or experimentation with unvalidated or irrational clinical practices.

References

1. List T, Axelsson S, Leijon G. Pharmacological interventions in the treatment of temporomandibular disorders, atypical facial pain, and burning mouth syndrome. A qualitative systematic review. J Orofac Pain 2003;17:301–310.

2. Ta LT, Phero JC, Pillemer SR, et al. Clinical evaluation of patients with temporomandibular joint implants. J Oral Maxillofac Surg 2002;60:1389–1399.

3. Magnusson T, Egermark-Eriksson I, Caarlson GE. Five-year longitudinal study of signs and symptoms of mandibular dysfunction in adolescents. Cranio 1986;4:338–344.

4. Speculand B, Goss AN, Hughes AO, Spence ND, Pilowsky I. Temporo-mandibular joint dysfunction: Pain and illness behaviour. Pain 1983;17:139–150.

5. Singer EJ, Dionne RA. A controlled evaluation of diazepam and ibuprofen for chronic orofacial muscle pain. J Orofac Pain 1997;11:139–147.

6. Gordon SM, Montgomery MT, Jones D. Comparative efficacy of piroxicam versus placebo for temporomandibular pain [abstract 876]. J Dent Res 1990;69(special issue):218.

7. Ta LE, Dionne RA. Treatment of painful temporomandibular joints with a cyclooxygenase-2 inhibitor: A randomized placebo-controlled comparison of celecoxib to naproxen. Pain 2004;111:13–21.

8. Walker JS, Lockton AI, Nguyen TV, et al. Analgesic effect of ibuprofen after single and multiple doses in chronic spinal pain patients. Analgesia 1996;2:93–101.

9. Walker JS, Levy G. Effect of multiple dosing on the analgesic actions of diflunisal in rats. Life Sci 1990;46:737–742.

10. Henry D, Drew A, Beuzeville S. Adverse drug reactions in the gastrointestinal system attributed to ibuprofen. In: Rainsford KD, Powanda MC (eds). Safety and Efficacy of Non-prescription (OTC) Analgesics and NSAIDs. London: Kluwer Academic, 1998:19–45.

11. Breder CD, Dewitt D, Kraig RP. Characterization of inducible cyclooxygenase in rat brain. J Comp Neurol 1995;355:296–315.

12. Cheng HF, Wang JL, Zhang MZ, et al. Angiotensin II attenuates renal cortical cyclooxygenase-2 expression. J Clin Invest 1999;103:953–61.

13. Leon CG, Marchetti J, Vio CP. Renal cyclooxygenase-2: Evidence for recruitment of thick ascending limb of henle cells in microdissected nephron segments. Hypertension 2001;38:630–634.

14. Lim H, Gupta RA, Ma WG, et al. Cyclo-oxygenase-2-derived prostacyclin mediates embryo implantation in the mouse via PPARdelta. Genes Dev 1999;13:1561–1574.

15. Houchen CW, Stenson WF, Cohn SM. Disruption of cyclooxygenase-1gene results in an impaired response to radiation injury. Am J Physiol Gastrointest Liver Physiol 2000;279:G858–G865.

16. Hawkey C, Laine L, Simon T, et al. Comparison of the effect of rofecoxib (a cyclooxygenase 2 inhibitor), ibuprofen, and placebo on the gastroduodenal mucosa of patients with osteoarthritis: A randomized, double-blind, placebo-controlled trial. The Rofecoxib Osteoarthritis Endoscopy Multinational Study Group. Arthritis Rheum 2000;43:370–377.

17. Schmassmann A. Mechanisms of ulcer healing and effects of nonsteroidal anti-inflammatory drugs. Am J Med 1998;104:43S–51S; discussion 79S–80S.

18. Reid KI, Dionne RA, Sicard-Rosenbaum L, Lord D, Dubner R. Evaluation of iontophoretically applied dexamethasone for painful pathologic temporomandibular joints. Oral Surg Oral Med Oral Pathol 1994;77:605–609.

19. Harkins S, Linford J, Cohen J, Kramer T, Cueva L. Administration of clonazepam in the treatment of TMD and associated myofascial pain: A double-blind pilot study. J Craniomandib Disord 1991;5:179–186.

20. Russell IJ, Fletcher EM, Michalek JE, McBroom PC, Hester GG. Treatment of primary fibrositis/fibromyalgia syndrome with ibuprofen and alprazolam. Arthritis Rheum 1991;34:552–560.

21. Dellemijn PLI, Fields HL. Do benzodiazepines have a role in chronic pain management? Pain 1994;57:137–152.

22. Elenbaas JK. Centrally acting oral skeletal muscle relaxants. Am J Hosp Pharm 1980;37:1313–1323.

23. Brown BR, Womble J. Cyclobenzaprine in intractable pain syndromes with muscle spasm. JAMA 1978;240:1151–1152.

24. Magni G. The use of antidepressants in the treatment of chronic pain: A review of the current evidence. Drugs 1991;42:730–748.

25. Onhenga P, Van Houdenhove B. Antidepressant-induced analgesia in chronic non-malignant pain: A meta-analysis of 39 placebo-controlled studies. Pain 1992;49:205–220.

26. Max MB, Gilron IH. Antidepressants, muscle relaxants, and N-methyl-D-aspartate recpetor antagonists. In: Loeser JD, Butler SH, Chapman CR, Turk DC (eds). Bonica's Management of Pain. Philadelphia: Lippincott, 2001:1710–1726.

27. Max MB, Culnane M, Schafer SC, et al. Amitriptyline relieves diabetic neuropathy pain in patients with normal or depressed mood. Neurology 1987;37:589–596.

28. Sharav Y, Singer E, Schmidt E, Dionne RA, Dubner R. The analgesic effect of amitriptyline on chronic facial pain. Pain 1987;31:199–209.

29. McQuay HJ, Carroll D, Glynn CJ. Low dose amitriptyline in the treatment of chronic pain. Anesthesia 1992;47:646–652.

30. McQuay HJ, Carroll D, Glynn CJ. Dose-response for analgesic effects of amitriptyline in chronic pain. Anesthesia 1993;48:281–285.

31. Zitman FG, Linssen ACG, Edelbrook PM, Stijnen T. Low dose amitriptyline in chronic pain: The gain is modest. Pain 1990;42:35–42.

32. Backonja M, Beydoun A, Edwards KR, et al. Gabapentin for the symptomatic treatment of painful neuropathy in patients with diabetes mellitus: A randomized controlled trial. JAMA 1998;280:1831–1836.

33. Rowbotham M, Harden N, Stacey B, et al. Gabapentin for the treatment of neuropathic neuralgia: A randomized controlled trial. JAMA 1998;280:1837–1842.

34. Solaro C, Lunardi GL, Capello E, et al. An open-label trial of gabapentin treatment of paroxysmal symptoms in multiple sclerosis patients. Neurology 1998;51:609–611.

35. Khan OA. Gabapentin relieves trigeminal neuralgia in multiple sclerosis patients. Neurology 1998;51:611–614.

36. Eckhardt K, Hufschmidt A, Feuerstein TJ. Treatment of chronic and neuropathic pain. MMW Fortschr Med 2000;142:29–30.

37. Nelson KA, Park KM, Robinovitz E, et al. High-dose oral dextromethorphan versus placebo in painful diabetic neuropathy and postherpetic neuralgia. Neurology 1997;48:1212–1218.

38. Backonja M, Arndt G, Gombar KA, et al. Response of chronic neuropathic pain syndromes to ketamine: A preliminary study. Pain 1994;56:51–57.

39. Felsby S, Nielsen J, Arendt-Nielsen L, et al. NMDA receptor blockade in chronic neuropathic pain: A comparison of ketamine and magnesium chloride. Pain 1996;64:283–291.

40. McQuay HJ, Carroll D, Jadad AR, et al. Dextromethorphan for the treatment of neuropathic pain: A double-blind randomised controlled crossover trial with integral n-of-1 design. Pain 1994;59:127–133.

CHAPTER 24

Physical Medicine

Jocelyne S. Feine and J. Mark Thomason

Chronic pain is resistant to many types of treatment and clinicians know that, unless the etiology can be confirmed and reversed by specific treatments, palliative and reversible therapies are more appropriate. Based on the notion that physical therapies and modalities could potentially provide relief to patients with chronic pain, clinicians have been recommending these types of procedures to patients with chronic temporomandibular disorder (TMD) pain. However, a previous review[1] revealed the lack of well-conducted, long-term studies on which to base solid conclusions about the value of these types of treatment. This chapter discusses these data and additional information obtained from more recent publications, as well as data from related studies in other parts of the body.

Physical therapies are widely used for the treatment of painful TMDs.[2,3] It is generally believed that these therapies are effective in reducing pain and other symptoms associated with these conditions. Empirically, it is known that most patients who undertake these procedures will report improvement in both their signs and symptoms, and many of these therapies are widely used to treat musculoskeletal conditions elsewhere in the body. However, of the many publications discussing these conditions, relatively few fulfill the criteria outlined for well-conducted clinical trials.[4] By the 1990s, many authors had commented on the poor methodologic quality of these studies.[5–12] Reviewing reports on biofeedback for the treatment of TMDs, Crider and Glaros[13] concluded that most trials had been undertaken with sample sizes of fewer than 20 subjects. They suggested that, although there is cumulative evidence of effectiveness when biofeedback was compared to controls, there remains a need for large-sample, controlled-outcome trials.

Other authors have noted that most studies have compared different forms of treatment[6,7] and that many treatment regimens included several forms of intervention. Disentangling the effects of the various phases of the intervention is difficult, which makes interpretations of the results open to question. As a result the validity of the claims of treatment efficacy remains unsettled.

In a review of the efficacy of physical therapies for painful TMDs, some authors have suggested that the use of such therapies is reasonable because they have been effective for other pain conditions.[7] Dahlström[14] highlighted the well-accepted observation that large numbers of patients with TMD pain have been treated conservatively with apparent success, although she concluded that no particular conservative treatment method is more effective than another.

These observations are supported by a meta-analysis of physical medicine treatments for other forms of chronic pain.[10] Although the researchers set low criteria for inclusion, only 109 studies published between 1950 and 1984 were of sufficient quality to be included. The authors looked at size of effect, percentage of improvement, type of pain, and type of outcome measure. They suggested that, despite the differences in the type of conditions, the measures used, and the patient's characteristics, the efficacy of the various treatments was uniform. The authors proposed that it is the similarities between these types of treatment rather than the differences that lead to similar outcomes. These shared characteristics include "the psychological factors that exaggerate pain, contact with an empathetic professional, and provision of hope for relief from symptoms."[10]

To evaluate specific treatment modalities and, where necessary, expand the field from problems of the temporomandibular region to musculoskeletal disorders in other parts of the body, a Medline search of the literature from 1997 to 2004 was carried out using the following terms: *myofascial pain syndromes* (n = 3,759) and *temporomandibular joint disorders* (n = 8,772). This basic data pool was then refined using a range of *physical therapies* (n = 99,463), *controlled or placebo or blind or randomized trial* (n = 469,754).

Table 24-1		Ultrasound and thermal therapies*			
Review	**Condition**	**Treatment**	**Meta-analysis**	**Summary**	
Clark et al[7]	TMD pain and other conditions of joint and muscle	Multiple therapies	No	Little research on TMDs. No evidence of efficacy for slowing progress of degenerative changes. All treatments seem to be effective in reducing pain.	
Chapman[6]	Musculoskeletal disorders	Thermal agents, ultrasound, short-wave diathermy, low-power laser	No	No evidence to support the use of cold, superficial heat, or ultrasound for long-term pain control. Cold and short-wave diathermy have short-term analgesic effects.	
Dahlström[14]	TMDs	Exercise, short-wave diathermy, ultrasound, thermal agents	No	No particular conservative treatment method appears superior to any other.	
Crider and Glaros[13]	TMDs	EMG, biofeedback	Yes	Majority of studies used sample sizes of fewer than 20 per condition. Studies of larger samples designed to estimate specific effects by direct within-study comparison needed.	

*EMG = electromyography.

Additional searches were carried out using several subcategories, including *fibromyalgia*, *back pain*, *headache*, and *spine*. Clinical trials and reviews of clinical trials written in French or English were accepted for inclusion. Studies that met few of the criteria of methodologic quality were eliminated.[4,15] Additional references cited in selected articles were used, including those in the article by Feine and Lund.[1] The findings are discussed in the following sections.

Ultrasound and Thermal Therapies

Ultrasound is often used in conjunction with stretching and other exercise therapies to treat chronic pain caused by TMDs.[16] However, it was not possible to find any publications on randomized clinical trials that have compared ultrasound to no treatment or placebo in patients with TMD pain. In the few studies comparing ultrasound singly or in combination with other modalities against placebo for the treatment of other chronic pain conditions, ultrasound was not found to be significantly more effective.[17–21] There were problems with the methodology or outcomes chosen in most of these studies. Nevertheless, in one well-designed study, no improvement was reported, either immediately or 2 months after ultrasound therapy, in subjects with knee joints that were painful as a result of osteoarthritis.[22]

One study tested the effect of ultrasound combined with massage and exercise against that of a placebo control therapy on myofascial trigger points in the neck and shoulder.[23] The numbers involved in the study suggested that it may have had sufficient statistical power, but this was not clarified by the authors, and there was no indication as to how the subjects were randomized. Although no differences were found between the study groups (ultrasound combined with massage and exercise versus sham ultrasound plus massage and exercise), both demonstrated a significant reduction in the number of myofascial trigger points. There was, however, no difference between the groups in pain at rest or on daily function, analgesic usage, or treatment satisfaction. Based on these results, the authors suggested that massage and exercise can reduce the number and intensity of myofascial trigger points but that ultrasound is not effective for that purpose.[23]

Application of heat or cold is often prescribed, but data on the effectiveness of these therapies are also limited. No studies that tested these thermal modalities in subjects with TMD pain were found. However, the effectiveness of local applications of cold and heat has been examined in conjunction with an exercise program to alleviate acute postsurgical knee pain.[24] The application of cold and exercise provided greater relief than heat and exercise or exercise alone. Swelling was also significantly reduced in the group that applied cold locally. These observations support the premise that cold can provide short-term relief and reduce inflammation.[6] However, in a small study, Williams et al[25] reported equal effectiveness between cold and exercise versus heat and exercise in patients with painful rheumatoid arthritis in the shoulder.

A summary of literature reviews of studies on ultrasound and thermal therapies is provided in Table 24-1.

Acupuncture

Acupuncture is believed to reduce pain by stimulating the release of endogenous opiates (endorphins). However, there is limited evidence for the effectiveness of acupuncture in patients with chronic musculoskeletal pain. Pain and drug intake were reduced to a greater degree in subjects with tension headaches receiving physiotherapy than in those receiving acupuncture, although no between-group comparisons were undertaken.[26]

In a study comparing acupuncture treatment for osteoarthritis of the knee to a nontreatment control, pain intensity was significantly reduced in the treatment group.[27] Assessment was undertaken over a 9-week period, and the authors reported that function was also improved. However, a similar study that included a sham control reported no between-group differences, although there were significant within-group improvements.[28] In a smaller study comparing acupuncture and diazepam in a placebo-controlled trial, the authors reported that all groups (including the group receiving the placebo) experienced significant reduction in pain "unpleasantness" between the pretreatment assessment and one made 2 hours later.[29]

In a randomized study of electroacupuncture versus sham acupuncture in patients with fibromyalgia, reductions in pain and stiffness and perceived general state were better in the treatment group.[30] However, the ratio of men to women was different in the two groups. Conflicting views emerge from two earlier meta-analyses of the use of acupuncture for the treatment of fibromyalgia.[31,32]

The effects of superficial and deep acupuncture have also been compared.[33] Forty-two subjects were randomly assigned to two groups for either superficial or deep acupuncture for the treatment of lumbar myofascial pain. At the end of treatment, there were no significant differences between groups. Surprisingly, the authors state in the opening of the discussion that "the power analysis conducted to evaluate the size of the sample showed 21 patients do not produce enough power." Nevertheless, both groups showed within-group improvements. At the 3-month follow-up, the patients who received deep stimulation had significantly better results than did those who received superficial acupuncture. Two of the same authors have reported broadly similar results in a comparable study involving myofascial pain in the shoulder, where again a significant posttreatment difference between groups was found.[34]

In a study of specific and nonspecific effects of acupuncture and heat on chronic myofascial neck pain, 46 patients were randomly assigned to one of three groups.[35] These were a relevant acupuncture group, an irrelevant acupuncture group (inappropriate acupuncture points), and a nonacupuncture control group receiving nonsteroidal anti-inflammatory drugs (NSAIDs). The relevant acupuncture group reported having had more previous acupuncture treatments, and after treatment they had significantly greater pretreatment-posttreatment pain differences than did the other two groups. The authors were unable to control for the previous acupuncture experience, because the subgroup size was small (and initial power was not stated). The authors also pointed out that both acupuncture groups were seen more often than the control group, which introduced a further problem for interpretation of the results.[1]

Limitations of statistical power again make interpretation difficult when placement of acupunture in classically recognized acupuncture points is compared with sham acupuncture (areas not recognized as acupuncture points) in patients with myofascial pain in the jaw muscles.[36] This study compared two groups of patients, with a total of 18 subjects, but the authors gave no indication as to the statistical power of the study. Both groups showed reductions in pain scores, but there were no significant between-group differences. Therefore the authors' conclusion that "pain reduction resulting from noxious stimulus (ie, needling) may not be specific to the location of the stimulus," is not well supported by their study results. Indeed, the lack of a difference may be real, but it may also simply reflect a lack of power in the study.

In addition to acupuncture needling, there is also a needling technique recommended for the treatment of myofascial trigger points. In reviewing the evidence for or against the efficacy of both wet (injecting substances) and dry needling therapies as an approach to myofascial trigger-point pain, Cummings and White[37] looked at a total of 23 articles. They suggested that "no trials were of sufficient quality or design to test the efficacy of any needling techniques beyond placebo in the treatment of myofascial pain." The nature of the injected substance made no difference in the outcome, and wet needling was not found to be superior to dry needling. They concluded by stressing the need for controlled trials to investigate whether such needling has an effect on myofascial trigger-point pain beyond that of placebo.

Comparing two groups of subjects with TMD pain treated with bite appliances or acupuncture, List and Helkimo[38] reported that the acupuncture group experienced greater relief than appliance wearers or controls, although direct between-group comparisons were not

Table 24-2	Acupuncture*		
Study	**Treatment groups**	**Site**	**Duration of treatment**
Raustia et al[40]; Raustia and Prohjola[41]	1: Acupuncture (n = 25) 2: Standard stomatognathic treatment (n = 25) 1 and 2: Occlusal appliances, and/or exercise, and/or counseling, and/or occlusal adjustment		1: 20-min sessions; 3 sessions over 1 mo
Johansson et al[39]	1: Acupuncture (n = 15) 2: Occlusal appliance (n = 15) 3: Nontreatment control (n = 15)	1: In painful sites and in classic sites	1: 30-min sessions; 6 sessions over an unspecified period
List et al[43]	1: Acupuncture, manual and electrical (n = 40) 2: Occlusal appliance (n = 34) 3: Nontreatment control (n = 22)	1: According to Haker and Lundeberg[47]	1: 30-min sessions; 1 session/wk over 6–8 wk 2: Appliances worn at night until evaluation at 6–8 wk
List and Helkimo[38] (follow-up to List et al[43])	1: Acupuncture (n = 22) 2: Occlusal appliance (n = 25) 3: Acupuncture and occlusal appliances (n = 5) 4: Additional treatments: physical therapy, occlusal adjustments, repositioning appliances, counseling (n = 20)	1: According to Haker and Lundeberg[47]	1: 30-min sessions; 1 session/wk over 6–8 wk 2: Appliances worn at night until evaluation at 6–8 wk
Goddard et al[36]	1: Acupuncture (n = 10) 2: Sham acupuncture (n = 8)	1: Right and left Hoku points, right and left stomach points 2: Sham points, right and left hand and 1 cm dorsal to stomach points	30 min

*ADL = Activities of daily living; VAS = visual analog scale.
†A = treatment compared to no treatment; D = more than one treatment group, unequal exposure to therapy.

made. The three groups differed in age and gender distribution, as well as the duration of the condition, and the acupuncture group was observed at more frequent intervals. After 1 year, the effect in the acupuncture group had decreased, while the improvement in the appliance group had increased. An earlier blind, randomized clinical trial examining the same treatment modalities failed to demonstrate differences between the treatment groups.[39] Similar findings were also reported earlier.[40,41]

In an attempt to identify practical recommendations for the use of acupuncture in the treatment of TMD pain, Rosted[42] reviewed the literature on the use of acupuncture for the treatment of such conditions. Initially he identified 14 articles that discussed acupuncture and

TMDs. Only six articles referred to blind randomized studies.[38–41,43,44] In all, three separate studies were reported in these six articles. Each of the studies used occlusal bite appliances as a control. List and Helkimo[38] used precise acupuncture points; however, this procedural aspect was less clear in the other articles. When contacted, the authors confirmed that logical points were selected as they were each in the same segment.

All of the articles gave clear information on the distant points used, including LI-4 (Hoku point). Subjects were seen between three and eight times for 20 to 30 minutes per visit. All the studies reported similar outcomes for acupuncture and appliance therapy. After review, Rosted[42] concluded that in all three of these randomized controlled studies,

Outcome variables	Posttreatment assessment	Results	Comments[†]
Pain, function, clinical signs (Helkimo dysfunction index)	1 and 3 mo	Both treatments reduced pain on function, but neither shown to be superior to other at 3 mo.	
Pain, perceived improvement, clinical signs (Helkimo dysfunction index)	1 and 2: At 3 mo 3: At 2 mo	1 and 2 significantly more improved than 3. In 1 and 2, pain decreased significantly and clinical dysfunction scores were lower than in 3. No differences between 1 and 2.	Test-retest interval longer for 1 and 2 than for 3. A, D
Pain, drug use, clinical signs (Helkimo dysfunction index), function (ADL), perceived improvement	At 6–8 wk	1 and 2 had significantly greater decrease in pain than 3. 1 had significantly greater improvement than other groups in ADL scores and in perceived improvement. No changes in drug use.	Groups significantly different for gender, age, and pain duration. A, D
Pain, drug use, clinical signs (Helkimo dysfunction index), function (ADL), perceived improvement	6 mo and 1 y	1 and 2 showed significant reduction in all variables at 1 y.	1 and 2 composed of subjects who had improved during treatment. 3 composed of nonresponders to appliance or acupuncture. 4 composed of nonresponders to appliance and acupuncture.
VAS of pain evoked to maximum tolerance; same force used posttreatment and VAS recorded again	Immediately after treatment	Both groups showed reduction in posttreatment pain scores.	Authors suggest that pain reduction from the needling may not be specific to the site at which undertaken; equally may reflect placebo effect and lack of power.

acupuncture proved to be effective. However, an article published 2 years earlier by Ernst and White[45] discussed the same six articles referring to the same three studies, but the interpretation of the results[45] differed considerably from that of Rosted.[42] Among other things, Ernst and White commented that the hypothesis that acupuncture is effective for TMD pain requires confirmation through more rigorous investigations, because none of the reviewed studies used blinded evaluators, and details of randomization procedures were not provided. In addition, because none of the studies was designed to control for a placebo effect, they concluded by questioning why trials with sham acupuncture controls have not been performed when, ethically, they are more justifiable than studies with nontreatment controls.[45]

The final report of the 1998 National Institutes of Health Consensus Development Conference on Acupuncture[46] stated that, although many studies have shown the potential usefulness of this modality, the results of the studies have often been equivocal. It was suggested that this was largely due to flawed study design and inadequate sample size. The report also emphasized that relatively few high-quality randomized controlled trials on the effects of acupuncture had been published and that future studies should be designed in a rigorous manner to allow evaluation of these effects.

The conference participants recognized that acupuncture has been used by millions of American patients and that promising results had emerged in the control of nau-

Table 24-3	Low-level laser therapy (LLLT)		
Study	**Treatment groups**	**Duration of treatment**	**Dose**
Bertolucci and Grey[54]	1: Low-intensity laser (n = 16) 2: Placebo (n = 16)	3 wk	1: 904 nm, 700 Hz, 27 W for 9 min; 3 times/wk for 3 wk 2: Sham laser
Conti[56]	1: Low-level laser therapy 2: Placebo n = 20 randomized to two groups, which were then divided	3 wk	830, 100 mW for 40 s versus no power for 40 s Once/wk for 3 wk
Kulekcioglu[57]	1: Daily exercise program and LLLT (n = 20) 2: Daily exercise program and sham LLLT (n = 15)	15 sessions	1: 904 nm, 1000Hz for 180 s 2: Not turned on for sham group

sea and vomiting as well as in the control of postoperative dental pain. In addition, the report commented on the potential value of acupuncture as an adjunctive or alternative therapy for other situations such as tennis elbow, osteoarthritis, low back pain, and myofascial pain.

However, the report emphasized that one major research complication lies in the inherent difficulty of providing appropriate controls, such as placebo or sham acupuncture groups. The vast majority of the acupuncture literature is composed of case reports, case series, or intervention studies with inadequate design. Sham acupuncture is the most widely used control, but contention about correct needle placement remains. Furthermore, placement of a needle in any position elicits a biologic response that may complicate interpretation, especially in studies investigating pain.

In addition, for all therapeutic interventions, nonspecific effects may account for a substantial proportion of the overall effectiveness. These effects may include the quality of the relationship between the clinician and the patient as well as a range of other factors. The conference document stressed that these confounding factors should not be "casually discounted."[46]

A summary of selected studies on acupuncture is provided in Table 24-2.

Low-Level Laser Therapy

In a meta-analysis of the literature from 1966 to 1990, Beckerman and colleagues[48] concluded that the efficacy of laser therapy for treating musculoskeletal pain seemed to be greater than that of placebo treatment. However, this conclusion was not supported by a similar review the following year.[49] In contrast, an earlier review suggested that it was not possible to draw conclusions because of the difference in the dosage and lasers used in the trials, as well as the outcomes, which differed widely.[50]

A well-designed, placebo-controlled trial studying the use of low-level laser therapy in cervical myofascial pain reported positive findings at both the 1- and 3-month reviews.[51] In contrast, Bulow et al[52] showed no between-group differences in knee pain between a low-power laser group and a placebo group over a 10-week treatment period. Moreover, in a crossover study of subjects with rheumatoid arthritis of the hand, pain was found to decrease in both the treatment and placebo arms of the study.[53] A reduction in pain and tenderness associated with degenerative disease of the TMJ has been reported.[54] However, the nature of the randomization procedure for this study is questionable, because the authors also presented the same data as part of a three-group randomized study.[55]

Unfortunately, a later study evaluating use of low-level laser therapy for TMD pain, using a more robust double-blind design, failed to give any indication of sample size estimation.[56] In addition, because the 20 patients were divided into four groups, the statistical power of this study is in question. Although the myogenous group reported alleviation of pain with treatment, no between-group analysis was undertaken, and the author was candid in concluding that further studies with greater statistical power are needed to elucidate the results.

More recently, in a study of 35 subjects,[57] all received a standard exercise program. Twenty were randomly

Outcomes variables	Posttreatment assessment	Results	Comments
Functional range of motion, deviations, pain	Throughout period of treatment	Significantly greater improvement with laser greater than placebo.	
Pain, function	5 min after each dosing	Improvement in pain in myogenous group. No significant difference between test and control groups.	Power of study?
Pain, joint motion, number of joint sounds, number of tender points	Immediately after and 1 mo after treatment	Significant reduction in pain in both groups. Active and passive mouth opening, lateral motion, and number of tender points only improved in 1.	

assigned to an active group that also received 15 sessions of low-level laser therapy. Fifteen were in the placebo group; they attended a similar number of sessions but the laser was not turned on. Analysis was undertaken by an investigator blinded to the treatment groups. A significant reduction in pain was observed in both groups, but the number of tender points was significantly reduced only in the active group. One month after treatment, significantly more improvement was noted in the active group in all parameters, apart from joint sound and pain intensity. These results offer some support for use of low-level laser therapy in conjunction with exercise therapy.

A summary of selected studies on low-level laser therapy is provided in Table 24-3.

Electrical Stimulation

There are many different stimulus regimens for the use of transcutaneous electrical nerve stimulation (TENS), and patients are often encouraged to experiment to find the one that best suits their condition. TENS treatment falls into two broad categories: conventional TENS and acupuncture-like TENS. Frequencies in the 100-Hz range are often used at low intensity, with the intention of producing pain-free paresthesia. It has been suggested that TENS is most useful in cases of acute and neurologic pain.[58] That review revealed that few studies included a follow-up and there was little evidence to suggest that true TENS was better than placebo, although most articles reported success. Despite being an advocate of TENS, Long,[59] in a 15-year review period, was able to find little

evidence of well-controlled studies that supported its use in patients with chronic musculoskeletal pain.

An improvement in pain scores was reported for all three treatment arms of a placebo-controlled study investigating TENS and anti-inflammatory drugs in patients with osteoarthritis.[60] Interestingly, the improvement was not confined to the active treatment period but began the week before treatment started. Similar results have been reported in TMD pain studies, but in an early study of this modality no significant difference was shown between a TENS group and a placebo group.[61] Similarly, testing an "interferential current" against a placebo produced no between-group differences for pain or maximum opening over a 3- to 9-day period, although both groups showed improvements.[62]

On the other hand, differences between a TENS group and an occlusal bite appliance group were reported by Linde et al[63]; there were significantly fewer subjects with a 50% reduction in their pain scores in the bite appliance group. Perhaps more interesting, however, were the similarities rather than the small differences between the treatments. More positive results of the use of TENS and low-power laser, as reported by Bertolucci and Grey,[54] have been mentioned earlier, but the problems concerning randomization still apply.

In a study comparing TENS with an occlusal bite appliance, 32 patients who exhibited bruxism participated in a randomly allocated crossover study.[64] Eight subjects were lost from the study, leaving 24 subjects. The authors' goal was to evaluate the effects of occlusal bite appliances and TENS on the manifestations of TMDs in patients with bruxism, and then further differentiate between those who grind and those who clench their teeth. Although the

Table 24-4	Therapy using electrical stimulation and pulsed electromagnetic fields*		
Study	Treatment groups	Site	Duration of treatment
Taylor et al[62]	1: TENS (n = 20) 2: Sham (n = 20)	Local	3 sessions, 23–72 h apart
Moystad et al[65]	1: TENS (n = 19) 2: Placebo (n = 19) 3: Acu-TENS (n = 13) 4: Acu-placebo (n = 13)	1 and 2: Local 3 and 4: Hegu points	1 to 4: 2 sessions; 30 min/session, 1 wk apart
Linde et al[63]	1: TENS (n = 16) 2: Occlusal appliance (n = 15)	TMJ	1: 30 min, 3 times/d, over 6 wk 2: Worn 24 h/d over 6 wk
Alvarez-Arenal et al[64]	1: TENS (n = 24) 2: Occlusal appliance (n = 24)	TMJ	TENS for 45–60 min for 15 sessions Appliance for 45 days
Al-Badawi et al[66]	1: PRFE (n = 20) 2: Sham PRFE (n = 20)	TMJ	6 applications over 2 wk

*TENS = transcutaneous electrical nerve stimulation; Acu-TENS = acupuncture-like transcutaneous electrical nerve stimulation; PRFE = pulsed radio frequency energy.

crossover design can be powerful, the authors did not include a calculation of statistical power. Hence, the study's power can be called into question based on the loss of subjects from the study, the division of such a small number of participants into subgroups, and the fact that some individuals who exhibit bruxism do not have a TMD.

Fifteen subjects presented with a TMD before treatment, but this rose to 19 after treatment. The study results suggested an association between bruxism and certain TMDs, because more than 60% of those who exhibited bruxism had a TMD. However, occlusal bite appliance therapy and TENS failed to reduce the signs or symptoms of TMD in these patients. It is difficult to extrapolate any other outcome from this study, but because the population with TMD symptoms was only 60% of a final population of 24, this is not surprising.

A summary of selected studies on therapies using electrical stimulation is provided in Table 24-4.

Pulsed Electromagnetic Fields

The use of pulsed electromagnetic fields (PEMFs) has been advocated as a noninvasive treatment for painful joints.[67–69]

Clinical studies have focused on delayed union in fractures[67,68] and osteoarthritis.[69] In a small randomized trial (n = 18) Smania et al[70] evaluated short- and medium-term effects of repetitive magnetic stimulation on myofascial pain. The treatment group showed a significant reduction in pain and in the disability related to pain, which was not observed in the placebo group. The resultant difference between groups was found to be significant.

Peroz and colleagues[71] undertook a multicenter, double-blind, placebo-controlled study to investigate the effect of PEMFs in patients with TMD pain. To effectively blind both the operator and the patients, active and placebo PEMF units were constructed. The groups differed only in that the placebo unit did not produce pulsed electromagnetic fields. Seventy-eight patients were randomized into two groups that underwent nine 1-hour sessions on consecutive days.

Most patients from both groups reported reduction in pain intensity and frequency and other assessment parameters.[71] Comparisons between groups were not significantly different for any of the parameters. The authors therefore concluded that PEMFs do not provide specific treatment effects for patients with TMD pain. However, although 78 patients entered the study and 99% completed it, there was no indication in the article as to the power of the study.

Dose	Outcomes variables	Posttreatment assessment	Results	Comments
1: 1–7 mA; 15 min, 90–100 Hz; 5 min 45–90 Hz	Pain, function	At 9 d	No significant between-group differences.	
1: 100 Hz, 0.15 ms, "sensation" 2: 2 Hz, 0.2 ms, "muscle contraction"s	Pain severity, tenderness	On treatment day	Significant treatment effects with all methods. Acu-TENS greater than placebo for pain during function (not specified).	No data shown. Crossover trial.
1: 90 Hz less than pain threshold 2: Worn 24 h/d	Pain, function, clinical signs	At 6 wk	Decrease in all scores over time. Pain less in 2. No significant between-group differences in other outcomes.	
0–25 mA	Pantographic reproducibility index	After each treatment	Neither occlusal appliance nor TENS significantly improved signs and symptoms of TMD in patients with bruxism.	Crossover design.
90-s exposure per visit	Pain, jaw function	Before and after each application, 1 wk and 2 wk	There was improvement in both groups.	No between-group comparison.

A recent study examined the efficacy of pulsed radiofrequency energy (PRFE) therapy in patients with TMD pain and dysfunction (see Table 24-4).[66] Forty subjects were randomly assigned to either the active treatment or the placebo group. The delivery machines were identical except that the one used for the sham therapy did not emit radiowaves. Treatment was delivered every other day for a total of six visits. Assessment was undertaken by a researcher who was blind to group assignment. Unfortunately, although both groups exhibited a significant improvement in mouth opening and lateral exclusion, there was no indication of the statistical power of the study for between-group differences.

Mixed Therapies

A number of authors have attempted to compare multiple and combination therapies, despite the added difficulties that this poses in terms of study design and required population size. In an attempt to compare the effects of acupuncture, steroid injections, and physiotherapy, Berry et al[72] developed a five-arm study including placebo physiotherapy and placebo injections, all of which were applied to a study population of 60 patients with shoulder rotator-cuff lesions over a 4-week period. Although no between-group difference was detected, pain intensity decreased significantly in all groups. Similar findings were reported in a study with similar group sizes comparing hot wax plus exercise, ultrasound plus exercise, and ultrasound plus hand baths in patients with rheumatoid arthritis in their hands.[73] In both of these studies, the lack of significant differences may reflect the limited statistical power offered by the small treatment groups, a problem that hinders much of the research in this area.

A series of articles have been published based on a large clinical trial comparing different therapies offered by different practitioners to patients with lower back and neck pain.[74–76] Unfortunately, there was an extremely large difference in the time that the subjects in each group spent with their therapist; in addition, mixed treatments and inappropriate outcome measures were used.[1] Differences between groups were small or insignificant, and the authors concluded that a substantial part of the treatment success represented a placebo effect. Subjects reported that medical practitioners were less effective than the other therapists, but these subjects only had a single visit with the medical practitioner while others spent several hours with the physical therapists. Indeed, patients did better

Table 24-5	Mixed therapies*		
Study	**Treatment groups**	**Duration of treatment**	**Outcome variables**
Talaat et al[79]	1: Pharmacologic 2: Short-wave diathermy 3: Ultrasound (n = 40 per group)	2 wk	Pain, function, joint sounds
Burgess et al[80]	1: Cold (ethyl chloride) + stretching (n = 10) 2: Resistance exercise (n = 11) 3: Nontreatment control (n = 8)	1 and 2: At home daily	Pain (MPQ), function, EMG activity
Nelson and Ash[82]	1: "Conventional TMJ therapy" plus heat 1 time/d (n = 19) 2: "Conventional TMJ therapy" plus heat 2–3 times/d (n = 8)	Heat applied at home, 20 min/d, 2–3 times/d, over 6 wk	Pain and function
McCreary et al[83]	1: Occlusal appliances plus physical therapy (exercise, thermal) and NSAIDs (n = 95) 2: Nontreatment control (n = 73)	Variable; mean 4.8 visits over 8 wk	Pain, psychological tests
Austin and Shupe[87]	1: Physical therapy (thermal, exercise, mobilization) (n = 24) 2: Nontreatment control (n = 26)	2 sessions/wk over 8 wk	Function
Gray et al[84]	1: Short-wave diathermy (n = 27) 2: Pulsed short-wave diathermy (n = 27) 3: Ultrasound (n = 30) 4: Low intensity laser (n = 29) 5: Sham laser (n = 26)	3 sessions/wk over 4 wk	Perceived improvement
Bertolucci and Grey[53]	1: TENS 2: Low-intensity laser 3: Placebo (n = 16 per group)	3 wk	Range of motion, jaw deviation, pain
Dworkin et al[85]	1: Usual treatment group 2: Self-care group	1: Usual treatment by dental specialists 2: One 75-min session, two 50- to 60-min sessions, and one telephone call with dental hygienist	Pain, pain-related activity interference, no. of dental visits, satisfaction with treatment
Carlson et al[86]	1: Physical self-regulation training (n = 22) 2: Standard dental care (n = 22)	50-min sessions at 3-wk intervals	Pain severity, life interference, perception of control, function, opening

*MPQ = McGill Pain Questionnaire; EMG = electromyography; NSAIDs = nonsteroidal anti-inflammatory drugs; TENS = transcutaneous electrical nerve stimulation.

†A = treatment compared to no treatment; B = treatment compared to placebo treatment; C = more than one treatment group, equal exposure to therapy; D = more than one treatment group, unequal exposure to therapy.

with frequent placebo physical therapy than with active treatment from a medical practitioner.

To compare the effects of ultrasound, short wave diathermy, and galvanic current treatment, plus the additional effects of NSAIDs, Svarcova et al[77] assessed their effects in subjects with osteoarthritis of the hip or knee over a 3-week period. Pain was rated with visual analog scales. Relief of symptoms was assessed by both the subject and the clinician at the fifth and last visit. There was no difference in pain reduction between the groups, but NSAIDs were found to be associated with greater pain relief than placebo.

Posttreatment assessment	Results	Comments[†]
At 2 wk, 6 mo, and 12 mo	2 and 3 reported reduced pain.	No statistical tests carried out.
After first treatment and at 3 wk	Pain in 1 and 2 significantly less after first treatment. At 3 wk, 1 significantly less pain than 2 and 3. No differences with other variables.	A, C
At random intervals during a 6-wk period	Pain and function significantly better in 1.	The results suggest no improvement with treatment 2. D
5–6 mo then 1–2 y	No significant between-group differences in function at 16 mo.	2 exhibited significantly more jaw dysfunction pretreatment. A
At 8 wk	1 achieved significantly greater maximal mouth opening.	Very unbalanced groups, nonrandomized. A
At 4 wk and 3 mo	At 4 wk, no significant between-group differences. At 3 mo, 1 to 4 improved significantly more than 5. No differences between other groups.	B, C
Throughout period of treatment	Changes with TENS and laser greater than changes with placebo.	Same data as Bertolucci and Grey.[54] How could some patients be randomized into three groups here but into two groups in other study?
Up to 12 mo posttreatment	Self-care group had lower levels of pain compared with treatment group at 12 mo, as well as fewer visits for TMD and higher levels of satisfaction.	
At 26-wk follow-up	Pain and life interference reduced in both groups at 6 wk. Greater improvement at 26 wk in 1.	

In a study comparing muscle training and more conventional physical therapies against a placebo control for the treatment of low back pain, researchers observed significant pain reduction in all groups during the pretreatment baseline period.[78] However, in the posttreatment assessment period (1, 6, and 12 months), the two treatment groups experienced significantly more pain relief than did the control group; no difference between the treatment groups was detected.

Reduction in pain and tenderness in TMD subjects over a 2-week period was reported with both ultrasonic therapy and short-wave diathermy, but not with pharmaceuticals. However, this result was not tested statistically.[79] Cold therapy plus stretching to passive resistance was also tested

Table 24-6	Jaw manipulation and exercise*		
Study	**Condition**	**Treatment groups**	**Duration of treatment**
Tegelberg and Kopp[97]	TMD, subdivided into RA and AS	1: Exercise: range of motion with and without resistance (n = 28) 2: Nontreatment control (n = 32)	Twice/d over 3 wk
Wright et al[101]	TMD	1: Posture training and TMD self-management instructions (n = 30) 2: TMD self-management instructions only (n = 30)	4 wk

*RA = rheumatoid arthritis; AS = ankylosing spondylitis.
†A = treatment compared to no treatment.

against nontreatment in subjects with myofascial pain and dysfunction.[80] Pain, measured with the McGill Pain Questionnaire, was significantly reduced in both groups. In a retrospective study, Braun[81] reported more postoperative pain in those who had only TMJ surgery compared to those who had surgery followed by an average of seven physical therapy sessions. However, mouth opening was the same in both groups at 6 and 12 months.

In a nonrandomized trial of patients with TMD-related myofascial pain, Nelson and Ash[82] concluded that the addition of moist heat therapy to occlusal bite appliance therapy improved the efficacy of the latter, despite the data showing that the group wearing the appliance showed little improvement over the 6-week study period.

Comparing a group with combined bite appliance and physical therapy with a group who refused treatment, McCreary et al[83] reported a significant difference between the groups at 16 months. However, some caution must be exercised in the interpretation of these results because this was not a randomized clinical trial and the baseline values for the two groups were significantly different. In another study, no differences were reported between groups in the ratio of improved to not improved patients at the end of 4 weeks of treatment or at the 3-month recall after the use of two forms of short-wave diathermy, ultrasound, or mixed placebos.[84]

Dworkin et al[85] compared the usual conservative treatment of TMD pain by specialists to a structured self-care intervention delivered by a dental hygienist. Subjects for the study were targeted using the Axis II assessments from the Research Diagnostic Criteria for Temporomandibular Disorders (see chapter 13) in order to recruit those who exhibited

minimal TMD-related psychosocial interference. The "usual treatment group" (UTG) was treated by six attending dentists who used their normal range of treatments for each patient's presenting conditions. These included (1) physiotherapy, consisting of passive and active jaw movement, stretching, and the application of hot and cold packs; (2) patient education concerning parafunctional oral behavior and diet; (3) medication that included muscle relaxants and analgesics; and (4) an intraoral flat plane occlusal bite appliance. There were no limitations to the number of visits or additional treatments that could be provided.

The "self-care group" (SCG) received a manual-based, individual three-session intervention emphasizing education and self-care for TMD pain and incorporating cognitive-behavioral methods. This was delivered by one of two dental hygienists in one 75-minute session, two 50- to 60-minute sessions, and during a 10-minute telephone contact. The manual-based program included education about the biopsychosocial model of TMD, chronic pain and self-management, guided reading with structured feedback, relaxation and stress management training, and the development of a "personal TMD self-care plan."

Sixty-one subjects were randomly allocated to the SCG and 63 subjects to the UTG. The study had an 80% power based on a group size of 56 patients. Pain levels in both groups dropped from baseline to posttreatment. The SCG continued with a more marked decline than that found in the UTG at 12 months posttreatment. The SCG reported significantly lower levels of characteristic pain than did the UTG at 12 months posttreatment. Similar results were found in the evaluation of pain-related activity interference. The SCG had significantly fewer visits to the dentist

Outcome variables	Posttreatment assessment	Results	Comments[†]
Pain, function, clinical signs (Helkimo dysfunction index)	At 3 wk	In the RA subgroup, pain relief was equal in 1 and 2; mouth opening was greater in 1 than 2. In the AS subgroup, pain relief was greater in 2 than 1; mouth opening was greater in 1 than 2.	A
Symptoms severity index Maximum pain-free opening Pressure algometer threshold Perceived symptoms	4 wk	1: Reported reduction in mean TMD and neck symptoms 2: No significant improvement	

during the 12-month follow-up period. Satisfaction with treatment received was also significantly greater in the SCG. The authors suggested that one reason for the difference between the two groups may be the fact that dentists may not pay careful attention to providing feedback and reinforcement for behavior change or management of relapse. They concluded that the encouragement of self-management may offer real benefits for a significant number of patients with a TMD.

Physical self-regulatory (PSR) training was also proposed to be effective in the short- and long-term management of TMDs by Carlson et al.[86] The intervention was presented in two 50-minute sessions by a dentist at 3-week intervals and was compared to standard dental care (SDC). SDC included the fitting and reevaluation of a bite appliance at the same time intervals and duration as the test group (impressions were taken for both groups at the initial visit). Forty-four subjects were randomized to one of the two test groups through the use of a random number table. Assessment was made by a dentist blinded to the study groups. Both groups had lower pain scores at the end of the 6-week study period, and their perception of the control of pain was increased. However, by 26 weeks, the PSR training group reported significantly less pain than the SDC group. These findings support the use of PSR training for both short- and long-term management of TMD pain. The authors also reported the cost effectiveness of this approach; there was an immediate 47% cost savings when the PSR training strategy was used instead of SDC, based on the current billing practice at the clinic where the study was undertaken.

A summary of studies on mixed therapies is provided in Table 24-5.

Jaw Manipulation and Exercise

There seems to be reasonable support for the concept that exercise and stretching can increase the range of movement in other parts of the body although the evidence for an effect on pain is less clear. No difference was found regarding change in pain between arthritis patients undertaking aerobic exercises (walking and swimming) and those performing exercises designed to improve range of movement at the 12-week assessment.[88] However, the aerobic group was significantly better with regard to physical activity, anxiety, and depression, as assessed with the Arthritis Impact Measurement Scale (AIMS). This difference was maintained 1 year following the intervention.

In another study of osteoarthritis patients following arthroplasty of the knee, a greater range of flexion at 12 weeks was observed in the exercise group than in an immobilized group, but no data regarding pain were presented.[89] However, a greater decrease in pain was reported in rheumatoid arthritis patients who exercised their hands than in those who received hot wax treatment or no treatment.[90] Hoenig et al[91] reported no differences in pain between groups treated with range of motion exercises, resistance exercises, or a combination of both and a nontreatment group over a 12-week period. However, the exercise groups did show greater grip strength compared to the control group. A study on supervised walking in patients with osteoarthritis appeared to reveal no advantage with regard to function or use of medication when compared with a nontreatment control.[92] However, the authors did report that patients exhibited significantly better walking ability and experienced less pain, as assessed by the AIMS instrument.

The effect of exercise in a self-managed exercise program in women with fibromyalgia was investigated by Burckhardt et al.[93] Treatment assignment was randomized and data were collected from the treatment and the control groups for 6 weeks using the Fibromyalgia Impact Questionnaire. No between- or within-group differences were found. However, there were between-group differences on the Self-Efficacy Scale (SELF) and the Quality of Life Scale (QOLS-S) apparently due to inequality in baseline scores.

Comparison of passive and active neck exercises against a control group in subjects with chronic neck pain has shown significantly greater pain relief in the active exercise groups; however, these groups also showed an imbalance in gender distribution.[94] Koes et al[9] were unable to offer positive support for the efficacy of exercise programs targeted for the back from their meta-analysis; however, support does come from other sources. In their study investigating TENS, Deyo et al[95] reported that the group including an exercise program showed improvements in self-reported pain scores at 1 month, together with reduced frequency of pain. Timm's comparison[96] of low-technology and high-technology exercise with other forms of therapy suggested that both exercise groups achieved significantly better results than did the other groups on functional measures and a composite disability score.

The positive effect of cold therapy when combined with exercise and stretching has already been discussed in regard to postoperative knee surgery patients.[24] In a parallel study comparing jaw exercises with a nontreatment control group in subjects with rheumatoid arthritis and ankylosing spondylitis, maximal mouth opening was significantly greater in the treatment groups for both conditions.[97] However, there were no differences between treatment groups for the subjective symptoms of pain and stiffness, although they were both better than the control group.

The type of exercise being evaluated must be carefully considered, as well as the group to which it is being delivered. Dao and colleagues[98] reported that after 3 minutes of chewing a piece of wax, TMD patients with high levels of pain at baseline showed some improvement, while those with low-level pain got worse.

The most positive evidence to support exercise comes from studies on general exercise. Treatment aimed at improving physical fitness seems to show positive outcomes for the condition under investigation.[12,88,96,99,100] In a study previously discussed,[23] the effect of exercise and massage was tested against a second exercise and massage group in which ultrasound therapy was added, as well as in a control group. Both exercise groups showed improvements compared to the control group, but the addition of ultrasound appeared to offer little advantage.

The effect of posture training as an adjunct to self-management instructions for patients with TMD pain was assessed in a randomized trial by Wright and colleagues.[101] The authors outlined the literature, suggesting that forward head posturing may contribute to such pain. Sixty patients who had experienced TMD pain for more than 6 months were randomized into two groups. All subjects were given self-management instructions; the trial group received three additional appointments with a physical therapist for posture exercises.

Significant improvements were found in the treatment group, but there was no significant improvement in the nontreatment group. As the authors commented, because each subject in the treatment group had three more appointments than the nontreatment group, the improvement in the treatment group may have been due to a placebo effect. This is clearly a weakness in the study. Unfortunately, the authors carried out no between-group comparisons.[101]

A summary of selected studies on jaw manipulation and exercise is provided in Table 24-6.

Summary

As concluded in earlier reports and summarized in this chapter, there is still no solid evidence to support claims of efficacy for any specific physical therapy or modality other than general exercise. However, as reported by Feine and Lund,[1] any noninvasive, reversible treatment is better than no treatment, and the longer the time spent in treatment, the better the outcome.

References

1. Feine JS, Lund JP. An assessment of the efficacy of physical therapy and physical modalities for the control of chronic musculoskeletal pain. Pain 1997;71:5–23.
2. Glass EG, McGlynn FD, Glaros AG. A survey of treatments for myofascial pain dysfunction. Cranio 1991;9:165–168.
3. Glass EG, Glaros AG, McGlynn FD. Myofascial pain dysfunction: Treatments used by ADA members. Cranio 1993;11:25–29.
4. Chalmers T, Smith HJ, Blackburn B, et al. A method for assessing the quality of randomized control trials. Control Clin Trials 1981;2:31–49.

5. Beckerman H, Bouter LM, van der Heijden GJ, de Bie RA, Koes BW. Efficacy of physiotherapy for musculoskeletal disorders: What can we learn from research? Br J Gen Pract 1993;43:73–77.

6. Chapman CE. Can the use of physical modalities for pain control be rationalized by the research evidence? Can J Physiol Pharmacol 1991;69:704–712.

7. Clark GT, Adachi NY, Dornan MR. Physical medicine procedures affect temporomandibular disorders: A review. J Am Dent Assoc 1990;121:151–162.

8. Deyo RA. Conservative therapy for low back pain. Distinguishing useful from useless therapy. JAMA 1983;250:1057–1062.

9. Koes BW, Assendelft BW, van der Heijden GJ, Bouter LM, Knipschild PG. Spinal manipulation and mobilisation for back and neck pain: A blinded review. Br Med J 1991;303:1298–1303.

10. Malone MD, Strube MJ, Scogin FR. Meta-analysis of nonmedical treatments for chronic pain. Pain 1988;34:231–244 [erratum 1989;37:128]; comment 1989;39:359–363.

11. Sturdivant J, Fricton JR. Physical therapy for TMD disorders and orofacial pain. Curr Opin Dent 1991;1:486–496.

12. Feine JS, Widmer CG, Lund JP. Physical therapy: A critique. Oral Surg Oral Med Oral Pathol Oral Radiol Endod 1997;83:123–1277; comment 1997;84:3.

13. Crider AB, Glaros AG. A meta-analysis of EMG biofeedback treatment of temporomandibular disorders. J Orofac Pain 1999;13:29–37.

14. Dahlström L. Conservative treatment methods in craniomandibular disorder. Swed Dent J 1992;16:217–230.

15. Fowkes FG, Fulton PM. Critical appraisal of published research: Introductory guidelines. BMJ 1991;302:1136–1140.

16. American Academy of Orofacial Pain, Okeson JP (ed). Orofacial Pain: Guidelines for Assessment, Diagnosis, and Management. Chicago: Quintessence, 1996.

17. Munting E. Ultrasonic therapy for painful shoulders. Physiotherapy 1978;64:180–181.

18. Nwuga VC. Ultrasound in treatment of back pain resulting from prolapsed intervertebral disc. Arch Phys Med Rehabil 1983;64:88–89.

19. Binder A, Hodge G, Greenwood AM, Hazleman BL, Page Thomas DP. Is therapeutic ultrasound effective in treating soft tissue lesions? Br Med J Clin Res Ed 1985;290:512–514.

20. Downing DS, Weinstein A. Ultrasound therapy of subacromial bursitis. A double blind trial. Phys Ther 1986;66:194–199.

21. Bromley J, Unsworth A, Haslock I. Changes in stiffness following short- and long-term application of standard physiotherapeutic techniques. Br J Rheumatol 1994;33:555–561.

22. Falconer, J, Hayes KW, Chang RW. Effect of ultrasound on mobility in osteoarthritis of the knee. A randomized clinical trial. Arthritis Care Res 1992;5:29–35.

23. Gam AN, Warming S, Larsen LH, et al. Treatment of myofascial trigger-points with ultrasound combined with massage and exercise—A randomised controlled trial. Pain 1998;77:73–79.

24. Hecht PJ, Bachmann S, Booth RE Jr, Rothman RH. Effects of thermal therapy on rehabilitation after total knee arthroplasty. A prospective randomized study. Clinical Orthop Relat Res 1983;Sep:198–201.

25. Williams J, Harvey J, Tannenbaum H. Use of superficial heat versus ice for rheumatoid arthritis shoulder: A pilot study. Physiother Can 1986;38:8–13.

26. Carlsson J, Fahlcrantz A, Augustinsson LE. Muscle tenderness in tension headache treated with acupuncture or physiotherapy. Cephalalgia 1990;10:131–141.

27. Christensen BV, Luhl IU, Vilbek H, Bulow HH, Dreijer NC, Rasmussen HF. Acupuncture treatment of severe knee osteoarthritis. A long-term study. Acta Anaesthesiol Scand 1992;36:519–525.

28. Takeda W, Wessel J. Acupuncture for the treatment of pain of osteoarthritic knees. Arthritis Care Res 1994;7:118–122.

29. Thomas M, Eriksson SV, Lundeberg T. A comparative study of diazepam and acupuncture in patients with osteoarthritis pain: A placebo controlled study. Am J Chinese Med 1991;19:95–100.

30. Deluze C, Bosia L, Zirbs A, Chantraine A, Vischer TL. Electroacupuncture in fibromyalgia: Results of a controlled trial. BMJ 1992;305:1249–1252.

31. Patel MS, Gutzwiller F, Pacaud FEA. A meta-analysis of acupuncture for the treatment of pain: A review of evaluative research. Pain 1986;24:15–40.

32. Reit T, Kleijnen J, Knipschild PG. Acupuncture and chronic pain: A criteria-based meta-analysis. J Clin Epidemiol 1990;43:1191–1199.

33. Ceccherelli F, Rigoni MT, Gagliardi G, Ruzzante L. Comparison of superficial and deep acupuncture in the treatment of lumbar myofascial pain: A double-blind randomized controlled study. Clin J Pain 2002;18:149–153.

34. Ceccherelli F, Bordin M, Gagliardi G, Caravello M. Comparison between superficial and deep acupuncture in the treatment of the shoulder's myofascial pain: A randomized and controlled study. Acupunct Electrother Res 2001;26:229–238.

35. Birch S, Jamison RN. Controlled trial of Japanese acupuncture for chronic myofascial neck pain: Assessment of specific and nonspecific effects of treatment. Clin J Pain 1998;14:248–255.

36. Goddard G, Karibe H, McNeill C, Villafuerte E. Acupuncture and sham acupuncture reduce muscle pain in myofascial pain patients. J Orofac Pain 2002;16:71–76.

37. Cummings TM, White AR. Needling therapies in the management of myofascial trigger point pain: A systematic review. Arch Phys Med Rehabil 2001;82:986–992.

38. List T, Helkimo M. Acupuncture and occlusal appliance therapy in the treatment of craniomandibular disorders. 2. A 1-year follow-up study. Acta Odontol Scand 1992;50:375–385.

39. Johansson A, Wenneberg B, Wagersten C, Haraldson T. Acupuncture in treatment of facial muscular pain. Acta Odontol Scand 1991;49:153–158.

40. Raustia AM, Pohjola RT, Virtanen KK. Acupuncture compared with stomatognathic treatment for TMJ dysfunction. 1. A randomized study. J Prosthet Dent 1985;54:581–585.

41. Raustia AM, Pohjola RT. Acupuncture compared with stomatognathic treatment for TMJ dysfunction. 3. Effect of treatment on mobility. J Prosthet Dent 1986;56:616–623.

42. Rosted P. Practical recommendations for the use of acupuncture in the treatment of temporomandibular disorders based on the outcome of published controlled studies. Oral Dis 2001;7:109–115.

43. List T, Helkimo M, Andersson S, Carlsson GE. Acupuncture and occlusal appliance therapy in the treatment of craniomandibular disorders. 1. A comparative study. Swed Dent J 1992;16:125–141.

44. Raustia AM, Pohjola RT, Virtanen KK. Acupuncture compared with stomatognathic treatment for TMJ dysfunction. 2. Components of the dysfunction index. J Prosthet Dent 1986;55:372–376.

45. Ernst E, White AR. Acupuncture as a treatment for temporomandibular joint dysfunction: A systematic review of randomized trials. Arch Otolaryngol Head Neck Surg 1999; 125:269–272.

46. NIH Consensus Conference. Acupuncture. JAMA 1998;280: 1518–1524.

47. Haker E, Lundeberg T. Laser treatment applied to acupuncture points in lateral numeral epicondylagia: A double-blind study. Pain 1990;43:243–247.

48. Beckerman H, de Bie RA, Bouter LM, De Cuyper HJ, Oostendorp RA. The efficacy of laser therapy for musculoskeletal and skin disorders: A criteria-based meta-analysis of randomized clinical trials. Phys Ther 1992;72:483–491.

49. Gam AN, Thorsen H, Lonnberg F. The effect of low-level laser therapy on musculoskeletal pain: A meta-analysis. Pain 1993;52:63–56.

50. Kitchen SS, Partridge CJ. A review of low level laser therapy. 1. Background, physiological effects and hazards. Physiotherapy 1991;77:161–168.

51. Ceccherelli F, Altafini L, Lo Castro G, Avila A, Ambrosio F, Giron GP. Diode laser in cervical myofascial pain: A double-blind study versus placebo. Clin J Pain 1989;5:301–304.

52. Bulow PM, Jensen H, Danneskiold-Samsoe B. Low power Ga-Al-As laser treatment of painful osteoarthritis of the knee. A double-blind placebo-controlled study. Scand J Rehabil Med 1994;26:155–159.

53. Heussler JK, Hinchey G, Margiotta E, et al. A double blind randomised trial of low power laser treatment in rheumatoid arthritis. Ann Rheum Dis 1993;52:703–706.

54. Bertolucci LE, Grey T. Clinical analysis of mid-laser versus placebo treatment of arthralgic TMJ degenerative joints. Cranio 1995;13:26–29.

55. Bertolucci LE, Grey T. Clinical comparative study of microcurrent electrical stimulation to mid-laser and placebo treatment in degenerative joint disease of the temporomandibular joint. Cranio 1995;13:116–120.

56. Conti PC. Low level laser therapy in the treatment of temporomandibular disorders (TMD): A double-blind pilot study. Cranio 1997;15:144–149.

57. Kulekcioglu S, Sivrioglu K, Ozcan O, Parlak M. Effectiveness of low-level laser therapy in temporomandibular disorder. Scand J Rheumatol 2003;32:114–118.

58. Meyerson BA. Electrostimulation Procedures: Effects, Presumed Rationale, and Possible Mechanisms, vol 5. New York: Raven Press, 1983.

59. Long DM. Fifteen years of transcutaneous electrical stimulation for pain control. Stereotact Funct Neurosurg 1991;56: 2–19.

60. Lewis B, Lewis D, Cumming G. The comparative analgesic efficacy of TENS and a non-steroidal anti-inflammatory drug for painful osteoarthritis. Br J Rheumatol 1994;33:455–460.

61. Block SL, Laskin DM. The effectiveness of TENS in the treatment of unilateral MPD syndrome [abstract]. J Dent Res 1980;59:519.

62. Taylor K, Newton RA, Personius WJ, Bush FM. Effects of interferential current stimulation for treatment of subjects with recurrent jaw pain. Phys Ther 1987;67:346–350.

63. Linde C, Isacsson G, Jonsson BG. Outcome of 6-week treatment with transcutaneous electric nerve stimulation compared with splint on symptomatic temporomandibular joint disk displacement without reduction. Acta Odontol Scand 1995;53:92–98.

64. Alvarez-Arenal A, Junquera LM, Fernandez JP, Gonzalez I, Olay S. Effect of occlusal appliance and transcutaneous electric nerve stimulation on the signs and symptoms of temporomandibular disorders in patients with bruxism. J Oral Rehabil 2002;29:858–863.

65. Moystad A, Krogstad BS, Larheim TA. Transcutaneous nerve stimulation in a group of patients with rheumatic disease involving the temporomandibular joint. J Prosthet Dent 1990;64:596–600.

66. Al-Badawi EA, Mehta N, Forgione AG, Lobo SL, Zawawi KH. Efficacy of pulsed radio frequency energy therapy in temporomandibular joint pain and dysfunction. Cranio 2004; 22:10–20.

67. Bassett CA, Schink-Ascani M. Long-term pulsed electromagnetic field (PEMF) results in congenital pseudarthrosis. Calcif Tissue Inf 1991;49:216–220.

68. Bassett CA. Beneficial effects of electromagnetic fields. J Cell Biochem 1993;51:387–393.

69. Trock D, Bollet A, Dyer R, Fielding L, Miner W, Markoll R. A double-blind trial of the clinical effects of pulsed electromagnetic fields in osteoarthritis. J Rheumatol 1993;20:456–460.

70. Smania N, Corato E, Fiaschi A, Pietropoli P, Agliotti SM, Tinazzi M. Therapeutic effects of peripheral repetitive magnetic stimulation on myofascial pain syndrome. Clin Neurophysiol 2003;114:350–358.

71. Peroz I, Chun YH, Karageorgi G, et al. A multicenter clinical trial on the use of pulsed electromagnetic fields in the treatment of temporomandibular disorders. J Prosthet Dent 2004;91:180–187.

72. Berry H, Fernandes L, Bloom B, Clark RJ, Hamilton EBD. Clinical study comparing acupuncture, physiotherapy, injection and oral antiinflammatory therapy in shoulder-cuff lesions. Curr Med Res Opin 1980;7:121–126.

73. Hawkes J, Care G, Dixon JS, Bird HA, Wright V. Comparison of three physiotherapy regimens for hands with rheumatoid arthritis. Br Med J Clin Res Ed 1985;291:1016.

74. Koes BW, Bouter LM, van Mameren H, et al. A blinded randomized clinical trial of manual therapy and physiotherapy for chronic back and neck complaints: Physical outcome measures. J Manipulative Physiol Ther 1992;15:16–23; comments 1992;15:406–507, 1992;15:332–333, 2001;24:143–144.

75. Koes BW, Bouter LM, van Mameren H, et al. Randomised clinical trial of manipulative therapy and physiotherapy for persistent back and neck complaints: Results of one year follow up. BMJ 1992;304:601–605; comment 1992;304:1309–1310, author reply 1310–1311, comment 1992;304:1176.

76. Koes BW, Bouter LM, van Mameren H, et al. The effectiveness of manual therapy, physiotherapy, and treatment by the general practitioner for nonspecific back and neck complaints. A randomized clinical trial. Spine 1992;17:28–35; comment 1993;18:169–170.

77. Svarcova J, Trnavsky K, Zvarova J. The influence of ultrasound, galvanic currents and shortwave diathermy on pain intensity in patients with osteoarthritis. Scand J Rheumatol Suppl 1987;67:83–85.

78. Hansen FR, Bendix T, Skov P, et al. Intensive, dynamic back-muscle exercises, conventional physiotherapy, or placebo-control treatment of low-back pain. A randomized, observer-blind trial. Spine 1993;18:98–108.

79. Talaat AM, el-Dibany MM, el-Garf A. Physical therapy in the management of myofascial pain dysfunction syndrome. Ann Otol Rhinol Laryngol 1986;95:225–228.

80. Burgess JA, Sommers EE, Truelove EL, Dworkin SF. Short-term effect of two therapeutic methods on myofascial pain and dysfunction of the masticatory system. J Prosthet Dent 1988;60:606–610.

81. Braun BL. The effect of physical therapy intervention on incisal opening after temporomandibular joint surgery. Oral Surg Oral Med Oral Pathol 1987;64:544–548.

82. Nelson SJ, Ash MM Jr. An evaluation of a moist heating pad for the treatment of TMJ/muscle pain dysfunction. Cranio 1988;6:355–359.

83. McCreary CP, Clark GT, Oakley ME, Flack V. Predicting response to treatment for temporomandibular disorders. J Craniomandib Disord 1992;6:161–169.

84. Gray RJ, Quayle AA, Hall CA, Schofield MA. Physiotherapy in the treatment of temporomandibular joint disorders: A comparative study of four treatment methods. Br Dent J 1994;176:257–261.

85. Dworkin SF, Huggins KH, Wilson L, et al. A randomized clinical trial using Research Diagnostic Criteria for Temporomandibular Disorders-Axis II to target clinic cases for a tailored self-care TMD treatment program. J Orofac Pain 2002;16:48–63.

86. Carlson CR, Bertrand PM, Ehrlich AD, Maxwell AW, Burton RG. Physical self-regulation training for the management of temporomandibular disorders. J Orofac Pain 2001;15:47–55.

87. Austin BD, Shupe SM. The role of physical therapy in recovery after temporomandibular joint surgery. J Oral Maxillofac Surg 1993;51:495–498 [erratum 1993;51:1058].

88. Minor MA, Hewett JE, Webel RR, Anderson SK, Kay DR. Efficacy of physical conditioning exercise in patients with rheumatoid arthritis and osteoarthritis. Arthritis Rheum 1989;32:1396–1405.

89. Johnson DP. The effect of continuous passive motion on wound-healing and joint mobility after knee arthroplasty. J Bone Joint Surg Am 1990;72:421–426.

90. Dellhag B, Wollersjo I, Bjelle A. Effect of active hand exercise and wax bath treatment in rheumatoid arthritis patients. Arthritis Care Res 1992;5:87–92.

91. Hoenig H, Groff G, Pratt K, Goldberg E, Franck W. A randomized controlled trial of home exercise on the rheumatoid hand. J Rheumatol 1993;20:785–789.

92. Kovar PA, Allegrante JP, MacKenzie CR, Peterson MG, Gutin B, Charlson ME. Supervised fitness walking in patients with osteoarthritis of the knee. A randomized, controlled trial. Ann Intern Med 1992;116:529–534; comments 1992;116:598–599, 1992;117:697–698.

93. Burckhardt CS, Mannerkorpi K, Hedenberg L, Bjelle A. A randomized, controlled clinical trial of education and physical training for women with fibromyalgia. J Rheumatol 1994;21:714–720.

94. Revel M, Minguet M, Gregoy P, Vaillant J, Manuel JL. Changes in cervicocephalic kinesthesia after a proprioceptive rehabilitation program in patients with neck pain: A randomized controlled study. Arch Phys Med Rehabil 1994;75:895–899.

95. Deyo RA, Walsh NE, Martin DC, Schoenfeld LS, Ramamurthy S. A controlled trial of transcutaneous electrical nerve stimulation (TENS) and exercise for chronic low back pain. New Engl J Med 1990;322:1627–1634; comment 1990;323:1423–1425.

96. Timm KE. A randomized-control study of active and passive treatments for chronic low back pain following L5 laminectomy. J Orthop Sports Phys Ther 1994;20:276–286.

97. Tegelberg A, Kopp S. Short-term effect of physical training on temporomandibular joint disorder in individuals with rheumatoid arthritis and ankylosing spondylitis. Acta Odontol Scand 1988;46:49–56.

98. Dao TT, Lund JP, Lavigne GJ. Pain responses to experimental chewing in myofascial pain patients. J Dent Res 1994;73:1163–1167.

99. Scientific approach to the assessment and management of activity-related spinal disorders. A monograph for clinicians. Report of the Quebec Task Force on Spinal Disorders. Spine 1987;12(suppl):S1–S59.

100. Fordyce WE. Back Pain in the Workplace: Management of Disability in Nonspecific Conditions. Seattle: IASP Press, 1995.

101. Wright EF, Domenech MA, Fischer JR Jr. Usefulness of posture training for patients with temporomandibular disorders. J Am Dent Assoc 2000;131:202–210; comment 2000;131:564, 566, 568.

CHAPTER 25

Oral Appliances

Glenn T. Clark and Hajime Minakuchi

Oral appliances are frequently used in patients with temporomandibular disorders (TMDs). This chapter discusses the various types of oral appliances and the indications for their use and reviews the scientific evidence for their effectiveness. It also reviews the complications that may be induced by chronic use of oral appliances.

Types of Oral Appliances

Oral appliances can be categorized into those that cover all the teeth (complete coverage) and those that cover only some of the teeth (partial coverage). They also can be categorized into those that deliberately attempt to reposition or realign the maxillomandibular relationship (repositioners) and those that do not seek to change this relationship (stabilizers or nonrepositioners). Moreover, most oral appliances are fabricated to attach to and cover only one arch (either maxillary or mandibular), although a few of them are fabricated as double-arch devices.

The specific symptoms these devices are supposed to treat and the presumed reasons underlying their use are listed in Table 25-1. This chapter discusses three types of oral appliance used in dental offices today: *(1)* nonrepositioning or stabilizing devices that provide complete coverage of the dental arch, *(2)* nonrepositioning devices that provide only partial arch coverage and *(3)* mandibular repositioning oral appliances of all types. Because most of the data in the literature involve the stabilization appliance, this review focuses mainly on the efficacy of that appliance.

Complete-Coverage Stabilizing Appliances

The complete-arch, hard acrylic resin stabilization appliance is best described as a nonrepositioning, flat-surface device that covers all the teeth in one arch and has equal, bilateral contact with all of the opposing teeth. Usually it provides anterior tooth guidance during any excursive movements, thereby creating disclusion of the posterior tooth contacts. It is commonly adjusted to the jaw closure position most akin to maximum intercuspation.[1] This position is also referred to as the *muscular contact position* or *centric occlusion.*

The primary purpose of the stabilization appliance when used in TMD patients for treatment of myalgia and/or arthralgia is not to change the existing maxillomandibular relationships, but instead to serve as a behavior-changing device that makes the patient aware of any oral parafunction. These appliances can be made for either the maxillary

Table 25-1	Reasons for use of oral appliances
Symptom or sign	**Indications for use of an oral appliance**
Masticatory myalgia	The myalgia is the result of sustained clenching and/or bruxism behaviors (either waking or sleeping) that cause a diminished circulation in the contracting muscles and ischemia-related muscle pain.
TMJ arthralgia or arthritis	There is localized arthralgia or arthritis that is caused by clenching and/or bruxism behavior or arthritis (either waking or sleeping), which causes TMJ surface damage, or the patient has a polyjoint arthralgia or arthritis and clenching and/or bruxism behavior that is irritating the damaged joint surface.
Atypical odontalgia	The patient has chronic tooth pain of unknown origin without evidence of cracks or dental-pulpal disease, and the teeth are sensitive to pressure.
TMJ dysfunction (eg, clicking and episodic locking)	The patient has chronic TMJ clicking and/or episodic locking of the TMJ, and it is suspected that the patient is clenching or grinding the teeth strongly and that this behavior is aggravating/causing the joint dysfunction.
Temporary occlusion	The occlusion is unstable (eg, tooth contacts on the posterior teeth are uneven or inadequate) and reconstruction is planned after a stable, comfortable jaw position is achieved. The occlusal instability could be the result of orofacial trauma, osteoarthritic changes in the TMJ, or iatrogenic changes to the dentition.
Cracked, chipped, or worn teeth	The patient has evidence of substantial attrition, cracking, or chipping of the teeth, presumably because of heavy bruxing or clenching.
Frequent headaches	The patient has episodic tension headache, migraine headache, or even chronic daily headache that is being triggered by masticatory myalgia or TMJ arthralgia induced by clenching and grinding of the teeth.

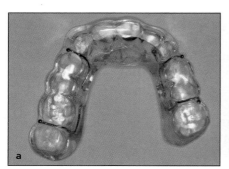 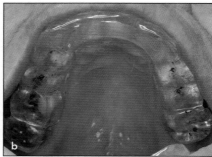 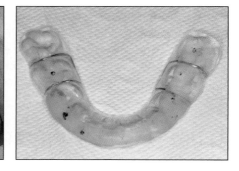

Fig 25-1 Maxillary complete-arch stabilization appliance. *(a)* Extraoral occlusal view. *(b)* Intraoral occlusal view.

Fig 25-2 Occlusal view of a mandibular complete-arch stabilization appliance.

or the mandibular arch (Figs 25-1 and 25-2). Because acrylic resin is far softer than enamel, single-arch complete-coverage oral appliances also have been used to reduce the chance of further wear, chipping, or cracking of the teeth in both arches. Stabilization appliances also can be used for management of an unstable occlusion, such as when a patient is missing multiple posterior tooth contacts bilaterally. Occasionally, they are used to lessen clenching-induced "earache" (also called *secondary otalgia*) and tooth pain as well as to alter certain types of headache patterns.[2–7] Finally, sta-

bilization appliances are sometimes used as an adjunct for managing symptoms associated with temporomandibular joint (TMJ) disc derangement.[8–11]

The basic theory explaining how these appliances work is a matter of considerable controversy, but certainly part of their effectiveness arises from the way that they assist patients to recognize and reduce clenching and tooth-grinding behaviors. The decision regarding which type of stabilization appliance to use (maxillary or mandibular) is based on several factors (Table 25-2).

Table 25-2	Factors determining choice of stabilization appliance (maxillary versus mandibular)
Problem	**Type of appliance indicated**
Patient appears to be clenching and/or grinding at night only and therefore the device is used predominately at night.	Maxillary: This allows more of the opposing teeth to contact on a flat surface, and the forces can be distributed across a greater surface area. The maxillary appliance is usually less likely to break, and it is easier to develop guidance in the canine region on a maxillary appliance than it is on a mandibular device.
Patient exhibits evidence of bruxism with wide excursive motions.	Maxillary: The appliance is wider so the teeth can travel farther laterally before going off the edge of the appliance.
Idiopathic tooth pain is present on specific teeth.	Either arch: Cover the arch in which the tooth pain is more prominent so individual pressure on the sore tooth can be avoided.
Patient shows evidence of chipping and cracking of teeth.	Maxillary: Often the chipped and cracked teeth are in the maxilla because this is the arch in which teeth are more likely to break.
Patient's third molars are erupted and in occlusion.	Maxillary: The appliance is easier to construct and is less likely to break in the posterior region.
Patient has unstable occlusion because of missing teeth, bad prior dental treatment, or TMJ destruction.	Either arch: Fabricate the appliance on the arch with the most missing teeth, so that it can oppose the more intact arch and provide occlusal stability.
Dental treatment is planned in near future, once a repeatable occlusal relationship is established.	Either arch: Select the arch in which the least amount of dental treatment is planned. This will allow the patient to use the appliance (with only minor adjustments)during and after the treatment period.
Patient is aware of daytime clenching or bracing habit.	Mandibular: Use this appliance for the patient who is aware of clenching during the day and wants to use the device as a reminder to prevent it. The mandibular appliance is easier to use in the day-to-day context because it does not interfere as much with speech.
Patient has a chronic cheek or lip biting habit.	Maxillary: Although patients can continue biting their cheek or lip even while wearing an oral appliance, it is more difficult with a maxillary appliance.
Patient has prior experience with an oral appliance.	Either arch: Use the arch on which the patient has successfully used an oral appliance before (assuming there are no contraindications for its use).

Stabilization appliances are generally worn during sleep and 1 to 2 hours during the day to allow the patient time to practice keeping the teeth apart. It is important to instruct patients not to bite or clench on the appliance when used during waking hours. Patients should reduce the amount of use of the appliance after their jaw pain has been relieved. However, if there is evidence of ongoing wear of the occlusal surface of the appliance, which indicates a strong bruxism habit, continued use at night is appropriate even over very long periods of time.

Assuming that the device is properly cleaned by the patient and that it is adjusted properly and checked periodically by a dentist, the only adverse consequence of using a complete-coverage stabilization appliance is that it may not be effective, so the time and expense of making the device will be for naught.

Partial-Coverage Appliances

A number of partial-coverage oral appliances are used by dentists for the treatment of TMD-related signs and symptoms.[12–17] The earliest form of these devices (anterior bite planes) were proposed as a method of preventing contact of the posterior teeth, because such "interfering" contacts were considered a major source of jaw pain and dysfunction.[18] Based on this concept, various designs of anterior bite planes were used to establish the "correct" relationship between the maxilla and mandible, presumably by allowing the mandible to seek its ideal horizontal position. It was assumed that once this maxillomandibular relationship was established, the jaw pain and dysfunction would fade and that the posterior teeth could be restored or adjusted to achieve interdigitation in this new position, thus preventing a recurrence of symptoms.

Although this theory may appear plausible, it has not been supported by the research. Instead, most authorities agree that, although occlusal interferences can produce local tooth pain and even tooth mobility, they have not been found to be strongly related to the development of myalgia or arthralgia.[19,20] Moreover, neither occlusal adjustment therapy nor occlusal reconstruction is currently considered to be a logical approach for the treatment of TMDs or related symptoms (see chapter 27). For these reasons, the anterior bite plane oral appliance, which had been widely used in the past, is currently not regarded by many dentists as a primary therapeutic appliance for most patients with TMDs. However, although there have been no randomized clinical trials to support the concept, the authors and many experts believe there is sufficient clinical evidence that the anterior bite plane appliance offers one advantage over a complete-coverage appliance: The anterior bite plane appliance can prevent clenching by physically separating the posterior teeth. Therefore, proponents believe that its use may be preferable in those patients who continue to clench hard with a stabilization appliance and thus continue to have myogenous pain. Because of the possibility of supereruption of the posterior teeth if the anterior bite plane is worn constantly, this appliance should only be worn at night.

In recent years, a new version of an old concept has evolved. It is based on the premise that patients who are able to clench or grind on only a few anterior teeth will produce less occlusal force. This theory has encouraged many dentists to use traditional as well as some new types of anterior bite plane appliance as a primary TMD treatment.[12–14,21] In one of the latest manifestations, the anterior bite appliance is a small device that fits over the maxillary central incisor teeth and contacts only one or two opposing mandibular anterior teeth. The published literature examining this "miniature anterior bite appliance" is discussed later in this chapter.

Another, somewhat older form of the partial-coverage oral device is one that covers only the posterior teeth. Sometimes these posterior coverage appliances are used to alter clenching habits or bruxism, and other times they are used to deliberately alter the mandibular position. Whether the appliance provides anterior tooth coverage or posterior tooth coverage (assuming that no deliberate repositioning is being produced), its mechanism of action is presumed to be that it encourages patients to reduce their clenching and grinding behaviors while it protects the teeth from attrition. The evidence regarding the ability of bite appliances of any kind to consistently and per-sistently alter clenching and bruxism behaviors is reviewed later in this chapter.

Mandibular Repositioning Appliances

The third major group of oral appliances comprises those that deliberately seek to alter the position of maximum intercuspation; these are referred to as *mandibular repositioning appliances*.[15,22–24] Although some advocates of these devices suggest that they be used to treat all or most signs and symptoms of TMDs, more often this type of appliance is used only in patients with painful clicking or intermittent TMJ locking. By holding the mandibular condyles in a more forward position, the appliance is supposed to "recapture" the displaced disc, that is, ensure that the disc is more properly aligned with the condyle. In successfully treated patients, the tendency of the TMJ to click or lock, as well as any secondary painful articular and muscular aspects of such internal derangements, will be decreased. This type of appliance generally works best when a small anterior positional change (less than 2 mm) can improve joint function.

The difficulty associated with the use of a repositioning device is that, once it is delivered to the patient, it requires constant monitoring (frequent office visits) to ensure that the altered jaw position prevents the disc-condyle displacement from recurring. Advocates for this device have suggested that this type of appliance must be worn 24 hours a day for at least 8 to 10 weeks, including when the patient is eating (if possible). The most common adverse effect associated with using the repositioning device in this fashion is permanent occlusal change.[25,26] The clinical implications of this effect are reviewed later in this chapter.

Efficacy of Oral Appliances

All therapies require that some basic principles of treatment be met:

1. It is essential to begin with a clear diagnosis.
2. It is necessary to prescribe the treatment that is most logical for the diagnosis and etiology.
3. The predicted effect of the treatment should be understood and monitored to confirm that it is actually occurring.
4. The treatment should be selected based on the scientific evidence.

Table 25-3	Scientific and professional society recommendations on treatments for TMDs*			
Treatment type	NIH-NOHIC	AAOP	AAOMS	AACFP
Home-based self-care procedures	Suggested	Suggested	Suggested	Suggested
Short-term use of oral appliances that do not change the occlusion	Suggested	Suggested	Suggested	Suggested
Short-term use of muscle relaxants and NSAIDs	Suggested	Suggested	Suggested	Not specified
Office-based physical medicine (including triggerpoint injections)	Not tested	Suggested, but triggerpoint injections not specific	Not specified	Not specified
Behavioral therapy (relaxation and stress management)	Not specified	Suggested	Suggested	Not specified
Restorative treatment (including long-term occlusal overlays)	Avoid	Avoid	Not specified	Suggested
Occlusal adjustment	Avoid	Avoid	Not specified	Suggested
Orthodontics	Not specified	Avoid	Not specified	Suggested
Open TMJ surgery (including surgery to repair the tissues)	Avoid	Avoid	Suggested; open surgery to repair if needed	If needed
Arthroscopic TMJ surgery	Not specified	Not specified	Suggested	Not specified
Alloplastic TMJ implants	Avoid	Not specified	Not specified	Not specified

*NIH-NOHIC = National Institutes of Health–National Oral Health Information Clearing House[27]; AAOP = American Academy of Orofacial Pain[28]; AAOMS = American Association of Oral and Maxillofacial Surgeons[29]; AACFP = American Academy of Craniofacial Pain[30]; NSAIDs = nonsteroidal anti-inflammatory drugs.

To better understand the scientific evidence, it is necessary view it from multiple perspectives. This chapter examines what the experts say to the public about oral appliances as well as what experts say to each other, as summarized in the conclusions of several recent literature reviews. This chapter also reviews what is known about complications from chronic use of the various oral appliances (stabilization, partial-coverage, and repositioning devices).

Scientific Evidence

Expert opinions about oral appliances

Various levels of scientific evidence can be used to assess the relative efficacy of any therapy. The first level is to compare and contrast what the experts are telling the general public (ie, patients) about oral appliances as well as other treatments commonly used for TMDs. This was done by examining the statements about treatment gathered from the websites of the National Institutes of Health–National Oral Health Information Clearing House (NIH-NOHIC)[27] and three other relevant professional dental societies in the United States: the American Academy of Orofacial Pain (AAOP),[28] the American Association of Oral and Maxillofacial Surgeons (AAOMS),[29] and the American Academy of Craniofacial Pain (AACFP).[30] These expert opinions are presented in a summary form in Table 25-3. Only two forms of treatment are uniformly endorsed by all four groups, namely, home-based self-care procedures and the short-term use of oral appliances that do not change the occlusion.

Table 25-4	Results of recent reviews on the use of oral appliances for TMDs	
Study	**Summary statements**	**Rating***
Lipton and Dionne[31]	"Although the more traditional forms of TMD therapy (eg, physical therapy and occlusal appliance therapy) are shown to be better than an inactive placebo condition, there is insufficient evidence to justify using them."	+/–
Marbach and Raphael[32]	"Most controlled studies conclude that appliances are not effective."	–
Dao and Lavigne[33]	"The results of controlled clinical trials lend support to the effectiveness (ie, the patient's appreciation of the positive changes which are perceived to have occurred during the trial) of the stabilization appliance in the control of myofascial pain."	+
Forssell et al[36]	"Splint therapy was found superior to 3 and comparable to 12 control treatments, and superior or comparable to 4 passive controls, respectively," and "The use of occlusal splints may be of some benefit in the treatment of TMD."	++
Forssell and Kalso[35]	"Occlusal splint studies yielded equivocal results. Even in the most studied area, stabilization splints for myofascial face pain, the results do not justify definite conclusions about the efficacy of splint therapy. Their clinical effectiveness to relieve pain also seems modest when compared with pain treatment methods in general."	+/–
Kreiner et al[25]	"Considering all of the available data (pro and con), we conclude that occlusal appliances do have sufficient evidence to support their use for the management of localized myalgia and/or arthralgia of the masticatory system. The likely mechanism of action for occlusal appliances is via a behavioral modification of jaw clenching."	++
Turp et al[34]	"Based on the currently best available evidence it appears that most patients with masticatory muscle pain are helped by the incorporation of a stabilization splint," and "A stabilization splint does not appear to yield a better clinical outcome than a soft splint, a non-occluding palatal splint, physical therapy, or body acupuncture."	++
Al-Ani et al[37]	"There is weak evidence to suggest that the use of stabilization splints for the treatment of pain dysfunction syndrome may be beneficial for reducing pain severity, at rest and on palpation, when compared to no treatment."	+/–

*++ = positive review; + = somewhat positive review; +/– = mixed review; – = negative review.

Published analytic reviews of oral appliances

In addition to the expert opinions previously listed, seven relevant review articles have been published since 1996. The first of these reviews is the position paper of the National Institutes of Health (NIH), which represents a summary of the existing scientific evidence that was available in 1996.[31] This document was produced following a "Technology Assessment Conference on Management of Temporomandibular Disorders" that was sponsored by the NIH. After 3 days of presentations and a massive amount of submitted documentation by numerous experts, the distinguished, independent NIH panel that was charged with summarizing the evidence concluded that "the preponderance of the data do not support the superiority of any method for initial management of most TMD problems. Moreover, their superiority to placebo controls or no-treatment controls remains undetermined."[31] They also stated that "the efficacy of most treatment approaches for TMD is unknown, because most have not been adequately evaluated in long-term studies and virtually none in randomized controlled group trials."[31]

One possible interpretation of this report is to conclude that until the more traditional forms of TMD therapy, such as occlusal appliances, are shown to be better than an inactive placebo, there is insufficient evidence to justify their use. However, since the NIH report in 1997, several additional reviews on the efficacy of occlusal appliances have been published.[25,32–37] Although the conclusions in these reviews are mildly favorable, some authors have still concluded that oral appliances are not valuable as a therapy. The stated conclusions of these various reports are presented in Table 25-4. To interpret these data, however, it is necessary to understand the difference between a nonspecific treatment control and a true placebo control.

True Placebo Control Versus Nonspecific Treatment Controls

In the broadest sense, a *placebo* is usually defined as "an intervention designed to simulate medical treatment, but it is not believed by the investigator to be a specific therapy for the target condition."[38] Placebos are typically used to control for observer bias as well as for the effect of time on the treatment intervention.

Sometimes it is discovered that the supposed "placebo treatment" is not an inert intervention at all. The usual explanation offered in such cases is that the patient's cognitive expectancy (or belief that the treatment will be effective) plays a vital role. When this happens, it turns the inert placebo into an active treatment. Such a response occurs most commonly when the patient can anticipate the expected outcome of the intervention, and when the outcome being measured is easily influenced by a behavioral change.[39,40] In fact, the effect of expectation-fulfillment can be so powerful that it can equal or overpower the active intervention.[41–43] The concept of expectation-fulfillment in a clinical trial is also called the *Hawthorne effect*, and this effect is defined as the tendency for people to change their behavior in a predicted direction because they are the focus of a study.[44] For all of these reasons, it may be necessary to consider that some placebo therapies (eg, nonoccluding oral appliances that are provided within the context of a formal research study) are active behavioral interventions, and study findings must be considered in this context.

Efficacy of Stabilization Appliances

Nonoccluding appliance–controlled studies

Several studies have compared an oral stabilization appliance to a nonoccluding appliance.[45–51] When the data from these studies are examined, the logical conclusion is that both a complete-coverage stabilization appliance and a nonoccluding control appliance can produce positive clinical responses in a significant percentage of the subjects. Overall, the "real" appliance is equal to or, at best, only slightly better than the control.

The most recent of these studies helps make sense of these facts, because it includes objective measurement data.[45] The investigators performed a crossover polygraphic (sleep laboratory) study to examine the efficacy and safety of oral appliances in tooth-grinding subjects. The nine subjects received either a complete-arch stabilization appliance or a nonoccluding appliance. All subjects first underwent sleep study that confirmed sleep bruxism. They then wore the assigned appliance for 2 nights and then underwent another sleep-recording session. This procedure was repeated with the second device after a 2-week washout period.

They found that both devices resulted in a statistically significant reduction in the number of sleep bruxism episodes and sleep bruxism bursts per hour (decreases of 40% and 41%, respectively; $P = .05$). Both devices also produced 50% fewer episodes of grinding noises ($P = .06$). It was concluded that both appliances reduced the muscle activity associated with sleep bruxism.[45]

Although the sample size was small, and there were more subjects with a bruxism habit than patients with symptomatic TMD problems, the data still are interesting. They provide strong support for the idea that the placebo or nonoccluding appliance condition is an active intervention. These results also confirm the findings from the earlier work by Clark et al,[52] who showed that stabilization appliances clearly decrease masseter muscle activity during sleep in a majority of subjects with myofascial pain, at least for a short period of time.

Considered in total, these data suggest that the clinical impact of an occlusal appliance is due to a combination of behavioral interventions and the mechanical effects produced by altering occlusal contacts and changing the rest position of the jaw. The unfortunate aspect about most of the randomized, placebo-controlled oral appliance studies (with some exceptions) is that few have measured whether their subjects had strong, ongoing, oral parafunctional behaviors, nor have most of these studies examined whether the appliance modified oral parafunction and, if so, for how long. Those studies that have measured masseter activity during sleep strongly suggest that at least a short-term change in clenching and/or bruxism behavior can be produced if a patient wears an oral appliance of any size and shape.

What is clearly needed at this time is collection of new sleep-period masseter electromyographic (EMG) data from a larger sample in which a random treatment assignment is made. It is essential in such a study to stipulate whether patients have active TMD symptoms (myalgia or arthralgia), idiopathic odontalgia, idiopathic otalgia, or episodic migraine headaches so that the effects of the oral appliances on these various patient subgroups can be assessed in a meaningful way. Without such data, the basic supposition that oral appliances work by altering bruxism or clenching patterns is still weak, especially because this effect may only be short lived. Such data also would clarify whether occlusal appliances work differently in patients with muscle pain induced by clenching or tooth grinding than they do in those with other types of jaw problem (eg, spontaneous daytime myofascial pain, localized osteoarthritis, and even derangements of the TMJ). In general, the use of disparate study samples and/or nonspecific definitions for study populations makes it difficult to know if occlusal appliance treatment would be more effective for one TMD subgroup than another. In addition, it is impossible to assess the confounding effect of involuntary sleep-state–dependent motor activation of the jaw system.

Randomized treatment comparison studies

Although most scientists consider nontreatment control group results less powerful than placebo-controlled data, it can be argued differently in the case of occlusal appliance research, because the so-called placebo occlusal appliances are not true placebos. In studies with a nontreatment control condition, the subjects have no expectations of improvement, so any changes seen are the simple effect of time on the symptoms.

Overall, these data consistently demonstrate that occlusal stabilization appliances impact the patients' symptom level far more than the mere passage of time. Furthermore, they seem to have efficacy similar to that of other forms of pain-relieving therapy, such as acupuncture and behavioral interventions (eg, relaxation therapy and biofeedback).[15,53–58] What these outcome data do not prove is whether this effect is strictly behavioral or some other specific appliance-related mechanism is being invoked.

Limitations and Complications of Oral Appliances

Stabilization Appliances

Several limitations and caveats must be discussed with a patient when the use of an oral stabilization appliance is contemplated. One concern is that some patients may actually clench their teeth more with an oral appliance than they do without the appliance.[52] This response is not the common reaction, but it can occur and should be considered when appliance effects are explained to the patient. Another concern with any appliance is that it is

possible to induce an inadvertent change in the occlusion. For this reason, most dentists do not recommend that patients use any of these appliances full time (24 hours a day, including meals); constant use can lead to an alteration in the position of the individual teeth or of the mandible to such a degree that the teeth no longer achieve intercuspation when the appliance is removed.

If indeed the stabilization appliance works by reducing the patient's bruxism behavior, this effect may only be short lived. The symptoms may be alleviated for a few weeks and then return in some patients. If the symptoms do not return, then success is declared and all is well. However, a careful review of the literature regarding bruxism and oral appliances strongly suggests that oral appliances do not stop side-to-side bruxism behavior; therefore, more data are needed to determine how these appliances change motor behavior of the jaw during waking and sleeping.

Several prospective studies have used clinical examination of the surface of the stabilization appliance as one outcome measure. One study contrasted appliance wear patterns to the subjective therapeutic effects of the appliance in patients with nocturnal bruxism and TMD symptoms.[59] The study group comprised 31 patients with clinically confirmed nocturnal bruxism. Based on their observations, the researchers concluded that, although sleep bruxism continued (from clinical evidence), the symptoms stopped or diminished with the long-term use of the occlusal appliance. They therefore suggested that the therapeutic value of the appliance is not dependent on whether it "stops" bruxism.

Another study examined the patterns of nocturnal bruxofacets on the occlusal surface of stabilization appliances in a series of TMD patients.[60] The researchers enrolled 26 subjects (22 female and 4 male, 16 to 54 years old) with TMD symptoms and gave each of them a stabilization appliance. Examinations were performed at multiple points across the 10-week study. They reported that 88% of the patients (n = 23) showed active shiny facets or scratches on the appliance during the study but that the pain was significantly decreased ($P < .001$) even though these patients had parafunctional activity that was not stopped by the oral device.

A far more quantitative study was done using a direct measurement of the surface of the appliance with a laser scanning method.[61] The measurements were made before and after 12 weeks of appliance use in bruxism patients who did not have TMD-related pain. The authors reported that ongoing wear of the appliance was occurring in a majority of these subjects.

Based on the results of these studies, it seems likely that no oral appliance will completely prevent a patient's bruxism behavior, but additional study of this issue is needed.

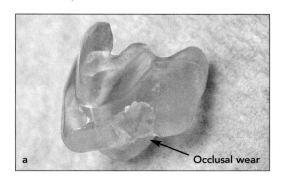
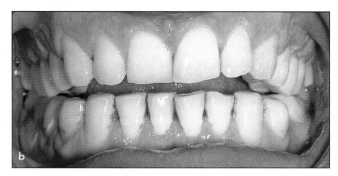

Fig 25-3 *(a)* Wear facets *(arrow)* on the occluding surface of a miniature anterior bite plane device after several weeks of use. *(b)* Anterior open bite induced by use of a partial-coverage, anterior contact–only appliance 24 hours a day over an extended period of time.

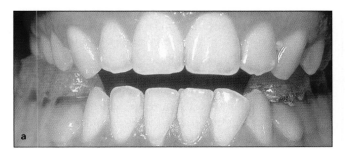
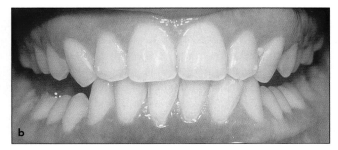

Fig 25-4 Use of a typical partial-coverage, posterior contact–only mandibular appliance. *(a)* The appliance in the mouth. *(b)* Bilateral posterior open bite induced by use of the appliance 24 hours a day for an extended period of time.

Partial-Coverage Appliances

Very few clinical trials have examined the efficacy of partial-coverage appliances for the treatment of TMD signs and symptoms. The best data regarding the efficacy of one type of anterior bite plane appliance come from a single study performed recently in Sweden.[21] Specifically, the study compared a miniature anterior bite plane device covering only the maxillary central incisors to a complete-arch stabilization device with regard to their effects on TMD signs and symptoms.

The study included 30 symptomatic TMD patients. A clinical examination was performed and subjective symptoms were registered before the start of treatment and after 3 and 6 months. Subjects were randomly assigned to one of the two appliances and instructed to use it nightly for 3 months. After 3 months, all participants were offered a change to the other type of appliance, in case there was no alleviation of their symptoms. One subject in each group was lost to follow-up early during the investigation.

At the 3-month follow-up, 4 patients who had received the miniature anterior bite plane appliance accepted the offer to change because there was no alleviation of their symptoms. No one in the stabilization appliance group accepted the offer to change treatment. At the 6-month follow-up, 7 of the remaining 10 subjects with miniature anterior bite plane appliances reported some (n = 1) or significant (n = 6) alleviation of symptoms, 2 reported no change, and 1 reported worsened symptoms. One subject treated with the miniature anterior bite plane appliance exhibited altered occlusion at the 6-month follow-up. All 14 subjects who had been treated with a stabilization appliance reported some (n = 2) or significant (n = 12) alleviation of symptoms. For all variables registered, the results were therefore more favorable for the stabilization appliance.[21]

An appliance-induced malocclusion is more likely to occur with partial-coverage appliances than with complete-coverage appliances, where it is rare unless the patient uses the device 24 hours per day (Figs 25-3 and 25-4). The mechanism for this change is controversial; some suggest that tooth intrusion or extrusion is responsible, but another explanation is that the TMJ can shift positions and the disc can change shape. This hypothesis is based in part on a study that examined the effect of a partial-coverage appliance (covering only the posterior teeth on one side) on the TMJ disc in adult rabbits.[62] The effect on the disc was to activate cellular proliferation on the appliance-covered side. This finding suggests that the adult mandibular disc may participate in compensatory change at a cellular level in response to altered loading.

These findings were confirmed in another study using young miniature pigs.[63] The authors examined the 2-month effect of two intraoral appliances (one that covered the posterior teeth bilaterally and a protrusive-bite appliance) against a nontreatment control condition. Confirming the data described in the earlier rabbit study, the results indicated that prolonged use of a partial-coverage and/or a repositioning appliance can induce remodeling and even injury of the TMJ tissues.

The previous data suggest that a partial-coverage appliance may be harmful to the jaw system and specifically to the TMJ itself. Of course, the animal studies only examined unilateral posterior contact and repositioning devices, and they did not specifically evaluate the effects of anterior bite plane devices. However, one recent study looked at the effect of anterior bite plane use in 10 healthy normal subjects (5 male and 5 female, aged 25 years) in whom EMG recordings of the masseter muscle during sleep were performed.[64] A silicone sensor was embedded in the appliance to measure bite force levels and patterns.

The peak occlusal forces on the anterior bite planes varied (3 to 80 N), and the average forces were between 5.5 and 24.0 N. The number of times that measurable force was applied to the sensor per night also varied from 39 to 558 times. These authors concluded that active intrusion of the anterior teeth is unlikely at this level of force. However, they also speculated that harmful effects could be produced by higher levels of force and that tooth movement could occur, especially in patients with periodontally compromised teeth.[64] Moreover, when these data are added to the information that animal studies have revealed about induced TMJ changes, the likelihood that partial-coverage devices have the potential to induce joint changes is increased.

The effect on the TMJ of biting on an anterior bite plane for a sustained period of time has been studied in a series of experiments in Japan.[65–67] The first of these studies examined the TMJ changes produced by unilaterally sustained biting on a positioned force transducer (molar clenching) at a force of 170 N held for 5 minutes.[65] The investigators took high-resolution computerized tomo-

graphic (CT) images of the TMJ before and after the clenching task and found that the joint space dimension was significantly reduced in the contralateral joint.

The second study examined the effects of sustained incisal clenching on the TMJ space using high-resolution CT images of the TMJ.[66] Nine subjects clenched on a bite force transducer for 10 minutes at a force of 49 N. The results were similar to those obtained with unilateral biting, namely, that the joint space dimension was significantly reduced and condylar position was significantly shifted upward after 10 minutes of biting.

Finally, another study examined the effect of biting on a repositioning appliance versus biting on a complete-coverage appliance.[67] This study had seven subjects perform maximum clenching, first on a stabilization appliance in intercuspal position and then on an anterior mandibular repositioning appliance, in each case maintaining strong clenching for as long as possible (usually about 60 seconds). The joint space was not changed when subjects were biting on the stabilization appliances, but it was significantly reduced when subjects were biting on the mandibular repositioning appliances.

Thus, it appears that partial-coverage appliances can be effective in reducing TMD symptoms, but they have the potential to produce a malocclusion and internal TMJ changes. Therefore, in the absence of data proving that they "stop" bruxism any better than complete-arch appliances, they do not seem to be a logical choice of therapy for TMD symptoms, except in those patients with definite and persistent clenching habits.

Repositioning Appliances

Repositioning appliances have also been used extensively to treat TMJ clicking since the early 1970s, when a repositioning appliance was first described to "recapture" anteriorly displaced discs.[68] Although these devices may reduce TMJ clicking in the short term, they often irreversibly change the occlusal relationship as well, thereby creating the need for major occlusal corrective procedures. This change might be acceptable if the condyle-disc derangement were permanently stabilized. However, data from long-term case report studies suggest that the TMJ clicking generally returns over time, and, even in the absence of audible joint sounds, most of the patients do not experience a normalization of the disc position as a result of the treatment.[69–79]

In 2002, one study examined the efficacy of the anterior repositioning appliance and used disc position on magnetic resonance imaging (MRI) as the primary outcome criterion.[80] The investigators examined 52 TMJs of

30 patients with TMJ derangement and found that 42 TMJs were abnormal (exhibiting anterior displacement without reduction [ADwoR], anterior displacement with reduction [ADwR], or osteoarthtitis). All 30 patients were given repositioning appliances, and images were taken before insertion of the appliance and immediately after insertion.

The postinsertion images revealed recapture of discs with a protrusive (repositioning) appliance in only 50% of the TMJ. If only those TMJs that had MRI-confirmed reducing disc displacements (ADwR) were counted, the recapture rate increased to 83% (15 of 18). However, the attempts to recapture the articular disc in those patients with ADwoR and with osteoarthritic changes were judged as uniformly unsuccessful.[80]

These results indicate why the treatment of so many patients with repositioning appliances has been unsuccessful at either eliminating joint sounds or improving TMJ mechanics. However, the remaining issue of long-term condyle-disc stability was not addressed in this study, because the investigators did not examine for joint sounds in the "successful" patients over time to see if the 15 recaptured discs were stable and joint sounds remained absent.[80]

In another study, reported in 2004, patients with an anterior repositioning appliance and a complete-arch maxillary stabilization appliance were compared to an untreated control group.[15] The study included 40 young patients (average age of 16.8 years; range 8.0 to 24.0 years) with confirmed internal derangement, joint pain, and joint noises in at least one TMJ for at least 2 months. The repositioning appliance was given to 20 subjects and the stabilization appliance to another 20 subjects. Ten untreated patients formed a control group. Visual analog scale ratings of pain intensity were collected monthly across the 8-month study period. The authors reported that pain was reduced significantly in the repositioning appliance group. However, the frequency of joint noises decreased over time in all three groups, and ultimately the authors concluded that the repositioning appliance was not better than the stabilization appliance for treating joint noises.

Therefore, because repositioning appliances can induce a major irreversible change in the patient's occlusion, and also because TMJ clicking frequently returns or is not substantially reduced following their use, these kinds of appliance are not a logical choice for treating TMJ disc derangement.

Conclusion

The reviewed studies suggest that occlusal appliances, when used for treating TMDs, function mainly as behavioral interventions and not as mechanical devices for altering the patients' maxillomandibular relationships. In fact, inducing a deliberate change in the vertical or horizontal position of the mandible with an oral appliance is likely to be problematic, because it usually requires a permanent change to be made in occlusal relationships afterward. Such iatrogenic changes generally should be avoided, especially when it has been demonstrated that reversible treatments (including appropriate oral appliances) can be equally effective for relieving pain and dysfunction in patients with TMDs (see chapter 14).

Support for the concept that oral appliances work as a behavioral intervention is derived from the repeated findings that patients who wear occlusal appliances clearly have better results than a wait-list control group but do not achieve better results than those using a credible nonocclusal appliance, which is itself a nonspecific behavioral therapy. If appliances are actually behavioral treatments, they are probably producing their therapeutic effect by changing jaw posture as well as motor activity, but this has not been proven conclusively. The limited short-term EMG data that are available suggest that sleep-related bruxism can be altered by a stabilization appliance as well as a nonoccluding appliance, but this effect may not be long lasting. In addition, what happens to daytime masticatory motor patterns when patients wear an appliance at night has not been determined.

When oral appliances were compared directly to a true behavior-modifying therapy such as biofeedback or relaxation therapy, they were shown to be essentially equal in efficacy. However, it must be acknowledged that an occlusal appliance certainly can function as a physical device that protects the teeth from attrition and high-force loading when worn. This benefit has not been contested in the literature and, when such a clinical situation exists, the prescription of an occlusal appliance is both reasonable and rational. Moreover, if the patient's teeth do not contact in a stable manner, occlusal appliances also can be used to provide a quick way of achieving a stable occlusal contact pattern until the occlusion is restored. Logic suggests that occlusal appliances might work best for those TMD patients who have parafunction-associated muscle, joint, or tooth pain. What is needed is additional information about which, if any, TMD subgroups would be most likely to benefit from an occlusal appliance.

Even in the absence of that information, it is clear that the stabilization-type oral appliance is an easily used, potentially long-term, and clinically effective treatment intervention with reasonable nightly patient compliance and good outcomes. Unless it is worn 24 hours a day, it has few potential complications. It is also reasonable to use a partial-coverage anterior bite appliance in those patients with a known tooth-clenching habit, because this habit cannot be controlled with a stabilization appliance. However, a confounder in almost all of the studies described in this chapter is that (with the exception of one study) none has confirmed that the experimental subjects were exhibiting oral parafunctional behavior during the study (eg, tooth clenching or grinding) or that any appliance altered this behavior.

Considering all of the available data, pro and con, it can be concluded that the oral stabilization appliance (one that does not strive to change the occlusion) has sufficient evidence to support its use for the management of localized myalgia and arthralgia of the masticatory system. It is much less likely to induce an inadvertent malocclusion, which is a strong negative consideration when the clinician is considering using either a repositioning or any partial-coverage oral appliance, especially over an extended period. Finally, the use of mandibular repositioning appliances to treat internal derangements of the TMJ is not supported by the scientific literature.

References

1. Okeson JP. Management of Temporomandibular Disorders and Occlusion, ed 4. St Louis: Mosby, 1998:474–502.
2. Biondi DM. Headaches and their relationship to sleep. Dent Clin North Am 2001;45:685–700.
3. Henrikson T, Nilner M. Temporomandibular disorders and the need for stomatognathic treatment in orthodontically treated and untreated girls. Eur J Orthod 2000;22:283–292.
4. Major PW, Nebbe B. Use and effectiveness of splint appliance therapy: Review of literature. Cranio 1997;15:159–166.
5. Bush FM. Tinnitus and otalgia in temporomandibular disorders. J Prosthet Dent 1987;58:495–498.
6. Andreasen JO, Andreasen FM, Mejare I, Cvek M. Healing of 400 intra-alveolar root fractures. 1. Effect of pre-injury and injury factors such as sex, age, stage of root development, fracture type, location of fracture and severity of dislocation. Dent Traumatol 2004;20:192–202.
7. Capp NJ. Occlusion and splint therapy. Br Dent J 1999;186:217–222.
8. Ekberg E, Vallon D, Nilner M. Treatment outcome of headache after occlusal appliance therapy in a randomised controlled trial among patients with temporomandibular disorders of mainly arthrogenous origin. Swed Dent J 2002;26:115–124.
9. Franco AA, Yamashita HK, Lederman HM, Cevidanes LH, Proffit WR, Vigorito JW. Frankel appliance therapy and the temporomandibular disc: A prospective magnetic resonance imaging study. Am J Orthod Dentofacial Orthop 2002;121:447–457.
10. Davies SJ, Gray RJ. The pattern of splint usage in the management of two common temporomandibular disorders. 1. The anterior repositioning splint in the treatment of disc displacement with reduction. Br Dent J 1997;183:199–203.
11. Linde C, Isacsson G, Jonsson BG. Outcome of 6-week treatment with transcutaneous electric nerve stimulation compared with splint on symptomatic temporomandibular joint disk displacement without reduction. Acta Odontol Scand 1995;53:92–98.
12. Shankland WE. Nociceptive trigeminal inhibition—Tension suppression system: A method of preventing migraine and tension headaches. Compend Contin Educ Dent 2002;23:105–108, 110, 112–113.
13. Shankland WE. Nociceptive trigeminal inhibition—Tension suppression system: A method of preventing migraine and tension headaches. Compend Contin Educ Dent 2001;22:1075–1080, 1082 [corrected and republished 2002;23:105–108, 112–113].
14. Shankland WE II. Migraine and tension-type headache reduction through pericranial muscular suppression: A preliminary report. Cranio 2001;19:269–278.
15. Tecco S, Festa F, Salini V, Epifania E, D'Attilio M. Treatment of joint pain and joint noises associated with a recent TMJ internal derangement: A comparison of an anterior repositioning splint, a full-arch maxillary stabilization splint, and an untreated control group. Cranio 2004;22:209–219.
16. Baar EH, Yarshansky OH, Ben Yehuda A. Intracoronal incisal splint. J Prosthet Dent 1993;70:491–492.
17. Kilpatrick SR. Use of the pivot appliance in the treatment of temporomandibular disorders. Cranio Clin Int 1991;1:107–121.
18. Becker I, Tarantola G, Zambrano J, Spitzer S, Oquendo D. Effect of a prefabricated anterior bite stop on electromyographic activity of masticatory muscles. J Prosthet Dent 1999;82:22–26.
19. Tsukiyama Y, Baba K, Clark GT. An evidence-based assessment of occlusal adjustment as a treatment for temporomandibular disorders. J Prosthet Dent 2001;86:57–66.
20. Gray RJ, Davies SJ, Quayle AA, Wastell DG. A comparison of two splints in the treatment of TMJ pain dysfunction syndrome. Can occlusal analysis be used to predict success of splint therapy? Br Dent J 1991;170:55–58.
21. Magnusson T, Adiels AM, Nilsson HL, Helkimo M. Treatment effect on signs and symptoms of temporomandibular disorders—Comparison between stabilisation splint and a new type of splint (NTI). A pilot study. Swed Dent J 2004;28:11–20.
22. Williamson EH, Rosenzweig BJ. The treatment of temporomandibular disorders through repositioning splint therapy: A follow-up study. Cranio 1998;16:222–225.

23. Sato H, Fujii T, Uetani M, Kitamori H. Anterior mandibular repositioning in a patient with temporomandibular disorders: A clinical and tomographic follow-up case report. Cranio 1997;15:84–88.

24. Kurita H, Ohtsuka A, Kurashina K, Kopp S. A study of factors for successful splint capture of anteriorly displaced temporomandibular joint disc with disc repositioning appliance. J Oral Rehabil 2001;28:651–657.

25. Kreiner M, Betancor E, Clark GT. Occlusal stabilization appliances. Evidence of their efficacy. J Am Dent Assoc 2001;132:770–777.

26. Widmalm SE. Use and abuse of bite splints. Compend Contin Educ Dent 1999;20:249–254, 256, 258–259.

27. National Institutes of Health–National Oral Health Information Clearing House [website]. Available at: http://www.nidcr.nih.gov/HealthInformation/SpecialCareResources/default.html. Accessed 16 Jan 2005.

28. American Academy of Orofacial Pain [website]. Available at: http://www.aaop.org. Accessed 16 Sept 2005.

29. American Association of Oral and Maxillofacial Surgeons [website]. Available at: http://www.aaoms.org. Accessed 6 Aug 2005.

30. American Academy of Craniofacial Pain [website]. Available at: http://www.aacfp.org. Accessed 27 June 2005.

31. National Institutes of Health Technology Assessment Conference on Management of Temporomandibular Disorders. Proceedings. Oral Surg Oral Med Oral Pathol Oral Radiol Endod 1997;83:49–183.

32. Marbach JJ, Raphael KG. Future directions in the treatment of chronic musculoskeletal facial pain: The role of evidence-based care. Oral Surg Oral Med Oral Pathol Oral Radiol Endod 1997;83:170–176.

33. Dao TT, Lavigne GJ. Oral splints: The crutches for temporomandibular disorders and bruxism? Crit Rev Oral Biol Med 1998;9:345–361.

34. Turp JC, Komine F, Hugger A. Efficacy of stabilization splints for the management of patients with masticatory muscle pain: A qualitative systematic review. Clin Oral Investig 2004;8:179–195.

35. Forssell H, Kalso E. Application of principles of evidence-based medicine to occlusal treatment for temporomandibular disorders: Are there lessons to be learned? J Orofac Pain 2004;18:9–22; discussion 23–32.

36. Forssell H, Kalso E, Koskela P, Vehmanen R, Puukka P, Alanen P. Occlusal treatments in temporomandibular disorders: A qualitative systematic review of randomized controlled trials. Pain 1999;83:549–560.

37. Al-Ani MZ, Davies SJ, Gray RJM, Sloan P, Glenny AM. Stabilisation splint therapy for temporomandibular pain dysfunction syndrome. The Cochrane Database of Systematic Reviews [website]. In: The Cochrane Library, Issue 1, 2004. Oxford, England: Update Software. Available at: http://www.mrw.interscience.wiley.com/cochrane/clsysrev/articles/CD002778/frame.html. Accessed 10 March 2005.

38. White L, Tursky B, Schwartz G. Placebo: Theory, Research and Mechanisms. New York: Guilford Press, 1985.

39. Smith TC, Thompson TL II. The inherent, powerful therapeutic value of a good physician-patient relationship. Psychosomatics 1993;34:166–170.

40. Thomas KB. General practice consultations: Is there any point in being positive? Br Med J (Clin Res Ed) 1987;294 (6581):1200–1202.

41. Wolf S. Effects of suggestion and conditioning on the action of chemical agents in human subjects; the pharmacology of placebos. J Clin Invest 1950;29:100–109.

42. Dinnerstein AJ, Halm J. Modification of placebo effects by means of drugs: Effects of aspirin and placebos on self-rated moods. J Abnorm Psychol 1970;75:308–314.

43. Dinnerstein AJ, Lowenthal M, Blitz B. The interaction of drugs with placebos in the control of pain and anxiety. Perspect Biol Med 1966;10:103–117.

44. Fletcher R, Fletcher S, Wagner E. Clinical Epidemiology: The Essentials, ed 2. Baltimore: Williams & Wilkins, 1988:137.

45. Dube C, Rompre PH, Manzini C, Guitard F, de Grandmont P, Lavigne GJ. Quantitative polygraphic controlled study on efficacy and safety of oral splint devices in tooth-grinding subjects. J Dent Res 2004;83:398–403.

46. Greene CS, Laskin DM. Splint therapy for the myofascial pain–dysfunction (MPD) syndrome: A comparative study. J Am Dent Assoc 1972;84:624–628.

47. Rubinoff MS, Gross A, McCall WD Jr. Conventional and nonoccluding splint therapy compared for patients with myofascial pain dysfunction syndrome. Gen Dent 1987;35:502–506.

48. Dao TT, Lavigne GJ, Charbonneau A, Feine JS, Lund JP. The efficacy of oral splints in the treatment of myofascial pain of the jaw muscles: A controlled clinical trial. Pain 1994;56:85–94.

49. Ekberg EC, Vallon D, Nilner M. Occlusal appliance therapy in patients with temporomandibular disorders. A double-blind controlled study in a short-term perspective. Acta Odontol Scand 1998;56:122–128.

50. Kuttila M, Le Bell Y, Savolainen-Niemi E, Kuttila S, Alanen P. Efficiency of occlusal appliance therapy in secondary otalgia and temporomandibular disorders. Acta Odontol Scand 2002;60:248–254.

51. Wassell RW, Adams N, Kelly PJ. Treatment of temporomandibular disorders by stabilising splints in general dental practice: Results after initial treatment. Br Dent J 2004;197:35–41; discussion 31.

52. Clark GT, Beemsterboer PL, Solberg WK, Rugh JD. Nocturnal electromyographic evaluation of myofascial pain dysfunction in patients undergoing occlusal splint therapy. J Am Dent Assoc 1979;99:607–611.

53. Dahlstrom L, Carlsson GE, Carlsson SG. Comparison of effects of electromyographic biofeedback and occlusal splint therapy on mandibular dysfunction. Scand J Dent Res 1982;90:151–156.

54. Okeson JP, Moody PM, Kemper JT, Haley JV. Evaluation of occlusal splint therapy and relaxation procedures in patients with temporomandibular disorders. J Am Dent Assoc 1983;107:420–424.

55. Johansson A, Wenneberg B, Wagersten C, Haraldson T. Acupuncture in treatment of facial muscular pain. Acta Odontol Scand 1991;49:153–158.

56. List T, Helkimo M, Andersson S, Carlsson GE. Acupuncture and occlusal splint therapy in the treatment of craniomandibular disorders. 1. A comparative study. Swed Dent J 1992; 16:125–141.

57. Turk DC, Zaki HS, Rudy TE. Effects of intraoral appliance and biofeedback/stress management alone and in combination in treating pain and depression in patients with temporomandibular disorders. J Prosthet Dent 1993;70:158–164.

58. Wright E, Anderson G, Schulte J. A randomized clinical trial of intraoral soft splints and palliative treatment for masticatory muscle pain. J Orofac Pain 1995;9:192–199.

59. Sheikholeslam A, Holmgren K, Riise C. A clinical and electromyographic study of the long-term effects of an occlusal splint on the temporal and masseter muscles in patients with functional disorders and nocturnal bruxism. J Oral Rehabil 1986;13:137–145.

60. Chung SC, Kim YK, Kim HS. Prevalence and patterns of nocturnal bruxofacets on stabilization splints in temporomandibular disorder patients. Cranio 2000;18:92–97.

61. Korioth TW, Bohlig KG, Anderson GC. Digital assessment of occlusal wear patterns on occlusal stabilization splints: A pilot study. J Prosthet Dent 1998;80:209–213.

62. Shaw RM, Molyneux GS. The effects of induced dental malocclusion on the fibrocartilage disc of the adult rabbit temporomandibular joint. Arch Oral Biol 1993;38:415–422.

63. Sindelar BJ, Edwards S, Herring SW. Morphologic changes in the TMJ following splint wear. Anat Rec 2002;266:167–176.

64. Wichelhaus A, Huffmeier S, Sander FG. Dynamic functional force measurements on an anterior bite plane during the night. J Orofac Orthop 2003;64:417–425.

65. Kuboki T, Azuma Y, Orsini MG, Takenami Y, Yamashita A. Effects of sustained unilateral molar clenching on the temporomandibular joint space. Oral Surg Oral Med Oral Pathol Oral Radiol Endod 1996;82:616–624.

66. Takenami Y, Kuboki T, Acero CO Jr, Maekawa K, Yamashita A, Azuma Y. The effects of sustained incisal clenching on the temporomandibular joint space. Dentomaxillofac Radiol 1999; 28:214–218.

67. Kuboki T, Takenami Y, Orsini MG, et al. Effect of occlusal appliances and clenching on the internally deranged TMJ space. J Orofac Pain 1999;13:38–48.

68. Farrar WB. Diagnosis and treatment of anterior dislocation of the articular disc. N Y J Dent 1971;41:348–351.

69. Clark GT. A critical evaluation of orthopedic interocclusal appliance therapy: Design, theory, and overall effectiveness. J Am Dent Assoc 1984;108:359–364.

70. Clark GT, Lanham F, Flack VF. Treatment outcome results for consecutive TMJ clinic patients. J Craniomandib Disord 1988;2:87–95.

71. Okeson JP. Long-term treatment of disk-interference disorders of the temporomandibular joint with anterior repositioning occlusal splints. J Prosthet Dent 1988;60:611–616.

72. LeBell Y, Kirveskari P. Treatment of reciprocal clicking of the temporomandibular joint using a mandibular repositioning splint and occlusal adjustment. Proc Finn Dent Soc 1985;81: 251–255.

73. Moloney F, Howard JA. Internal derangements of the temporomandibular joint. 3. Anterior repositioning splint therapy. Aust Dent J 1986;31:30–39.

74. Anderson GC, Schulte JK, Goodkind RJ. Comparative study of two treatment methods for internal derangement of the temporomandibular joint. J Prosthet Dent 1985;53:392–397.

75. Lundh H, Westesson PL, Kopp S, Tillstrom B. Anterior repositioning splint in the treatment of temporomandibular joints with reciprocal clicking: Comparison with a flat occlusal splint and an untreated control group. Oral Surg Oral Med Oral Pathol 1985;60:131–136.

76. Lundh H, Westesson PL. Long-term follow-up after occlusal treatment to correct abnormal temporomandibular joint disk position. Oral Surg Oral Med Oral Pathol 1989;67:2–10.

77. Hersek N, Uzun G, Cindas A, Canay S, Kutsal YG. Effect of anterior repositioning splints on the electromyographic activities of masseter and anterior temporalis muscles. Cranio 1998;16:11–16.

78. Tallents RH, Katzberg RW, Macher DJ, Roberts CA. Use of protrusive splint therapy in anterior disk displacement of the temporomandibular joint: A 1- to 3-year follow-up. J Prosthet Dent 1990;63:336–341.

79. Summer JD, Westesson PL. Mandibular repositioning can be effective in treatment of reducing TMJ disk displacement. A long-term clinical and MR imaging follow-up. Cranio 1997;15:107–120.

80. Eberhard D, Bantleon HP, Steger W. The efficacy of anterior repositioning splint therapy studied by magnetic resonance imaging. Eur J Orthod 2002;24:343–352.

Biobehavioral Therapy

Richard Ohrbach

The extent of psychological distress and psychosocial dysfunction is the same in individuals with chronic pain from a temporomandibular disorder (TMD) as it is in those with any other chronic pain condition. Consequently, knowledge about chronic pain in general should be applied to the evaluation and treatment of persistent TMD pain. A biobehavioral evaluation will reveal the behavioral, psychological, and psychosocial information relevant to an individual's pain problem (see chapter 13). That evaluation, performed in an escalating manner dependent on each patient's level of need, leads to an understanding of individual differences in how patients present with chronic pain. This, in turn, leads to the development of a tailored treatment program. An integration of the findings from a biobehavioral evaluation into a problem-oriented assessment (such as "stress responses," "depressed mood," "inability to relax," and "high level of treatment seeking") will point toward the types and extent of biobehavioral treatments likely to be helpful for each individual.

This chapter addresses the scope of these treatments, their relevance for TMD-related pain and dysfunction, and the link between biobehavioral treatments and the customary physical treatments. The primary thrust can be summarized succinctly: All pain is real, conventional physical treatments for TMD pain produce substantial nonspecific therapeutic effects, and integrative treatment (ie, appropriately combining physical and biobehavioral treatments) increases the likelihood of better outcomes as pain becomes more chronic and more pervasive in its impact on the individual.

The physical diagnosis of a chronic TMD pain problem, in contrast to that of a carious tooth, for example, does not provide a basis for an accurate prediction of treatment outcome. This problem of poor prediction of treatment outcome for patients with chronic TMD pain is exemplified by the frequently observed inconsistency between the physical findings (or functional status) and the levels of reported pain, pain behavior, and disability.[1] Herein lies the rationale for biobehavioral treatment: Within a given range of clinical symptoms (eg, related to TMD pain), there may be a wide range of psychosocial functioning.

Often, a particular disorder is expected to be responsive to a specific treatment, the implication being that the treatment will resolve the particular problem. When there is no improvement, the patient may be referred to a psychologist; obviously, the pain must not be real, because the treatment specific for that disorder did not work. An evaluation that includes a clear consideration of both the biobehavioral and biomedical treatment domains at the outset will improve predicted treatment outcomes. Furthermore, it will prevent subsequent problems associated with treatment failure, such as a psychological referral made *after* the physical treatment has failed, which implies that the patient's pain is not real.

Treatments for TMDs that are oriented to address only the physical diagnosis do not work reliably for the following reasons:

1. They ignore behavior (eg, motor behavior or frequently observed habits) and its impact on the masticatory system.
2. They ignore the patient's psychological status as an influence on both behavior and pain reporting.
3. They ignore the influence of the patient's psychological status on treatment response within the physical domain.
4. They ignore the interaction between environmental factors (for example, stress, substance abuse, or chronic sleep problems) that precipitate or aggravate pain episodes and the patient's role in maintaining that environment.

Prerequisites for Success

Before biobehavioral treatment approaches for chronic TMD pain are discussed, three issues central to the context for providing that treatment must be addressed. The first issue is how to conceptualize the vast array of information potentially available from a patient's history, including attention to the psychosocial realm.[2–5] The way that a clinician conceptualizes such information has an impact on which biobehavioral treatments are selected, how they will be presented to the patient, and how they will be implemented. The second issue is mind-body relations, which provides the large context for all biobehavioral and biomedical treatment for TMD pain. Patients seem to accept that the body and the mind interact when that concept is presented in a nonthreatening way. The third issue is the development of a collaborative relationship; a biobehavioral treatment model can easily subsume biomedical approaches to treatment but not the reverse. All three of these issues are connected.

Positive Conceptualization of Patients' Needs

Significant biobehavioral findings should be referred to as *problems* rather than given psychiatric labels. Although thinking in terms of psychiatric diagnosis may be useful at the level of assessment, this approach is less useful when the clinician is linking assessment to treatment. When used to describe the psychosocial functioning of a particular individual, psychiatric labels such as *major depression*, *somatization*, and *hypochondriasis* tend to be confrontational to the patient who is presenting with pain as the primary complaint. Rather, the obtained information should be integrated at a descriptive level.

Certainly, specific constellations of psychosocial data do occur in patients with chronic pain, leading to appropriate psychiatric diagnoses (eg, major depression). However, because of the elusiveness of clear physical signs of a disease, patients with chronic pain are often labeled with psychiatric terms in an attempt to explain their symptoms. Such patients often feel dismissed because no one takes their complaints seriously, or they believe that their complaints are viewed as "imaginary" or "all in the head." Although certain psychiatric terms, such as *somatization* or *major depression*, are often theoretically correct as an explanation for an individual's symptoms, his or her biobehavioral data should be integrated as *problems* as close to the behavioral level as possible; consequently, the pain problem remains in the foreground. This approach leads logically to the types of treatment available, and patients seem to exhibit better acceptance. Further, a behavioral formulation or conceptualization based on common-sense terms is more appropriate for the practitioner who is not trained in mental health interviewing and diagnosis.

Acknowledgment of Mind-Body Relations

The relationship between pain and psychological factors is commonly viewed only as the impact of pain on psychological functioning (eg, depression or other mood changes, marital or family dysfunction, substance abuse, employment problems, or social dysfunction). With chronicity, however, psychological factors exert a multidimensional impact on the pain. When this concept is stated clinically, the patient typically responds, "but *my* pain is real." That is, when talking about emotional or psychological issues in conjunction with TMD pain, many people (both healthcare providers and patients) immediately jump to the implication that emotional and psychological factors are causal to the pain. Accordingly, and unfortunately, a dichotomy is formed: The pain must be *either* psychological *or* physical in origin.

In contrast to this dualist view, the empirical evidence demonstrates a reciprocal dynamic relationship: There is a psychological context within which chronic pain develops and is maintained, and that context is linked inherently to the pain itself. That is, chronic pain is not some external thing that attacks a person. Every physical sensation has an emotional aspect (attraction or aversion) and a cognitive aspect (search for meaning or understanding); when someone feels a sting to the skin and says, "Oh, it is a mosquito," the person is also expressing relief that it is not something else that is presumably more sinister.

When a patient experiences pain in the face but is not able to see the source of the pain, and when healthcare providers are not able to find the source of the pain, it is not uncommon to feel worse: The experienced pain *and* reported pain escalate because of the patient's fear of a serious, potentially life-threatening problem. In this case, the pain, the fear, and the prior experience of others expressing views about the legitimacy of the pain all must be considered when the specifics about a particular individual are evaluated. Such patients present with mind-body problems. These beliefs have to be explored as part of the treatment.

Although not specifically trained in providing biobehavioral treatment, the dentist has a very important role in helping people with chronic pain. By providing explanations and treatments from both domains, ie, biobehavioral as well as biomedical, the dentist can help the patient bridge the dichotomy between body and mind. Presented with a suggestion that psychological factors are involved with their pain, patients often respond with an exaggerated style reflecting disagreement or with flat-out denial by contending that their pain is "real pain." The most important person who can address this dualism is the patient's general practitioner (dentist or physician). The dentist can avoid getting trapped into taking sides with the physical domain—that is, trying to find the hidden physical cause for such clinical problems to please the patient—by following these recommendations: Use valid and reliable diagnostic tests, escalate diagnostic testing appropriately, maintain a long-term commitment to the patient, and remain sensible.

Development of a Collaborative Relationship

The most critical issue emerging from the past 20 years of research and clinical treatment involving the person with chronic pain is the importance of self-management in treatment. This holds true regardless of whether the primary treatment is biomedical or whether it is biobehavioral. All the treatments advocated in this book require the active participation of the patient to be effective, although some therapies require less participation than others. For example, proper surgical management of a joint problem requires postsurgical mobility exercises. The standard belief implied by the biomedical model is that if the correct diagnosis is identified and the correct treatment is selected, the patient's disease will be cured. However, in patients with chronic disease and illness, such as chronic TMD pain, behavioral and psychological adaptation has occurred during the development of the clinical problem. These adaptive changes will often interfere with the expected outcome from the biomedical treatment. Thus, all treatments benefit from the use of a biobehavioral approach.

Linked to the importance of self-management is the readiness of the patient to embrace the commitment to self-management.[6,7] Participation by the patient is often termed *compliance*. However, the definition of this term implies that the patient does exactly what the dentist or physician has prescribed. For self-management–based treatments to be effective, a different type of relationship is advocated, one that the biobehavioral model provides: in this relationship, the provider and patient work together and make decisions in consultation with one another.

One problem encountered in the delivery of any kind of treatment is that the provider's explanatory model regarding how disease and illness are remedied says that the patient *should* comply fully with the provider's treatment prescription. However, the patient's explanatory model regarding illness may say that full compliance with the provider's prescription is important but, then again, it may not be. Many patients do not agree with following "doctor's orders," and they will often not follow the prescription and will not let the provider know that the treatment has been scuttled. This phenomenon is well known in the area of medication treatment for serious diseases, such as cardiac problems; patients systematically take less medication than prescribed, and they often do not tell their providers about this because they know that their provider will disapprove and perhaps even be angry. Such an interaction between patient and provider exemplifies the problems inherent to approaching treatment from a purely biomedical perspective: a provider-patient collaboration has not been achieved.

Thus, the conceptualization of behavioral and psychosocial complications associated with chronic pain as mind-body problems, and the application of that concept to a collaborative treatment process that identifies the patient as central to treatment delivery, are both essential to all treatments that are provided to patients with TMDs. This perspective begins with patient assessment and not with treatment.

Treatment Approaches

Biobehavioral treatments can be extremely effective for chronic TMD pain. These treatments are generally not standardized, which means that they are most effective when tailored specifically to the individual. Although they require extensive specialized training in order to be implemented optimally, particularly for the patient who has a serious illness, there are levels at which these techniques can be used by a provider who is not trained specifically in their optimal use.

Counseling

Counseling can be defined as communication of recommendations or advice by the provider to the patient. Counseling may take on a more active role after an adequate biobehavioral evaluation has been performed, because then the dentist will have much greater information available about the patient and his or her functioning. At that point, the dentist's ability to have some influence on the patient's behavior would presumably increase. However, counseling by itself has little effect overall in the treatment of pain. Receiving comforting advice, well-intended recommendations, or polite platitudes about healthy living from the dentist can certainly feel pleasant to the patient, but the comfort is generally short lived, particularly for the psychosocially dysfunctional patient.

Counseling, as a modality, is quite limited because it does not provide a structured context by which the patient can acquire new knowledge and skills. It is new skills that many patients need, particularly when active coping and perceived control are low and when depression, anxiety, and somatization are high. In other words, it is the patient's behavior that ultimately must be modified to a more adaptive stage. Therefore, counseling can only be considered as successful when it helps the patient to see changes across time with respect to symptoms (and how they are linked to lifestyle factors).

Stress Management

There are few medical disorders or illnesses that do not worsen in the presence of stress.[8] Stress is a common reason accepted by patients with chronic TMD pain for considering biobehavioral treatment, and stress management is a treatment concept familiar to such patients. Stress management is generally considered to be short-term therapy focusing on skill building (much like that described in the section on cognitive-behavioral treatment of pain).

To the extent that there are particular skills that can be taught and that can be generally helpful for the individual who has difficulty in coping with stress, such short-term therapy may be useful. However, many other factors, such as prior beliefs, manner of conducting interpersonal relationships, and the interaction of stress and pain, commonly underlie the stress experience in patients with chronic pain but are not necessarily addressed by stress management approaches. These issues should be considered when the clinician selects the type and extent of any biobehavioral treatment that is likely to be best for a given patient. Nevertheless, stress management is often an excellent first step toward a more comprehensive or inclusive biobehavioral treatment approach.

The similarity between stress and pain, in terms of mechanism, also suggests that treatment for stress should often be considered from a broader perspective. For example, the more general term *distress* (rather than *stress*) includes all of the mood changes and other forms of unhappiness that seem to be important. Just as the model of nociception presents pain as a neural process initiated by a potentially damaging stimulus (pressure, heat, or inflammation), stress likewise is often initiated by a stimulus, usually an event.[9] As a stimulus, an event

can be internal (that is, intrapsychic or created in the individual's mind, such as a worry or a memory of something that happened yesterday) or external (such as a recurring marital fight or dealing with a difficult employer). However, even an external event, like nociception following activation from a receptor in response to external injury, becomes transduced via the appropriate sense organs and enters into perception and appraisal, just as nociception can become pain. The behavior that the person exhibits in response to such events contributes powerfully to the impact that the event has and will continue to exert on him or her. Thus, stress includes the individual's experience of the event, as well as his or her style of coping with it, all of which will have consequences for the individual.

From this perspective, the kind of skill training needed for pain management is the same kind of skill training needed for stress management. Therefore, the patient with severe stress-related problems as well as pain should have both managed simultaneously, because failure to address the severe stress-related reactions can interfere with the appropriate biomedical treatment for the pain. This is particularly true because chronic pain is not only a significant cause of stress but often the most significant cause.

One special form of stress reaction is anger, including its more specific forms, such as frustration or rage. Anger reactions are typically characteristic of the individual. They generally represent nonproductive ways of coping with challenging or threatening events. The psychophysiologic process associated with anger typically escalates musculoskeletal pain through increased bodily guarding behaviors and diminished resilience. It is difficult to teach relaxation skills to someone who experiences frequent anger reactions.[10] Consequently, anger must be addressed at the outset of biobehavioral treatment.

Biofeedback

Biofeedback is probably the best known of the therapies that approach the mind-body union. Biofeedback for muscular pain and tension uses a measurement device, commonly electrodes that are attached to the skin overlying muscle and connected to an amplifier. This device produces a visual or auditory signal that is based on the amount of motor unit activation. The theory is that, if the patient can gain a sense of the input strength, he or she can learn to control the behavior that produces the input signal. When used for chronic TMD pain, the electrodes are generally attached to the masseter or temporalis muscle and the patient uses the feedback (tone, light, or meter indicator) from the amplifier to learn how to control the level of muscle contraction as well as to integrate a kinesthetic perception of the level of muscle tonus.

This treatment was popular for several decades, declined in popularity, and is now undergoing resurgence. Although much research had shown that biofeedback treatment for muscle pain is efficacious,[11] the theory was significantly challenged when experiments showed that pain decreased regardless of whether a patient increased or decreased the level of muscle activity.[12] Although all of those studies focused on headache, the negative results contributed to the decline in the popularity of biofeedback for the treatment of chronic TMD pain.

Nevertheless, clinical trials indicate that biofeedback continues to be useful for teaching certain TMD patients how to regulate their body tension.[11,13–15] This is particularly the case when other, more behavioral methods have failed. The mechanism then appears to be less that of learning muscle relaxation per se but more that of learning motor control. Indeed, relaxation of the muscles can be learned much quicker than continuous intentional control over the state of muscle activation. A single trial of biofeedback, consisting of assessment and instruction in control and perception, can often be quite powerful when accompanied by appropriate behavioral follow-up.

The following is one of many possible approaches to biofeedback therapy.[16] Electrodes are attached to the skin overlying the painful muscle, following the method recommended by the amplifier manufacturer, and the gain is set appropriately. While the feedback indicator is shielded from the patient's view, the patient is given 5 minutes to relax; the baseline level and 5-minute level of muscle tension are assessed. During the relaxation period, the starting and ending levels of muscle tension are observed.

If the level started high and stayed high 5 minutes later, biofeedback could be very helpful in teaching the patient how to relax the muscles. If the level started high and ended low, the patient is able to relax the muscles but may need help in learning how to do it more quickly and under less serene circumstances or in identifying his or her ability to relax the muscles. If the level started low and ended low, then the provider should first suspect that the behavior observed in the office is not representative of the behavior emitted in other environments. This finding is common in patients with parafunctional behaviors. For these patients, biofeedback is not likely to be useful.

A reasonable resting level of masseter muscle contraction is 1 to 3 μV, although patients can easily learn to decrease resting levels consistently to less than 2 μV with a relatively small amount of practice. Patients appear to report substantial reductions in pain and subjective jaw tension.

Patients who are asked to relax the jaw often do not know what that means and hence cannot comply. A method useful in teaching relaxation, after a baseline level is established, is to ask the patient to *increase* the tension up to a certain level and hold it for 5 to 10 seconds; the amount of increase requested can be as small as 1 μV or much greater, depending on the patient's capability. The patient is then asked to lower the tension level back to the baseline level. Next, the patient is asked to raise the level again and to then lower it. Then the patient is encouraged, after the tension level is raised and lowered again to baseline, to continue to lower the level even beyond the initial baseline and to hold the tension at that level, now the new baseline. Cycles are alternated in this way, and a new baseline might be established on alternate trials, depending on how fast the patient learns to relax. The entire session might last about 20 to 30 minutes, including rest periods.

Interspersed with cycles of increasing tension and release, while the patient is paying attention to the feedback signal and always working toward increasingly lower baseline resting levels, it is important to add trials without the feedback. First, while the patient is increasing and decreasing the level of muscle contraction with feedback, he or she should be asked to also notice the internal sensations accompanying the changing levels of muscle tension. That is, the patient is asked to rely on internal proprioception instead of the external monitoring. Using these sensations as feedback, the patient is then asked to increase contraction and hold, and then decrease contraction to the previous baseline level and hold, using the proprioception that has been developed during the preceding trial. The patient then returns to the feedback trials to check the level of relaxation produced by the newly calibrated proprioception versus the external signal. Several biofeedback sessions spaced 1 to 2 weeks apart should be adequate for the patient to learn the appropriate muscle control and relaxation skills. Home practice of these skills is strongly emphasized.

Monitoring of the internal state is essential for the patient to rapidly generalize from the clinic to the natural environment. Further generalization includes considering the influence of environmental factors (for example, marital strain) on postural activity of the jaw. Although this can be addressed simultaneously with the biofeedback treatment, it is not expected that the dentist will have that kind of therapy skill. Instead, this aspect of treatment might be addressed by referral to an appropriate specialist or within a cognitive-behavioral treatment program (discussed in the next section).

Before biofeedback is implemented, the patient should first be taught a behavioral method of jaw postural control that avoids muscle overuse, because a behavioral approach is generally all that is needed for most patients. For patients who have difficulty in learning to monitor their internal state or in interpreting the proprioceptive signals, the progress achieved with biofeedback therapy is much quicker if they have already been learning the essential behavioral skills. In addition, the previous practice of these skills facilitates their home practice after each biofeedback session.

Cognitive-Behavioral Approach to Pain Treatment

The behavioral model says that an individual's behavior can be changed if the right contingencies or conditions are set up. Essentially, these conditions allow for the acquisition of new skills at a behavioral level. The clinician can foster development of these new skills by modeling certain behavioral responses for the patient, by providing appropriate reinforcements for desired behaviors or withdrawal of previous reinforcements for undesired behaviors, by teaching spouses how to respond to operant pain complaints, and, most importantly, by teaching relaxation skills.

Despite these very useful targets of behavioral change, however, the cognitive model emerged because the behavioral model alone was found to be inadequate based on outcomes research. The cognitive model asserts that cognition—how people think and what they think about—is an important mediator in the pathway to behavior and that altering cognition will alter behavior. Generally, the studies of cognitive treatment for disorders such as depression have shown that cognition can be altered and new behaviors can emerge with a simultaneous reduction in symptoms.[17–19] The same is true for studies of cognitive treatment of pain, which have shown that the experience of pain is influenced strongly by both cognitive and behavioral processes.[20,21]

However, the sufficiency of the cognitive-behavioral model for treating pain is currently being challenged by other psychological theories.[22] One strong set of theories says that an individual's internal representations of important events and people, and the emotions associated with these representations, have a profound impact on cognition itself and that failure to attend to those representations and emotions will result in a poor treatment outcome from a purely cognitive-behavioral treatment perspective. Other strong theories propose that interpersonal relationships, and what they mean to people, are also profound mediators that underlie behavior and that failure to address these aspects of functioning will interfere with attempts to alter cognition.

Because both human relationships and internal representations are critical aspects of healthy functioning, the possible limits of the cognitive-behavioral approach to the treatment of pain should be acknowledged. Clini-

cally, more comprehensive psychotherapy is often indicated for the person whose life has been significantly impacted by chronic pain, but only after basic coping skills have been successfully acquired and the pain has come under better control.

Although the cognitive-behavioral model can look deceptively simple, significant specialized training beyond the typical training of a dentist or physician is required to use the model with high efficacy. The cognitive-behavioral model has been empirically implemented at two levels for the treatment of chronic TMD pain: administered by a trained dental hygienist for the patient with only mild pain-related disability[23] or by a trained psychologist for the patient with moderate to severe pain-related disability.[24] The evidence from these two studies indicates that both models are more efficacious than some of the usual dental treatments (bite appliance, medications, and jaw exercises) for the respective clinical groups.

Both the simple and complex versions of the cognitive-behavioral model are composed of a variety of procedures and tactics. These include relaxation skills training, self-monitoring of problematic behaviors and symptoms, a self-disciplined approach for introducing new behaviors, and exercises that incorporate new proprioceptive learning and alter dysfunctional behavioral patterns. In addition, the clinician must use strategies for alteration of cognitions, including psychoeducation regarding pain and mind-body relations. All of these approaches require sufficient guidance, feedback, and support from the provider. The level of implementation varies, depending on the provider and consequently on the need. Several manuals and texts more fully describe this information.[21,25–27]

Relaxation

Relaxation is the cornerstone of the biobehavioral treatment of most individuals with chronic pain, and there is substantial evidence of its efficacy.[13,28,29] This holds for almost any pain condition, but it is especially true for those individuals with muscle- and joint-related problems. The primary reason that relaxation is so strongly advocated is that it provides an opportunity for the individual to reduce not only physical but also mental tension. In that process, the perception of pain and related body sensations is modified. The modification of perception is facilitated by an approach to relaxation that is based on mindfulness.[30] Biofeedback or hypnosis can also be used to facilitate such changes.[31]

Many patients with chronic muscle pain either are aware that relaxation might be useful, but have never tried it, or have tried it and found that it helped but have never pursued it diligently. Some patients with chronic muscle pain have tried to learn to relax, found that it was difficult, and decided that they were not the kind of person who can learn to relax. When relaxation training is taught within the context of a biobehavioral model, even patients who believe that it is impossible to learn to relax are often surprised to notice how relaxed they can become.

There are several complications to the teaching of relaxation techniques. One common difficulty in learning how to relax is high anxiety (which is the condition most in need of, and most likely to benefit from, relaxation practice). Anxiety leads to preoccupation with the bodily state, and any change in that state, such as via relaxation, can be frightening; thus, a paradoxical increase in anxiety accompanies relaxation in highly anxious patients when they first learn how to relax. Rather than let this paradoxical increase in anxiety further reinforce for the patient that he or she cannot learn how to relax, the clinician has several options: Using relaxation methods that focus very directly on bodily sensations, adding hypnosis into the mix, or referring the patient to a behavioral medicine specialist.

A second complication is that individuals with the strongly fixed belief that a prior injury is solely responsible for the chronicity of their pain will often, after discovering that relaxation can be profoundly helpful in the reduction of their pain, completely reject further biobehavioral treatment. Paradoxically, it seems that positive experiences of self-directed pain reduction can be profoundly disturbing to an individual's prior causal attributions, leading to a challenge to the patient's sense of control. If control and responsibility for pain reduction have been transferred to the provider, then it can be daunting to the patient's self-identification to reclaim that responsibility.

These difficulties in acquiring relaxation skills, something that should be relatively simple and ultimately natural, can lead to very complex clinical situations that require high levels of provider skill. This problem is much better addressed by the dentist and psychologist working together. Illness beliefs can be very powerful, and teaching effective relaxation skills often throws the provider (and the patient) into the vortex of those beliefs.

Current evidence and theory hold that one primary means by which relaxation occurs is via modulation of attention.[32,33] Given that the existence of pain is generally attributed to a bodily cause, attention to the body is exactly the appropriate way to teach relaxation. Although many might find that idea paradoxical, it is the patient's concern regarding the body that prompts so much distress and illness behavior; thus, further attention to the body in the form of relaxation training and other exercises actually allays the patient's fears and concerns.

Many methods exist for teaching relaxation. Although progressive muscle relaxation (which involves systematic contraction, holding the contraction, and then release of the muscles in each part of the body) has become very popular over the years in general behavioral medicine and psychotherapy, a method that more closely resembles yoga or meditation has emerged as a clear alternative.[34,35] It seems counterproductive for individuals who are in pain because of purported muscle tension to substantially contract the muscle further to relax it. (The method advocated under the section on biofeedback uses only very small increases in muscle tension, not the large increases required with progressive muscle relaxation, which is done without any external monitoring.)

Within this general framework of relaxation, there are many ways to teach it, none inherently superior. Rather, the critical element is the practitioner's own practice of that method and thus the personal understanding of the process. From personal understanding, the provider can teach the method in a way that allows it to be highly individualized for that patient, and it allows the provider to respond usefully to the inevitable questions and problems that emerge in the practice of the method. The provider's own understanding allows him or her to bridge the ideal of the practice to the exigencies of real life and to become an ally in the patient's attempts to learn new skills.

In the relaxation approach, two particular aspects are emphasized: abdominal breathing and general bodily relaxation. In abdominal breathing, the patient is taught to monitor the breath by allowing it to move into the lower part of the lungs, thus forcing the abdomen out. Observations have frequently been made that pain patients practice shallow breathing and use only the top portion of the lungs; it is suspected that such breathing may lead to increased anxiety. A standard regimen is to practice abdominal breathing at least 5 to 10 minutes twice per day. In conjunction with the regular practice, patients can also use what is called a *signal breath*, turning their attention to their breathing and inducing abdominal breathing for a few cycles whenever distressed or upset, as a method of short-circuiting automatic cognitive, autonomic, and behavioral reactions.

One method to teach general bodily relaxation is to train the patient and simultaneously make a personalized audiotape for home practice. Although standardized tapes (either commercial or the practitioner's own version) are also useful, the relaxation literature supports greater efficacy for custom tapes.[36] The patient is directed to attend to the body, one segment at a time (eg, first the left foot, then the left lower leg), noticing all of the normal sensations in that part of the body, observing for any tension, observing for any sensations of relaxation, and allowing any part to become less tense, if possible, but without expectation. Such an approach will require about 20 to 30 minutes, depending on the depth of relaxation desired. Patients are asked to practice this relaxation technique at least once per day with the tape and, as skills develop, to practice without the tape to generalize the skills.

One caveat about relaxation practice is that considerable discipline is required for time management and environmental control so that the practice can be pursued. Often, for individuals with significant demands on their time (which induce stress responses), gaining control of those demands is the major hurdle. The resolution of these problems is fundamentally critical for individuals to begin to master their stress responses. For many individuals, the problems inherent in resolving those demands, so that they can even begin to practice relaxation, are sufficiently serious that referral to a behavioral medicine specialist might be the only alternative in order to continue with biobehavioral treatment. This issue cannot be emphasized enough: It is critical that an individual be able to make time for self-care.

Self-monitoring

Both success and compliance with these biobehavioral modalities must ultimately be assessed by the clinician, but to do so he or she will need detailed progress information from the patient. Therefore, patients are asked to maintain a daily log for as long as necessary to record symptoms and associated behaviors, affects, and cognitions. Generally, the practice of self-monitoring is self-explanatory as the individual develops insight into his or her situation.

The clinician provides support for the patient to perform this task. The use of custom forms is highly recommended because they facilitate the patient's activity; however, for simple recording tasks, index cards also serve well. Patients will be more responsive when the instructions regarding what to do are concrete. Patients should start off with just one or two things to record at a time, and they should be monitored for compliance; that is, the clinician must evaluate what the patient did and discuss it for the patient to want to continue. The patient is asked to record every time an exercise is done, every time relaxation is practiced, and every time a specific technique is used. The process of recording both symptoms and self-management skills reinforces the learning of the new skills. The self-monitoring process and recording of skill utilization may also help minimize relapse.

People who are too busy to record their adherence and progress are generally too busy to perform at a level necessary for progress to occur. People who are unable to modify their existing schedule (itself often an adaptation to the existence of chronic pain) to adhere to treatment seldom progress with skill building. The observation of such behavioral signs suggests the need for reassessment in terms of a possible personality disorder that impacts medical care.[37,38]

Exercise

Exercises accomplish several aims simultaneously: They are used as another method for training attention in general; they are used to restructure the patient's experience of illness associated with malfunction of the body; and they are used to rehabilitate limitations in function. Clearly, patients may perform exercises in such a way that only the last aim is pursued. Often this happens because the patient, finding the exercises boring, will do them only while driving the car or watching television.

Much is potentially lost in terms of possible benefits when therapeutic exercise is performed in an unconscious manner. Exercise can invoke intentional behavior and, with attention to the new behavioral pattern, further changes are possible within the brain's motor programs, sensory perception and appraisal processes, and in beliefs about self.[39] The power of sustained attention to the development of new motor skills, which includes physical rehabilitation, has been repeatedly observed by athletes perfecting their craft. Similarly, patients need to learn control, self-discipline, and healthy proprioception and appraisal.

Primary therapeutic exercises (see chapter 24) are also part of a cognitive-behavioral program; an exercise that increases range of motion also becomes a cognitive-behavioral practice. Whether the exercise is to increase range of motion of the jaw, to correct dysfunctional movement patterns of the jaw, or to correct tight limitations in the cervical area, all exercises should be performed with this type of attention. Efforts by the patient to focus on the pain and to work within the range of movement imposed by the pain will contribute to increased self-efficacy.[40]

One of the major goals of the cognitive-behavioral model, when applied to chronic TMD pain conditions, is to correct the misperception that pain automatically signals damage to the body. When bodily damage is their main concern, patients often develop a behavioral avoidance pattern, which means that any activity that causes pain (such as moving the jaw within a normal range) will be inhibited, leading to more and more physical limitation and altering central neural patterns. To overcome this concern, the patient is asked to engage in the exercises with conscious and intentional awareness so that the exercise will help restructure experience and beliefs. Pain that signals bodily damage must be discriminated from pain as an experience.

A second form of exercise is whole body movement, which can also be increased to an aerobic level. For example, a walking exercise, whether aerobic or not, becomes a cognitive-behavioral treatment when used consciously by the patient.

Cognition

At the intellectual level, biobehavioral therapy is aimed at helping individuals transform distorted patterns of thought, which may be a complex undertaking. Without professional training in the application of psychotherapeutic and cognitive therapy skills, the dentist should not try to provide a formal version of these treatments. However, with the right self-directed educational materials, patients can make some significant improvements on their own in terms of correcting thinking patterns that increase pain. When this approach is used, underlying belief systems probably will not change, but more superficial thought patterns, which are often significantly potent in their effect on current suffering, can be altered surprisingly well by the patient. Many good self-direction guides are available.[41]

More complex dysfunctional thought patterns, which can contribute significantly to pain chronicity, require direct therapy. One common pain-related dysfunctional belief, well-identified in persons with back pain, is kinesophobia: the belief that movement (ie, using the involving organ system) will result in (re)injury.[42,43] Although no research on this critical pain cognition and associated behavioral consequence has been performed yet in the chronic TMD pain population, pain avoidance in the form of guarding is commonly observed in these patients, and such behaviors appear to cause pain.[44] While a behavioral approach to such guarding behavior should be sufficient, it often is not. As a result, the patient's beliefs about reinjury are capable of preventing therapeutic exercise as well as postural control practices from accomplishing their goal.

The importance of cognitive therapy for the treatment of chronic pain is frequently underestimated. Instead, incorrect belief systems about a particular illness state frequently are accepted as fact by both patient and provider. In frustration, both may get swept into escalation of other diagnostic tests and treatments simply because progress with biobehavioral treatment is slow and often indirect. Unfortunately, in the domain of behavioral therapies, dose response is not as simple as the response to potent analgesic medications. Biobehavioral therapies require calendar time for efficacy to emerge, which means that the patient needs support and encouragement to pursue such treatments. In addition, the patient often needs repeated assurances that the diagnosis is correct (ie, that no malignant or progressive disease is present) and that the provided treatments ultimately can be efficacious.

Psychoeducation

Psychoeducation is the use of educational materials about the disease and the illness. Numerous studies have shown that such materials can produce changes in patients' understanding of a disease or of themselves.[21] Both written and audiovisual materials can provide a basic introduction to the various TMDs (anatomy of joint and muscle, basic theory of pain, role of behaviors, etc); teach abdominal and general relaxation skills and provide an introduction to stress theory and how stress affects the body. They can also expose patients to the cognitive issues associated with chronic pain and illness; discuss relapse and how to minimize it; and address patients' direct responsibility for self-care and how that interacts with their communication with their healthcare providers. This can be supplemented by other materials that give patients information about depression, anxiety, sleep hygiene, nutrition, and so on. The goal is to increase knowledge and awareness of the factors that affect pain, transferring control to the patient in terms of making choices from a broad selection of options.

Guidance

In this structured cognitive-behavioral approach, the dentist's role is often that of providing guidance, acting as a collaborator with patients and helping to support them in the acquisition of new skills. In reality, the patients are teaching themselves the new skills. However, the dentist's role as an understanding clinician who helps patients to integrate self-learning with the traditional biomedical treatments is critical to this process. Rather than taking on the role of authority, the dentist can be more helpful by assisting patients to question existing patterns and behaviors in order to guide them toward a sustainable and sensible series of self-management skills and practices.

Psychotherapy

The term *psychotherapy* refers to therapeutic approaches that address in more fundamental ways the overall functioning of a patient, and this is not restricted to issues directly associated with pain. The phrase "not directly associated" is used to emphasize that almost any personal issue for a person with pain can be tied in one way or another to that person's pain. For example, childhood experiences that did not foster mastery for the individual will exert effects throughout life; for persons with chronic pain, that lack of self-mastery will influence their ability to take an active role in self-management. Simultaneously, that lack of self-mastery will exert effects on the person's social skills, thus negatively affecting social support as well as the person's ability to learn new skills. These skill deficits may, in turn, lead to decreased self-esteem, which leads to depression, which makes pain worse. All of these factors, in turn, will affect the person's pain response.

In other words, everything in a person's life is interrelated at some level, so to partition chronic pain into some kind of separate category may be artificial at the least and damaging to the patient at the worst. If the practitioner ignores the psychosocial aspects of a patient's pain problem, the result may be that effective psychotherapeutic options are ignored, delayed, disparaged, or minimized.

Thus, for individuals who have serious problems across multiple life dimensions, in addition to problems with chronic pain, the type of treatment that will foster solid gains and minimize relapse probably should include psychotherapy to address the multitude of issues that may be present. For such a patient, however, it may not be wise to initially recommend treatment in that direction, because psychotherapy does not necessarily foster development of the kinds of skills that are described under the self-management model and that are needed by persons with chronic pain. For these patients, it is essential that they first acquire solid skills that will help their pain and reduce their pain-related suffering. Such success in self-management is helpful to the patient's self-image, which ultimately helps the dentist in providing biomedical treatments. Thus, psychotherapy for the person with chronic pain is generally more appropriately considered to be a second step after cognitive-behavioral treatment for the pain.

Before deciding whether to refer a patient for psychotherapy, the clinician should monitor the outcome of treatment via the self-management approach coupled with appropriate biomedical approaches. If there is a priori psychosocial information that might suggest relapse, that concern should be shared up front with the patient; should relapse occur, the reasons for relapse can be explored. For example, does the patient simply need a booster session of the self-management model, or would the patient be better served by an explanation of the causal relations within the patient's lifestyle that may have precipitated the relapse? If these issues can be identified, would the patient like to address them or continue to ride a roller coaster of cycles of improvement and relapse?

Hypnosis

Hypnosis can be a very powerful technique for helping people learn to modulate nociception and pain. It can also be misused if too much emphasis is placed on it as a panacea without considering that, for conditions such as chronic TMD pain, it is best used within an overall biobehavioral treatment context. Although many dentists learn hypnosis to manage acute procedural pain during dental treatment, the use of hypnosis for chronic TMD and facial pain typically requires other skills as well because pain modulation is usually not the only issue to target. Thus, in such cases, hypnosis is more effectively used when other psychotherapeutic skills can be applied as well. This should not be construed as a recommendation that dentists not use hypnosis on such patients but only as a caution.

Sometimes, chronic TMD pain is related to nociception problems (eg, centrally mediated pain) that cannot be managed biomedically without the use of drugs that have unacceptable side effects or by invasive neuroablative surgery. In such cases, hypnosis should be considered. However, although hypnosis is often considered a treatment of last resort to be used only after all biomedical treatments have failed, it might be more appropriate in some cases to consider hypnosis earlier.[45]

The body has an amazing capacity to heal itself and to modulate its nociceptive signals to the central nervous system, but sometimes it needs some help and hypnosis can be that type of help. Although some would argue that hypnosis does not eliminate the nociception, that complaint seems irrelevant if the goal is to reduce pain and suffering in such patients,[46] which hypnosis can do without the complications and side effects of medications or surgical procedures.[47] The techniques for use of hypnosis are well described in many textbooks.[48]

Finally, among the biobehavioral treatments, hypnosis may have potentially specific effects on the treatment of nocturnal bruxism. The evidence is solely anecdotal at this point,[49] but the notion that hypnosis may be helpful for this condition makes it unique. So far, no other biobehavioral treatment has been shown to be efficacious for reducing nocturnal bruxism, especially when it exists as a solitary condition in the absence of all other aggravating factors involved in chronic pain.

Today it is widely recognized that nocturnal bruxism is best construed as a sleep disorder; if the symptoms are not responsive to the usual mechanical treatment (intraoral appliance), it may well represent a more severe form of central dysregulation. Hypnosis has the known capacity to work effectively at that level of brain activity. This is one area where randomized controlled trials are strongly needed to evaluate alternative treatments as well as to explore theoretical considerations regarding bruxism.

Summary

Many treatment approaches for chronic TMD pain that fit within the biobehavioral model have been described, and there are certainly more that could be described and used. However, the ones presented in this chapter form a critical mass of approaches that can be used successfully with most patients. The structured, short-term, cognitive-behavioral self-management program, when used in its entirety, provides a sampling of a number of different approaches that allows patients to find what works best for them. It also exposes patients to new insights regarding different possible treatments and how these treatments can be effective at different levels.

For the dentist wishing to embark on using biobehavioral treatment approaches, the acquisition of additional training is desirable. To this end, professional supervision can be sought from a licensed behavioral medicine practitioner. Alternatively, should dentists wish to refer a patient for such treatment, the approaches described in this chapter should help them in finding the kind of treatment that can make a difference for patients with chronic TMD pain.

For biobehavioral treatment to be successful, it cannot be regarded as the treatment of last resort. Patients sent for consultation in that circumstance are often resentful toward the consulting psychologist. These kinds of patients have had many encounters with the medical system in which they were repeatedly told that their problem (pain) was real as long as there were treatment options but were told their problem was psychogenic when the options were exhausted. The consequence is that many patients with chronic TMD pain have developed a need to prove the reality of their problem (pain).

To avoid this unfortunate and unnecessary state of affairs, better integration of medical and biobehavioral treatments (ie, treatments that address both mind and body) is urgently needed. TMD-related pain often is recurrent, and many patients seek repeated treatment. However, when there is a choice between the physical and the psychological or behavioral approaches, psychological or behavioral treatment is quickly advocated by the practitioner for the "resistant" cases. Treatment problems inherent in a reliance on biomedical treatments can be avoided by the use of a broad-based approach to management; the clinician can accomplish this goal by using valid and reliable diagnostic tests to evaluate the biobehavioral and the physical domains, using a moderated approach to escalation of diagnostic evaluations, making a long-term commitment to the patient, and by being sensible about the overall patient management.

References

1. Ohrbach R, Dworkin SF. Longitudinal changes in TMD: Relationship of changes in pain to changes in clinical and psychological variables. Pain 1998;74:315–326.
2. Ohrbach R. History and clinical examination. In: Zarb GA, Carlsson GE, Sessle BJ, Mohl ND (eds). Temporomandibular Joint and Masticatory Muscle Disorders. Copenhagen: Munksgaard, 1994:406–434.
3. Mohl ND, Ohrbach R. Decision making in TMD. J Dent Educ 1992;56:823–833.
4. Mohl ND, Ohrbach R. The dilemma of scientific knowledge versus clinical management of TMD. J Prosthet Dent 1992; 67:113–120.
5. Ohrbach R, Burgess J. Temporomandibular disorders and craniofacial pain. In: Rakel R (ed). Conn's Current Therapy. Philadelphia: Saunders, 1999:997–1004.
6. Jensen MP, Nielson WR, Turner JA, Romano JM, Hill MP. Readiness to self-manage pain is associated with coping and with psychological and physical functioning among patients with chronic pain. Pain 2003;104:529–537.
7. Jensen MP, Nielson WR, Romano JM, Hill ML, Turner JA. Further evaluation of the pain stages of change questionnaire: Is the transtheoretical model of change useful for patients with chronic pain? Pain 2000;86:255–264.
8. Melmed RN. Mind, Body, and Medicine. New York: Oxford University Press, 2001.
9. Ohrbach R, Blascovich JJ, Gale EN, McCall WD Jr, Dworkin SF. Psychophysiological assessment of stress in chronic pain: A comparison of stressful stimuli and response systems. J Dent Res 1993;77:1840–1850.
10. Hazaleus SL, Deffenbacher JL. Relaxation and cognitive treatment of anger. J Consult Clin Psychol 1986;54:222–226.
11. Flor H, Birbaumer N. Comparison of the efficacy of electromyographic biofeedback, cognitive-behavioral therapy, and conservative medical interventions in the treatment of chronic musculoskeletal pain. J Consult Clin Psychol 1993; 61:653–658.
12. Borgeat F, Elie R, Larouche LM. Pain response to voluntary muscle tension increases and biofeedback efficacy in tension headache. Headache 1985;25:387–391.
13. National Institutes of Health Technology Assessment Conference on Integration of Behavioral and Relaxation Approaches into the Treatment of Chronic Pain and Insomnia. Bethesda, MD: National Institutes of Health, 1995.
14. Flor H, Schugens MM, Birbaumer N. Discrimination of muscle tension in chronic pain patients and healthy controls. Biofeedback Self-Regul 1992;17:165–177.

15. Gessel AH, Alderman MM. Management of myofascial pain dysfunction syndrome of the temporomandibular joint by tension control training. Psychosomatics 1971;12:302–309.

16. Glaros AG, Lausten L. Temporomandibular disorders. In: Schwartz MS, Andrasik F (eds). Biofeedback: A Practitioner's Guide. New York: Guilford, 2003:349–368.

17. Rudy TE, Kerns RD, Turk DC. Chronic pain and depression: Toward a cognitive-behavioral mediation model. Pain 1988;35:129–140.

18. Whisman MA. Mediators and moderators of change in cognitive therapy of depression. Psychol Bull 1993;114:248–265.

19. Teasdale JD, Segal Z, Williams JMG. How does cognitive therapy prevent depressive relapse and why should attentional control (mindfulness) training help? Behav Res Ther 1995;33:25–39.

20. Jensen MP, Romano JM, Turner JA, Good AB, Wald LH. Patient beliefs predict patient functioning: Further support for a cognitive-behavioral model of chronic pain. Pain 1999;81:95–104.

21. Turner JA, Keefe FJ. Cognitive-behavioral therapy for chronic pain. In: Max M (ed). Pain 1999—An Updated Review. Seattle: IASP Press, 1999:523–533.

22. Grzesiak RC, Ury GM, Dworkin RH. Psychodynamic psychotherapy with chronic pain patients. In: Gatchel RJ, Turk DC (eds). Psychological Approaches to Pain Management. New York: Guilford, 1996:148–178.

23. Dworkin SF, Huggins KH, Wilson L, et al. A randomized clinical trial using Research Diagnostic Criteria for Temporomandibular Disorders–Axis II to target clinic cases for a tailored self-care TMD treatment program. J Orofac Pain 2002;16:48–63.

24. Dworkin SF, Turner JA, Mancl L, et al. A randomized clinical trial of a tailored comprehensive care treatment program for temporomandibular disorders. J Orofac Pain 2002;16:259–276.

25. Dworkin SF, Massoth DL, Wilson L, Huggins KH, Truelove E. Guide to Temporomandibular Disorders: A Self-Management Approach. 1. Patient's Manual. Seattle: University of Washington, 1997.

26. Dworkin SF, Huggins KH, Massoth DL, Truelove E. Guide to Temporomandibular Disorders: A Self-Management Approach. 2. Dental Hygienist's Manual. Seattle: University of Washington, 1997.

27. Skevington SM. Psychology of Pain. Chichester, NY: Wiley, 1995.

28. Linton SJ, Götestam KG. A controlled study of the effects of applied relaxation and applied relation plus operant procedures in the regulation of chronic pain. Br J Clin Psychol 1984;23:291–299.

29. Mizes JS, Doleys DM, Dolce J. The psychophysiological effects of the relaxation component of a comprehensive pain program: A clinical descriptive study. Clin J Pain 1986;2:87–92.

30. Kabat-Zinn J. Full Catastrophe Living: Using the Wisdom of Your Body and Mind to Face Stress, Pain, and Illness. New York: Delacorte, 1990.

31. Barber TX, Hahn KW. Hypnotic induction and "relaxation." Arch Gen Psychiatry 1963;8:107–112.

32. Goleman DJ, Schwartz GE. Meditation as an intervention in stress reactivity. J Consult Clin Psychol 1976;44:456–466.

33. Kutz I, Borysenko JZ, Benson H. Meditation and psychotherapy: A rationale for the integration of dynamic psychotherapy, the relaxation response, and mindfulness meditation. Am J Psychiatry 1985;142:1–7.

34. Kabat-Zinn J. An outpatient program in behavioral medicine for chronic pain patients based on the practice of mindfulness meditation: Theoretical considerations and preliminary results. Gen Hosp Psychiatry 1982;4:33–37.

35. Kabat-Zinn J, Lipworth L, Burney R. The clinical use of mindfulness meditation for the self-regulation of chronic pain. J Behav Med 1985;8:163–190.

36. Borkovec TD, Sides JK. Critical procedural variables related to the physiological effects of progressive relaxation: A review. Behav Res Ther 1979;17:119–125.

37. Kight M, Gatchel RJ, Wesley L. Temporomandibular disorders: Evidence for significant overlap with psychopathology. Health Psychol 1999;18:177–182.

38. Kinney RK, Gatchel RJ, Ellis E, Holt C. Major psychological disorders in chronic TMD patients: Implications for successful management. J Am Dent Assoc 1992;123:49–54.

39. Stroud MW, Thorn BE, Jensen MP, Boothby JL. The relation between pain beliefs, negative thoughts, and psychosocial functioning in chronic pain patients. Pain 2000;84:347–352.

40. Jensen MP, Turner JA, Romano JM. Self-efficacy and outcome expectancies: Relationship to chronic pain coping strategies and adjustment. Pain 1991;44:263–269.

41. Caudill MA. Managing Pain Before it Manages You. New York: Guilford, 1995.

42. Vlaeyen JWS, Kole-Snijders AMJ, Boeren RGB, Van Eek H. Fear of movement/(re)injury in chronic low back pain and its relation to behavioral performance. Pain 1995;62:363–372.

43. Vlaeyen JWS, Seelen HAM, Peters M, et al. Fear of movement/(re)injury and muscular reactivity in chronic low back pain patients: An experimental investigation. Pain 1999;82: 297–304.

44. Glaros AG, Tabacchi KN, Glass EG. Effect of parafunctional clenching on TMD pain. J Orofac Pain 1998;12:145–152.

45. Holroyd J. Hypnosis treatment of clinical pain: Understanding why hypnosis is useful. Int J Clin Exp Hypn 1996;44:33–51.

46. Rainville P, Carrier B, Hofbauer RK, Bushnell MC, Duncan GH. Dissociation of sensory and affective dimensions of pain using hypnotic modulation. Pain 1999;82:159–171.

47. Ohrbach R, Patterson DR, Carrougher G, Gibran N. When medication fails—A case study of hypnosis for pain control in a burn ICU. Clin J Pain 1998;14:167–175.

48. Barber J. Hypnotic analgesia: Clinical considerations. In: Barber J (ed). Hypnosis and Suggestion in the Treatment of Pain. New York: Norton, 1996:85–120.

49. LaCross MB. Understanding change: Five-year follow-up of brief hypnotic treatment of chronic bruxism. Am J Clin Hypn 1994;36:276–281.

Management of Dental Occlusion

Christian S. Stohler

The relationship between the dental occlusion and the function of the masticatory system has been of great interest for at least the past 50 years. During this time, the field of occlusion experienced explanatory shifts as the scientific and practicing communities strove to obtain a better match between clinical observations and theoretical predictions. It has been especially challenging to explain patients' variable responses to clinical interventions such as occlusal adjustments, fixed partial dentures, and occlusal appliances. Unlike many other subject matters in dentistry, this topic has often generated acrimonious and arguably counterproductive discussions.

During the past 15 years, however, a mounting body of evidence has emerged that challenged past thinking about the role of the dental occlusion in the various temporomandibular disorders (TMDs). In particular, the clinical decision-making process for using occlusal treatment for the various TMDs, which historically was the fundamental reason for dentistry's involvement in the management of these conditions, must be reconsidered. Dentistry as a discipline is increasingly required to recognize and reevaluate the uncomfortable factual irregularities that do not fit the prevailing explanatory models.

An understanding of the occlusal requirements for restoring dentitions still constitutes core knowledge of the dental curriculum, and the skills necessary to manage the dental occlusion are essential to any kind of dental care. By no means should this body of knowledge and the corresponding skills necessary to achieve comfort in jaw function be regarded as a trivial matter. However, for patients in whom the function of the masticatory apparatus is compromised by disease or pain, additional complexity enters the clinical decision-making process

regarding the dental occlusion, calling for actions that often differ from those applied in routine dentistry.

Conventional wisdom suggests that there is a significant relationship between diseases of the masticatory system and the dental occlusion. For example, inflammatory periapical processes can cause hypereruption of affected teeth that, in turn, influences the patient's occlusal comfort and can disrupt the interplay between the maxillary and mandibular dentitions. Similar phenomena can occur in states of acute periodontal disease. Alternatively, changes in the temporomandibular joint (TMJ), such as loss of articular tissue or swelling due to intracapsular exudation, can also affect the relationship and dynamic interplay between the opposing arches. Anterior open bites and lateral open bites can result from these kinds of intracapsular conditions.

Irrespective of the underlying disease process responsible for positional change in a particular dental or condyle-fossa relationship, patients recognize changes in their dental occlusion, stressing that their bite no longer feels the same. As far as the clinician is concerned, these occlusal complaints may be attributable to a specific pathologic condition (eg, degenerative joint disease, acute traumatic arthritis, or advanced stages of dental pulpitis), but sometimes it is difficult to determine the underlying cause of a patient's sudden occlusal awareness (Fig 27-1).

Although altered occlusal perception is often encountered in patients' histories, modern classification systems for diseases affecting the function of the masticatory system do not routinely call for inspection and analysis of the dental occlusion as a criterion for diagnostic assignment. On the other hand, there is little doubt in a patient

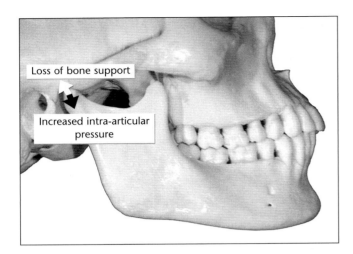

Fig 27-1 Alterations in the relationship between the condyle and the glenoid fossa have a bearing on the dental occlusion. Increased intra-articular pressure can result in loss of contact of posterior teeth. On the other hand, loss of articular bone support can cause an anterior open bite and heavy contacts on posterior teeth.

with rheumatoid arthritis of the TMJ that the dramatic changes of the occlusion (anterior open bite) are of diagnostic value with respect to the severity of loss of articular bone support.[1] Whether occlusal relationships should be routinely considered as an important part of diagnostic reasoning in patients with TMDs continues to be a point of contention for many practicing clinicians, with some wanting them to be the major focus while others want to ignore them.

This omission also confuses patients, because their occlusal complaint does not seem to get the necessary attention; they may wonder, "Why is my dentist not paying attention to my bite? It bothers me all the time. " In fact, complaints that the occlusion "does not feel right" are not surprising, in view of the exquisite, low-threshold mechanosensitivity of the periodontal apparatus. Unlike during normal chewing, during a conscious biting task extremely small discrepancies in the dental occlusion are reliably recognized by subjects.[2]

TMJ Classification Systems and Dental Occlusion

Patients' perceptions and clinicians' observations of the dental occlusion receive little attention in the classification

of TMDs.[3] There is only one classification system that recognizes, in a systematic fashion, changes in occlusal relationships of teeth imposed by the various TMDs, including both objective findings as well as changes reported by patients.[4] In fact, patients' occlusal awareness represents a unique property of Bell's classification system[4] because it emphasizes the symptom over "objective" findings obtained with articulating paper or an articulator. Not only does this classification distinguish between the same major subsets of TMD as the Research Diagnostic Criteria for Temporomandibular Disorders (RDC/TMD),[5] but it also recognizes subjective disease attributes such as pain, restriction of or interference with mandibular movement, and occlusal awareness.

Thus, Bell's system is unique for including perceived changes in the dental occlusion in a biologically plausible conceptual framework, placing greater emphasis on their presence as a symptom than a sign. Given that all diagnostic systems for TMDs tend to be overly sensitive with respect to the diagnostic validity of so-called objective signs, putting greater importance on patients' reports is scientifically justified. With respect to complaints about the occlusion, Bell[4] introduced the term *acute malocclusion*, referring to a symptom and not a sign, to capture the type of occlusal complaints associated with the various subsets of TMDs (Table 27-1).

Working with dental casts mounted on an articulator during the first 2 years of the dental curriculum makes it obvious to any dental student that minor changes in the TMJ articulation have a profound effect on the dental occlusion. Less obvious is the effect of painful jaw muscle disorders on the dental occlusion, although perceived occlusal changes and decreased range of motion are often reported by patients with masticatory muscle pain. However, there is experimental evidence that muscle pain indeed can cause systematic changes in subjective and objective measures of the occlusion and altered jaw function.[6] For example, tonic muscle pain induced by infusion of an algesic solution into the central portion of the superficial masseter muscle, when compared with administration of isotonic saline as a control (the subjects were blinded to the type of substance given), had significantly different effects on the mandibular range of motion. The pain also affected the subject's ability to close in centric relation, as shown by the change in the position of the apex of the Gothic arch tracing in the anterior and transverse directions (Fig 27-2). Moreover, subjects described shifts in their occlusion and restrictions in range of motion in the presence of jaw muscle pain, which disappeared after resolution of the pain.[7]

Table 27-1	Explanatory model linking occlusal complaints to the various TMDs
Bell's TMJ subsets[4]	**Nature of associated occlusal changes[†]**
Acute muscle disorders*	Acute malocclusion is muscle induced.
Disc interference disorders*	Acute malocclusion, if any, is due to fracture or protracted dislocation of the articular disc.
Inflammatory TMJ disorders*	Acute malocclusion, if any, is due to intracapsular fluid, intracapsular swelling, or bone loss.
Chronic mandibular hypomobilities	There is no acute malocclusion.
Growth disorders	Acute malocclusion, if any, is due to rapid osseous change.

*Subdivisions based on clusters of symptoms also identified by the Research Diagnostic Criteria for Temporomandibular Disorders.[5]
[†]Acute malocclusion: A change in the occlusal relationship of the teeth recognized as being imposed by a TMD and of which the patient is consciously aware.[4]

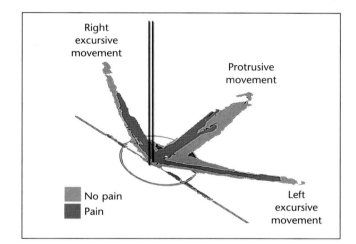

Fig 27-2 Gothic arch tracings show the maximum protrusive and lateroexcursive range of mandibular motion in the presence and absence of experimental jaw muscle pain. The most posterior position from which lateral movements can be made is located farther anteriorly (< 1 mm) in the presence of pain than in the absence of pain.[7]

Controversial Issues

Occlusal Causation Revisited

Although the pitfalls of relying on correlation data in making decisions about causal relationships are well known, it took the dental profession almost 20 years to diminish the purported role of the dental occlusion in the pathogenesis of the various TMDs (see chapter 14). If Sackett's rules of evidence are applied,[8] the available data with respect to cause-and-effect conclusions[9] make it clear that the risk that occlusal features will lead to development of a TMD must be judged as being low to very low (Table 27-2). On the other hand, the evidence favors the view that conditions affecting TMJ morphology, as well as those producing musculoskeletal pain, can affect the dental occlusion, causing patients to observe changes in their occlusion. Thus, the occlusal changes are the result of the disease or disorder as opposed to being the cause of the disease or disorder.

If perceived changes of the occlusion are the consequence of a TMD rather than the cause of the problem, the rationale in support of occlusal treatment for various TMDs changes in a significant way, especially if the condition is reversible.[7] In addition, preventive occlusal treatment, notably comprehensive occlusal adjustment, cannot be justified in terms of lowering the risk that a TMD will develop, which means that routine occlusal adjustments

Rule of evidence	Literature consistent with causation	Literature opposing causation
Table 27-2 Summary of available epidemiologic evidence supporting or rejecting the causal role of occlusal factors in the development of various TMDs*		
Strength of statistical association	Low to moderate levels of statistical association are reported in epidemiologic studies.	Levels of reported statistical associations are too low to support a causal role.
Consistency of observation	—	Reports of statistically significant associations are inconsistent and vary from study to study.
Temporal relationship	Experimental occlusal interferences can, but are not necessarily sufficient to, cause symptoms.	Changes in the occlusion are the result of altered maxillomandibular relationships caused by changes in the TMJ and/or the effect of pain on jaw muscle function.
Gradient effect	—	There is no evidence of any gradient effect.
Biologic plausibility	—	Explanatory models are inconsistent with general orthopedic knowledge.

*Data from Stohler.[9]

are clearly a therapeutic approach of the past. Caution is also indicated in the presence of TMJ disease, because disease activity, including pain, can produce further occlusal instability with time. Taken together, these facts lead to the inevitable conclusion that irreversible occlusal treatments are contraindicated in most TMD patients; instead, the preponderance of available evidence supports symptom management by means of a low-technology, high-prudence approach that consists of reversible measures, including occlusal appliances such as stabilization splints[10] (see chapter 25).

Success of Active and Placebo Therapies

An estimated 75% to 95% of primary care patients with various TMDs benefit from currently offered interventions that are administered by an array of healthcare professionals, including dentists; family physicians; ear, nose, and throat specialists; chiropractors; osteopaths; rheumatologists; neurologists; physical therapists; acupuncturists; psychiatrists; and psychologists. Not surprisingly, given the range of healthcare providers involved, therapies encompass a wide variety of modalities, including occlusal appliances, occlusal equilibration, thermal pads, a host of pharmacologic interventions, orthodontics, prosthodontic treatments, surgery, physical therapy, relaxation training, acupuncture, biofeedback, and psychological and diet counseling.[11] Troublesome is the fact that no single remedy appears to produce a substantially better outcome than any of the other forms of therapy, although each approach appears to have its own underlying rationale and presumably unique mechanism of action.

It makes a great deal of sense to ask why outcomes are so remarkably similar, especially when it appears that offered therapies distinguish themselves only in terms of safety but not efficacy. It also is difficult to explain the fact that well-executed clinical trials often show no difference between interventions, even for situations with and without the presumably active ingredient. For example, one study used a parallel, randomized, controlled, and blind design and assigned study participants to one of three groups: (1) passive control (complete occlusal appliance worn only 30 minutes at each appointment); (2) active control (palatal appliance worn 24 hours a day); and (3) treatment (complete occlusal appliance worn 24 hours a day). Pain ratings decreased significantly with time, and the quality of life improved for all three groups. However, there were no significant differences between groups in any of the outcome measures during the trial duration of 10 weeks.[12] The fact that the efficacy of "inactive" treatments (placebos) does not differ from that of "real" treatments in some well-controlled clinical trials deserves further discussion.

The placebo response is conceptualized as a change in health status that results from the symbolic significance attributed by the patient to the interaction with a healthcare professional. Recent evidence points to the fact that this effect is mediated, at least in part, by the brain's opioidergic reward system and is linked to the subject's expectation of clinical benefit.[13] If so, the clinical benefit induced by placebos must depend on the subject's perceived likelihood of clinical benefit with respect to the offered therapeutic intervention, which in turn may be influenced by factors that influence the involved brain circuits, such as the subject's emotional state and conditioning.

The extent to which the placebo response is influenced by the therapeutic environment has been recognized for some time in the field of TMD research.[14–16] There is reason to believe that the likelihood that any type of intervention will produce a substantial improvement in health status diminishes with the number of unsuccessfully rendered treatments, suggesting that neither active treatments nor placebos are effective in those patients whose conditions are described as chronic. In fact, a condition is considered chronic if treatments—typically more than two—do not result in the resolution of symptoms. This raises the question of whether patients who are unresponsive to an array of treatments exhibit traits that diminish the likelihood of their experiencing improvement with any of these treatments, including placebos.

Historically, strong conviction about the occlusal etiology of the various TMDs encouraged a narrowly defined scope of inquiry and excluded other research avenues. However, no longer can the increasing body of evidence about the true nature of these conditions be ignored, especially insofar as it highlights the major deficits of explanatory models that assign primary etiologic significance to the dental occlusion. Although success rates of up to 95% have been reported for occlusal therapies, tending to endorse a sense of certainty, it becomes increasingly difficult to overlook newer data that support alternative disease constructs to explain the variance in TMD patients' vulnerability to disease as well as their response to treatment, including placebos. Regardless of how uncomfortable such discussions may be for the dental community, they are necessary to obtain better congruence between treatment response and theoretical models.

Unequal Susceptibility and Response

Clinical empirics and epidemiologic data suggest that individuals are not equally susceptible to developing a TMD. For example, men and women younger than 50

years represent the majority of those seeking care. While less likely in later life, these conditions can still occur in the elderly, although at much lower prevalence rates.[17]

The case-defining physical attributes of TMDs appear to be comparable among patients encountered in primary and tertiary care settings, but significant differences concerning severity, persistence, and impact exist between these patient pools. The proportion of women increases from 50% to 60% in community-based observations to more than 90% in primary and tertiary care settings.[18,19] In this respect, the various TMDs are no different from many other pain conditions in which the personally most devastating and clinically most challenging forms occur in females in much greater number than in males.[20] In children and prepubertal adults, however, gender differences do not appear to be present.[21,22]

Regarding race and ethnicity, according to the 1989 National Health Interview Survey, the prevalence rates for facial and jaw pain are 7% for whites and 5% for blacks.[23]

In addition to demographic factors, such as age, sex, and race, distinct genotypes are relevant in many medical conditions. For example, particular genotypes are linked to characteristic activation patterns of the body's pain-stress response system, resulting in case-specific sensory, affective, neuroendocrine, and autonomic messages that contribute to a patient's distinct symptom complex.

Recently, the hunt for vulnerability genes moved TMD research to a new frontier with far-reaching implications for the management of disease, increasingly shifting emphasis from one-size-fits-all management strategies to treatments based on molecular fingerprinting. For example, when subjected to experimentally induced sustained jaw muscle pain that is matched in terms of perceived pain intensity, it was found that sensory and affective pain experiences depend on subjects' activation level of the endogenous, pain-suppressing μ-opioid system.[24]

Activation of the μ-opioid system, in turn, is influenced by the catechol-O-methyltransferase (COMT) gene polymorphism, which is responsible for variations in enzyme activity because of the valine-methionine substitution.[25] The fact that COMT activity is also 20% to 30% lower in women than in men[26–29] may further explain both the greater prevalence and severity of TMDs among women. The suppressing effect of estrogen on COMT activity is consistent with data showing that the likelihood that treatment for a TMD would be sought by women increased by 77% in the 1990s; this coincided with the popular use of supplemental estrogen in the postmenopausal years during that period.[30]

However, the clinical reality is far more complex and cannot be attributed to the function of a single gene. Instead, symptoms (including pain) should be conceptu-

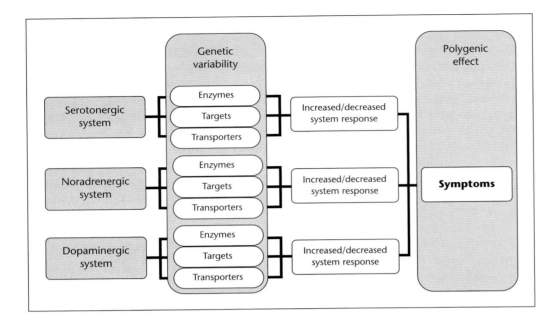

Fig 27-3 Symptoms, including pain, appear to be shaped by the function of many genes. For example, genes such as those affecting the function of key neurotransmitter systems (serotonin, noradrenaline, and dopamine) may influence the threshold of symptom awareness and the perceived level of symptom severity.

alized as the consequence of many genes that increase or decrease a person's vulnerability to develop symptoms, influence symptom severity, or both (Fig 27-3).

Pathogenesis, Causation, and Treatment

Ideally, knowledge of the pathogenesis and causation of the various TMDs should be the basis for the selection of appropriate therapies. Similarly, it would be nice to have more concrete data about both the specificity and efficacy of the available treatments. Taken together, this would define the scope for the ideal management of these conditions. However, not all of this information is available at this time.

While prevention focuses on measures to reduce exposure to the causative agent, "cures" aim to significantly suppress or eliminate the cause. Definitive therapies target the underlying pathogenesis, affecting pathways that lead to the development of symptoms. Symptom management, on the other hand, refers to a series of low-technology approaches that seem to be useful in reducing symptom severity while having no known influence on the underlying cause of disease (Fig 27-4).

Although the TMD literature is full of theories and speculations regarding causation, including many heated arguments about the role of dental occlusion, it is reasonable to conclude that future explanatory models of these disorders will differ in major ways from past thinking. With a high level of confidence, however, it is safe to infer today that occlusal features have few characteristics of what is expected from a causal agent. Because occlusal phenomena, such as premature or balancing contacts, can no longer be regarded as causal, the elimination of such features by means of occlusal adjustment cannot be justified as a preventive measure for the various TMDs, as suggested by some authors.[31] In addition, because perceived changes of the occlusion are more likely the consequence rather than the cause of disease, occlusal therapy should be considered only to address TMD patients' discomfort with their occlusion. In some cases, the structural and functional consequences of the TMD may persist, and this will have bearing on future dental treatment.

In the future, owing to rapid advances in biotechnology, the scientific community will increasingly understand the reasons why some subjects develop symptoms and will develop technologies to assess a person's vulnerability. The foundation of individualized care will most likely be based on molecular individuality.

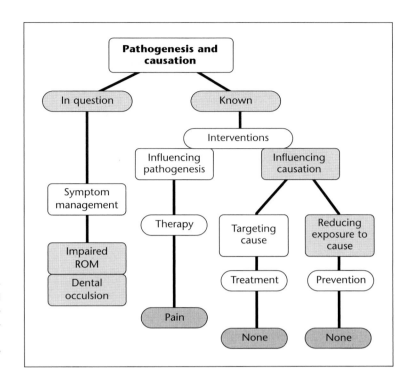

Fig 27-4 Hierarchy of therapeutic interventions for the various TMDs. Low-technology approaches are used for symptom management. With respect to pain, some pharmacologic therapies target specific aspects of the underlying pathogenesis of pain. At present, no causal or preventive treatments are established. (ROM) Range of motion.

Spatial Involvement and Chronicity

Local disease involvement tends to be addressed by local, site-specific means. On the other hand, systemic treatments constitute the main thrust of the care offered to patients with generalized symptoms. Although the case features of the various TMDs focus on the craniofacial complex, critical information outside the local region of interest can be relevant to treatment decisions. However, this kind of information is often insufficiently acknowledged by the dental community, thereby biasing both systemic and locally administered therapies, including occlusal treatments.

Experienced clinicians recognize that pain in TMD patients is not always limited to the face, and studies have shown that individual pain distributions can fall into one of three case clusters based on involvement of (1) trigeminal dermatomes (V_1–V_3), (2) trigeminal and upper cervical (C_2–C_6) dermatomes, and (3) pain sites in addition to the aforementioned ones.[32] Pain conditions that overlap with the various TMDs include systemic arthritides, headaches, regional myofascial neck and shoulder pain, and widespread pain, also known as *fibromyalgia syndrome* (see chapter 22). TMJ arthritides

can occur in isolation, or they may be part of a systemic joint disease. With respect to fibromyalgia, the overlap with the various TMDs among patients encountered in academic referral centers is substantial,[33,34] but the current classification systems do not help clinicians to decide where the treatment should be focused.

Epidemiologic data are also suggestive of a significant overlap among the various TMDs and the tension-type and migraine headaches.[35] Because these headaches are often accompanied by pericranial tenderness, more among patients with tension-type headache than migraine headache,[36,37] it becomes clear that the diagnostic boundaries are blurred by this overlap. On the other hand, treatments are quite different, depending on the diagnostic assignment and/or the treating practitioner.

Besides pain distribution, case severity and chronicity represent critical factors in the decision-making process. Severe pain intensity may limit occlusal treatments to the most conservative occlusal appliances, but some patients with unremitting pain may almost beg to undergo occlusal therapy in the hope that alignment of the teeth and/or jaws may resolve their pain and jaw dysfunction. Some patients with a TMD may have a significant malocclusion that would be corrected with prosthodontic therapy, orthodontics, or orthognathic surgery. However, experience teaches that treatment of such patients has to focus

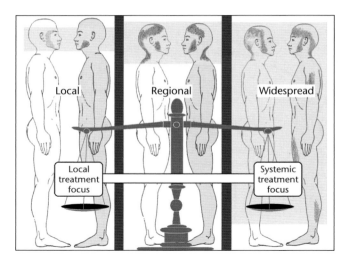

Fig 27-5 Determination of the focus of care. Local disease involvement is addressed by locally administered means, while systemic treatments constitute the main thrust of the care offered to patients with generalized symptoms. For those patients, local treatments may be added to achieve desirable outcomes.

on pain as the primary concern and that any consideration of reconstructive treatment has to be postponed until the status of the patient has improved.

Chronicity that is exemplified by the lack of a favorable response to many interventions calls for a treatment focus broader than the alignment of teeth and jaws by means of occlusal therapy. Notably, the presence of comorbid conditions (eg, sleep disturbances; cardiovascular, gastrointestinal, and reproductive system complaints; weight loss or weight gain; swelling, numbness, sweating and flushing; and concerns regarding loss of libido, drive, attention, and memory) points to the dysregulation of vital body systems, which suggests the need for a treatment focus that is multidisciplinary and patient oriented and not targeted only at specific symptoms or findings.

Framework for the Decision-Making Process

A structured decision-making process helps the clinician to reach reasonable choices with respect to therapy for any condition, so that the scope of care is defined by the extent to which the condition manifests itself locally or

systemically. Systemic involvement should be viewed not only as a matter of pain distribution but also in terms of the activation of the autonomic and affective systems (Fig 27-5).

If uncontrolled pain and disease are present, there is little justification for reconstructive dental treatment. If any occlusal treatment is indicated for the patient's comfort, it should be limited to the use of conservative occlusal appliances. On the other hand, a previous TMD may have left the patient with a significant malocclusion that is in need of correction for functional or esthetic reasons. The timing of such corrective occlusal treatment is determined by an assessment of the risk-benefit ratio for treatment in comparison to continued observation. Because high-level evidence in the form of tested decision trees is not available, prudence represents the guiding principle.

Because case severity, chronicity, and complexity shape clinical decisions and actions, their assessment constitutes a clinical necessity The gradual nullification of theories regarding the causal contribution of occlusal disharmonies to TMDs has come from a large body of research over a period of 20 years, which has fundamentally changed both the rationale and justification for occlusal treatments for these disorders (see chapter 14). Although occlusal treatments in dentistry today cover a broad range, from reversible occlusal appliances to irreversible procedures such as equilibration, prosthodontics, orthodontics, and orthognathic surgery, most of them are not directly relevant to the presentation or treatment of the various TMDs. In those few cases in which both the TMD and the occlusion must be dealt with, the prudent clinician will first deal with the pain and later with the occlusal problem.

References

1. Boering G, Dibbets J. Effect of arthropathia deformans of the temporomandibular joint in young people on the growth of the mandible [in German]. Fortschr Kiefer Gesichtschir 1980; 25:49–51.
2. Owall B, Moller E. Oral tactile sensibility during biting and chewing. Odontol Rev 1974;25:327–346.
3. Ohrbach R, Stohler CS. Current diagnostic systems. In: Dworkin SF, LeResche L (eds). Research Diagnostic Criteria for Temporomandibular Disorders: Review, criteria, examinations and specifications, critique. J Craniomandib Disord 1992;6:307–317.
4. Bell WE. Classification of TM disorders. In: Laskin D, Greenfield W, Gale E, et al (eds). The President's Conference on the Examination, Diagnosis and Management of Temporomandibular Disorders. Chicago: American Dental Association, 1983:24–29.

5. Dworkin SF, LeResche L. Research Diagnostic Criteria for Temporomandibular Disorders: Review, criteria, examinations and specifications, critique. J Craniomandib Disord 1992;6:301–355.

6. Lund JP, Donga R, Widmer CG, Stohler CS. The pain-adaptation model: A discussion of the relationship between chronic musculoskeletal pain and motor activity. Can J Physiol Pharmacol 1991;69:683–694.

7. Obrez A, Stohler CS. Jaw muscle pain and its effect on gothic arch tracings. J Prosthet Dent 1996;75:393–398.

8. Sackett DL, Haynes RB, Guyatt GH, Tugwell P. Clinical Epidemiology. A Basic Science for Clinical Medicine, ed 2. Boston: Little, Brown, 1991.

9. Stohler CS. Occlusal therapy in the treatment of temporomandibular disorders. Oral Maxillofac Surg Clin North Am 1995;7:129–139.

10. Stohler CS, Zarb GA. On the management of temporomandibular disorders: A plea for a low-tech, high-prudence therapeutic approach. J Orofac Pain 1999;13:255–261.

11. Turp JC, Kowalski CJ, Stohler CS. Treatment-seeking patterns of facial pain patients: Many possibilities, limited satisfaction. J Orofac Pain 1998;12:61–66.

12. Dao TT, Lavigne GJ, Charbonneau A, Feine JS, Lund JP. The efficacy of oral splints in the treatment of myofascial pain of the jaw muscles: A controlled clinical trial. Pain 1994;56:85–94.

13. Zubieta JK, Bueller JA, Jackson LR, et al. Placebo effects mediated by endogenous opioid activity on the μ-opioid receptors. J Neuroscience 2005;25:7754–7762.

14. Greene CS, Laskin DM. Splint therapy for the myofascial pain–dysfunction (MPD) syndrome: A comparative study. J Am Dent Assoc 1972;84:624–628.

15. Shipman WG, Greene CS, Laskin DM. Correlation of placebo responses and personality characteristics in myofascial pain–dysfunction (MPD) patients. J Psychosom Res 1974;18:475–483.

16. Laskin DM, Greene CS. Influence of the doctor-patient relationship on placebo therapy for patients with myofascial pain–dysfunction (MPD) syndrome. J Am Dent Assoc 1972;85:892–894.

17. Hiltunen K, Schmidt-Kaunisaho K, Nevalainen J, Narhi T, Ainamo A. Prevalence of signs of temporomandibular disorders among elderly inhabitants of Helsinki, Finland. Acta Odontol Scand 1995;53:20–23.

18. Von Korff M, Dworkin SF, Le Resche L, Kruger A. An epidemiologic comparison of pain complaints. Pain 1988;32:173–183.

19. Von Korff M, Wagner EH, Dworkin SF, Saunders KW. Chronic pain and use of ambulatory health care. Psychosom Med 1991;53:61–79.

20. Unruh AM. Gender variations in clinical pain experience. Pain 1996;65:123–167.

21. Riolo ML, Brandt D, TenHave TR. Associations between occlusal characteristics and signs and symptoms of TMJ dysfunction in children and young adults. Am J Orthod Dentofac Orthop 1987;92:467–477.

22. Pilley JR, Mohlin B, Shaw WC, Kingdon A. A survey of craniomandibular disorders in 800 15-year-olds. A follow-up study of children with malocclusion. Eur J Orthod 1992;14:152–161.

23. Lipton JA, Ship JA, Larach-Robinson D. Estimated prevalence and distribution of reported orofacial pain in the United States. J Am Dent Assoc 1993;124:115–121.

24. Zubieta JK, Smith YR, Bueller JA, et al. Regional μ opioid receptor regulation of sensory and affective dimensions of pain. Science 2001;293(5528):311–315.

25. Zubieta JK, Heitzeg MM, Smith YR, et al. COMT val158met genotype affects mu-opioid neurotransmitter responses to a pain stressor. Science 2003;299(5610):1240–1243.

26. Fahndrich E, Coper H, Christ W, Helmchen H, Muller-Oerlinghausen B, Pietzcker A. Erythrocyte COMT-activity in patients with affective disorders. Acta Psychiatr Scand 1980;61:427–437.

27. Floderus Y, Saaf J, Ross SB, Wetterberg L. Catechol-O-methyltransferase activity in human erythrocytes: Methodological aspects. Upsala J Med Sci 1981;86:309–318.

28. Floderus Y, Ross SB, Wetterberg L. Erythrocyte catechol-O-methyltransferase activity in a Swedish population. Clin Genet 1981;19:389–392.

29. Boudikova B, Szumlanski C, Maidak B, Weinshilboum R. Human liver catechol-O-methyltransferase pharmacogenetics. Clin Pharmacol Ther 1990;48:381–389.

30. LeResche L, Saunders K, Von KM, Barlow W, Dworkin SF. Use of exogenous hormones and risk of temporomandibular disorder pain. Pain 1997;69:153–160.

31. Kirveskari P, Jamsa T, Alanen P. Occlusal adjustment and the incidence of demand for temporomandibular disorder treatment. J Prosthet Dent 1998;79:433–438.

32. Turp JC, Kowalski CJ, O'Leary TJ, Stohler CS. Pain maps from facial pain patients indicate a broad pain geography. J Dent Res 1998;77:1465–1472.

33. Hedenberg-Magnusson B, Ernberg M, Kopp S. Symptoms and signs of temporomandibular disorders in patients with fibromyalgia and local myalgia of the temporomandibular system. A comparative study. Acta Odontol Scand 1997;55:344–349.

34. Korszun A, Papadopoulos E, Demitrack M, Engleberg C, Crofford L. The relationship between temporomandibular disorders and stress-associated syndromes. Oral Surg Oral Med Oral Pathol Oral Radiol Endod 1998;86:416–420.

35. Agerberg G, Carlsson GE. Functional disorders of the masticatory system. 2. Symptoms in relation to impaired mobility of the mandible as judged from investigation by questionnaire. Acta Odontol Scand 1973;31:337–347.

36. Forssell H, Kangasniemi P. Mandibular dysfunction in patients with migraine. Proc Finn Dent Soc 1984;80:217–222.

37. Forssell H, Kangasniemi P. Mandibular dysfunction in patients with muscle contraction headache. Proc Finn Dent Soc 1984;80:211–216.

Indications and Limitations of TMJ Surgery

Daniel M. Laskin

The conditions affecting the temporomandibular joint (TMJ) can be divided into those that are managed only medically, those that are treated only surgically, and those that are initially treated medically but that may be treated surgically if a medical approach is unsuccessful. Thus, surgery can play an important role in the primary or secondary management of many TMJ problems. It is therefore essential for clinicians treating such problems to understand when surgery is and is not indicated and to know which operations are most successful, especially because different surgical approaches for treating the same condition are often recommended in the literature.

Conditions Requiring Primary Surgical Management

Conditions that are always treated surgically involve problems of overdevelopment or underdevelopment of the mandible resulting from alterations of condylar growth, mandibular ankylosis, and benign and malignant tumors of the TMJ.

Mandibular Growth Disturbances

Those conditions causing mandibular overgrowth include unilateral condylar hyperplasia and mandib-ular prognathism, and those resulting in absent or deficient mandibular growth include condylar agenesis and condylar hypoplasia. The congenital and developmental conditions that produce mandibular growth disturbances are discussed in chapter 2. Although congenital hypoplasia can occur, mandibular underdevelopment is most often a result of postnatal causes. These include trauma, infection, and radiation therapy. The extent of the deformity will be determined not only by the severity of the etiologic factor but also by the time of occurrence. Thus, the effect will be more extreme early in life when condylar growth activity is the greatest.

Treatment of condylar hypoplasia depends on the age at which the patient condition is diagnosed. Because the facial deformity usually develops slowly, patients in whom there is no associated jaw dysfunction may be at an age at which growth has stopped or nearly stopped before concern about their appearance causes them to seek care. For these patients, orthodontics and various forms of orthognathic surgery are generally used to correct the malocclusion and the facial deformity. In addition, genioplasty and facial augmentation grafts or implants may be needed to provide a better esthetic result. In patients who are still growing, restoration of ramal height and replacement of the deficient condylar growth site can be accomplished by placement of a costochondral graft or use of distraction osteogenesis (see chapter 29).

Box 28-1	Causes of ankylosis of the mandible

I. Congenital
II. Traumatic (direct or indirect; local and regional)
  A. At birth
  B. Later
    1. Accidental (fractures, including depressed
      fracture of the zygomatic arch; hemarthrosis)
    2. Surgical (scarring)
III. Inflammatory
  A. Local
  B. Regional
    1. Otitis media and mastoiditis
    2. Osteomyelitis of mandible, dental and
      parotid abscesses, etc
    3. Radionecrosis (soft tissue and bone)
    4. Noma
  C. Hematogenous
    1. Osteomyelitis
    2. Scarlet fever
    3. Gonorrhea
  D. Systemic
    1. Rheumatoid arthritis
IV. Neoplastic
  A. Local
  B. Regional, including osteochondroma of the
    coronoid process
V. Idiopathic, including enlarged coronoid processes

Ankylosis

TMJ ankylosis can be classified as congenital, traumatic, inflammatory, or neoplastic in origin (Box 28-1). All these types of ankylosis are treated by surgery except the inflammatory group, which is often managed medically initially and then treated surgically, if necessary.

Four basic principles are involved in the surgical treatment of TMJ ankylosis:

1. In a growing child, the treatment should be initiated as early as feasible, and an autogenous costochondral graft should be placed to reestablish mandibular growth and prevent severe facial deformity.
2. In the adult, the new joint should be created at the most superior aspect of the ramus possible to maintain the maximum ramal height, minimize the postoperative shift of the mandible in patients undergoing unilateral surgery, and prevent an open bite in patients undergoing bilateral surgery.
3. A biocompatible material should be placed in the new joint space to prevent fusion of the parts.
4. Vigorous postoperative physical therapy is essential to maintaining the surgically established range of mandibular movement.

Tumors of the TMJ

Benign tumors of the TMJ are always treated surgically, just as in any other region. Most of the malignant tumors of the TMJ are not radiosensitive and therefore are also managed in this manner (see chapter 35).

Conditions Involving Secondary Surgical Management

In addition to the inflammatory conditions affecting the TMJ, other conditions that usually involve surgery only secondarily include the various forms of arthritis, fractures of the condyloid process, anterior disc displacement with or without reduction, and mandibular dislocation.

Arthritis

The TMJ is affected by all of the forms of arthritis that involve other joints in the body (see chapters 9 and 15). As in these other regions, the most common types of arthritis are infectious, traumatic, rheumatoid, and degenerative. In addition to medical management with antibiotics, infectious arthritis may require aspiration or incision and drainage of the joint as well as possible secondary sequestrectomy. On the other hand, traumatic arthritis uncomplicated by the presence of a fracture is totally managed medically. Rheumatoid arthritis is also treated medically unless ankylosis develops; this condition requires surgical management. Whereas the primary treatment for degenerative joint disease is medical, just as it is in other joints, surgery has been used when such treatment is not effective (see chapter 31).

Fractures of the Condyloid Process

It is generally agreed that fractures of the condyloid process with minimal or no displacement are managed nonsurgically by closed reduction and short-term maxillomandibular fixation (see chapter 18). The unilaterally fractured, dislocated condyloid process is also often managed in the same manner. However, there does not appear to be any agreement regarding other types of condyloid process fractures. Bilateral fractures with dislocation, particularly when the patient is edentulous or there is an associated fracture of the maxilla, are often managed by open surgical reduction and fixation. Likewise, when the malpositioned condyloid process interferes with motion of the jaw, or when no occluding teeth are present on the side of the fracture, surgery is often recommended.

The following factors should be considered when making a decision about open or closed reduction of condyloid process fractures: (1) the age of the patient, (2) whether the fracture is unilateral or bilateral, (3) whether the patient has an adequate number of teeth for achieving fixation, (4) the level at which the condyloid process is fractured, (5) whether or not the fragments are in contact, and (6) whether the condyle is in the glenoid fossa. The general condition of the patient, as well as the time that has elapsed since the injury occurred, must also be considered.

Anterior Disc Displacement with Reduction

There is general agreement that the clicking or popping sounds that occur when an anteriorly displaced disc reduces to its normal position on mouth opening requires no treatment unless it is so loud that it is socially unacceptable or it is accompanied by pain. In the former instance, the joint noise can only be eliminated by surgically repositioning the disc to its normal anatomic position (discoplasty). In the latter instance, however, the treatment is aimed only at nonsurgical elimination of the pain (see chapters 23 and 25). It has been shown that, when the painful aspects of the internal derangement are addressed, very few patients have further problems,[1] even though the clicking may still persist. For the small percentage of patients in whom the pain cannot be controlled nonsurgically, discoplasty is the recommended treatment (see chapter 32).

Anterior Disc Displacement Without Reduction

Various nonsurgical treatments, used alone or in combination, have been recommended for the management of nonreducing anterior disc displacement (closed lock). These include nonsteroidal anti-inflammatory drugs,[2] occlusal appliances,[3] exercise therapy,[4,5] and manual manipulation.[6] However, in those instances where such treatments are unsuccessful, minor intracapsular interventions or open surgery become alternative solutions.

The initial treatment involves lysis of adhesions and lavage of the joint either by arthrocentesis or arthroscopy. If such therapy is ineffective, open joint surgery with discoplasty is indicated (see chapter 32). Such treatment should not be delayed, because it may be impossible to salvage the disc when it has undergone further degenerative or atrophic changes or when there is a large perforation in the disc or retrodiscal tissue.

Mandibular Dislocation

Acute mandibular dislocation is usually managed nonsurgically by manually pressing the mandible downward to stretch the spastic elevator muscles and then backward to relocate the condyle within the glenoid fossa. Although this can sometimes be accomplished without medicating the patient, generally it is necessary to use a sedative, such as intravenous diazepam. Following reduction, the patient should voluntarily limit use of the jaw for at least a week. However, in many patients this may not be feasible; instead, the clinician will need to immobilize the mandible with a head-chin strap or maxillomandibular fixation to facilitate repair of the stretched capsule and ligaments and to prevent redislocation while these tissues are still lax.

If the joint was relatively normal at the time that the dislocation occurred, this treatment should be adequate. If the dislocation occurred because the tissues were already very lax, however, there may be a tendency for repeated episodes (chronic recurrent dislocation). Under such circumstances, more definitive treatment is usually indicated.

Five basic surgical methods have been recommended for correction of chronic recurrent mandibular dislocation: (1) mechanical tightening of the capsule (capsulorrhaphy), (2) fastening of parts of the joint or mandible to adjacent fixed structures, (3) creation of mechanical interferences in the condylar path, (4) elimination of interference with the condylar path (eminectomy), and (5) reduction of lateral pterygoid muscle pull. Relatively good success has been reported with most of these surgical procedures except those that attempt to limit jaw movement by anchoring the mandible to adjacent fixed structures.

The reason that such diverse methods are effective is related to one common factor: All of these procedures are intra-articular operations that produce capsular scarring and therefore limit the range of mandibular motion. However, because a similar effect can be produced more easily and safely by the injection of a sclerosing solution (sodium morrhuate or sodium tetradecyl sulfate) into the joint capsule, such treatment is preferable to surgery in most cases.[7]

The sclerosing technique and the various surgical procedures sometimes fail because of the persistence of the condition that initially caused looseness of the capsule and ligaments. For example, the patient with uncontrollable epileptic seizures, severe parkinsonism, or orofacial dyskinesia will continue to stretch these structures and eventually

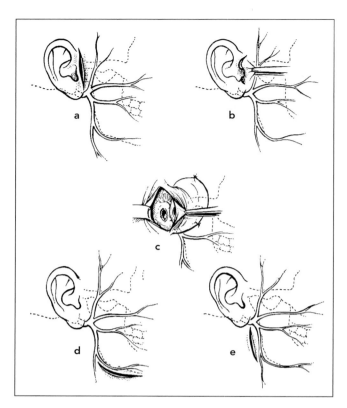

Fig 28-1 Surgical approaches to the TMJ. *(a)* Standard preauricular approach; *(b)* endaural approach; *(c)* postauricular approach; *(d)* submandibular approach; *(e)* retromandibular approach.

Surgical Approaches to the TMJ

There are four main surgical approaches to the TMJ, all of which are designed to provide adequate access while avoiding injury to the facial nerve: the preauricular, postauricular, retromandibular, and submandibular (Fig 28-1). An endaural approach has also been described,[12] but it provides limited access and also may cause meatal stenosis.

Preauricular Approach

The preauricular approach is the one most commonly used to expose the TMJ. There are relatively few complications, and it provides excellent esthetic results. Because the approach is made in the gap between the buccal and marginal mandibular branches of the facial nerve, injury to the nerve is not a common occurrence. The incision starts in front of the ear at the level of attachment of the auricle and follows the anterior border of the ear until it reaches the point of attachment of the lobule (Fig 28-2a).

For even better esthetics, the incision can be modified so that when it reaches the upper aspect of the tragus, it is continued along the crest of the tragus and then exited onto the skin in a vertical direction until the point of attachment of the lobule (Fig 28-2b). An oblique extension from the superior end of the incision ("hockey stick incision") is used only when it is necessary to expose a portion of the temporalis fascia and muscle, because it provides no additional access to the joint. When it is used, this incision should be made parallel to the temporal branch of the facial nerve to avoid injury to that structure.

Once the preauricular incision is carried through the skin and subcutaneous tissues, a small mosquito hemostat is used to spread the tissues in the upper end laterally to expose the temporalis fascia. This establishes the plane for further dissection. The hemostat is then used to create a tunnel along the anterior border of the ear to the inferior aspect of the incision, and this layer of tissue is detached from the auricle with a small scissors. This tissue layer, which contains the parotid gland, facial nerve, superficial temporal artery and vein, and the auriculotemporal nerve, is bluntly reflected forward with a periosteal elevator to expose the joint capsule (Fig 28-3).

When a discoplasty or a discectomy is to be performed (see chapter 32), the disc is isolated by parallel incisions through the capsule extending into the upper and lower joint spaces. When the TMJ is being treated for an ankylosis or some other form of condylar pathosis, the routine preauricular approach is also used until the capsule is encountered. The joint is then exposed by a T-shaped inci-

dislocation will recur. In such patients, bilateral lateral pterygoid myotomy, which limits anterior condylar translation, is an effective form of treatment.[8,9] More recently, injection of botulinum toxin into the lateral pterygoid muscle has been suggested as an alternative treatment.[10,11] Although this procedure has been shown to be effective for relatively short periods, its long-term effectiveness has not been established, and, in most cases reported, the injections have had to be repeated.

Occasionally a patient's acute mandibular dislocation is not reduced immediately, and simple manual reduction becomes impossible because of muscular contraction, severe fibrosis, or bony changes in the condyle and fossa. Such persistent dislocation can sometimes be treated by manual manipulation aided by traction wires placed through the angles of the mandible while the patient is under general anesthesia. If this procedure fails, temporal myotomy performed through an intraoral vertical incision over the anterior border of the coronoid process is generally effective in allowing the condyles to be repositioned in the glenoid fossae.[8]

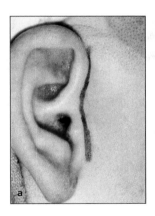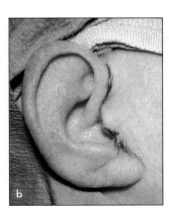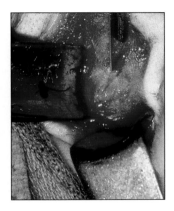

Fig 28-2 Preauricular incisions used to access the TMJ. *(a)* Standard incision made just in front of the auricle; *(b)* modified preauricular incision that extends over the crest of the tragus rather than anterior to it.

Fig 28-3 Incision of the joint capsule after anterior reflection of the parotid gland. The access provided by this small incision is adequate.

sion, so that the horizontal component extends beneath the zygomatic arch in the upper joint space and the vertical component extends inferiorly along the middle of the condylar neck.

Postauricular Approach

The postauricular approach to the TMJ entails an incision made behind the ear, followed by division of the cartilaginous auditory canal and reflection of the entire auricle.[13] The articulation is then exposed from behind. The incision, which is made about 3.0 to 5.0 mm posterior to the auricular flexure and extended in depth to the level of the mastoid fascia, begins near the superior aspect of the ear and continues to the tip of the mastoid process. Blunt and sharp dissection in an anterior direction is then used to expose approximately two thirds of the external auditory canal. Superiorly, the dissection is extended along the temporalis fascia from the base of the zygomatic arch to approximately the junction of its posterior and middle thirds. An incision is then made through the cartilaginous auditory canal and the auricle is reflected forward. The TMJ is exposed by making a longitudinal incision along the lower half of the posterior third of the zygomatic arch and then extending it vertically over the condyle anteriorly.

Although it is reported that the postauricular approach to the TMJ is more advantageous than the preauricular approach because there is negligible intraoperative bleeding, less chance of developing a salivary fistula or a sialocele, no facial nerve paresis, less postsurgical edema, and better esthetics,[13] comparison studies supporting these claims have never been completed. Moreover, the potential complications of stenosis of the external auditory canal, infection of the auditory canal and cartilaginous framework of the ear, paresthesia of the external ear, and deformity of the auricle are more serious than those complications associated with the preauricular approach and do not justify any possible esthetic advantage the postauricular approach may have.

Retromandibular Approach

The retromandibular approach provides direct access to the neck of the condyloid process and is therefore the preferred method for performing a condylectomy or open reduction of subcondylar fractures and for placing condylar prostheses or grafts. Because children have short rami, this approach also provides sufficient access to the TMJ for treating ankylosis in such patients, thus avoiding the need for a second (submandibular) incision when a graft is to be placed. Because the retromandibular incision is located in the shadow of the mandible, the resulting scar is very inconspicuous.

A 3.0- to 3.5-cm incision is made through the skin and subcutaneous tissues just posterior and parallel to the posterior border of the ascending ramus, extending from a point just below the level of the lobule of the ear infe-

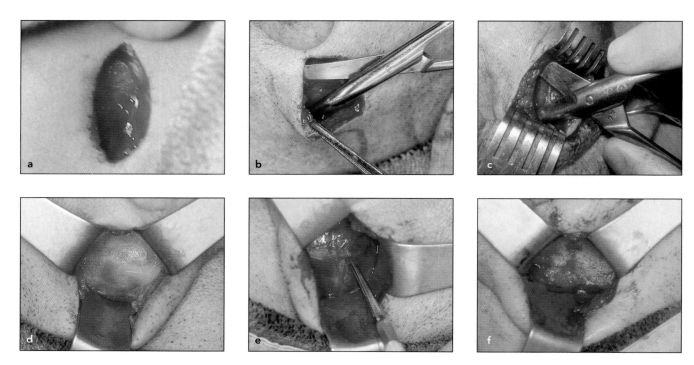

Fig 28-4 Retromandibular approach to TMJ surgery. *(a)* Retromandibular incision. *(b)* Undermining of the skin to permit free movement of the tissues in all directions. *(c)* Vertical splitting of the fascia at the anterior border of the parotid gland. *(d)* Masseter muscle after the posterior retraction of the parotid gland. *(e)* Incision of the masseter muscle. *(f)* Fracture of the condyloid process exposed via the retromandibular approach.

riorly to a point just above the angle of the mandible (Figs 28-1e and 28-4a). A pair of scissors is used to undermine the skin in all directions so that it can be moved freely and facilitate exposure of all aspects of the surgical site (Fig 28-4b). The wound margins are then retracted to expose the parotideomasseteric fascia and the parotid capsule. After the depression marking the anterior border of the tail of the parotid gland is identified, a Metzenbaum scissors is inserted into the depression and the fascia is opened in a vertical direction (Fig 28-4c). The parotid gland is then retracted posteriorly, exposing the masseter muscle (Fig 28-4d), which is incised at its posterior border as far superiorly and inferiorly as possible (Fig 28-4e). The masseter is then reflected with a periosteal elevator, exposing the lateral aspect of the mandibular ramus and the condyloid process to the level of the joint capsule (Fig 28-4f).

Submandibular Approach

Because of its distant location from the TMJ, this approach provides the poorest access to the region. However, it can be used for open reduction of low subcondylar fractures and as part of the approach for the placement of condylar prostheses and grafts, although the retromandibular incision provides better access and results in a more esthetic, less obvious scar.

The initial incision, which is about 3.0 cm long, is made through the skin and subcutaneous tissues to the level of the platysma muscle. It is placed either 1.0 or 2.0 cm below and parallel to the lower border of the mandible or slightly lower so that it is located in or parallel to a skin crease. The lower location generally produces a less conspicuous scar.

Once the platysma is exposed, it is undermined with a small, curved hemostat and incised parallel to the skin incision, revealing the underlying superficial layer of the deep cervical fascia. This fascial layer is undermined and incised in the lower aspect of the wound to avoid damage to the marginal mandibular branch of the facial nerve. However, if the incision extends anteriorly into the region of the antegonial notch, the facial artery and vein must be located, isolated, and ligated before the entire fascial layer is opened. A submandibular lymph node (node of Stahr) is usually present in the region of the antegonial notch, and it can serve as a landmark for finding the facial vessels, which are located anterior and deep to it. Once the cervical fascia is completely incised, the upper wound margin is retracted superiorly to expose the mandibular angle.

The pterygomandibular sling is then incised and the masseter muscle and underlying periosteum are reflected and retracted superiorly to expose the lateral aspect of the ramus and the condyloid process.

Effectiveness of TMJ Surgery

It is essential to understand not only when surgery is or is not indicated for the management of certain TMJ disorders but also what is the best procedure for treating a particular patient when surgery is appropriate. In some instances, there are long-standing protocols that have been shown to be clinically effective. However, in other situations, several operations are often recommended for the same condition, and the surgeon is faced with determining which is the most effective. Ideally, the clinician should be able to find well-designed, randomized clinical trials reported in the literature to help in making such decisions. Unfortunately, such studies do not exist in most instances. At best, the literature encompasses mainly retrospective studies with small sample sizes, unclear inclusion and exclusion criteria, short-term follow-up, and varying, mainly subjective outcome measures, making comparisons between reports difficult if not impossible. Therefore, before adopting any new procedures, clinicians should proceed cautiously until there is sufficient long-term evidence for their relative effectiveness.

References

1. Greene CS, Laskin DM. Long-term status of TMJ clicking in patients with myofascial pain and dysfunction. J Am Dent Assoc 1988;117:461–465.
2. Yuasa H, Kurita K. Randomized clinical trial of primary treatment for temporomandibular joint disk displacement with reduction and without osseous changes: A combination of NSAIDs and mouth-opening exercise versus no treatment. Oral Surg Oral Med Oral Pathol Oral Radiol Endod 2001;91:671–675.
3. Lundh H, Westesson PL, Eriksson L, Brooks SL. Temporomandibular joint disk displacement without reduction. Treatment with a flat occlusal splint versus no treatment. Oral Surg Oral Med Oral Pathol 1992;73:655–658.
4. Minakuchi H, Fuboki T, Matsuka Y, Maekawa K, Yatani H, Yamashita A. Randomized controlled evaluation of nonsurgical treatments for temporomandibular joint disk displacement without reduction. J Dent Res 2001;80:924–928.
5. Minakuchi H, Kuboki T, Maekawa K, Matsuka Y, Yatani H. Self-reported remission, difficulty, and satisfaction with nonsurgical therapy used to treat anterior disc displacement without reduction. Oral Surg Oral Med Oral Pathol Oral Radiol Endod 2004;98:435–440.
6. Foster ME, Gray RJM, Davies SJ, Macfarlane TV. Therapeutic manipulation of the temporomandibular joint. Br J Oral Maxillofac Surg 2000;38:641–644.
7. Laskin DM. Surgical management of diseases of the temporomandibular joint. In: Hayward J (ed). Oral Surgery. Springfield, IL: Thomas, 1976:173–190.
8. Laskin DM. Myotomy for management of recurrent and protracted mandibular dislocation. In: Kay L (ed). Oral Surgery. Copenhagen: Munksgaard, 1972:264–268.
9. Sindet-Pedersen S. Intraoral myotomy of the lateral pterygoid muscle for treatment of recurrent dislocation of the mandibular condyle. J Oral Maxillofac Surg 1988;46:445–449.
10. Ziegler CM, Haag C, Muhling J. Treatment of recurrent temporomandibular joint dislocation with intramuscular botulinum toxin injection. Clin Oral Investig 2003;7:52–55.
11. Martinez-Perez D, Garcia Ruiz-Espiga P. Recurrent temporomandibular joint dislocation treated with botulinum toxin: Report of 3 cases. J Oral Maxillofac Surg 2004;62:244–246.
12. Davidson AS. Endaural condylectomy. Br J Plast Surg 1956;8:64–67.
13. Alexander RH, James RB. Postauricular approach for surgery of the temporomandibular articulation. J Oral Surg 1975;33:346–350.

Congenital and Developmental Anomalies

Maria J. Troulis and Leonard B. Kaban

Understanding and managing congenital and developmental deformities of the temporomandibular joint (TMJ) require a three-dimensional analysis of the abnormal anatomy and consideration of the fourth dimension, that is, growth over time. Moreover, in addition to the primary anomaly, development of secondary deformities of the contiguous and contralateral facial skeletal structures over time must be considered. Furthermore, the surgeon must try to determine the effects of an early operation on facial growth and body image development in growing patients.

To understand the effects of various congenital syndromes, it is also essential to be familiar with the related embryology. The branchial or pharyngeal arches appear at 4 weeks in embryonic development. Each pharyngeal arch consists of endodermal, mesodermal, and ectodermal tissue layers. Within the core of each arch are neural crest cells that form the skeletal components of the face. The first pharyngeal arch progresses via intramembranous ossification to form the maxilla, mandible, palatine bone, vomer, and zygoma and the tympanic portion of the temporal bone. Also, two of the ossicles (malleus and incus) of the middle ear are formed in the first pharyngeal arch, although they are derived from Meckel cartilage. The muscles of mastication (temporalis, masseter, and medial and lateral pterygoids), anterior belly of the digastric, mylohyoid, tensor tympani, and tensor palatini muscles are all derived from the first arch. The nerve of the first pharyngeal arch is the trigeminal nerve (cranial nerve V).

The second pharyngeal arch forms the stapes (the most proximal middle ear ossicle), the styloid process of the temporal bone, and the lesser horn of the hyoid bone. The stylohyoid ligament also develops from this arch. The muscles of the second arch include the stapedius, stylohyoid, and posterior belly of the digastric, as well as the muscles of facial expression. The nerve of the second arch is the facial nerve (cranial nerve VII).

This chapter discusses the diagnosis and management of several congenital (hemifacial microsomia [HFM], bilateral craniofacial microsomia, and Treacher Collins syndrome [TCS]) and developmental (condylar hyperplasia) first and second pharyngeal arch defects that can affect the TMJ.

Congenital Anomalies

Hemifacial Microsomia

Hemifacial microsomia is a variable, progressive, and asymmetric congenital craniofacial deformity.[1] It involves the skeletal, neural, and muscular tissues and soft tissue envelope of the first and second pharyngeal arches, and it is the second most common congenital facial deformity (affecting 1 in 5,600 live births) after cleft lip and palate.[2–4]

Although the actual mechanism by which HFM develops in humans is unknown, Poswillo[5] has developed and described an animal phenocopy in mice in which hemorrhage from the developing stapedial artery produces a hematoma in the area of the first and second pharyngeal arches. The size of the hematoma and resultant tissue destruction explains the morphology and variability of HFM, at least in the experimental model.[4] Johnston and

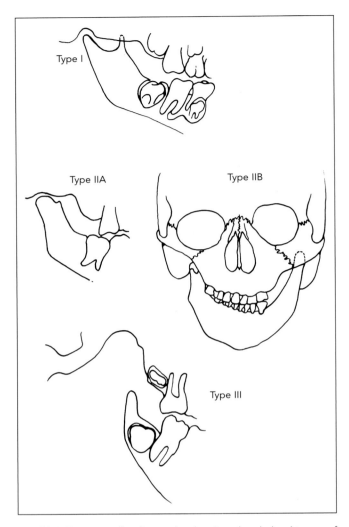

Type I

Type IIA

Type IIB

Type III

Fig 29-1 Tracings of radiographs showing the skeletal types of hemifacial microsomia.

Bronsky[6] have replicated deformities similar to HFM by the administration of retinoic acid to pregnant mice. Retinoic acid is known to destroy neural crest cells and interfere with their movement and dispersal. This may explain the wide spectrum of phenotypes exhibited by patients with HFM.[7]

Facial growth

The earliest *skeletal* manifestation of HFM is the asymmetric mandible. The newborn with HFM usually has symmetric orbits. The nose (alar bases), labial commissures, and maxillary occlusal plane are parallel to each other but on a tangent to a line across the superior orbital rims and to the true horizontal (Frankfort plane). The mandible is short on the affected side and, with asymmetric growth, the ipsilateral alveolar ridge becomes

canted upward on the affected side. The mandibular and maxillary alveolar ridges contact prematurely on the affected side, and there is an open bite on the unaffected side. The chin is deviated toward the short side. Asymmetric mandibular growth and the hypoplastic muscles and soft tissues of the first and second pharyngeal arches contribute to the progressive deformity of the ipsilateral and contralateral facial skeleton.[2]

Normally, the mandible grows downward and forward in relation to the cranial base by growth of the condylar cartilage as well as bone deposition and resorption on its periosteal and endosteal surfaces.[4,8] This pattern of growth determines the eventual size and shape of the mandible and also plays an important role in the three-dimensional relationships of the mandible, maxilla, midface, and cranial base. The ramus increases in height because of growth of the condylar cartilage and by bone deposition on the posterior-inferior surface and resorption on the anterior surface. Resorption on the medial surface and deposition on the lateral surface account for the shape and width of the mandible in the transverse plane.[4,8] In patients with HFM, mandibular growth on the affected side is impaired, and the resultant mandible is short (in the vertical dimension), retrusive in the sagittal plane, and narrow in the horizontal (transverse) plane.

The maxilla normally grows inferiorly (downward) and anteriorly (forward) as a result of bone resorption on the superior (nasal) and anterior surfaces and deposition of bone on the inferior (palatal) surface.[4,8] In patients with HFM, the abnormal mandibular growth pattern blocks the normal downward (vertical) growth of the maxilla and midface. This results in a short maxilla with an occlusal cant (upward on the abnormal or affected side); the orbit may be inferiorly displaced.[1–4,9,10]

Classification

Skeletal deformity

The skeletal deformities of HFM are classified according to the anatomy of the mandibular ramus and TMJ (Fig 29-1).[3,10,11] A type I skeletal deformity consists of a normally shaped but small mandible and TMJ with all structures present (ie, condyle, sigmoid notch, coronoid process, glenoid fossa, muscles of mastication, and disc). The range of motion—rotation, translation, and lateral excursion—is usually normal.

A type II skeletal deformity consists of a small and abnormally shaped mandibular ramus and TMJ. This group is further subdivided into types IIA and IIB. In type IIA, the degree of TMJ hypoplasia is mild and the joint is located in an acceptable position. The muscles of mastication are hypoplastic but do provide for some transla-

Fig 29-2 Teenage patient with left skeletal type IIB hemifacial microsomia. (Reprinted from Kaban[4] with permission.) *(a)* Frontal view demonstrating the typical physical findings of end-stage hemifacial microsomia: Marked contour asymmetry resulting from soft tissue deficiency on the left side; left epibulbar dermoid; macrostomia; canting of the alar base and labial commissures upward toward the left; and marked deviation of the chin to the left. The ear is low set but normal in morphology. *(b)* Anteroposterior cephalometric tracing showing the medial and inferior location of the TMJ and ramus, deviation of the chin point, cant of the occlusal plane, and orientation of a plane formed by the mandibular dental and skeletal midlines. *(arrows)* Direction of movement necessary to correct the deformity.

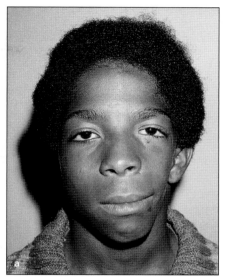

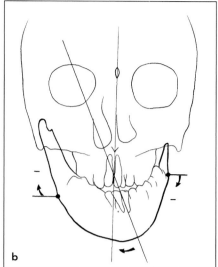

tion, rotation, and lateral excursive movements. In patients with a type IIB defect, the TMJ is hypoplastic and displaced far medially, anteriorly, and inferiorly in relation to the normal side. These patients are functionally similar to those with a type III deformity.

Type III HFM is characterized by complete absence of the mandibular ramus and TMJ.[2–4,12–16] The muscles of mastication are severely hypoplastic or absent, as is the articular disc. Although maximal interincisal opening is usually normal in the HFM patient, lateral excursion and protrusion of the jaw are progressively diminished on the affected side as the severity of the skeletal deformity increases.[17]

The end-stage skeletal deformity of HFM consists of a short, medially displaced mandibular ramus and TMJ. The abnormal side of the mandible is flat and the chin point is deviated toward the affected side. A plane drawn between the mandibular dental and skeletal midlines is rotated so that the upper end (dental) is shifted toward the normal side and the lower end (skeletal) is shifted toward the affected side (Fig 29-2). The midface is short, resulting in a canted occlusal plane in which the distance among the infraorbital rim, piriform aperture, and maxillary alveolus is decreased. The zygomatic bone is flat, and the orbit is sometimes inferiorly displaced.[2,3]

Soft tissue defects

The soft tissue defects are analyzed by physical examination and review of frontal, lateral, oblique, and submental photographs. Components of the soft tissue to consider include the bulk of subcutaneous soft tissue; the

muscles of mastication and facial expression; the presence or absence of macrostomia, skin tags, and facial clefts; the external ear anatomy; cranial nerve function (particularly nerve VII); and soft palate function.[3,10,12]

The deformity consists of a decrease in mass of subcutaneous tissue ranging from mild to severe; the degree of soft tissue hypoplasia usually, though not always, correlates with the severity of the skeletal defect. The muscles of mastication and facial expression are hypoplastic. The patient may have macrostomia, and skin tags may be present along a line from the tragus to the commissure of the lips.

Patients with minimal subcutaneous and muscle hypoplasia, absence of or slight macrostomia, and a normal or mild auricular deformity (preauricular tags may be present) are classified as mild HFM. Those with severe subcutaneous tissue and muscle hypoplasia, facial clefts, severe ear anomaly, and macrostomia are classified as severe HFM. Patients with an intermediate degree of soft tissue deformity are classified as moderate.[3,10,12]

The external ear anomaly is documented with the system described by Meurman[18]:

- Grade 1: Mild hypoplasia and mild cupping but all structures present
- Grade 2: Absence of the external auditory canal and variable hypoplasia of the concha
- Grade 3: Absent auricle and anteriorly and inferiorly displaced lobule; conductive hearing loss because of hypoplasia of the ear ossicles[3,12]

Table 29-1	Progression of facial asymmetry in patients with hemifacial microsomia*					
	Primary dentition (< 6 y)		Mixed dentition (6 to 13 y)		Permanent dentition (> 13 y)	
	Group I[†]	Group II[‡]	Group I[†]	Group II[‡]	Group I[†]	
Piriform rim angle (degrees)	7.0 ± 3.6	9.5 ± 3.5	7.7 ± 3.8	11.7 ± 4.7	8.4 ± 3.0	
Maximum occlusal plane angle (degrees)	4.3 ± 3.0	6.2 ± 4.3	5.0 ± 3.5	7.6 ± 3.8	6.6 ± 4.5	
Intergonial angle (degrees)	4.4 ± 2.4	5.3 ± 3.8	4.3 ± 2.8	8.0 ± 3.4	6.1 ± 3.6	
Mean age (y)	4.1 ± 0.9	3.4 ± 1.4	8.6 ± 2.3	8.0 ± 1.7	20.9 ± 8.9	

*Data from Kearns et al.[1]
[†]Group I consisted of a total of 38 patients with Type I or IIA deformities.
[‡]Group II consisted of a total of 29 patients with Type IIB or III deformities.

Analysis of the neuromuscular defects are included in the soft tissue evaluation. More than 25% of the patients have cranial nerve abnormalities, usually consisting of facial nerve palsy (VII) or deviation of the soft palate toward the affected side with motion. Palatal deviation is due to a combination of muscle hypoplasia and cranial nerve weakness (cranial nerves V and X). The presence or absence of seventh nerve palsy correlates with the severity of the ear defect and not the skeletal defect. The most common facial nerve weakness involves the marginal mandibular branch, followed by the branch to the frontalis muscle. Rarely, a patient will have total seventh nerve weakness, a sensory deficit in the fifth nerve distribution, or both.[19,20]

OMENS classification

Vento et al[21] and Mulliken et al[22] have described the OMENS classification of hemifacial microsomia, which is an acronym for the structures involved: orbit, mandible (and TMJ), ear, nerves, and soft tissues. The orbit is designated as normal (score 0), abnormal in size (1), abnormal in position (2), or both (3). The mandible may be normal (score 0), type I (1), type IIA (2A), IIB (2B), or type III (3). The ear anomaly is classified to correspond to Meurman's system and is designated E0 to E3. The facial nerve defect is described as N0 to N3 to correspond to no facial nerve involvement, upper branch involvement, lower branch involvement, or all branches involved, respectively. The soft tissue deficiency is classified as normal (0), mild (1), moderate (2), or severe (3).

This is a rigorous system that forces the clinician to evaluate and document all aspects of the hemifacial

microsomia anomaly in each patient. In addition, there is some evidence that a summation of the OMENS score in the different categories has some predictive value for the presence of additional anomalies, eg, skeletal, renal, and cardiac. Patients who have an OMENS score of greater than 7 should undergo an abdominal ultrasound, skeletal survey, and cardiac evaluation.[23]

Treatment

Skeletal deformity

Accurate classification of the skeletal defect is critical in developing a treatment plan. The skeletal type determines the rate of progression of the asymmetry and the end-stage distortion of the contiguous and contralateral skeletal structures (Table 29-1).[1,7,17,24,25]

Nongrowing patients. Surgical correction in the nongrowing patient begins with clinical examination, routine radiographs, and computerized tomographic (CT) scans to classify the end-stage deformity. The treatment strategy for three-dimensional correction of the end-stage deformity of hemifacial microsomia depends on the skeletal type.

The first steps are to level the midface (below the infraorbital rims), piriform apertures (floor of the nose), and alveolar portion of the maxilla in the coronal plane; correct the position of the maxilla in the sagittal plane (advancement as required); and correct any residual width deficiency and the maxillary dental midline (horizontal or transverse plane). Usually a Le Fort I osteotomy is sufficient. However, at times, a higher midface or orbital osteotomy may be required.

If the height of the midfacial skeleton relative to the upper lip is normal, then the center of rotation to level the maxillary occlusal plane is in the midline. The net result is a combination of lengthening the short side and shortening the long side to level the maxilla and to maintain the relationship of the maxillary anterior teeth to the upper lip. In patients with HFM types I and IIA, once the maxilla is repositioned, bilateral mandibular osteotomies are used to correct the mandibular deformity. In patients with HFM types IIB and III, construction of the ramus-condyle unit (RCU), and sometimes the glenoid fossa and zygomatic arch, is required to complete the correction. Contour defects in the skeleton are managed with onlay bone or allografts; the soft tissue and ear defects are usually corrected later, after skeletal symmetry has been achieved.

The new RCU is constructed from a costochondral and, when necessary, an iliac crest graft. The glenoid fossa is constructed from full-thickness rib, iliac crest, or calvarial bone. The bone is secured in place with screws or plates and screws lateral to the existing zygomatic arch or lateral to the cranium, if no zygomatic arch is present. A glenoid fossa is hollowed out of this graft and lined with perichondrium or temporalis fascia and muscle, if present.[12,20]

Growing patients. The overall goals of early correction of HFM in growing children are to achieve and maintain optimal facial symmetry and improved function. Thus, treatment is directed toward *(1)* increasing the size of the underdeveloped and malformed mandible and associated soft tissues; *(2)* creating an articulation between mandible and temporal bone, when absent; *(3)* promoting vertical maxillary growth and therefore correcting or preventing secondary deformities of the maxilla; and *(4)* establishing a functional occlusion.

A child with HFM must be in the mixed dentition to benefit from early management. Success depends on the potential for vertical growth of the midface as the primary teeth are shed and the permanent teeth erupt. The operation consists of elongation, rotation, and advancement of the hypoplastic mandible to bring the chin point to the midline and to create an open bite on the affected side.[4] In type I, type IIA, and some type IIB deformities, this is achieved by mandibular osteotomy with or without bone grafting, as indicated (Fig 29-3), or by distraction osteogenesis (DO) (Fig 29-4). In the majority of patients with type IIB and all patients with type III deformities, the operation consists of construction of the RCU and glenoid fossa, if necessary.

A major goal of early surgical correction of HFM is to achieve a symmetric maxilla and midface with a level occlusal plane and level alar bases (piriform angle). Failure to understand this rationale leads to inadequate attention to creation and management of the open bite. The open bite space must be maintained by an orthodontic appliance (occlusal bite block) for a period of at least 3 to 6 months while the osteotomized or constructed ramus heals. Then the maxillary teeth can be allowed to erupt by a combination of passive movement and orthodontic forces, thereby leveling the occlusal plane. If the open bite space is not maintained adequately during this crucial period, it closes rapidly by a combination of supraeruption of the teeth and resorption and deformation of the lengthened ramus under the compressive forces of the occlusion. Thus, the desired effect of early treatment is lost.[26]

Treatment must proceed stepwise, beginning with presurgical orthopedic management of the mandible. A functional appliance is constructed to hold the affected side of the mandible in a lowered and forward position. The appliance stimulates bone apposition in the RCU by substituting for the normal translatory motion produced by the lateral pterygoid muscle. This treatment is applied routinely for children during the presurgical growth management phase.

Response to this functional therapy is beneficial, particularly for patients with HFM types I and IIA. A study of 15 type I patients showed that, during treatment with a functional appliance, the affected side grew more than the contralateral side in four children, grew by an amount equal to the contralateral side in another four, and grew slightly less than the contralateral side in the remaining seven subjects. There was no significant group mean difference in growth of the two sides in this sample.[27] A similar response to this type of treatment was documented by Melsen and coworkers.[28]

The results of treatment of HFM in childhood have periodically been analyzed at Boston Children's Hospital.[13,26] Kaban et al[13] evaluated 20 patients classified as type I or IIA (group 1, n = 10) and type IIB or III (group 2, n = 10). They were treated by the protocol previously described. The mean follow-up times were 50.9 months (group 1) and 45.0 months (group 2). In all children, the midface grew vertically to close the surgically created open bite and the occlusal plane was leveled without maxillary osteotomy. Among patients who had type I or IIA HFM and who were followed to completion of growth (n = 9 of 10), none required a maxillary osteotomy or a second operation on the mandible. In patients with type IIB or III HFM (n = 4), who were operated on during the primary dentition stage (younger than 5 years), the affected mandible required a second elongation procedure in the late mixed dentition or early teen years. No patients needed a midfacial osteotomy

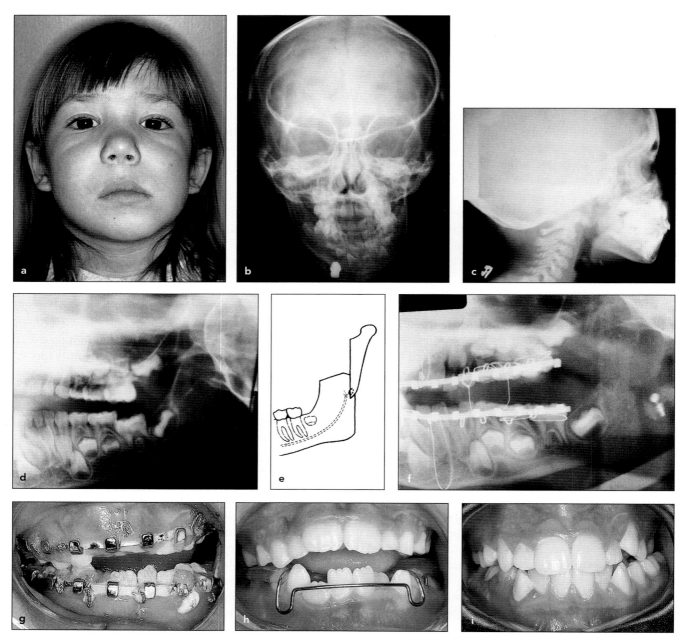

Fig 29-3 Girl with left type IIA hemifacial microsomia. (Reprinted from Kaban[4] with permission.) *(a)* Frontal photograph of the patient at 5 years, demonstrating deviation of the chin point. *(b)* An anteroposterior cephalogram revealing deviation of the chin point, a short ramus, and deviation of the mandibular dental midline. *(c)* Lateral cephalogram demonstrating the double images of the short and long sides of the asymmetric mandible. *(d)* Panoramic radiograph of the hypoplastic and abnormally shaped left ramus, a type IIA deformity. *(e)* Diagrammatic representation of the elongation of the left ramus with a vertical osteotomy. *(f)* Immediately postoperative panoramic radiograph of the lengthened ramus and the surgically created open bite. *(g)* Immediately postoperative intraoral view demonstrating the surgically created open bite. *(h)* Intraoral view 5 months postoperatively with the intraoral appliance in place. The appliance is progressively adjusted to allow eruption of the maxillary dentition and vertical growth of the maxilla. The open bite closes over an 18- to 24-month period postoperatively. *(i)* Intraoral photograph taken 5 years postoperatively, revealing closure of the open bite and coincident midlines. The patient will now begin conventional orthodontic treatment to correct her crowded dentition.

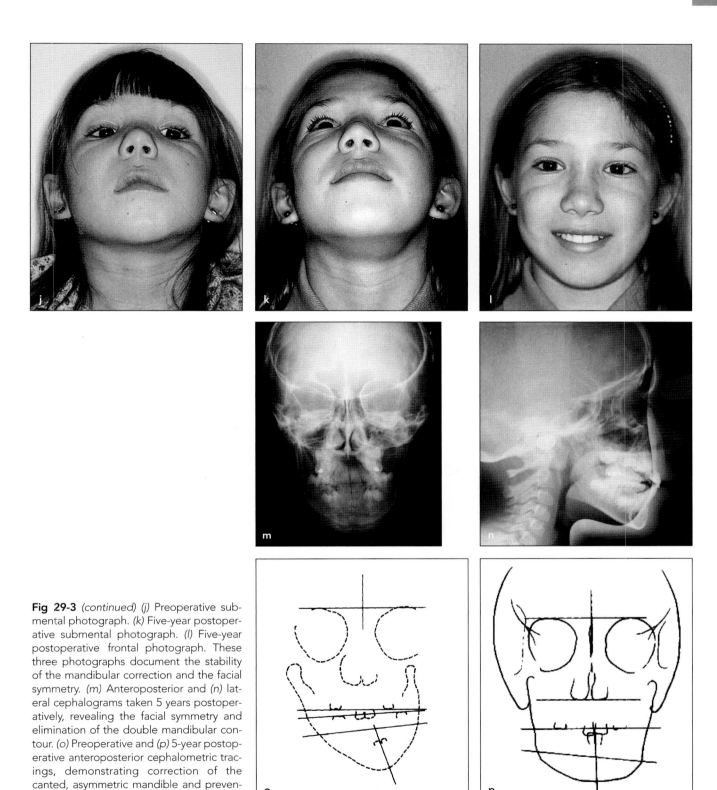

Fig 29-3 *(continued) (j)* Preoperative submental photograph. *(k)* Five-year postoperative submental photograph. *(l)* Five-year postoperative frontal photograph. These three photographs document the stability of the mandibular correction and the facial symmetry. *(m)* Anteroposterior and *(n)* lateral cephalograms taken 5 years postoperatively, revealing the facial symmetry and elimination of the double mandibular contour. *(o)* Preoperative and *(p)* 5-year postoperative anteroposterior cephalometric tracings, demonstrating correction of the canted, asymmetric mandible and prevention of midfacial asymmetry.

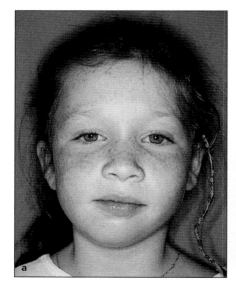

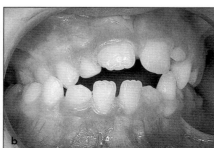

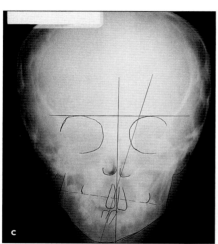

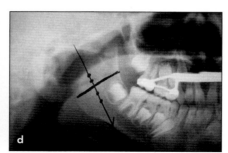

Fig 29-4 Right-side type IIA hemifacial microsomia. (Reprinted from Kaban[4] with permission.) *(a)* Frontal and *(b)* intraoral photographs of a child in the mixed dentition stage, revealing deviation of the chin point to the right and slight canting of the alar bases and commissures. The unilateral crossbite is being treated by maxillary expansion with a removal device. *(c)* Anteroposterior cephalogram and overlay tracing showing deviation of the chin point, the short ramus, and deviation of the mandibular dental midline. The piriform apertures and occlusal plane are canted upward to the right. *(d)* Panoramic radiograph demonstrating the type IIA mandible and the location of the osteotomy. *(arrow)* Vector of movement of the jaw. *(e)* Immediately postoperative anteroposterior cephalogram taken with the distraction device in place. *(f)* Anteroposterior cephalogram at the end of distraction, revealing the amount of mandibular lengthening. *(g)* Lateral photograph showing separation of the proximal and distal mandibular segments (separation of the pins) at the end of distraction.

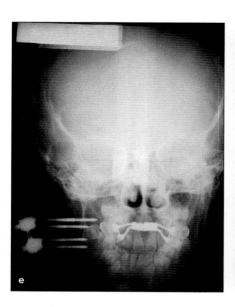

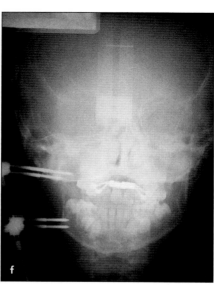

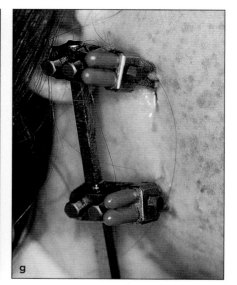

Fig 29-4 *(continued)* *(h)* Frontal photograph of the patient 1 year after DO, demonstrating that the chin point is coincident with the facial midline and symmetry is improved. *(i)* Intraoral view revealing the remaining surgically created open bite that will be progressively closed by eruption of the maxillary teeth. This will level the occlusal plane and maintain mandibular position. *(j)* Frontal, *(k)* lateral, and *(l)* intraoral views of the patient 4 years after distraction. Note the maintenance of facial symmetry and closure of the open bite. *(m)* Panoramic radiograph and *(n)* anteroposterior cephalogram 4 years after distraction, revealing mandibular symmetry and level piriform apertures and occlusal plane.

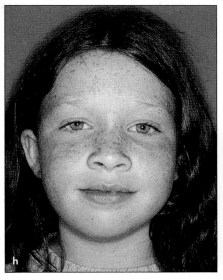

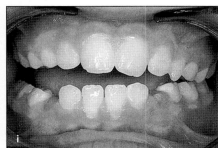

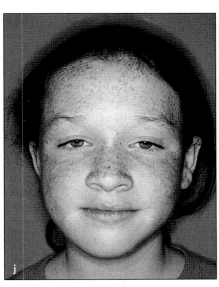

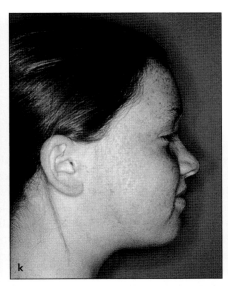

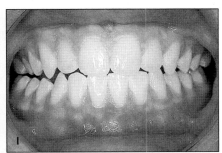

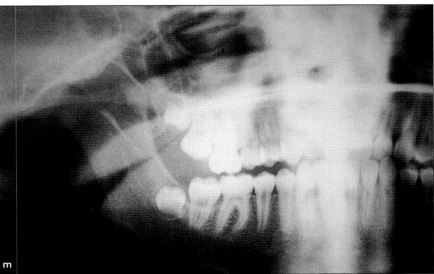

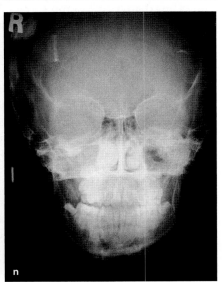

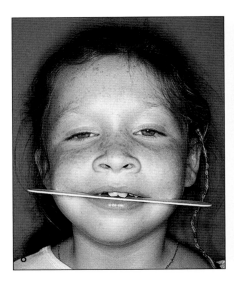 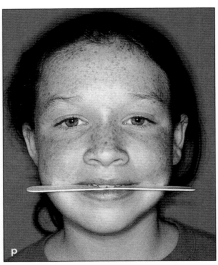

Fig 29-4 *(continued) (o)* Preoperative and *(p)* 4-year postoperative frontal views with a tongue depressor in the mouth, demonstrating the change in the occlusal plane.

in this series. In a sense, the patients were converted from type IIB or III to type IIA.

Padwa et al[26] evaluated 33 children who underwent costochondral graft construction for types IIB (n = 19) and III (n = 14) HFM. Mean age at operation was 6.2 years, and the mean follow-up was 5.5 years. Stability of the results was judged on the basis of maintenance of the occlusal cant correction. Based on previously published data,[25] an occlusal cant of less than 5 degrees was considered a successful outcome (group I), a cant equal to or greater than 5 and less than 8 degrees was acceptable (group II), and a cant equal to or greater than 8 degrees was a failure (group III).

The severity of the deformity, as reflected by the OMENS score, and the age at operation affected the outcome. The patients who had a successful result (group I) had a mean OMENS score significantly lower than did those in groups II and III (6.3, 6.8, and 7.8, respectively) and were operated on at an older age (6.7, 6.3, and 5.8 years, respectively). Furthermore, the occlusal cants in group I improved (decreased) with age, whereas the cants remained stable in group II and worsened with time in group III. The authors concluded that, after construction of the RCU in patients with types IIB and III HFM, vertical midfacial growth occurred secondary to a combination of midfacial and alveolar growth.[26]

Vargervik et al[27] reported continual growth of the lengthened mandibular ramus in the majority of 10 patients who were operated on early and followed until growth was completed. In 3 patients, however, growth of the affected side did not keep pace with the contralateral side and asymmetry recurred, requiring a second surgical procedure that also involved maxillary leveling. The maxilla was corrected orthodontically in all these patients.

Soft tissue defects

Treatment of the soft tissue abnormalities, such as removal of skin tags, may begin during infancy. Significant macrostomia is usually repaired during the first year of life. The external ear deformity is usually left untreated until after the skeletal correction is completed.[12] This is to ensure that the ear will be placed in its correct position. Furthermore, ear growth is completed at around the age of 6 years, and there is sufficient donor cartilage by that age. The ear construction is carried out with autogenous tissue and the techniques described by Tanzer[29] and refined by Brent and Byrd.[30,31]

The deficiency of subcutaneous tissues is also corrected after the skeletal correction. Occasionally, the contour defect can be corrected with onlay bone or allografts, but in patients with moderate and severe soft tissue deficiency augmentation with soft tissue is necessary. The most common method involves the use of free vascularized tissue transfer. This provides the most natural soft tissue texture without the disadvantage of gravitational sag.

Bilateral First and Second Pharyngeal Arch Defects

The two most common bilateral first and second pharyngeal arch deformities are Treacher Collins syndrome and bilateral craniofacial microsomia. Patients with TCS (mandibulofacial dysostosis) and bilateral craniofacial microsomia have a characteristic constellation of anomalies that include hypoplastic TMJs, short mandibular rami, and decreased posterior face height. It is only recently that the importance of decreased posterior face height in the evolution of the end-stage deformity has been appreciated.[4,32]

Treacher Collins syndrome

With an incidence of 1:10,000 live births, TCS is an autosomal-dominant trait with incomplete penetrance and variable expressivity.[4,33] It has been recently discovered that the genetic basis for TCS resides in mutations in the *TCOF1* gene loci 5q32-q33.1.[32]

The clinical features of this syndrome were described by Thomson[34] in 1847, Berry[35] in 1889, and Treacher Collins[36] in 1900. Franceschetti and Klein[37] called it *mandibulofacial dysostosis*. Clinical features of the syndrome are variable, with a wide spectrum of anomalies that are characteristically bilateral and symmetric.[38] There is a downward cant of the palpebral fissures, with or without a coloboma at the corner of the eyelids (usually lower), and pathognomonically an absence of eyelashes along the medial third of the lower lid. The external ears are low set and small. There is usually a conductive hearing loss in association with abnormalities of the external and middle ear. The inner ear, not being formed from the first or second pharyngeal arch, develops normally. There tends to be an extension of temporal hair onto the cheek. The nose is large, and the zygomatic bones and arches are hypoplastic.[32,34–49]

Bilateral craniofacial microsomia

Patients with bilateral craniofacial microsomia have the bilateral form of hemifacial microsomia and therefore some characteristics similar to those of individuals with TCS. The defects are asymmetric; in addition, the patients have eyelashes on the medial third of the lower eyelids, and they may have unilateral or bilateral facial nerve deficits and macrostomia, both of which are not the case in persons with TCS. TCS is inherited as an autosomal-dominant trait, but bilateral craniofacial microsomia is not hereditary.[39,40]

Treatment

The orbital deformities of TCS are corrected with bone grafts to the zygomas and orbital floors and recontouring of the supraorbital rims. The lateral canthi are elevated, and the soft tissue defects around the eyelids are usually corrected with local flaps. Secondary zygomatic augmentation is often accomplished with alloplastic materials, such as Medpor (Porex Surgical Products), as the child grows.

Common to both TCS and bilateral craniofacial microsomia is the short posterior facial height. Correction of the skeletal deformity in both syndromes consists of elongation of the mandibular rami and advancement of the mandible. In the adult patient with an end-stage deformity, this also involves an operation on the maxilla, at the Le Fort I or II level. The posterior maxilla is rotated downward to lengthen the posterior face; the center of rotation is at the nasofrontal region or anterior nasal spine. An interpositional bone graft is placed in the gaps. The mandibular ramus is then lengthened with a sagittal split osteotomy, with a ramus osteotomy and bone graft, or by construction of a new ramus and TMJ.[33]

In the growing child, the mandibular ramus is elongated and the body is advanced and rotated counterclockwise to close any existing anterior open bite. The mandible is placed in a prognathic relationship to the maxilla, and a bilateral posterior open bite is created. The open bite is regulated and progressively reduced with an orthodontic appliance, allowing the maxilla and midface to grow vertically and maintain the increase in posterior facial height. However, in certain cases, the mandible must be elongated and advanced for airway considerations at an age too early to perform a Le Fort osteotomy. These patients will require a Le Fort I or II osteotomy at a later date. The maxillary procedure may sometimes be avoided in patients with bilateral facial microsomia, as it is in some individuals with hemifacial microsomia.

Developmental Anomalies

Unilateral Condylar Hyperplasia

Unilateral condylar hyperplasia is the most common postnatal growth abnormality of the TMJ. It occurs more frequently in females than in males, and it is the result of a hyperactive growth center in the affected condyle. The condition must be differentiated from mild HFM on the opposite side (ie, condylar hypoplasia) and from a generalized asymmetric growth pattern (mandibular hemihypertrophy), which are not accompanied by a localized hyperactive condylar region.[41–44]

Children with unilateral condylar hyperplasia are typically born with a symmetric jaw. They and their families recall the first sign of asymmetry as occurring during the onset of puberty. Asymmetric jaw growth progresses simultaneously with the rapid increase in overall body size. After a variable period of time, the abnormal growth center becomes quiescent and progression of the deformity ceases. This cycle of abnormal growth generally continues over a period of several years. Approximately two thirds of patients who present to the surgeon or orthodontist for evaluation are stable, in the quiescent phase of condylar hyperplasia.[43]

TMJ symptoms, such as noise in the joint or discomfort with function, are uncommon. Patients may exhibit limitation of motion, particularly an inability to translate forward and backward, because the condyle is disproportionately large in relation to the glenoid fossa.

There are two growth patterns in this disorder[4]: In the first pattern, excessive mandibular growth occurs in a predominantly vertical direction. The patients always exhibit increased height of the ramus and often of the mandibular body. Intraorally, there is an open bite on the affected side; there is usually no crossbite on the unaffected side. As the abnormal ramus grows excessively, the chin point and dental midline become slightly deviated toward the normal side.

The second growth pattern is rotational. Not only is a vertically long ramus present on the affected side, but also the mandibular body is convex and the chin point and dental midline are significantly deviated toward the normal side. Intraorally, there is a crossbite on the unaffected side. The clinical appearance of patients with this form often resembles that of patients with end-stage hemifacial microsomia.

Diagnosis

History and physical examination

The diagnosis of condylar hyperplasia is made if the history indicates that progressive mandibular asymmetry has developed after birth. Although the asymmetry is most commonly noticed during or after the onset of puberty, it can be manifest between the ages of 4 and 7 years, when the mandible is also growing rapidly. Physical examination demonstrates one of the two growth patterns previously described. In patients with the vertical pattern, there may be an occlusal cant downward on the affected side. This occurs with time as dental compensations (ie, supraeruption of the teeth) result in spontaneous closure of the open bite (Fig 29-5).

Condylar hyperplasia is differentiated from mild HFM on the opposite side by the absence of ear anomalies, soft tissue contour deficiency, seventh cranial nerve paresis, and soft palatal deviation during palatal muscle contraction with function (all manifestations of first and second branchial arch defects). Patients with condylar hyperplasia often have a Class III occlusion on the affected side and Class I occlusion on the unaffected side, whereas those with HFM may have Class II occlusion on both sides. In addition, the mandibular asymmetry of HFM is almost always accompanied by secondary abnormality in the midface. This is because the anomaly is present at birth and mandibular hypoplasia has a profound effect on vertical growth of the midface.

Imaging studies

Panoramic and TMJ radiographs of patients with condylar hyperplasia demonstrate asymmetry in the condylar head and neck regions. The condyle is larger and the neck is longer on the affected side. The unaffected ramus-condyle unit is normal in morphology. Skeletal scintigraphy using technetium 99m methylene diphosphonate is a useful diagnostic tool.[3,4,43–51] Patients with condylar hyperplasia will exhibit greater uptake in the affected condyle than will control subjects.[43,44]

With this technique, it is possible to (1) differentiate the normal from the abnormal side of the mandible (Is the small side hypoplastic or the large side hyperplastic?); (2) determine the presence of an abnormal condylar growth center versus generalized asymmetric mandibular growth; and (3) differentiate between an actively progressive condition versus a stable growth abnormality.[43,44] Pogrel and coworkers[52] have also correlated increased uptake in the affected condyle with condylar hyperplasia using technetium 99m uptake in single photon emission CT scans.

Treatment

To develop a treatment plan, the surgeon must determine whether the abnormal condylar growth is progressive or has stopped. Patients in the active phase can be observed until the growth cycle is complete or may be offered a growth-arresting procedure (high condylectomy). The latter is most advantageous when carried out early, prior to the development of dental compensations, to avoid the need for bimaxillary orthognathic surgery. Patients who present with both active condylar hyperplasia and secondary deformities requiring correction will benefit from simultaneous high condylectomy and orthognathic surgery (Fig 29-6).[53–55]

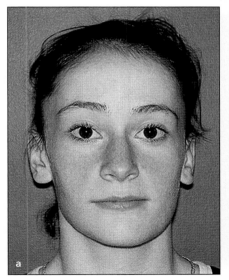

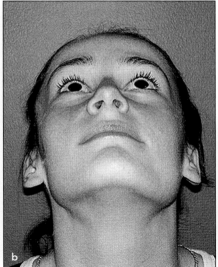

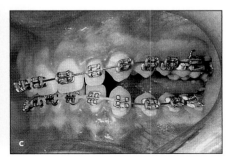

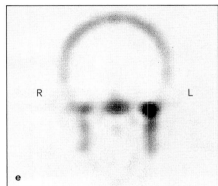

Fig 29-5 Uncompensated vertical pattern condylar hyperplasia. (Reprinted from Kaban[50] with permission.) *(a)* Frontal and *(b)* submental views of a 15-year-old girl with a left mandibular ramus that has been elongated by condylar hyperplasia. *(c)* Intraoral view showing the left posterior open bite prior to the development of dental compensations. *(d)* Axial technetium 99m scan showing the increased uptake on the left side. *(e)* Coronal view showing the hyperactive left condyle.

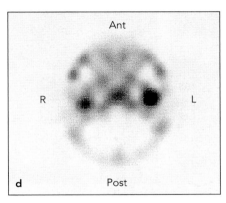

High condylectomy is performed through a standard preauricular incision; the hyperplastic condylar region is usually well demarcated and easily identified as a soft, marrowlike cap on the condylar head. This is excised (high condylectomy), leaving the normal condylar stump in place.

Recently, Troulis and Kaban[54] have described a minimally invasive endoscopic technique for high condylectomy. A 1.5-cm submandibular incision is used to expose the mandible and create an optical cavity. The hyperplastic condylar head can then be identified and the abnormal region removed. Bimaxillary correction of the jaw asymmetry is completed in the standard fashion using Le Fort I and mandibular osteotomies.

Patients with a clinically stable deformity, confirmed by a normal bone scan, are treated by orthodontic decompensation of the teeth and standard orthognathic surgical correction. In these patients, high condylectomy is not performed unless there are TMJ symptoms such as decreased motion, pain, or marked deviation on opening because of mechanical interference by the large condylar head.

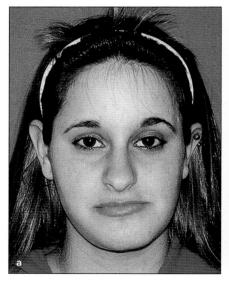
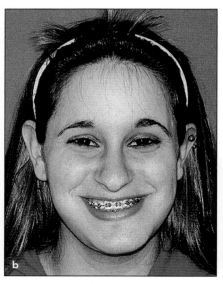
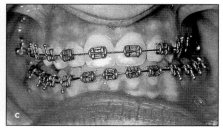
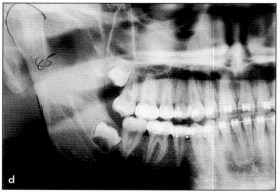
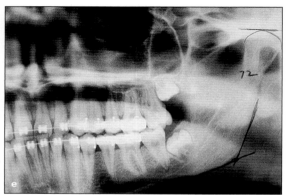
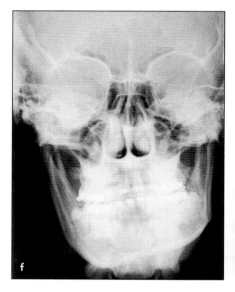
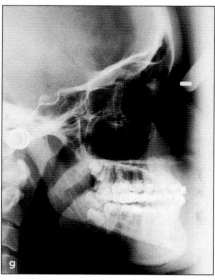

Fig 29-6 Compensated condylar hyperplasia. (Reprinted from Kaban[50] with permission.) *(a and b)* Frontal and *(c)* intraoral preoperative photographs. *(d)* Right and *(e)* left preoperative panoramic views. *(f)* Anteroposterior and *(g)* lateral cephalograms revealing marked asymmetry.

Fig 29-6 *(continued)* *(h)* Intraoperative view of Le Fort I osteotomy with rigid fixation. The right side was shortened and the left side slightly elongated and stabilized with a bone graft. The center of rotation of the movement was determined by measurements to ensure the proper relationship of the maxillary anterior teeth to the upper lip. *(i)* Segment of the right ramus and condylar head. A right vertical ramus osteotomy was performed endoscopically, the ramus segment was removed, and the hyperplastic condylar head (marked in pencil) was then excised. The segment was replaced and rigidly fixed. The left side was treated with a rigidly fixed sagittal split osteotomy. *(j)* Inferior border ostectomy outlined. *(k)* Mandibular symmetry after the segment was removed. *(l)* Anteroposterior cephalogram, *(m)* lateral cephalogram, *(n)* right panoramic radiograph, and *(o)* left panoramic radiograph showing correction of the asymmetry. Note the elimination of the cant, the leveling of the occlusal plane, the midline position of the chin, the correction of the double shadow of the inferior mandibular borders, and the symmetry of the right and left ramus lengths.

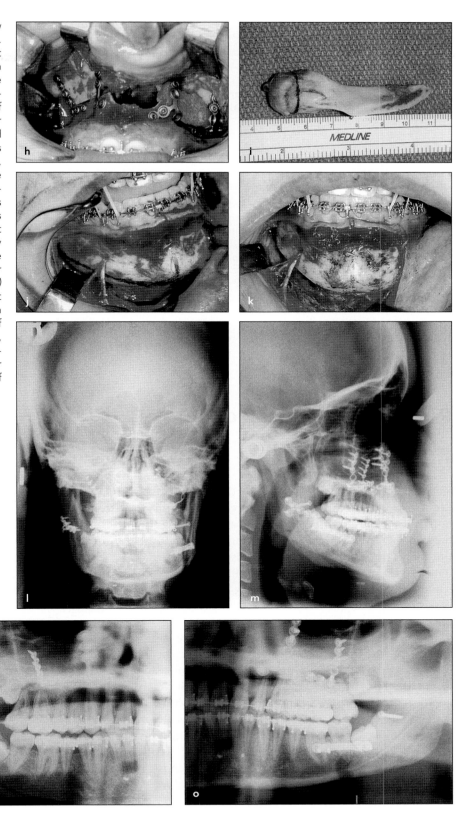

Table 29-2	Use of distraction osteogenesis (DO) in patients with hemifacial microsomia*	
	Treatment methods	
Skeletal type	**Adult end-stage (fixed or static) deformity***	**Growing children**
I or IIA	Bimaxillary orthognathic surgery or bimaxillary DO Correction of chin-contour asymmetry Secondary bimaxillary DO in patients who are inadequately corrected	Mandibular DO only Conventional osteotomy (mandible only) Orthodontics to maintain open bite Mandibular DO in patients who are inadequately corrected
IIB or III	Construction of RCU +/- TMJ construction Bimaxillary orthognathic surgery Correction of chin-contour asymmetry Secondary bimaxillary DO in patients who are inadequately corrected	Construction of RCU +/- TMJ construction Orthodontics to maintain open bite Mandibular DO in patients who are inadequately corrected

*RCU = ramus-condyle unit; +/- = with or without.

Role of Advanced Technology

Distraction Osteogenesis

Since Codivilla[56] first reported on the technique of distraction osteogenesis in 1905, there have been a large numbers of studies published on skeletal expansion using this method. DO is a technique of bone lengthening that uses the body's inherent healing mechanisms to form new bone. As described and popularized by Ilizarov,[57–59] a corticotomy is made in the bone, leaving the marrow and endosteal blood supply intact. A rigid device is fixed to the bone across the gap and, after a latency period, the device is activated at a rate of 1 mm per day. When the desired expansion is achieved, the bone is rigidly fixed for a period of days approximately twice the number of millimeters of distraction. Bone fill is documented by routine radiographs and/or ultrasound. The distraction protocols currently used in the craniomaxillofacial region are derived from various clinical and experimental studies in the long bones and face of both humans and animal models.[57–64]

DO is a useful technique for bone lengthening in patients with HFM, TCS, and bilateral craniofacial microsomia.[65–70] Surgeons using this technique must follow the treatment principles and guidelines described previously in this chapter, with DO substituted for the indicated osteotomies, acute movements, and bone grafts.

However, the technique is only applicable for correction in patients who meet the following criteria: (1) Enough bone stock must be present in the mandibular RCU to allow the corticotomy and placement of the distraction device and (2) the skeletal movements required to correct the deformity must be possible by DO. For example, the majority of HFM patients with an end-stage deformity require a combination of lengthening of the short side and shortening the long side of the mandible to correct the asymmetry. This type of three-dimensional, bilateral correction cannot be accomplished by DO, which can only be used to lengthen the skeleton (Table 29-2). However, if a patient with an end-stage type I or IIA deformity happens to have a long upper lip and/or a normal vertical midface length on the unaffected side (with normal to inadequate tooth show), bimaxillary distraction of the short side is possible. For patients with types IIB or III deformity, the bone stock is usually inadequate and the RCU must be constructed.

In the growing child with a type I or IIA deformity, DO of the short side, used in accordance with the previously described guidelines for early treatment, is feasible. Growing children with a type IIB deformity usually require construction of the RCU, and those with a type III deformity always do (see Table 29-2).

DO is particularly useful in patients with TCS who have severe micrognathia, decreased posterior facial height and tracheostomy-dependent airway obstruction. It is the only technique that allows RCU lengthening and counterclockwise rotation of the mandible of the magnitude required in these children. Skeletal stability has been satisfactory and prevention or elimination of the tracheostomy has been documented.[71–77] DO is used for the same reason in other syndromic and nonsyndromic cases of severe micrognathism.

Three-dimensional Treatment Planning

CT and magnetic resonance imaging of the human body have had an enormous impact on the practice of medicine and surgery during the past 20 years. Three-dimensional data acquisition allows visualization and analysis of complex craniomaxillofacial anomalies.[78,79] Application of three-dimensional imaging for surgical treatment planning and navigation[80,81] is crucial for guiding minimally invasive reconstructive techniques, such as DO. The success of most craniomaxillofacial surgical corrections depends on careful analysis and planning based on a variety of diagnostic information, eg, clinical examination, photographs, radiographs, and articulated dental casts. The lateral cephalogram has been a valuable tool for conventional planning and for outcome evaluation. However, this radiograph has its limitations because it only represents a composite of the sagittal plane and does not account for asymmetry, which is often present.[81–85] Advances in minimally invasive surgical techniques (including and especially DO) further heighten the need for accurate treatment planning.[83–90]

In collaboration with the Harvard Surgical Planning Laboratory, a three-dimensional treatment planning system called Osteoplan has been developed. The software uses CT data to produce three-dimensional images for visualization of the craniomaxillofacial skeleton and allows the operator to simulate osteotomies and to move the resultant bony fragments. The software also allows the insertion of landmarks, measurement of angles and distances between landmarks, simulation of osteotomies, repositioning of bones and bone fragments, detection of virtual bone collisions, superposition and comparison of preoperative and postoperative CT scans and comparison of postoperative (actual) and predicted skeletal movements.

The visual superimposition of two casts can be used for qualitative and quantitative comparisons. With the three-dimensional models and landmarks registered to a standard orientation, the software provides a potential tool for measuring cephalometric distances and angles. Finally, the program calculates the vector of the proposed skeletal movement and provides a prescription for the location of the osteotomy and for the design of a distraction device to accomplish the movement. Ultimately, this system will also incorporate accurate dental and surface (skin) data.[81–87]

Summary

This chapter presents an evidence-based summary of current knowledge about clinical characteristics, diagnosis, and treatment of congenital and developmental TMJ anomalies. The important concept of progression of the deformity with time and growth is emphasized. The purpose of treatment in the growing child is to enhance the growth potential of the mandible, maxilla, and developing dentition. In addition, early treatment can decrease or prevent secondary deformity in contiguous and contralateral facial skeletal structures, and improve body image development.

Acknowledgment

The material in this chapter has been adapted from Kaban.[4,50]

References

1. Kearns GJ, Padwa BL, Mulliken JB, Kaban LB. Progression of facial asymmetry in hemifacial microsomia. Plast Reconstr Surg 2000;105:492–498.
2. Kaban LB, Mulliken JB, Murray JE. Three-dimensional approach to analysis and treatment of hemifacial microsomia. Cleft Palate J 1981;18:90–99.
3. Murray JE, Kaban LB, Mulliken JB. Analysis and treatment of hemifacial microsomia. Plast Reconstr Surg 1984;74:186–199.
4. Kaban LB. Congenital abnormalities of the temporomandibular joint. In: Kaban LB, Troulis MJ (eds). Pediatric Oral and Maxillofacial Surgery. Philadelphia: Saunders, 2004:302–339.
5. Poswillo D. The pathogenesis of first and second branchial arch syndrome. Oral Surg Oral Med Oral Pathol 1973;35:302–328.
6. Johnston MC, Bronsky PT. Animal models for human craniofacial malformations. J Craniofac Genet Dev Biol 1991;11:277–291.
7. Kaban LB, Padwa BL, Mulliken JB. Surgical correction of mandibular hypoplasia in hemifacial microsomia: The case for treatment in early childhood. J Oral Maxillofac Surg 1998;56:628–638.
8. Enlow OH. Handbook of Facial Growth. Philadelphia: Saunders, 1975.
9. Moss ML. Twenty years of functional cranial analysis. Am J Orthod 1972;61:479–485.

10. Murray JE, Kaban LB, Mulliken JB, Evans CA. Analysis and treatment of hemifacial microsomia. In: Caronni EP (ed). Craniofacial Surgery. Boston: Little, Brown, 1985:377–391.

11. Pruzansky S. Not all dwarfed mandibles are alike. Birth Defects 1969;1:120.

12. Mulliken JB, Kaban LB. Analysis and treatment of hemifacial microsomia. Clin Plast Surg 1987;14:91–100.

13. Kaban LB, Moses ML, Mulliken JB. Correction of hemifacial microsomia in the growing child. Cleft Palate J 1986;23 (suppl 1):50–52.

14. Kaban LB, Moses ML, Mulliken JB. Surgical correction of hemifacial microsomia in the growing child. Plast Reconstr Surg 1988;821:9–19.

15. Kaban LB, Mulliken JB, Murray JE. Facial growth after early correction of hemifacial microsomia. Presented at the 68th annual meeting of the American Association of Oral and Maxillofacial Surgeons, New Orleans, 24–28 September 1986.

16. Moses MH, Kaban LB, Mulliken JB, Evans CA, Murray JE. Facial growth after early correction of hemifacial microsomia. Presented at the 64th Annual Meeting of the American Association of Plastic Surgeons, San Diego, 1 May 1985.

17. Vargervik K, Kaban LB. Management of hemifacial microsomia in the growing child. In: Bell W (ed). Modern Practice in Orthognathic and Reconstructive Surgery. Philadelphia: Saunders, 1991:1533–1560.

18. Meurman Y. Congenital microtia and meatal atresia; observations and aspects of treatment. AMA Arch Otolaryngol 1957;66:443–463.

19. Kaban LB, Evans C, Mulliken JB, et al. Analysis and treatment of hemifacial microsomia. In: Shelton DW, Irby WB (eds). Current Advances in Oral and Maxillofacial Surgery: Orthognathic Surgery, ed 5. St Louis: Mosby, 1986:288–315.

20. Bennun RD, Mulliken JB, Kaban LB, Murray JE. Microtia: A microform of hemifacial microsomia. Plast Reconstr Surg 1985;76:859–863.

21. Vento AR, LaBrie RA, Mulliken JB. OMENS classification of hemifacial microsomia. Cleft Palate J 1989;28:68–76.

22. Mulliken JB, Ferraro NF, Vento AR. A retrospective analysis of growth of the constructed condyle-ramus in children with hemifacial microsomia. Cleft Palate J 1989;26:312–317.

23. Horgan JE, Padwa BL, LaBrie RA, Mulliken JB. OMENS-plus: Analysis of craniofacial and extracraniofacial anomalies in hemifacial microsomia. Cleft Palate Craniofac J 1995;32: 405–412.

24. Posnick J. Surgical correction of mandibular hypoplasia in hemifacial microsomia: A personal perspective. J Oral Maxillofac Surg 1998;56:639–650.

25. Padwa BL, Kaiser MO, Kaban LB. Occlusal cant in the frontal plane as a reflection of facial asymmetry. J Oral Maxillofac Surg 1997;55:811–816.

26. Padwa BL, Mulliken JB, Maghen A, Kaban LB. Midfacial growth after costochondral graft construction of the mandibular ramus in hemifacial microsomia. J Oral Maxillofac Surg 1998;56:122–127.

27. Vargervik K, Ousterhout DK, Farias M. Factors affecting long-term results in hemifacial microsomia. Cleft Palate J 1986;23(suppl 1):53–68.

28. Melsen B, Bjerregaard J, Bundgaard M. The effect of treatment with functional appliance on a pathologic growth pattern of the condyle. Am J Orthod Dentofacial Orthop 1986;90:503–512.

29. Tanzer RC. Total reconstruction of the auricle. The evolution of a plan of treatment. Plast Reconstr Surg 1971;47:523–533.

30. Brent B. The correction of microtia with autogenous cartilage grafts: I. The classic deformity. Plast Reconstr Surg 1980;66:1–12.

31. Brent B, Byrd HS. Secondary ear reconstruction with cartilage grafts covered by axial, random, and free flaps of temporoparietal fascia. Plast Reconstr Surg 1983;72:141–152.

32. Cohen MM Jr. Malformations of the craniofacial region: Evolutionary, embryonic, genetic and clinical perspectives. Am J Med Genet 2002;115:245–268.

33. Tulasne JF, Tessier PT. Results of the Tessier integral procedure for correction of Treacher Collins syndrome. Cleft Palate J 1986;23(suppl 1):40–49.

34. Thomson A. Notice of several cases of malformation of the external ear, together with experiments on the state of hearing in such persons. Month J Med Sci 1847;7:420.

35. Berry GA. Note on a congenital defect (coloboma) of the lower lid. R Lond Ophthalmol Hosp Rep 1889;12:255.

36. Treacher Collins E. Case with symmetrical congenital notches in the outer part of each lower lid and defective development of the malar bones. Trans Ophthalmol Soc UK 1900;20:190.

37. Franceschetti A, Klein D. Mandibulofacial dysostosis: A new hereditary syndrome. Acta Ophthalmol 1949;27:143.

38. Stovin JJ, Lyon JA Jr, Clemmens RL. Mandibulofacial dysostosis. Radiology 1960;74:225–231.

39. Kaban LB, Mulliken JB, Murray JE. Craniofacial deformity. In: Welch KJ (ed). Pediatric Surgery. Chicago: Year Book, 1986: 233–248.

40. Kaban LB. Congenital and acquired growth abnormalities of the temporomandibular joint. In: Keith DA (ed). Surgery of the Temporomandibular Joint. Boston: Blackwell, 1988: 55–90.

41. Hovell JH. Condylar hyperplasia. Br J Oral Surg 1963;47: 105–111.

42. Walker RV. Condylar hyperplasia. In: Bell WH, Proffit WR, White RB (eds). Surgical Correction of Dentofacial Deformities. Philadelphia: Saunders, 1980:951–953.

43. Cisneros G, Kaban LB. Computerized skeletal scintigraphy for assessment of mandibular asymmetry. J Oral Maxillofac Surg 1985;42:513–520.

44. Kaban LB, Treves ST. Skeletal scintigraphy for assessment of mandibular growth and asymmetry. In: Treves ST (ed). Pediatric Nuclear Medicine. New York: Springer, 1985:49–58.

45. Matteson SR, Proffit WR, Terry BC, Staab EV, Burkes EJ Jr. Bone scanning with 99m technetium phosphate to assess condylar hyperplasia. J Oral Maxillofac Surg 1985;60: 356–367.

46. Gray RJ, Sloan P, Quayle AA, Carter DH. Histopathological and scintigraphic features of condylar hyperplasia. Int J Oral Maxillofac Surg 1990;19:65–71.

47. Pogrel MA. Quantitative assessment of isotope activity in the temporomandibular joint regions as a means of assessing unilateral condylar hypertrophy. J Oral Maxillofac Surg 1985;60:15–17.

48. Robinson PD, Harris K, Coghlan KC, Altman K. Bone scans and the timing of treatment for condylar hyperplasia. Int J Oral Maxillofac Surg 1990;19:243–246.

49. Gray RJ, Horner K, Testa HJ, Lloyd JJ, Sloan P. Condylar hyperplasia: Correlation of histological and scintigraphic features. Dentomaxillofac Radiol 1994;23:103–107.

50. Kaban LB. Acquired abnormalities of the temporomandibular joint. In: Kaban LB, Troulis MJ (eds). Pediatric Oral and Maxillofacial Surgery. Philadelphia: Saunders, 2004:340–376.

51. Harris SA, Quayle AA, Testa HJ. Radionuclide bone scanning in the diagnosis and management of condylar hyperplasia. Nucl Med Commun 1984;5:373–380.

52. Pogrel MA, Kopf J, Dodson TB, Hattner R, Kaban LB. A comparison of single-photon emission computed tomography and planar imaging for quantitative skeletal scintigraphy of the mandibular condyle. J Oral Maxillofac Surg 1995;80:226–231.

53. Wolford LM, Mehra P, Reiche-Fischel O, Morales-Ryan CA, Garcia-Morales P. Efficacy of high condylectomy for management of condylar hyperplasia. Am J Orthod Dentofacial Orthop 2002;121:136–150.

54. Troulis MJ, Kaban LB. Endoscopic approach the ramus/condyle unit: Clinical applications. J Oral Maxillofac Surg 2001;59:503–509.

55. Bertolini F, Bianchi B, DeRiu G, DiBlasio A, Sesenna E. Hemimandibular hyperplasia treated by early high-condylectomy: A case report. Int J Adult Orthodon Orthognath Surg 2001; 16:227–234.

56. Codivilla A. On the means of lengthening, in the lower limbs, the muscles and tissues which are shortened through deformity. 1904. Clin Orthop Relat Res 1994;301:4–9.

57. Ilizarov G. The tension-stress effect on the genesis and growth of tissues. Part I. The influence of stability of fixation and soft-tissue preservation. Clin Orthop Relat Res 1989;238:249–281.

58. Ilizarov G. The tension-stress effect on the genesis and growth of tissues. Part II. The influence of the rate and frequency of distraction. Clin Orthop Relat Res 1989;239:263–285.

59. Ilizarov G. The principles of the Ilizarov method. 1988. Bull Hosp Dis 1997;56:49–53.

60. Snyder CC, Levine GA, Swanson HM, Browne EZ Jr. Mandibular lengthening by gradual distraction. Preliminary report. Plast Reconstr Surg 1973;51:506–508.

61. Michieli S, Miotti B. Lengthening of mandibular body by gradual surgical-orthodontic distraction. J Oral Surg 1977; 35:187–192.

62. Costantino PD, Shybut G, Friedman CD, et al. Segmental mandibular regeneration by distraction osteogenesis. An experimental study. Arch Otolaryngol Head Neck Surg 1990;116:535–545.

63. Klotch DW, Ganey TM, Slater-Haase A, Sasse J. Assessment of bone formation during osteogenesis: A canine model. Otolaryngol Head Neck Surg 1995;112:291–302.

64. Troulis MJ, Glowacki J, Perrott DH, Kaban LB. Effects of latency and rate on bone formation in a porcine mandibular distraction model. J Oral Maxillofac Surg 2000;58: 507–514.

65. McCarthy JG, Schreiber J, Karp N, Thorne CH, Grayson BH. Lengthening the human mandible by gradual distraction. Plast Reconstr Surg 1992;89:1–8.

66. Perrott DH, Berger R, Vargervik K, Kaban LB. Use of a skeletal distraction device to widen the mandible: A case report. J Oral Maxillofac Surg 1993;51:435–439.

67. Chin M, Toth BA. Distraction osteogenesis in maxillofacial surgery using internal devices: Review of five cases. J Oral Maxillofac Surg 1996;54:45–53.

68. Chin M, Toth BA. LeFort III advancement with gradual distraction using internal devices. Plast Reconstr Surg 1997; 100:819–830.

69. Ortiz Monasterio F, Molina F, Andrade L, Rodriguez C, Sainz Arregui J. Simultaneous mandibular and maxillary distraction in hemifacial microsoma in adults: Avoiding occlusal disasters. Plast Reconstr Surg 1997;100:852–861.

70. Padwa BL, Kearns GJ, Todd R, Troulis M, Mulliken JB, Kaban LB. Simultaneous maxillary and mandibular distraction osteogenesis with a semiburied device. Int J Oral Maxillofac Surg 1999;28:2–8.

71. Steinbacher DM, Kaban LB, Troulis MJ. Treatment of tracheostomy-dependent children with severe micrognathia. J Oral Maxillofac Surg 2005;63:1072–1079.

72. Moore MH, Guzman-Stein G, Prodman TW, Abbott AH, Netherway DJ, David DJ. Mandibular lengthening by distraction for airway obstruction in Treacher-Collins syndrome. J Craniofac Surg 1994;5:22–25.

73. Williams JK, Maull D, Grayson BH, Longaker MT, McCarthy JG. Early decannulation with bilateral mandibular distraction for tracheostomy-dependent patients. Plast Reconstr Surg 1999;103:48–57; discussion 1999;103:58–59.

74. Denny AD, Talisman R, Hanson PR, Recinos RF. Mandibular distraction osteogenesis in very young patients to correct airway obstruction. Plast Reconstr Surg 2001;108:302–311.

75. Morovic CG, Monasterio L. Distraction osteogenesis for obstructive apneas in patients with congenital craniofacial malformations. Plast Reconstr Surg 2000;105:2324–2330.

76. Sidman J, Sampson D, Templeton B. Distraction osteogenesis of the mandible for airway obstruction in children. Laryngoscope 2001;111:1137–1146.

77. Cohen SR, Ross DA, Burstein FD, et al. Skeletal expansion combined with soft-tissue reduction on the treatment of obstructive sleep apnea in children: Physiologic results. Otolaryngol Head Neck Surg 1998;119:476–485.

78. Vannier MW, March JL, Warren JD. Three-dimensional CT reconstruction images for craniofacial surgical planning and evaluation. Radiology 1984;150:179–184.

79. Levy RA, Edwards WT, Meyer JR, Rosenbaum AE. Facial trauma and 3-D reconstructive imaging: Insufficiencies and correctives. AJNR Am J Neuroradiol 1992;13:885–892.

80. Ayoub AF, Wray D, Moos KF, et al. Three-dimensional modeling for modern diagnosis and planning in maxillofacial surgery. Int J Adult Orthodon Orthognath Surg 1996;11: 225–233.

81. Bill JS, Reuther JF, Dittmann W, et al. Stereolithography in oral and maxillofacial operation planning. Int J Oral Maxillofac Surg 1995;24:98–103.

82. Seldin EB, Troulis MJ, Kaban LB. Evaluation of a semiburied fixed-trajectory curvilinear distraction device in an animal model. J Oral Maxillofac Surg 1999;57:1442–1446.

83. Troulis MJ, Everett P, Seldin EB, Kikinis R, Kaban LB. Three-dimensional treatment planning system based on computed tomographic data. Int J Oral Maxillofac Surg 2002; 31:349–357.

84. Gateno J, Teichgraeber JF, Aguilar E. Computer planning for distraction osteogenesis. Plast Reconstr Surg 2000;105:873–882.

85. Everett P, Seldin EB, Troulis M, Kaban LB, Kikinis R. A 3-D system for planning and simulating minimally-invasive distraction osteogenesis of the facial skeleton. In: Delp SL, DiGioia AM, Jaramaz B (eds). MICCAI 2000. Proceedings of the 3rd International Conference on Medical Image Computing and Computer-Assisted Intervention. New York: Springer, 2000:1029–1039.

86. Gateno J. Accuracy of custom stereolithographic templates for the installation of an external multiplanar distractor. J Oral Maxillofac Surg 1999;57:96.

87. Gateno J, Teichgraber JF, Aguilar E. Distraction osteogenesis: A new surgical technique for use with the multiplanar mandibular distractor. Plast Reconst Surg 2000;105:883–888.

88. Xia J, Ip HHS, Samman D, et al. Computer-assisted three-dimensional surgical planning and simulation: 3D virtual osteotomy. Int J Oral Maxillofac Surg 2000;29:11–17.

89. Cohen MM Jr. Variability versus "incidental findings" in the first and second branchial arch syndrome: Unilateral variants with anophthalmia. Birth Defects Orig Artic Ser 1971;7: 103–180.

90. Harvold EP, Vargervik K, Chierici G. Treatment of Hemifacial Microsomia. New York: Liss, 1983.

Medical Management of TMJ Arthritis

Sigvard Kopp

Treatment of the temporomandibular joint (TMJ) arthritides is directed toward the different mechanisms causing or amplifying the inflammatory process in the joint. The TMJ is basically similar to other synovial joints and is therefore subject to the same arthritic processes and the same treatment principles. This chapter presents an overview of the possibilities and shortcomings of medical and pharmacologic management of these various conditions.

Although osteoarthritis (OA) is considered a degenerative process primarily affecting the articular surfaces, it has secondary inflammatory components that are associated with many of its symptoms and signs. The systemic primary inflammatory joint diseases, on the other hand, originate in the synovial tissues and then cause bone and cartilage destruction. Although there are several different arthritides that involve the TMJ, including OA, rheumatoid arthritis (RA), gout, ankylosing spondylitis, and psoriatic arthritis, their treatment has much in common because it is directed toward reducing and, if possible, eliminating the inflammatory process. This involves systemic, local, and intra-articular approaches.

Systemic Treatments

Analgesics

Acetaminophen, also known as *paracetamol* (Tylenol, McNeil; Alvedon, AstraZeneca), is an analgesic drug with an antipyretic effect, but it lacks inhibitory effects on prostaglandin synthesis and inflammation as well as on blood clotting. It was introduced as a substitute for aspirin because it causes less irritation of the gastrointestinal tract. The pain-relieving effect is equal to that of aspirin. Although acetaminophen is not used to treat arthritis, it has been recommended as the drug of choice for mild or moderate pain in OA.[1]

Nonsteroidal Anti-inflammatory Drugs

A large variety of nonsteroidal anti-inflammatory drugs (NSAIDs) can be used to reduce TMJ inflammation and the associated pain. They should be used at an early stage before any other treatment. However, they are not a long-term remedy for TMJ arthritis.

Cyclooxygenase inhibitors

There is evidence that NSAIDs have a stabilizing effect on lysosomal membranes and an inhibitory effect on leukocyte migration. The main effect, however, is inhibition of the production of prostaglandins and thromboxanes by blocking the enzyme cyclooxygenase (COX), which explains the reduction of inflammation and pain (Fig 30-1). Two COX isoforms have been identified: COX-1, which is expressed constitutively in most tissues, and COX-2, which is expressed constitutively in the brain and kidney but can be induced in other tissues and at sites of inflammation. The older NSAIDs block both isoforms. However, NSAIDs with a specific blocking effect on the enzyme isomer COX-2 (coxibs) have been developed recently.

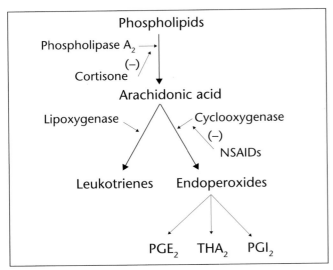

Fig 30-1 Prostaglandin biosynthesis. Cortisone has an inhibitory effect (–) on the enzyme phospholipase A₂, and nonsteroidal anti-inflammatory drugs (NSAIDs) have an inhibitory effect on cyclooxygenase. (PGE₂) prostaglandin E₂; (THA₂) thromboxane A₂; (PGI₂) prostaglandin I₂.

The pain-relieving effect of the coxibs is good and similar to high doses of the traditional NSAIDs, according to studies in patients with RA[2] and OA.[3] The adverse effects are the same, except for a significantly lower frequency of stomach ulcers.[4] Gastrointestinal ulcers occur in 15% to 20% of patients taking traditional NSAIDs, and 70% of these ulcers occur in the stomach.[5] There is good scientific evidence for the effects of the traditional NSAIDs,[6] but the short- and long-term effects or side effects of the coxibs are not yet sufficiently documented. NSAIDs are known to produce a wide variety of effects on metabolism, similar to those produced by glucocorticosteroids (eg, an antianabolic effect), and their long-term use is therefore questionable. This is also true for the specific COX-2 blockers.

The oldest NSAID is acetylsalicylic acid (ASA), or aspirin, which has analgesic, anti-inflammatory, and antipyretic effects. It is well known that headache, arthralgia, and muscular aches respond to ASA. Its modest anti-inflammatory effect is exerted at a relatively high dose (3 to 5 g), which often creates gastrointestinal symptoms or bleeding (30% to 45% of patients). These side effects can be reduced by the use of enteric-coated preparations, but the analgesic effect is delayed.

Indomethacin (Indocin, Merck) is frequently used as an anti-inflammatory agent at night to prevent morning stiffness and pain in patients with RA. It is quite effective against arthritis but may produce peptic ulcers, which limits its usefulness. Among the newer NSAIDs, naproxen sodium (Naprosyn, Roche), ibuprofen (Advil, Wyeth; Motrin, McNeil), diclofenac (Voltaren, Novartis), and meloxicam (Mobic, Boehringer Ingelheim) are well-known drugs that have been used extensively as analgesics for patients with OA and RA and should therefore be suitable alternatives.

The coxibs (COX-2 blockers), which included celecoxib (Celebrex, Pfizer), rofecoxib (Vioxx, Merck), valdecoxib (Bextra, Pfizer), and etoricoxib (Arcoxia, Merck), have been popular because they produce less upper gastrointestinal toxicity. However, because of the evidence that long-term use of certain COX-2 inhibitors can cause an increased risk of stroke and heart attack, most have been taken off of the market. This raises the question of whether the other selective COX-2 inhibitors will also eventually be shown to have such adverse side effects after long-term use. However, when the coxibs are used for short periods, they do not appear to cause an increased risk of adverse cardiovascular events.

Some of the classic NSAIDs currently on the market have also been shown to be somewhat COX-2 selective, and theoretically these may cause less gastrointestinal toxicity than the nonselective NSAIDs, such as ibuprofen and others. These include diclofenac (Voltaren), etodolac (Lodine, Ayerst), meloxicam (Mobic), and nabumetone (Relafen, GlaxoSmithKline). However, there are no clinical data to show that these NSAIDs actually cause fewer gastrointestinal complications.

When gastrointestinal protection is necessary, use of drugs such as misoprostol (Cytotec, Searle), the proton pump inhibitor omeprazole (Prilosec, AstraZeneca; and others), and the H₂-receptor antagonists (Zantac, GlaxoSmithKline) has been recommended, but there is no convincing evidence that they can prevent serious NSAID-related gastrointestinal complications in the long term.

Nutraceuticals

Glucosamine sulfate (Glucosine, Recip; Artrox, Pfizer) is an endogenous substance that is synthesized in cartilage. Animal studies have suggested that exogenous administration increases the proteoglycan synthesis in cartilage and thereby reduces its breakdown, while clinical studies have indicated that it provides pain relief and improves mobility in patients with mild to moderate OA.[7] Glucosamine and chondroitin preparations are often effective and have few side effects. Meta-analysis has shown evidence of their benefit for patients with OA in the knee and hip joints,[7,8] and a randomized placebo-controlled trial has shown less progression of OA in the knee over a 3-year period.[9] However, further high-quality, independent studies are needed.

Treatment Guidelines

The following guidelines are recommended for the systemic treatment of the TMJ arthritides:

1. The NSAIDs are indicated for patients with exacerbations of TMJ involvement with painful degenerative, inflammatory, or traumatic joint conditions. These drugs can be combined with an analgesic such as acetaminophen. However, effort should be made to find even better means for further local treatment.
2. There is evidence for short-term benefit of the analgesic and anti-inflammatory effects of the coxibs in the arthritides such as OA and RA.[10] However, the indications for coxibs in TMJ treatment are limited. They are recommended for short-term treatment in patients with increased risk for, or history of, stomach bleeding.
3. Glucosamine sulfate is included in the Evidence-Based Medicine (EBM) guidelines for treatment of OA,[1] but there are no clinical trials to verify a specific effect on TMJ arthritides.

Cytokine Inhibitors

Infliximab (Remicade, Centocor) is a chimeric monoclonal antibody (cA29) that binds to tumor necrosis factor α and thereby neutralizes its biologic actions, eg, by reduction of C-reactive protein release. Systemic treatment with infliximab is effective in reducing disease activity in patients with rheumatoid arthritis[11]; the drug has an acceptable safety profile and leads to improvement in radiographic scores. However, larger and longer studies are required to detect rare adverse events.

According to results from a study in our clinic, infliximab results in a significant reduction in both general joint pain and local TMJ and knee joint pain within 2 weeks; these effects last for at least 22 weeks.[12] Pain reduction was associated with a decreased level of the proinflammatory interleukin 6 in the synovial fluid, while recurrence of pain was associated with increased levels. The use of local intra-articular treatment has not yet been tried.

Immunosuppresive Drugs

Immunosuppresive drugs are sometimes used in the managemant of severe, active RA to reduce inflammation and slow the progression of the disease.[13] During the last few years, sulfasalazine and methotrexate have become the drugs of choice, to be used in combination with other drugs to obtain a greater effect than is possible with single-drug therapy. Systemic corticosteroid therapy, which usually relieves inflammatory symptoms quickly in RA, is given in the smallest effective dose (5.0 to 7.5 mg daily), often while the patient awaits the effect of slow-acting, disease-modifying antirheumatic drugs such as sulfasalazine and methotrexate.[14] There are investigations suggesting that corticosteroids prevent the development of joint erosion.[15]

Tumor necrosis factor α blockers are also used in combination with sulfasalazine and methotrexate when the inflammatory activity is moderate to high.

Local Treatments

Physical Therapy for the TMJ

Restricted mouth opening is frequently associated with acute arthritis of the TMJ because of the painful synovitis and intra-articular effusion. Traumatic arthritis and other inflammatory joint diseases involve the creation of a fibrin network by the inflammatory process and a risk for development of fibrous adhesions between the joint components. Restricted mandibular mobility also is a common finding in patients with chronic RA and is mainly caused by restricted translation in the joint. The jaw muscles are also often affected by TMJ arthritis. They may develop increased tension because of the articular pain, as in OA, or may be more directly involved by the inflammatory process, as in RA.

Irrespective of whether reduced mandibular mobility is caused by intra-articular restriction or by muscular dysfunction, physical exercises are beneficial to prevent formation of intra-articular adhesions and to increase the blood flow and strength of the jaw muscles. Physical therapy is therefore a valuable adjunct to other treatments for TMJ arthritis aimed at normalizing the functional capability of the temporomandibular system.

Effects

The short-term effects of a self-administered physical training program on temporomandibular disorders in patients

Box 30-1	Patient instructions for TMJ exercise program

1. Relax and lower your shoulders.
2. Let your lower jaw relax and make the M sound. Make sure that the teeth do not contact. Relax your tongue.
3. Make small, relaxed, up-and-down and side-to-side movements without tooth contact to warm up the muscles.
4. Open and close your mouth as much as you can without pain or discomfort. Move your lower jaw as far forward as possible and then back again. Make similar movements toward each side and then relax.
5. Make the same movements as in exercise 4 but against resistance with your hand. Press with your fist below the chin during mouth opening. Push your thumb against the point of your chin during forward movement and against the right and left sides of your chin during lateral movements. Keep your lower jaw at the extreme point of each movement for a few seconds.
6. Open your mouth as wide as possible and then try to close while you resist this movement by pushing downward against your lower front teeth with your fingers. Hold the jaw in this position for a few seconds.
7. Open your mouth as wide as you can. Then stretch further by pushing with your fingers against the upper and lower front teeth.
8. While looking in the mirror, try to move your lower jaw straight up and down. Avoid deviations as well as movements that produce clicking or locking of the jaw.
9. End the exercise program by resting on your back for 5 to 10 minutes.

with RA and ankylosing spondylitis have been compared to no treatment.[16] All patients, including those not subjected to local physical training, reported reduced severity of symptoms at follow-up. Clinically, however, only those who performed physical exercises showed improvement. In patients with RA, the improvement was greatest among those with initial restriction in TMJ translatory mobility. They showed a significant increase in maximum voluntary mouth opening. None of the patients reported an impaired condition at follow-up. In patients with ankylosing spondylitis, the clinical improvement was greatest among those with high disease activity, as reflected by high values of the serum concentration of C-reactive protein. Another finding was that lack of occlusal support was a negative prognostic factor in the ankylosing spondylitis group.

Indications

When the acute inflammatory process has subsided, physical therapy is indicated for all forms of arthritis of the TMJ to mobilize the joint and prevent adhesions as well as to normalize the muscle function and blood circulation and thereby to restore the bite force.[17] The effect of physical training on the radiographic progression of RA, however, remains uncertain. Especially in

patients with chronic arthritides, continued exercises are valuable to maintain acceptable function in the temporomandibular system.

Technique

The self-administered physical training program is a modification of exercises that have evolved through use in many clinics throughout the world (Box 30-1). The exercises involving mouth opening and laterotrusion and protrusion of the mandible are first performed without resistance (exercises 1 to 4) and then, if allowed with respect to pain or other discomfort, against resistance to recruit the greatest possible number of muscle motor units (exercises 5 to 7). The last part of the program is especially indicated to restore strength in atrophied muscles.

It is most important that the patient receive a thorough explanation and a practical demonstration of the exercise program. To ensure full cooperation, which is essential, the aims and goals of the treatment must also be explained. During the demonstration and while the patient is exercising, the use of a mirror is valuable to give feedback about the movements performed.

Each exercise should be performed about 10 times, and the whole training program should be performed twice a day, unless otherwise prescribed. Movements that cause pain should be avoided. Local application of heat over the TMJs and cheeks often makes the exercise easier and more comfortable to perform because heat increases elasticity of the tissues and local blood circulation. It is important to evaluate the effects of the program at follow-up, to reinstruct and motivate the patient, if necessary, and to check for improvement in symptoms and signs and in maximum mandibular movement capacity.

Prognosis

The prognosis is quite good for physical therapy in patients with TMJ arthritis. Persistent, severe pain and locking, however, are factors that might reduce the applicability of jaw exercises. In advanced cases of TMJ arthritis with complete or partial ankylosis (eg, in RA and ankylosing spondylitis), little improvement in mandibular mobility can be expected.

Acupuncture

Acupuncture has been used as an adjunct to other therapies for pain relief in patients with RA. Acupuncture is a traditional Chinese method in which thin needles are inserted into specific body points believed to represent concentrations of body energy. A small electrical impulse may be added through the needles. The needles have been shown to cause systemic release of endorphins and subsequent local or general analgesia.

There is no research-based evidence from controlled trials in patients with RA that shows an effect superior to sham needling or other placebo treatment.[18] A review of treatment of RA[19] concluded that acupuncture or electroacupuncture cannot be recommended based on the present evidence. Furthermore, acupuncture has no effect on joint pain and tenderness or on the acute phase reactants and disease activity.

Iontophoresis

Iontophoresis is a technique to enhance the transport of drug ions across a tissue barrier. A weak current carries the drug ions through the skin into the deeper tissues, where the drug exerts its effect. Iontophoretic devices are used for treatment of inflammatory conditions in skin, muscles, tendons, and joints (eg, TMJ). One of the main applications for iontophoresis is cortisone treatment of superficial local inflammation. Only cortisone in a water-soluble, injectable form may be used.

A dexamethasone solution for injection, 5 mg/mL, is recommended for the Phoresor device (IOMED). This medication has a negative charge, and the cathode is thus connected to the medication electrode. The local tissue concentration of dexamethasone after iontophoretic administration over the elbow joint was studied in rhesus monkeys and was found to be higher than that after systemic administration but lower than that obtained by local injection.[20]

The effects of iontophoretically applied dexamethasone in combination with lidocaine were evaluated in patients with painful TMJ disc displacement, with or without reduction, and in patients with OA.[21] The results suggest that iontophoretically applied dexamethasone is no more effective than a saline placebo in providing pain relief in these patients. A randomized clinical trial studied the short-term effects of iontophoretic delivery of dexamethasone and lidocaine for treatment of TMJ disc displacement without reduction and concurrent capsulitis.[22] Iontophoretically delivered dexamethasone was effective in improving mandibular function (mobility) but not in reducing pain. This result suggests that intra-articular injections are probably more effective.

Phonophoresis

Phonophoresis is another method for drug delivery through the skin, using ultrasound instead of an electric current. There are few studies of the use of this treatment modality in the TMJ. However, one randomized clinical trial of the effect of indomethacin phonophoresis on TMJ pain has been performed.[23] Pain was decreased and the pressure pain threshold was increased in the experimental group but not in the control group. However, the nature or diagnosis of the pain was not defined. Evidence is lacking for this treatment modality in general and for TMJ arthritis in particular.

Topical Ointments

Topical administration of ointments containing capsaicin and NSAIDs has been used for treatment of arthritis. The effectiveness of topically applied capsaicin has been investigated in a meta-analysis, where it was found to be better than placebo to provide pain relief in OA.[24] In a double-blind trial in OA and RA patients, significantly more pain relief was reported by the capsaicin-treated patients than the placebo-receiving patients. After 4 weeks of treatment, the RA and OA patients demonstrated reductions in pain of 57% and 33%, respectively.[25]

The potential role of topical capsaicin in the management of pain in the TMJ region also has been discussed by Hersh and colleagues.[26]

There is evidence that topical NSAIDs are significantly more effective than placebo and as effective as oral NSAIDs in the treatment of both acute and chronic musculoskeletal pain.[27] It is believed that this route reduces the adverse gastrointestinal events caused by NSAIDs because systemic involvement is decreased. Current guidelines recommend topical NSAIDs as an effective treatment of OA, and a systematic review confirmed that topical NSAIDs are superior to placebo treatment during 2 weeks of chronic pain from OA and tendinitis.[28] The authors concluded that no studies had the design and power to provide definite evidence but, until adequate studies are available, the topical NSAIDs should be considered effective and safe. However, in a meta-analysis of randomized clinical trials on the efficacy of topical administration of NSAIDs for the treatment of osteoarthritis, the authors concluded that there is no evidence of efficacy superior to placebo after 2 weeks and that no data exist to support their long-term use.[29]

Bite Appliances

Muscular hyperfunction or occlusal trauma can be a primary cause of OA, and these factors might also be detrimental and accelerate tissue destruction in the case of systemic inflammatory joint disease involving the TMJ. Treatment with occlusal bite appliances has been advocated mainly in patients with pain of muscular origin due to muscle hyperfunction or tension.[30,31] The effect of such devices for the treatment of TMJ arthritis is less known, and such patients frequently respond better clinically to intra-articular injections of glucocorticosteroid than to occlusal treatment (occlusal appliances or occlusal adjustment).[32]

There is an urgent need for carefully controlled clinical trials in this field. In a systematic review of randomized controlled trials of occlusal treatments in patients with temporomandibular disorders, Forsell and colleagues[33] concluded that appliance therapy was superior to ultrasound, palliative treatment, and a palatal splint. However, this review refers to treatment of temporomandibular disorders, which is a nonspecific term covering all the conditions that involve the temporomandibular system. There is no evidence of the efficacy of treating TMJ arthritis with an occlusal appliance.[34]

Intra-articular Treatments

Glucocorticosteroids have been used for a long time as anti-inflammatory drugs for intra-articular use, while sodium hyaluronate and morphine have been tried more recently.

Glucocorticosteroids

The anti-inflammatory effects on synovial tissues of the glucocorticosteroids given systemically or intra-articularly are well documented. Intra-articular corticosteroids have proved to be useful in alleviating pain, swelling, and dysfunction in patients with inflammatory diseases of joints, such as RA and gout, as well as in those with primarily noninflammatory joint diseases, such as OA.

Mechanism of action

The mechanism by which glucocorticosteroids exert their anti-inflammatory action is not entirely understood. They have been reported to stabilize the membrane of the lysosomes of damaged cells and thereby to prevent the release of proteolytic enzymes and to inhibit the enzymes already released. Mast cell activity, histamine activity, and the cellular response to inflammatory mediators are also inhibited by glucocorticosteroids.

In a study in the TMJ, intra-articular administration of glucocorticosteroid caused a short-term decrease in the level of neuropeptide Y in the synovial fluid in patients with specific inflammatory joint disease, mainly RA; at the same time, the pain and hyperalgesia in the joint decreased (Figs 30-2a to 30-2c).[35] These findings indicate that part of the analgesic effect of glucocorticosteroid is due to blocked neuropeptide release from nerve terminals involved in neurogenic inflammation. The synthesis of prostaglandin E is reduced because glucocorticosteroid inhibits production of arachidonic acid from cellular phospholipids (see Fig 30-1).

Side effects

Glucocorticoid also inhibits the synthesis of proteoglycans and collagen; that is, it has an antianabolic effect and thus may impair the healing process. This factor is important with prolonged systemic use but not with a limited number of intra-articular injections. In addition, limited use does not produce general side effects such as iatrogenic Cushing syndrome, osteoporosis, or inhibition of corticotropin production, although a single injection

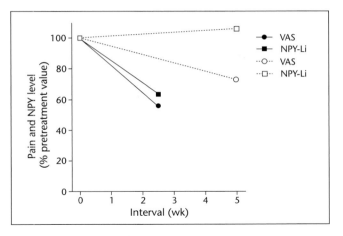

Fig 30-2a Changes in visual analog scale (VAS) reports of TMJ pain and TMJ synovial fluid aspirate levels of neuropeptide Y–like (NPY-Li) immunoreactivity of the assay, *(solid lines)* 2 to 3 weeks (11 patients) or *(dotted lines)* 4 to 6 weeks (10 patients) after intra-articular glucocorticoid injections for specific general inflammatory joint disease. Changes over time are shown in percentage of pretreatment values. At 2 to 3 weeks, the differences in VAS scores ($P < .01$) and NPY levels ($P < .05$) were statistically significant. At 4 to 6 weeks, the difference in VAS scores was statistically significant ($P < .05$); the difference in NPY levels was not significant. (From Alstergren et al.[35] Reprinted with permission.)

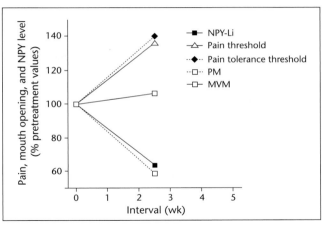

Fig 30-2b Changes in TMJ aspirate level of neuropeptide Y–like (NPY-Li) immunoreactivity of the assay, pressure pain threshold, pressure pain tolerance threshold, pain on mandibular movement (PM), and maximum voluntary mouth opening capacity (MVM), 2 to 3 weeks after intra-articular glucocorticoid treatment in eight patients (11 joints) with specific general inflammatory joint disease. Changes over time are shown in percentage of pretreatment values. The differences in pain threshold ($P < .05$), pain tolerance threshold ($P < .05$), and PM ($P < .01$) were statistically significant. The difference in MVM was not significant. (From Alstergren et al.[35] Reprinted with permission.)

may have a systemic effect on general joint symptoms in patients with RA. There are many new synthetic glucocorticosteroids that are more potent than cortisone and hydrocortisone, but their side effects are greater as well.

Local side effects of intra-articular injection of glucocorticosteroids, such as destruction of articular cartilage, infection, and progression of already manifested joint disease, have been reported.[36] The cause of these deleterious effects has not been fully explained and adequate controls are lacking. In an experimental study of intra-articular glucocorticosteroid treatment on induced arthritis in the guinea pig knee, the drug did not cause any macroscopic or microscopic damage on control knees in which arthritis had not been induced.[37] A clinical study indicated that intra-articular glucocorticoid injections resulted in less release of proteoglycan into the joint fluid than before treatment.[38,39] Recurrence of symptoms coincided with an increase of proteoglycan release.

Besides the glucocorticosteroid, other factors such as infection, trauma in association with the actual injection, and the suspension medium are likely causes of the deleterious effects, at least when a limited number of injections have been made. Another adverse effect that occasionally occurs is local skin atrophy, which is due to accidental intracutaneous or subcutaneous injection of the drug.

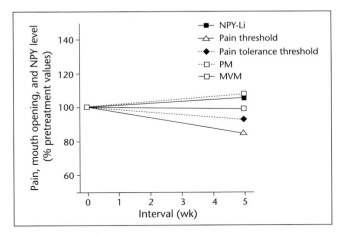

Fig 30-2c Changes in TMJ aspirate level of neuropeptide Y–like (NPY-Li) immunoreactivity of the assay, pressure pain threshold, pressure pain tolerance threshold, pain on mandibular movement (PM), and maximum voluntary mouth opening capacity (MVM) 4 to 6 weeks after intra-articular glucocorticoid treatment in eight patients (10 joints) with specific general inflammatory joint disease. The changes over time are shown in percentage of pretreatment values. The differences were not statistically significant. (From Alstergren et al.[35] Reprinted with permission.)

Efficacy

Patients with long-standing local pain and dysfunction from arthritis of the TMJ have been subjected to intra-articular glucocorticosteroid injections following failure of more conservative treatment.[31] The results showed that intra-articular injections of glucocorticosteroid combined with a local anesthetic agent have a good long-term palliative effect on subjective symptoms and clinical signs in this joint. However, the long-term prognosis is poor in patients with advanced radiographic signs of OA or when systemic joint disease is present. Patients have been followed for 8 years after glucocorticosteroid treatment of the TMJ,[36] and the subjective symptoms and the clinical signs have remained very slight or absent. TMJ clicking and crepitation, however, did not decrease significantly. No radiographic signs of erosion of the cortex of the joint were found in any of the patients 8 years after treatment.

In another long-term study that included treatment with glucocorticosteroid, a significant effect was found on subjective symptoms and clinical signs such as joint tenderness, maximum voluntary mouth opening, and bite force.[40] Neither joint crepitation nor muscle tenderness was affected by the treatment. In a clinical trial in patients with RA of the TMJ, methylprednisolone acetate (Depo-Medrol, Pfizer) had a significant short-term effect that exceeded the effect of saline on both subjective symptoms and clinical signs.[41]

A randomized, double-blind trial investigated the long-term safety and efficacy of intra-articular glucocorticoid injections (triamcinolone acetonide, 40 mg), given every 3 months for up to 2 years, for OA of the knee.[42] There was no difference in radiographic progression of OA with triamcinolone acetonide or with saline injection, but knee pain and stiffness were significantly alleviated after glucocorticoid injection but not after injection of a placebo.

Intra-articular injections of glucocorticosteroids into the TMJ have been advocated for patients with acute synovitis secondary to OA and for patients with acute exacerbations of inflammatory joint disease, such as RA. This recommendation is supported by substantial evidence,[1,6] and the treatment is associated with minimal risk.[43] The American College of Rheumatology guidelines[44] state that intra-articular glucocorticoid injections are of value in the treatment of acute knee pain in patients with OA, particularly in patients with signs of local inflammation and joint effusion. Besides being effective for RA and OA, intra-articular glucocorticosteroid injections are also effective in inflamed joints associated with psoriatic arthropathy, ankylosing spondylitis, gout, chondrocalcinosis, Reiter syndrome, and rheumatic fever.[45–49]

Forms

There are many glucocorticosteroid preparations available for intra-articular injection. These include cortisone and hydrocortisone, which rapidly diffuse out of the joint, and the new synthetic steroid esters, which are poorly soluble in aqueous media and are administered as microcrystalline suspensions. The disodium phosphate ester of betamethasone, which is readily soluble and thereby has a quick therapeutic effect, is used together with its acetate ester, which has a sustained release and prolonged effect (Celestone, Schering-Plough).

The duration of these long-acting preparations seems to be directly related to the insolubility of the ester. Methylprednisolone acetate (Depo-Medrol) has an intermediate solubility and duration, while triamcinolone acetonide (Kenacort, Bristol-Myers Squibb) and especially triamcinolone hexacetonide (Lederspan, Wyeth) have very low solubility and long duration. The crystals of the triamcinolone hexacetonide are retained in the joint for up to 6 weeks. The EBM guidelines recommend methylprednisolone for smaller joints.[50]

The long-acting glucocorticosteroids may produce an acute postinjection flare because of their crystalline nature. This reaction occurs in about 2% of injections and is reversible. It usually begins several hours after injection and subsides spontaneously in 24 to 72 hours. Varying degrees of pain may be noted by the patient. Glucocorticosteroid is often injected together with a local anesthetic agent to counteract some of these adverse local effects.

A long-acting preparation, methylprednisolone acetate (Depo-Medrol), or a combination of betamethasone acetate and betamethasone disodium phosphate (Celestone) are the drugs of choice for intra-articular injection of the TMJ. The dose of the specific drug is determined according to its individual clinical potency. An appropriate dose of methylprednisolone is 20 mg in a 0.5- to 1.0-mL suspension, which corresponds to 3 mg of betamethasone. If not used prior to the injection, a local anesthetic (0.5 mL) can be added to the steroid suspension to reduce the discomfort that may occur shortly after the injection.

If the therapeutic effect of the steroid injection is unsatisfactory, it can be repeated after 4 weeks. The maximum number of injections per year and per joint is dependent on the dose given. The EBM guidelines[50] recommend no more than three injections per year and not more frequently than once a month for weight-bearing joints (the knee and the wrist); smaller joints may be injected more frequently.

The subjective and clinical short- and long-term results, as well as the long-term radiographic progression in the TMJ, were favorable after a series of three injections with 1-week intervals.[32,36] Clinical side effects of a severe nature were very rare, but slight, temporary stiffness or pain was reported by some patients.

The long-term prognosis for steroid treatment of TMJ arthritides is less favorable if radiographic signs of severe destruction of the TMJ and general joint symptoms are present.[32] Crepitation of the TMJ has also been found to be a negative prognostic factor in the treatment of degenerative and traumatic arthritis.[51] Generally the most pronounced effect is obtained in patients with severe clinical symptoms.

Morphine

Mechanism of action

The peripheral opioid receptors have been reported to be upregulated in inflamed tissues,[52] and locally applied opioids may have antinociceptive and anti-inflammatory actions. Intra-articular administration of morphine most probably activates the opioid receptors on the peripheral afferent nerve terminals. These receptors are synthesized in the trigeminal caudal subnucleus in the brainstem, from which they are transported axonally toward the nerve terminals, where they are activated by exogenous agonists or endogenous opioids expressed in inflammatory cells.[53]

Efficacy

The evidence for an analgesic effect of intra-articular morphine is weak at present, but Kalso et al[54] concluded that intra-articular administration of morphine may have some effect on postoperative pain. However, no dose-response relationship has been shown and further study is needed. A later randomized, double-blind crossover study on chronic pain from OA of the knee found that patients reported significantly greater pain relief from intra-articular morphine than from intra-articular saline.[55] A single-dose intra-articular injection of 0.1/1.0 mg of morphine was tried in a randomized, multicenter, double-blind study in patients with arthralgia or OA of the TMJ,[56] but no evidence of an analgesic effect was found. This result is in agreement with a randomized double-blind study of postoperative analgesia following TMJ arthroscopy.[57]

In a study including patients with both OA (knee joint) and RA of chronic character, intra-articular morphine was reported to be as effective as dexamethasone, which might be explained by a better response among the RA patients, who had a more pronounced inflammatory pathophysiology.[58] There is no evidence to support low-dose intra-articular administration of morphine for the treatment of TMJ arthritides such as OA and RA.

Sodium Hyaluronate

Sodium hyaluronate, which is prepared from natural high–molecular weight hyaluronate, may be used as an anti-inflammatory drug or for viscosupplementation. It is commonly referred to as *hyaluronic acid,* but at normal physiologic pH the acid can only occur as a sodium salt. When dissolved in isotonic sodium chloride, the long hyaluronate molecules form random coils that become entangled with other hyaluronate molecules. At a concentration of 1%, the viscosity is almost 500,000 times greater than that of physiologic saline, and at 10% it becomes solid and can be formed into balls or sheets.

Mechanism of action

Hyaluronate is characterized by its high viscosity and elasticity. Clinical research suggests that high molecular weight and high concentration are important features of hyaluronate with respect to its anti-inflammatory properties and its ability to enhance wound healing.[59] The mode of action in arthritis is not fully known, but it has been proposed that sodium hyaluronate normalizes the biochemical conditions in the joint by replacing the low–molecular weight hyaluronate of the inflamed joint with high–molecular weight hyaluronate. It might thereby restore soft tissue lubrication, resulting in reduced friction, relief of pain, and improved joint mobility; it would also reestablish the synovial barrier function, which inhibits invasion by leukocytes and enzymes and, in addition, restores the nutrition of the articular cartilage. More specific effects of both a physiochemical and a cellular biologic nature are the prevention of adhesions and the enhancement of cellular migration during tissue repair by stimulating fibroblastic proliferation. It also seems to reduce postoperative ectopic bone formation.

Intra-articularly administered hyaluronate disappears from the joint within 72 hours, but it is reported that it stimulates the synthesis of endogenous hyaluronate by the fibroblasts of the synovial membrane of the joint.[60]

Efficacy

Intra-articular injections of high–molecular weight hyaluronate have been tried with encouraging results in patients with severe clinical signs of TMJ osteoarthritis and traumatic arthritis not responding to more conservative treatment. Hyaluronate has a therapeutic effect similar to that of glucocorticosteroid in this patient category.[39,50] Hyaluronate is therefore a therapeutic alternative to glucocorticosteroid in patients affected with TMJ inflammation caused by advanced OA.

Intra-articular administration of hyaluronate has also been tried in patients with symptomatic RA of the TMJ. In general, it had less short-term effect on signs and symptoms than did intra-articular glucocorticosteroid.[41]

Intra-articular injections of hyaluronate have also been tried with promising results in human knee joints with OA.[61] Several recent clinical studies have indicated a beneficial effect of hyaluronate in patients with OA, although most of these trials lacked adequate placebo control.[62,63] The mechanism behind its pain-relieving effect must be considered largely unknown.

Hyaluronate and glucocorticosteroid by the intra-articular route have been reported to show similar long-term effects on chronic nonsystemic arthritis of the TMJ.[64] Intra-articular hyaluronate might be the better alternative because of the minimal risk of side effects. However, according to a recent review there is insufficient evidence to either support or refute the use of hyaluronate for treatment of patients with TMJ problems.[655] On the other hand, it is beneficial for patients with advanced OA, for whom glucocorticosteroids seem to be less effective, and is included in the EBM guidelines for treatment of OA.[1] Intra-articular hyaluronate was superior to glucocorticosteroid in the knee joint with OA, but intra-articular hyaluronate in combination with dexamethasone was superior to hyaluronate alone.[66,67] There is no indication for the use of hyaluronate in patients with chronic systemic arthritis, eg, RA.

Forms

Synvisc (Genzyme) is a preparation of high–molecular weight (7×10^3 kD) sodium hyaluronate extracted from rooster combs. It contains 0.8% sodium hyaluronate (8 mg/mL) dissolved in a phosphate buffer with added sodium chloride. Arzt AstraZeneca is a preparation of sodium hyaluronate (10 mg/mL) that also is extracted from rooster combs but has a lower average molecular weight than Synvisc (1000 kD). A similar preparation is Hyalgan (10 mg/mL; Sanofi-Aventis), which has a molecular weight of 500 to 700 kD.

Sodium hyaluronate in a concentration of 1% can be injected intra-articularly with a 23-gauge needle. At least two injections at 1-week intervals should be given for treatment of arthritis of the TMJ.

Technique for Intra-articular Injection

Before intra-articular injection, the joint should be carefully palpated during mandibular movements to locate the condyle and the mandibular fossa. The fossa is felt as a depression anterior to the tragus on mouth opening. Hair over the joint is shaved, and any hair in the vicinity of the joint is held aside with adhesive tape. A head cap can then be used to cover the remaining hair. The skin area 4 to 5 cm around the injection site is cleansed with benzalkonium chloride (0.1%), iodine (5%), or alcohol (70%).

A surgical drape with a 6-cm hole in the center is placed over the joint to maintain a sterile area. The operator should wear gloves and a face mask. A mouth prop makes maintaining the mouth opening during the injection more comfortable for the patient.

A sterile 2-mL syringe should be used with a disposable 23-gauge (0.6-mm) needle that is 1.0 to 1.5 inches (25 to 40 mm) long. Use of a smaller diameter creates a risk that the needle will bend underneath the skin, and a wider diameter results in a larger puncture wound that increases the risk of bleeding. The syringe should be filled with a local anesthetic. While the patient's mouth is open, the needle is inserted in the fossa 2 to 3 mm beneath the zygomatic arch and 8 to 10 mm anterior to the anterior border of the tragus (Fig 30-3). These landmarks may vary, so palpation of the condyle and fossa is imperative. The needle is directed slightly upward and forward to account for the angulation of the condyle.

If resistance is felt, or the needle is stuck, it might have penetrated the disc and not the upper joint space proper. This might occur in patients with restricted condylar translation. The needle should not be forced further but withdrawn, and the insertion should be tried again. Scratching of the articular surfaces by the needle should be avoided.

When properly positioned, the needle should have penetrated 20 to 30 mm beneath the skin surface. One milliliter of the local anesthetic is then injected, and aspiration is performed. If the joint space is accurately penetrated, the local anesthetic in the syringe can be injected and aspirated repeatedly. The syringe is then detached, another syringe containing the drug to be used is attached, and the injection is made.

The needle is removed and pressure is maintained with a gauze dressing over the injection site for 1 to 2 minutes. Usually, there is no need for a dressing over the injection site when the patient leaves, because bleeding is very uncommon. Antibiotics are unnecessary because infection following an intra-articular injection is extremely rare. Gray et al[68] have calculated the risk to be less than 1:20,000.

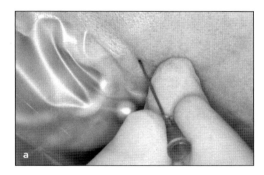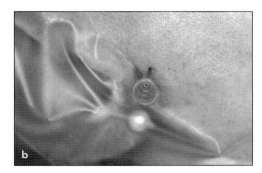

Fig 30-3 *(a)* Insertion of the needle into the upper compartment of the temporomandibular joint. *(b)* Final intra-articular position of the needle. Final intra-articular position of the needle.

Conclusion

The choice of treatment for TMJ arthritis depends on many factors, such as disease activity (acute or chronic), stage (early or late), and whether permanent joint damage is present. The various treatments described can be used to permit most patients to function well in a relatively pain-free manner. For those who do not respond after a reasonable period of treatment, surgical management may be indicated in some instances (see chapter 28).

References

1. Treatment of osteoarthritis. Evidence-Based Medicine Guidelines [website]. 9 Apr 2004:ebm00396. Available at: http://www.ebm-guidelines.com. Accessed 26 May 2004.

2. Simon LS, Weaver AL, Graham DY, Kivitz AJ, Lispky PE, Hibard RC. Anti-inflammatory and upper gastrointestinal effects of celecoxib in rheumatoid arthritis. A randomized controlled trial. JAMA 1999;282:1921–1928.

3. Saag K, Fischer C, McKay J, Ehrich E, Zhao PL, Bolognese J. MK-0966, a specific COX-2 inhibitor, has clinical efficacy comparable to ibuprofen in the treatment of knee and hip osteoarthritis (OA) in a 6 week controlled clinical trial [abstract]. Arthritis Rheum 1998;41(suppl):S196.

4. Langman MJ, Jensen DM, Watson DJ, et al. Adverse upper gastrointestinal effects of rofecoxib compared with NSAIDs. JAMA 1999;282:1929–1933.

5. Madhok R, Kerr H, Capell HA. Clinical review—Recent advances in rheumatology. Br Med J 2000;321:882–885.

6. Pispati PK. Evidence-based practice in rheumatology. APLAR J Rheumatol 2003;6:44–49.

7. McAlindon TE, LaValley MP, Gulin JP, Felson DT. Glucosamine and chondroitin for treatment of osteoarthritis. JAMA 2000;283:1469–1475.

8. Glucosamine in the treatment of osteoarthritis [evidence summary]. Evidence-Based Medicine Guidelines [website]. 9 Apr 2004:evd01028. Available at: http://www.ebm-guidelines.com. Accessed Aug 2004.

9. Reginster JY, Deroisy R, Paul I, et al. Glucosamine sulfate significantly reduces progression of knee osteoarthritis over 3 years: A large randomized, placebo-controlled, double-blind, prospective trial [abstract]. Arthritis Rheum 1999;42 (suppl):1975.

10. Garner S, Fidan D, Frankish R, et al. Rofecoxib for rheumatoid arthritis. The Cochrane Database of Systematic Reviews [website]. In: The Cochrane Library, Issue 3, 2003. Oxford, England: Update Software. Available at: http://www.mrw .interscience.wiley.com/cochrane/clsysrev/articles/CD0036 85/frame.html. Accessed 26 May 2004.

11. Infliximab for rheumatoid arthritis [evidence summary]. Evidence-Based Medicine Guidelines [website]. 4 Feb 2003: evd03501. Available at: http://www.ebm-guidelines.com. Accessed 26 May 2004.

12. Kopp S, Alstergren P, Ernestam S, Nordahl S, Morin P, Bratt J. Reduction of temporomandibular joint pain after treatment with a combination of methotrexate and infliximab is associated with changes in synovial fluid and plasma cytokines in rheumatoid arthritis. Cells Tissues Organs 2005;180:22–30.

13. Drug treatment of rheumatoid arthritis. Evidence-Based Medicine Guidelines [website]. 29 Mar 2004:ebm00456. Available at: http://www.ebm-guidelines.com. Accessed 26 May 2004.

14. Dixon A, Graber J. Local Injection Therapy in Rheumatic Diseases, ed 3. Basel: Eular, 1989.

15. Hickling P, Jacoby RK, Kirwan JR. Joint destruction after glucocorticoids are withdrawn in early rheumatoid arthritis. Br J Rheum 1998;37:930–936.

16. Tegelberg Å, Kopp S. Short-term effect of physical training on temporomandibular disorder in individuals with rheumatoid arthritis and ankylosing spondylitis. Acta Odontol Scand 1988;46:49–56.

17. Physical activity and rheumatoid arthritis [evidence summary]. Evidence-Based Medicine Guidelines [website]. 20 Apr 2004:evd02356. Available at: http://www.ebm-guidelines.com. Accessed 16 Sept 2004.

18. Acupuncture as a symptomatic treatment for osteoarthritis [evidence summary]. Evidence-Based Medicine Guidelines [website]. evd00028. Available at: http://www.ebm-guidelines.com. Accessed 16 Sept 2004.

19. Casimiro L, Barnsley L, Brosseau L, et al. Acupuncture and electroacupuncture for the treatment of RA. The Cochrane Database of Systematic Reviews [website]. In: The Cochrane Library, Issue 3, 2003. Oxford, England: Update Software. Available at: http://www.mrw.interscience .wiley.com/cochrane/clsysrev/articles/CD003788/frame.html. Accessed 16 Sept 2004.

20. Glass JM, Stephen RL, Jacobson SC. The quantity and distribution of radiolabeled dexamethasone delivered to tissue by iontophoresis. Int J Dermatol 1980;19:519–525.

21. Reid KI, Dionne RA, Sicard-Rosenbaum L, Lord D, Dubner R. Evaluation of iontophoretically applied dexamethasone for painful pathologic temporomandibular joints. Oral Surg Oral Med Oral Pathol 1994;77:605–609.

22. Schiffman EL, Braun BL, Lindgren BR. Temporomandibular joint iontophoresis: A double-blind randomized clinical trial. J Orofac Pain 1996;10:157–165.

23. Shin SM, Choi JK. Effect of indomethacin phonophoresis on the relief of temporomandibular joint pain. Cranio 1997;15:345–348.

24. Zhang WY, Li Wan Po A. The effectiveness of topically applied capsaicin. A meta-analysis. Eur J Clin Pharmacol 1994;46:517–522.

25. Deal CL, Schnitzer TJ, Lipstein E, et al. Treatment of arthritis with topical capsaicin: A double blind trial. Clin Ther 1991;13.383–395.

26. Hersh EV, Pertes RA, Ochs HA. Topical capsaicin-pharmacology and potential role in the treatment of temporomandibular pain. J Clin Dent 1994;5:54–59.

27. Topically applied non-steroidal anti-inflammatory drugs [evidence summary]. Evidence-Based Medicine Guidelines [website]. evd03148. Available at: http://www.ebm-guidelines .com. Accessed 12 Oct 2004.

28. Moore RA, Tramer MR Caroll D, Wiffen PJ, McQuay HJ. Quantitative systematic review of topically applied non-steroidal anti-inflammatory drugs. BMJ 1998;316:333–338 [erratum 1998;316:1059].

29. Lin J, Zhang W, Jones A, Doherty M. Efficacy of topical non-steroidal anti-inflammatory drugs in the treatment of osteoarthritis: Meta-analysis of randomised controlled trials. BMJ 2004;329:324–335.

30. Major PW, Nebbe B. Use and effectiveness of splint appliance therapy: Review of literature. Cranio 1997;15:159–166.

31. Ekberg E, Vallon D, Nilner M. The efficacy of appliance therapy in patients with temporomandibular disorders of mainly myogenous origin. A randomized, controlled, short-term trial. J Orofac Pain 2003;17:133–139.

32. Kopp S, Wenneberg B. Effects of occlusal treatment and intra-articular injections on temporomandibular joint pain and dysfunction. Acta Odontol Scand 1981;39:87–96.

33. Forsell H, Kalso E, Koskela P, Vehmanen R, Puukka P, Alanen P. Occlusal treatments in temporomandibular disorders: A qualitative systematic review of randomized controlled trials. Pain 1999;83:549–560.

34. Al-Ani MZ, Davies SJ, Gray RJM, Sloan P, Glenny AM. Stabilisation splint therapy for temporomandibular pain dysfunction syndrome. The Cochrane Database of Systematic Reviews [website]. In: The Cochrane Library, Issue 2, 2004. Oxford, England: Update Software. Available at: http://www.mrw.interscience.wiley.com/cochrane/clsysrev/articles/CD002778/frame.html. Accessed 16 Sept 2004.

35. Alstergren P, Appelgren A, Appelgren B, Kopp S, Lundeberg T, Theodorsson E. The effect on joint fluid concentration of neuropeptide Y by intra-articular injection of glucocorticoid in temporomandibular joint arthritis. Acta Odontol Scand 1995;54:1–7.

36. Wenneberg B, Kopp S, Gröndahl HG. Long-term effect of intra-articular injections of a glucocorticosteroid into the TMJ: A clinical and radiographic 8-year follow-up. J Craniomandib Disord 1991;5:11–18.

37. Mejersjö C, Kopp S. Effect of corticosteroid and sodium hyaluronate on induced joint lesions in the guinea-pig knee. Int J Oral Maxillofac Surg 1987;16:194–201.

38. Saxne T, Heinegård D, Wollheim FA. Proteoglycans in synovial fluid: The effect of intra-articular corticosteroid injections. Br J Rheumatol 1985;24:221.

39. Saxne T, Heinegård D, Wollheim FA. Therapeutic effects on cartilage metabolism in arthritis as measured by release of proteoglycan structures into the synovial fluid. Ann Rheum Dis 1986;45:491–497.

40. Kopp S, Carlsson GE, Haraldson T, Wenneberg B. Long-term effect of intra-articular injections of sodium hyaluronate and corticosteroid on temporomandibular joint arthritis. J Oral Maxillofac Surg 1987;45:929–935.

41. Kopp S, Åkerman S, Nilner M. Short-term effects of intra-articular sodium hyaluronate, glucocorticoid, and saline injections on rheumatoid arthritis of the temporomandibular joint. J Craniomandib Disord 1991;5:231–238.

42. Raynauld JP, Buckland-Wright C, Ward R, et al. Safety and efficacy of long-term intra-articular steroid injections in osteoarthritis of the knee: A randomized, double-blind, placebo-controlled trial. Arthritis Rheum 2003;48:370–377.

43. Buckwalter J. Intra-articular corticosteroids: Beneficial effects in managing OA of the knee. Medscape [website]. 29 June 2001. Available at: http://www.medscape.com/viewarticle/416506_21. Accessed March 2004.

44. Guidelines for the management of rheumatoid arthritis—American College of Rheumatology Subcommittee on Rheumatoid Arthritis Guidelines, Arthritis Rheum 2002;46:328–346.

45. Psoriatic arthropathy. Evidence-Based Medicine Guidelines [website]. 3 Apr 2000:ebm00444. Available at: http://www.ebm-guidelines.com. Accessed 26 May 2004.

46. Ankylosing spondylitis. Evidence-Based Medicine Guidelines [website]. 18 Feb 2004:ebm00443. Available at: http://www.ebm-guidelines.com. Accessed 26 May 2004.

47. Gout. Evidence-Based Medicine Guidelines [website]. 28 Apr 1999:ebm00451. Available at: http://www.ebm-guidelines.com. Accessed 26 May 2004.

48. Chondrocalcinosis (pseudogout). Evidence-Based Medicine Guidelines [website]. 1 June 1998:ebm00453. Available at: http://www.ebm-guidelines.com. Accessed 26 May 2004.

49. Reactive arthritis and rheumatic fever. Evidence-Based Medicine Guidelines [website]. Feb 2004:ebm00450. Available at: http://www.ebm-guidelines.com. Accessed 26 May 2004.

50. Local corticosteroid injections in soft tissues and joints. Evidence-Based Medicine Guidelines [website]. 17 May 2001: ebm00465. Available at: http://www.ebm-guidelines.com. Accessed 26 May 2004.

51. Kopp S, Wenneberg B, Haraldson R, Carlsson GE. Short-term effect of intra-articular injections of sodium hyaluronate and corticosteroid on temporomandibular joint pain and dysfunction. J Oral Maxillofac Surg 1985;3:429–435.

52. Schafer M, Imai Y, Uhl GR, Stein C. Inflammation enhances peripheral mm-opioid receptor-mediated analgesia, but not mm-opioid receptor transcription in dorsal root ganglia. Eur J Pharmacol 1995;279:165–169.

53. Stein C. The control of pain in peripheral tissue by opioids. N Engl J Med 1995;332:1685–1690.

54. Kalso E, Tramèr MR, Caroll D, McQuay HJ, Moore RA. Pain relief from intra-articular morphine after knee surgery: A qualitative systematic review. Pain 1997;71:127–134.

55. Likar R, Schäfer M, Paulak F, et al. Intra-articular morphine analgesia in chronic pain patients with osteoarthritis. Anesth Analg 1997;84:1313–1317.

56. List T, Tegelberg Å, Haraldson T, Isacsson G. Intra-articular morphine as analgesic in temporomandibular joint arthralgia/osteoarthritis. Pain 2001;94:275–282.

57. Bryant CJ, Harrison SD, Hopper C, Harris M. Use of intra-articular morphine for postoperative analgesia following TMJ arthroscopy. Br J Oral Maxillofac Surg 1999;37:391–396.

58. Stein A, Yassouridis A, Szopko C, Helmke K, Stein C. Intra-articular morphine versus dexamethasone in chronic arthritis. Pain 1999;83:525–532.

59. Laurent C, Hellström S, Fellenius E. Hyaluronan improves the healing of experimental tympanic membrane perforations—A comparison of preparations with different rheological properties. Arch Otolaryngol 1988:114:1435–1441.

60. Smith MM, Ghosh P. The synthesis of hyaluronic acid by human synovial fibroblasts is influenced by the nature of the hyaluronate in the extracellular environment. Rheumatol Int 1987;7:113–122.

61. Namiki O, Toyoshima H, Morisaki N. Therapeutic effect of intra-articular injection of high molecular weight hyaluronic acid on osteoarthritis of the knee. Int J Clin Pharmacol Ther Toxicol 1982;20:501–507.

62. Balazs EA, Denlinger JL. Viscosupplementation: A new concept in the treatment of osteoarthritis. J Rheumatol 1993;20:3–9.

63. Lussier A, Cividino AA, McFarlane CA, Olszynski WP, Potashner WJ, de Médicis R. Viscosupplementation with hyaluronate for the treatment of osteoarthritis: Findings from clinical practice in Canada. J Rheumatol 1996;23:1579–1585.

64. Hyaluronate for temporomandibular joint disorders [evidence summary]. Evidence-Based Medicine Guidelines [website]. 2 Oct 2003:evd04227. Available at: http://www.ebm-guidelines.com. Accessed 26 May 2004.

65. Shi Z, Guo C, Awad M. Hyaluronate for temporomandibular joint disorders. The Cochrane Database of Systematic Reviews [website]. In: The Cochrane Library, Issue 2, 2004. Oxford, England: Update Software. Available at: http://www.mrw.interscience.wiley.com/cochrane/clsysrev/articles/CD002970/frame.html. Accessed 26 May 2004.

66. Pharmacological therapy in osteoarthritis of the knee [evidence summary]. Evidence-Based Medicine Guidelines [website]. evd02339. Available at: http://www.ebm-guidelines.com. Accessed 26 May 2004.

67. Towheed TE, Hochberg MC. A systematic review of randomized controlled trials of pharmacological therapy in osteoarthritis of the knee, with an emphasis on trial methodology. Semin Arthritis Rheum 1997;26:755–770.

68. Gray RG, Tennenbaum J, Gottlieb NL. Local corticosteroid injection treatment in rheumatic disorders. Semin Arthritis Rheum 1981;10:231–254.

Surgical Management of TMJ Arthritis

Louis G. Mercuri

Statistics indicate that the incidence of arthritis worldwide is 3.2% of the population. These conditions affect females more often than males (2.7:1) and lead to joint destruction and disability in 10% to 15% of afflicted patients. Arthritic disease is the second most frequent cause of complaints among outpatients with chronic diseases.[1]

Although arthritis has many causes, the common end result is deterioration of the affected joint surfaces, resulting in loss of joint function. If the cause can be determined, that information will help the clinician to anticipate the clinical characteristics and the rate of deterioration of the joint surfaces for any given arthritic condition.

One of the most difficult problems for patients with arthritis to accept is that the disease is chronic, with little likelihood of spontaneous remission. People with arthritis must live with their disease, because they will not die from it. Therefore, appropriate management of the results of the disease is critical to maintaining the quality of life for these patients. For example, Voog et al[2] studied the impact of temporomandibular joint (TMJ) pain on daily living in patients with rheumatoid arthritis and found that pain or discomfort from the TMJ in these patients was greatest on the performance of physical exercise and jaw movements, while it was least during the performance of hobbies and eating. Thus, a management plan must be developed that addresses the specific problems faced by the patient. This includes the use of appropriate regimens of rest, exercise, diet, medications, and oral appliances. In some cases, it also requires the use of the various physical and surgical modalities to increase and maintain masticatory function, return form to the face, decrease the need for further, more complex management, and relieve pain.

A critical factor in all management plans is education of the patients about their disease process, the management modalities to be used, the principles of joint protection from overuse, and energy conservation. If patients understand the management rationale, they are more likely to comply with the regimen. Providing them with information about reasonable functional goals and limitations of jaw function will result in greater long-term success.

Principles of Surgical Management

Management of arthritic conditions can be divided into noninvasive (see chapter 30) and invasive (surgical) approaches. The decision to manage any form of TMJ arthritis surgically must be based on evaluation of the patient's response to noninvasive management, the patient's mandibular form and function, and the effect the condition has on the patient's quality of life.

The management goals for patients with TMJ arthritis should be:

1. Relief of pain, swelling, and fatigue
2. Improvement of joint function
3. Prevention of further joint damage
4. Prevention of disability and disease-related morbidity

When the clinician is considering surgical management of TMJ arthritis, the following factors also should be taken into account:

1. The medications the patient is taking (nonsteroidal anti-inflammatory drugs, cyclooxygenase inhibitors, corticosteroids, etc) can affect blood coagulation and wound healing.

Table 31-1 Classification of TMJ arthritis, based on symptoms, signs, and imaging, with management options*

Stage	Symptoms	Signs	Imaging	Management options
I. Early disease	Joint/muscle pain Limited function Crepitation	Little or no occlusal or facial esthetic changes	Mild to moderate erosive changes of condyle, fossa, and eminence	Minimally invasive procedures (first) Soft tissue procedures (second)
II. Arrested disease	Little or no joint pain Muscle pain Some joint dysfunction Crepitation	Class II malocclusion Apertognathia	Flattened condyle and eminence	Bone and joint procedures (first) Salvage procedures (second)
III. Advanced disease	Joint/muscle pain Loss of function Crepitation present or absent Progressive retrognathia	High-angle Class II malocclusion Apertognathia Developing fibrosis/ankylosis	Gross erosive changes Loss of condyle and eminence height Ankylosis Hypertrophy of coronoid process	Salvage procedures (first) Bone and joint procedures (second)

*Modified from Steinbrocker et al[4] and Kent et al.[5]

2. Positioning the patient for a prolonged anesthesia may lead to pressure necrosis of overlying fragile skin because of joint deformities.
3. Cervical spine involvement and the potential for cervical myelopathy in arthritic patients require that critical care be taken in the positioning of the head for surgical access, because improper positioning can add to the risk of cervical cord injury.[3]

The evidence-based discussion of the surgical management of arthritis of the TMJ presented in this chapter is based on a classification scheme involving the clinical signs and symptoms and imaging findings, modified from that developed by Steinbrocker et al[4] and Kent et al[5] (Table 31-1).

The surgical procedures available for management of each stage of disease can be divided into four main categories:

1. Minimally invasive procedures such as intra-articular injections, arthrocentesis, and arthroscopy (see chapters 30 and 32)
2. Soft tissue procedures, such as synovectomy

3. Bone and joint procedures, including arthroplasty and orthognathic surgery
4. Salvage procedures, such as total autogenous or alloplastic joint reconstruction.

The first two categories can be considered as preventive and the latter two as reparative in nature. The stage of the disease in each patient will dictate which of these procedures will be used for management.

The use of various noninvasive modalities of management, including medications, bite appliances, and especially physical therapy,[6–8] may be indicated as adjunctive treatments with each of the surgical procedures described above[7] (see chapter 24). Physical modalities can reduce inflammation and pain. Superficial moist heat, deep heat, or localized cold applications may relieve pain sufficiently to permit exercise. Therapeutic exercises are designed to increase muscle strength, reduce joint contracture, and maintain a functional range of motion. Ultrasound, electrogalvanic stimulation, and massage techniques are also helpful in reducing inflammation and pain. In pursuing physical therapy, patients should avoid heavy loading exercises that compress the joint. For this reason, the majority of muscle-strengthening exercises are best done isometrically in a position that does not cause pain. Assisted, passive range of motion exercises, such as with the Therabite Jaw Exerciser (Therabite), are also recommended.[9] Maxillomandibular fixation has no role in the management of arthritic TMJ disease and leads to joint contractures and masticatory muscle atrophy and fibrosis.

A soft diet and the use of an oral appliance can aid in decreasing the load across the articulating surfaces of the joint. A flat-plane processed acrylic resin maxillary bite appliance should to be worn 24 hours per day for 1 month, except while the patient is eating, during any acute phase, then at night thereafter. This appliance should provide complete coverage, opening the bite 2 to 3 mm posteriorly. It should allow freedom of movement in all excursions of the mandible with a canine rise or group function in lateral excursions and incisal guidance in protrusion. In those cases in which advanced arthritis has produced significant occlusal changes, reconstruction of the occlusion to provide bilateral occlusal stability will decease the potential for unilateral joint overload, and therefore it may be recommended after the active osteoarthritic process has "burned out."

Low-Inflammatory Arthritis

The low-inflammatory arthritic disorders include degenerative arthritis and posttraumatic arthritis. The following are various treatments that have been used for these conditions.

Arthrocentesis

Nitzan and Price[10] reported a 20-month follow-up study of 36 patients (38 joints) who had not responded to nonsurgical management to determine the efficacy of arthrocentesis in restoring functional capacity to osteoarthritic joints. They found that 26 joints (68%) responded favorably to arthrocentesis. Subjective pain and dysfunction scores significantly decreased and objective measurements (maximum interincisal opening and lateral excursions) significantly increased. These authors concluded that arthrocentesis is a rapid and safe procedure that may enable the osteoarthritic TMJ to return to a functional state. However, the failure of arthrocentesis (in one third of the cases) suggests that painful limitation of TMJ function might be the result of fibrous adhesions or osteophytes that require arthrotomy for management. The limitations of this study are the small sample size, the inability to generalize the results to a male population because the overwhelming majority of the patients were female, the lack of a control group, the influence of concomitant use of anti-inflammatory or other analgesic agents, and the short follow-up.

Arthroscopy

The value of TMJ arthroscopy is primarily based on its relatively conservative nature, as well as the fact that it provides a direct three-dimensional view of the joint. This permits both earlier diagnosis and simpler management of arthritic processes affecting the TMJ, which could prevent the late-stage complications of open bite and ankylosis.[11–13]

Holmlund[11] described the arthroscopic picture as varying widely, depending on the stage of the arthritic process when the procedure is performed and whether disease-modifying therapeutic agents have been given. For example, in rheumatoid arthritis, early features of synovial involvement may be increased vascularity and capillary hyperemia; the more severe the disease, the more features that will be found. The same is true of the cartilage, in which the findings may vary from early superficial changes, such as localized areas with fibrillation, to lesions and exposure of subchondral bone. Late-stage marked fibrosis or ankylosis makes arthroscopy impossible and negates its usefulness.

Arthroplasty

Condylotomy

Henny and Baldridge[14] described this procedure (also known as a *high condylar shave*) as a limited removal of the damaged articular surface of the condyle that maintains the height of the ramus, the articular disc, and the surrounding soft tissues, including the lateral pterygoid muscle attachment. Its use was advocated in patients with severe, unremitting degenerative joint disease. Reshaping of the articular surfaces to eliminate osteophytes, erosions, and irregularities found in degenerative joint disease refractory to other modalities of treatment was also described by Dingman and Grabb.[15] Although both techniques reportedly provided pain relief, concerns about the resultant mandibular dysfunction, dental malocclusion, facial asymmetry, and the potential for development of further bony articular degeneration, disc disorders or loss, and ankylosis also led to the development of techniques for interposing autogenous tissues or alloplastic materials.

The need for replacement of the articular disc in such cases remains controversial.[16] The literature on TMJ anatomy and function suggests that the articular disc serves many functions (see chapters 1 and 2).[17] These include shock absorption, maintaining congruency between the articulating surfaces of the condyle-fossa-eminence complex, facilitation of jaw movements, distribution of functional loads, and dispersion of synovial fluid. To date, however, there is little scientific evidence to substantiate many of these inferences. Therefore, it is impossible to objectively define the ideal properties and requirements of a disc replacement material.[18] According to Moriconi et al,[19] TMJ replacement materials should fulfill the following criteria: biologic compatibility, adequate strength, good biomechanics, and resistance to the adverse affects of the biologic environment.

Autogenous disc replacement

A number of different autogenous tissues have been advocated as a replacement for the TMJ articular disc.[20] However, the literature on the use of the vascularized temporalis muscle flap appears to present the data most applicable to the management of the arthritic TMJ.[21–28] The advantages of the temporalis muscle flap are its reliable blood supply[29,30] and its proximity to the TMJ. Feinberg and Larsen[23] stated that one of the most important roles of the temporalis muscle flap is the maintenance of functional movements. Because the flap is attached to the coronoid process, when the mandible translates, the movement of the mandible pulls the muscle flap in an anterior direction, simulating the natural functional movements of the disc. Investigators who performed follow-up studies on patients with temporalis muscle replacement have demonstrated the presence of viable muscle tissue within the joint.[21,22,31]

Tong and Tideman[32] reported the re-formation of a disclike interpositional structure 18 months after use of the pedicled temporalis muscle flap in four discectomized rhesus monkeys with osteoarthritis. They also reported that a milder degree of osteoarthritis was observed histologically in the joints in which the graft survived (three of the four monkeys).

Henry and Wolford[33] have suggested the following contraindications to the use of the temporalis muscle and fascia graft: patients with failed Proplast-Teflon (Vitek) or Silastic (Dow Corning) implants and a continuing foreign-body giant cell reaction,[34–36] rheumatoid arthritis or other high-inflammatory connective tissue disease,[33] progressive osteoarthritis,[33] or two or more prior TMJ surgeries.[37,38]

Alloplastic hemiarthroplasty

Placement of an alloplastic bearing surface articulating with bone, either diseased or normal, has been used in orthopedic surgery for fractures of the hip and shoulders in geriatric patients. This surgery can be quite successful in such patients, in whom functional demands are low. However, under normal functional loading, a metal articulation will cause breakdown of articular cartilage, leading to failure of the hemiarthroplasty, pain, and progression to total joint replacement.[39–41] For this reason, hemiarthroplasty should generally not be performed in young patients or in patients with osteoarthritis.[42,43]

In low- and high-inflammatory arthritic conditions, except juvenile rheumatoid arthritis, both articulating components of a joint are involved; in such cases, orthopedists recommend total joint replacement, not hemiarthroplasty. Comparison studies have demonstrated that total joint replacement has significantly better outcomes than hemiarthroplasty with regard to pain, stability, function, failure rates, and requirement for further revision.[44–47]

A number of different implantable alloplastic materials have been advocated for hemiarthroplasty of the TMJ.[48] Among these were Silastic and Proplast-Teflon, both of which have been determined to be inappropriate for use in the TMJ because of their poor wear characteristics and the resultant foreign-body giant cell osteolysis they cause.

Park et al[49] reported an 8-year retrospective pilot study on the use of a metal alloplastic hemiarthroplasty in advanced TMJ degenerative joint disease in 108 joints. The mean follow-up was 3 years. The authors concluded that their findings of significant pain relief and increased TMJ function warranted further investigation of this treatment.

However, in light of the poor long-term orthopedic experience with hemiarthroplasty in patients with arthritic disease, it would appear logical that use of this concept for the management of TMJ arthritis might lead to the same outcome. Therefore, it should not be recommended until further long-term, well-designed clinical trials with larger populations have demonstrated the safety and efficacy of hemiarthroplasty for the management of TMJ arthritis.

Orthognathic Surgery

Patients with active TMJ disease and either concomitant or resultant maxillofacial skeletal discrepancies that are treated only with orthognathic surgery often experience poor outcomes and significant relapse.[50–57]

High-Inflammatory Arthritis

The high-inflammatory arthritic conditions include infectious arthritis as well as rheumatoid arthritis and the rheumatoid-like conditions (adult and juvenile rheumatoid arthritis, gout, psoriatic arthritis, lupus erythematosus, ankylosing spondylitis, Reiter syndrome, and arthritis associated with ulcerative colitis). The following treatments have been used for these conditions.

Arthrocentesis

Trieger et al[58] evaluated the objective and subjective changes in 12 patients with documented rheumatoid arthritis 6 weeks after TMJ arthrocentesis. They concluded that this procedure resulted in a statistically significant short-term improvement in pain and enhanced function. Yara et al[59] replicated these findings in a later study. It has been suggested that the relief of symptoms is the result of removal of debris and other inflammatory products.[60] The major limitations of these studies are the small sample sizes, the lack of control groups, the influence of concomitant use of anti-inflammatory or other analgesic agents, and the short follow-up periods.

Arthroscopy

In early-stage rheumatoid disease, arthroscopic lysis and lavage have been reported to alleviate symptoms in the TMJ.[61,62] A possible explanation for the relief of symptoms is that inflammatory breakdown products and cytokines are removed.[60] In patients with only minor areas of synovial inflammation, sometimes found in those with early-stage rheumatoid disease, subsynovial injection of small volumes of corticosteroids and/or sodium hyaluronate during arthroscopy also has been reported to be helpful in reducing symptoms and increasing function.[63,64]

Advanced arthroscopic surgical techniques have been used to perform synovectomy in more advanced rheumatoid disease when hypertrophic synovium or granulation tissue is present. The removal of such tissue may arrest the disease process in the joint. These techniques demand considerable skill and must always be performed under direct vision. Bleeding often obscures the visibility, and these procedures should be limited to patients with well-defined lesions and performed only by highly skilled arthroscopists.[11,65]

Although diagnostic and surgical arthroscopic procedures have reduced morbidity and avoided the cost of more invasive TMJ procedures, it is essential to understand that there are limitations to their use. In certain stages of TMJ arthritis, it is inappropriate or even contraindicated to attempt to inset an arthroscope, for example, when fibrosis or bony ankylosis has resulted in marked clinical impairment of mobility. Such TMJs, as well as those showing imaging consistent with pronounced granulation tissue or suspected villus formation, are best managed by open arthrotomy procedures.[11,66,67]

Synovectomy

Surgical management of rheumatoid arthritis involves either preventive or reconstructive procedures.[68] Preventive surgery, in the form of synovectomy and tenosynovectomy, is performed when pain and functional impairment persist in the face of good medical management and minimal or no bone involvement is demonstrable radiographically.[69]

The synovial membrane has been removed experimentally in animals, and the rapid regeneration of a fairly normal synovial membrane has been observed repeatedly.[70] The new membrane is somewhat less vascularized and somewhat more fibrous than the original membrane, but the changes are small. In humans, it has been possible to remove the diseased synovial membrane by a refinement of the technique that was developed over the last few decades.

When the diseased synovial membrane is removed as completely as possible, a new one regenerates, very often with few or no signs of inflammation. The new membrane is produced in 60 to 90 days and is surprisingly resistant to new attacks of inflammation.[71] Even in the presence of histologic signs of inflammation in the new membrane, the pathologic process in the joint seems to be retarded to a considerable degree. According to Moberg,[72] this is probably not a question of true recurrence but rather a new expansion of granulation tissue not completely removed during the primary operation. Radical, meticulous removal is therefore recommended. When performed early in the disease process, synovectomy can alleviate pain and restore function of the joint as well as arrest the progression of the disease; results last 5 years or more in a high percentage of patients.[69] However, most of the clinical studies of synovectomy have involved joints other than the TMJ.

Haanæs et al[73] reported a 3-year follow-up of discectomy and synovectomy in the TMJ of one patient with rheumatoid arthritis. During the first year postoperatively, a moderate anterior open bite developed, along with a posterior movement of the mandible. They managed these changes with an anterior repositioning appliance that resulted in good overjet and overbite after 3 years. These authors concluded that, because of the anatomy of the TMJ, it is difficult to remove the synovial membrane completely. When patients with rheumatoid arthritis are treated, the clinician must consider the possible variations in the activity of the disease. Extensive, irreversible occlusal treatment should be avoided until the disease is in an inactive period.

Bjornland et al[74] reported the results of discectomy and synovectomy in 29 joints afflicted with various inflammatory arthritic conditions. Pain relief was reported in 85% of the patients 3 months postoperatively and in 79% of the patients 12 months postoperatively. The authors concluded that most patients with high-inflammatory arthritic disease and TMJ involvement are not candidates for discectomy and synovectomy because of the fluctuations of this disease's activity and because TMJ problems may have a lower priority in these patients than other joints that are more severely involved. Further, they stated that the short-term results they reported, while encouraging, necessitate further studies on the long-term effect on pain, function, and the progression of the disease in this joint. This group also presented similar results and conclusions in a later publication.[65]

There is little difference between the synovitis found in rheumatoid arthritis and that occurring in other high-inflammatory diseases such as psoriatic arthritis and ankylosing spondylitis. However, there have been no reports on the surgical management of these conditions in the TMJ, so it is not known whether synovectomy can be a helpful procedure.

Salvage Procedures for Total Joint Reconstruction

Autogenous Procedures

Several autogenous tissues have been used to reconstruct the mandibular condyle in order to regain facial form and restore mandibular function, but most of the patients in these reports have been treated for developmental abnormalities, postneoplastic or posttraumatic discontinuity defects, and ankylosis. However, some studies, although not specifically related to the treatment of arthritis of the TMJ, have included such cases.

Wolford et al[75] reported on the long-term results in 38 cases, followed for a mean of 45 months (range, 10 to 84 months), in which autogenous sternoclavicular grafts were used, 10 of which were in patients with documented inflammatory arthritis. The results showed that autogenous sternoclavicular joint TMJ reconstruction had excellent subjective and objective outcomes when used to manage joints not affected by prior failed TMJ alloplastic devices (Proplast-Teflon or Silastic) or inflammatory

arthritis. According to the subjective and objective criteria used for the study, the procedure was successful in only 50% of the patients who were affected by either of those contraindications. Ankylosis requiring reoperation and reconstruction with an alloplastic total TMJ prosthesis was the typical course for these failed autogenous replacements in patients with inflammatory arthritis.

Lindqvist et al[76] reported a clinical 10-year mean follow-up study of 16 of 60 patients with costochondral grafts that they had previously described.[77] All of these patients were affected unilaterally, and 4 had the preoperative diagnosis of "severe TMJ arthritis." There was no indication as to whether these 4 patients had low- or high-inflammatory arthritis; however, based on the pathophysiology of these diseases processes, it seems likely that these patients had a low-inflammatory TMJ arthritic disease (osteoarthritis), because this type of arthritis is more commonly unilateral than are the high-inflammatory forms of TMJ arthritis. The authors concluded that the long-term clinical results of autogenous costochondral TMJ reconstruction in adult patients are "fairly good."

MacIntosh[20,78,79] discussed a rationale and provided clinical examples for the use of autogenous costochondral grafting for the management of the functional and esthetic consequences of osteoarthritis, rheumatoid arthritis, and juvenile arthritis. He advocated disc preservation in patients with early-stage high-inflammatory arthritic disease. In patients with late-stage high-inflammatory arthritis, he first performed a two-stage autogenous temporalis flap (stage 1, fossa) and then an autogenous costochondral (stage 2, condyle-ramus) graft. However, he did not provide any data with which to evaluate the results of these recommendations. MacIntosh[20] concluded:

> Absolute guidelines for determining the appropriate time to operate on the rheumatoid arthritis patient do not exist. The author has found a quiescent period of 2 years, during which the number of affected body articulations remain stable (although not normal), and imaging of the temporomandibular joint and status of jaw position-occlusion remain unchanged, to offer reasonable expectations for postsurgical stability.

However, no data are presented to support this observation.

Perrott et al[80] reported a retrospective study of 26 patients, 7 growing and 19 nongrowing, with a mean follow-up of approximately 4 years. One of the nongrowing patients had a pre-reconstruction diagnosis of "autoimmune arthritis" and 2 others had diagnoses of "degenerative joint disease" (osteoarthritis). When the data are reviewed, it can be seen that the follow-up radiographic measurement of the patient with "autoimmune arthritis" (high-inflammatory arthritis) revealed a significant total bilateral loss of posterior mandibular vertical dimension, and this was the only patient with a decrease in maximum interincisal opening. However, the follow-up data for the 2 patients with degenerative joint disease shows that their radiographic measurements and maximum interincisal opening corresponded with the pre-reconstruction findings. These authors concluded that the results indicated that costochondral grafting may be used to successfully construct or reconstruct the ramus-condyle unit.

Freitas[81] et al reported on 12 arthritic nongrowing patients (24 joints) requiring total TMJ reconstruction. Six were managed with autogenous sternoclavicular or costochondral grafts and 6 with total alloplastic TMJ prostheses. The groups were followed for a mean of 48.8 and 58.5 months, respectively. The authors reported that, based on the criteria established for the study, the patients who underwent alloplastic TMJ reconstruction had statistically significant better subjective and objective outcomes than did those who underwent reconstruction with autogenous bone. They concluded, in light of these results and the fact that the alloplastic reconstruction avoids the need for another operative site, reduces potential morbidity, decreases operating room time, and allows simultaneous mandibular advance-ment with predictable long-term results and stability,[82] that a total alloplastic TMJ reconstruction is the appropriate treatment for patients with low- as well as high-inflammatory arthritis.

Saeed and Kent[83] retrospectively reviewed 76 costochondral grafts (57 patients) after a mean follow-up of 53 months (range, 24 to 161 months). Nine patients (3 with ankylosis and 6 without ankylosis) had a preoperative diagnosis of arthritis, but the authors never stated whether it was a low- or a high-inflammatory arthritic condition. They concluded that, in patients with no previous TMJ surgery, arthritic disease, or congenital deformity, the costochondral graft performed well. A preoperative diagnosis of ankylosis was associated with a high complication rate, suggesting that use of autogenous costochondral grafting should be approached cautiously in arthritic patients.

The use of autogenous costochondral grafting in the growing patient with juvenile rheumatoid arthritis (American Rheumatism Association), also known as *juvenile chronic arthritis* (European League Against Rheumatism), has been studied more extensively than its use in adults with rheumatoid arthritis.[84,85] When replacement of a seriously damaged arthritic condyle is required in a child with juvenile rheumatoid arthritis, autogenous costochondral reconstruction provides considerable growth

potential for the mandible, good mandibular function, early esthetic improvement, and a low morbidity rate.

Juvenile rheumatoid arthritis affects the lower compartment rather than the upper compartment of the TMJ, and this may account for the success with costochondral grafting in such patients.[86] The other high-inflammatory arthritic conditions affect both the upper and lower compartments of the TMJ, and this may account for the poor performance and ankylosis of autogenous tissue often experienced in these cases.

Alloplastic Procedures

Resection arthroplasty, introduced in the 1960s, was an uncertain procedure after which recurrent deformity and limited motion were common complications. It was for this reason that joint prostheses were developed.[87] Early problems of material failure have been resolved and most designs involve the use of a convex metal (cobalt-chrome) surface against a concave ultrahigh–molecular weight polyethylene surface.

Alloplastic reconstruction of the TMJ has been discussed at length.[48,88–92] All of these authors agree that when the mandibular condyle is extensively damaged, degenerated, or lost, as in patients with arthritic conditions, replacement with either an autogenous graft or an alloplastic implant is an acceptable approach to achieve optimal symptomatic and functional improvement. However, dissatisfaction with some of the facets of autogenous costochondral grafting, particularly in patients with high-inflammatory arthritic disease and ankylosis, led to the development and use of total alloplastic TMJ devices. Nevertheless, it was not until 1986, when Zide et al[93] and Kent et al[5] published their comprehensive reviews of rheumatoid arthritis and its surgical management, that the subject was specifically addressed. Despite the fact that the latter article discusses management with devices that are no longer available, the authors provided a paradigm for the management of TMJ arthritic conditions (see Table 31-1).

In a subsequent publication, Kent et al[94] described 57 cases of degenerative joint disease and 14 cases of rheumatoid arthritis that were treated by either partial or total alloplastic reconstruction. Unfortunately, their results are difficult to interpret and apply because the partial and total alloplastic prostheses all contained Proplast-Teflon, which caused a severe foreign-body reaction.

In 1994, Kent and Misiek[89] provided a comprehensive review of partial and total TMJ reconstruction. They concluded that when a patient exhibits a significantly reduced vertical dimension, loss of the disc and entire condylar

Table 31-2	Demographics of all patients in the TMJ Concepts/Techmedica Database				
Patients (No.)	**Joints (No.)**	**Sex (No.)**	**Age (y)**	**Duration of problem (y)**	**Txs***
494	835 (678 bilateral; 157 unilateral)	448 female 46 male	Mean, 40.9 SD, 9.19 Range, 15–77	Mean, 12 SD, 6.63 Range, 1–44	Mean, 5.6 SD, 4.44 Range, 0–48

*Txs = number of prior TMJ surgeries.

Table 31-3	Demographics of the patients in the TMJ Concepts/Techmedica Database with low- or high-inflammatory arthritic conditions					
Condition	**Patients (No.)**	**% of total**	**Sex (No.)**	**Age (y)**	**Duration of problem (y)**	**Txs***
Low-inflammatory arthritis	60	12%	58 female 2 male	Mean, 40.3 SD, 12.1	Mean, 10.5 SD, 7.33	Mean, 3.9 SD, 4.43
High-inflammatory arthritis	27	5%	22 female 5 male	Mean, 37.8 SD, 12.8 Range, 18–65	Mean, 14.3 SD, 10.9 Range, 1–44	Mean, 2 SD, 2.49 Range, 0–9

*Txs = number of prior TMJ surgeries.

head, chronic pain, hypomobility, and malocclusion, as occurs in advanced arthritic conditions, total joint reconstruction with an alloplastic prostheses is indicated.

In 2000, Speculand et al[95] published a report of 86 total alloplastic joints (27 VK II, Vitek; 59 TMJ Implant System, TMJ Implants) used to reconstruct patients with degenerative joint disease and rheumatoid arthritis. The median follow-up was 14.5 months (range, 1 to 120 months). Using the subjective (pain and diet) and objective (interincisal opening) criteria they established for this study, the authors reported an overall success rate of 94%. However, 4 patients required replacement of the VK II devices due to foreign-body giant cell reactions caused by the Teflon-Proplast implant.

In a 2001 publication, Saeed et al[96] reported on 7 patients with rheumatoid arthritis in whom the TMJs were replaced with TMJ Implant System devices. After a mean follow-up of 30 months (range, 8 to 50 months), they reported improved subjective (pain and diet) and objective (interincisal opening) scores in these patients. They[96] concluded that alloplastic total joint reconstruction should be considered for patients with severe rheumatoid arthritis affecting the TMJ, to restore some normal function and appearance.

Mishima et al[97] reported on 6 patients with rheumatoid arthritis in whom they performed total alloplastic TMJ reconstructions to improve respiratory status and correct occlusal discrepancies. After surgery, symptoms of day-time sleepiness and nighttime snoring diminished, and each patient's ability to masticate solid foods improved significantly. Postoperative cephalograms revealed that both posterior airway space and ramal height were significantly increased and dental occlusion was significantly improved. Mean oxygen saturation levels significantly increased 1 month after reconstruction, but the apnea and hypopnea indices did not change significantly.

A number of long-term follow-up studies have included patients with diagnoses consistent with low- and high-inflammatory arthritis of the TMJ in their total alloplastic reconstruction datasets,[92,96,98–102] but to date only the studies previously discussed[95–97] have directly examined the results of alloplastic reconstruction in patients with arthritic disease affecting the TMJ. Therefore, the prospective patient registry files of TMJ Concepts/Techmedica were analyzed to determine the outcomes of total TMJ alloplastic reconstruction with the computer-generated total TMJ reconstruction system in patients with low- and high-inflammatory arthritic conditions. The details of this system have been described elsewhere.[99–101] Of the 494 patients in the dataset reviewed, 60 (12%) had diagnoses consistent with low-inflammatory TMJ arthritis, and 27 (5%) had diagnoses consistent with high-inflammatory TMJ arthritis (Tables 31-2 and 31-3).

After a mean follow-up period of 31.8 months (range, 2 to 48 months), the data revealed a significant improvement ($P < .0003$) in the subjective variables of pain, function, and

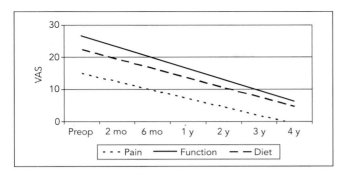

Fig 31-1 Subjective variable (pain, function, and diet) trend lines in patients with high-inflammatory arthritic conditions managed with total alloplastic TMJ prostheses. (VAS) visual analog scale; (Preop) preoperative score.

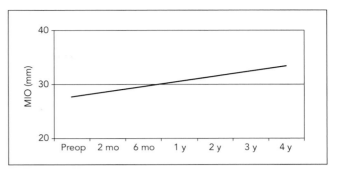

Fig 31-2 Objective variable (maximum interincisal opening [MIO]) trend line in patients with high-inflammatory arthritic conditions managed with total alloplastic TMJ prostheses. (Preop) preoperative measurement.

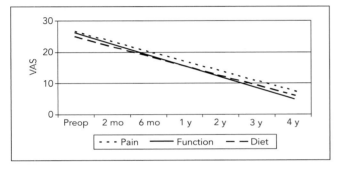

Fig 31-3 Subjective variable (pain, function, and diet) trend lines in patients with low-inflammatory arthritic conditions managed with total alloplastic TMJ prostheses. (VAS) visual analog scale; (Preop) preoperative score.

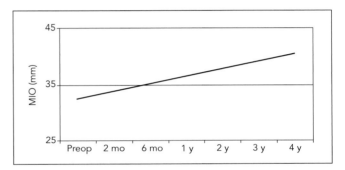

Fig 31-4 Objective variable (maximum interincisal opening [MIO]) trend line in patients with low-inflammatory arthritic conditions managed with total alloplastic TMJ prostheses. (Preop) preoperative measurement.

diet, and improvement in measured maximum interincisal opening ($P < .161$) in the high-inflammatory diagnosis group (Figs 31-1 and 31-2). There was also a significant improvement in pain, function, and diet ($P < .005$) and in measured maximum interincisal opening ($P < .05$) in the low-inflammatory diagnosis group (Figs 31-3 and 31-4).

In light of these findings, previously published reports in both the orthopedic and oral and maxillofacial surgery literature, and the studies comparing autogenous and alloplastic total TMJ replacement in arthritic conditions, it appears that total alloplastic TMJ reconstruction should be considered appropriate management for advanced stage arthritic disease of the TMJ (Fig 31-5).

Scott and Frew[102] reported a situation that all surgeons must account for when reconstructing lost posterior vertical dimension resulting from severe condylar degeneration, especially in patients with chronic TMJ arthritic disease. There is a reciprocal relationship between the clockwise rotation of the mandible and the lengthening of the coronoid process because of the effect of that movement on the tendon of the temporalis muscle. This will cause the coronoid process to elongate over time as the anterior apertognathia develops. Therefore, reconstruction by osteotomy, autogenous tissue, or alloplastic materials must also involve a coronoidectomy to ensure maximum mandibular function after reconstruction.

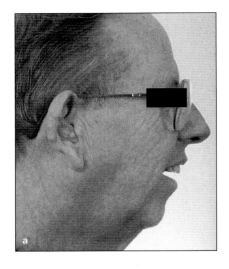

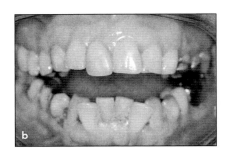

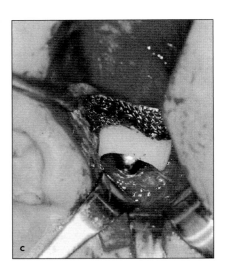

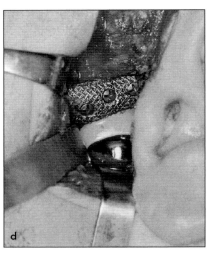

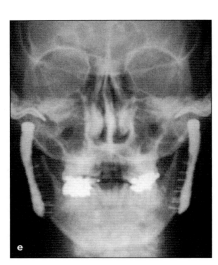

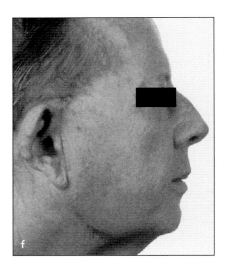

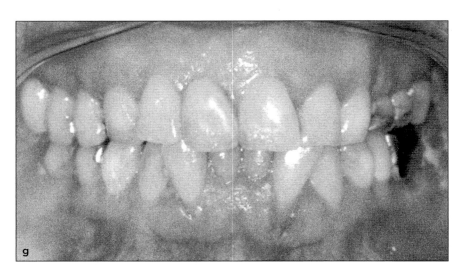

Fig 31-5 Total alloplastic TMJ reconstruction in a patient with Stage III high-inflammatory arthritic joints. *(a)* Preoperative profile. *(b)* Preoperative occlusion. *(c)* Right TMJ alloplastic reconstruction. *(d)* Left TMJ alloplastic reconstruction. *(e)* Postoperative posteroanterior cephalometric image. *(f)* Postoperative profile. *(g)* Postoperative occlusion.

Box 31-1 Treatment of TMJ arthritis

Low-Inflammatory Arthritic Disease
- Degenerative joint disease (osteoarthritis)
  - Early disease: Nonsurgical management (see chapter 30)
  - Moderate disease: Arthrocentesis, arthroscopic lysis and lavage
  - Advanced disease: Autogenous/alloplastic hemiarthroplasty, total autogenous/alloplastic reconstruction
- Posttraumatic arthritis
  - Early disease: Nonsurgical management
  - Moderate disease: Arthrocentesis, arthroscopic lysis and lavage
  - Advanced disease: Autogenous/alloplastic hemiarthroplasty, total autogenous/alloplastic reconstruction

High-Inflammatory Arthritic Disease
- Infectious arthritis
  - Early disease: Incision and drainage, arthrocentesis
  - Arrested disease: Arthroscopic lysis and lavage if there is fibrosis (adhesions) affecting function
  - Advanced disease: Autogenous/alloplastic hemiarthroplasty, total autogenous/alloplastic reconstruction, if there is considerable joint destruction
- Adult rheumatoid arthritis
  - Early disease: Nonsurgical management (see chapter 30)
  - Progressive disease: Arthrocentesis, arthroscopic lysis, and lavage
  - Advanced disease: Total alloplastic reconstruction
- Juvenile rheumatoid arthritis
  - Early disease: Nonsurgical management
  - Arrested disease: Osteotomy
  - Advanced disease: Total autogenous reconstruction with costochondral graft
- Other high-inflammatory arthritic conditions (gout, psoriatic arthritis, arthritis associated with lupus erythematosus, ankylosing spondylitis, arthritis associated with Reiter syndrome, arthritis associated with ulcerative colitis)
  - Early disease: Nonsurgical management (see chapter 30)
  - Moderate disease: Arthrocentesis, arthroscopic lysis and lavage
  - Advanced disease: Total alloplastic reconstruction

Conclusion

Based on the evidence in the literature and the symptoms, signs, and imaging characteristics for the stages of each disease process outlined in Table 31-1, the paradigms shown in Box 31-1 are currently being recommended for the management of arthritic conditions affecting the TMJ. However, longer-term clinical trials on larger patient populations are needed to substantiate their use.

Early diagnosis is the key to successful management of these conditions, because it generally permits the use of nonsurgical means or minimally invasive procedures. However, in late-stage disease, total joint replacement may enable many patients to attain an improved quality of life with less pain and improved function.

References

1. Rodrigo JJ, Gershwin ME. Management of the arthritic joint. In: Chapman MW (ed). Chapman's Orthopaedic Surgery, ed 3. Philadelphia: Lippincott, Williams & Wilkins, 2001:2551–2572.
2. Voog U, Alstergren P, Leibur E, Kallikorm R, Kopp S. Impact of temporomandibular joint pain on activities of daily living in patients with rheumatoid arthritis. Acta Odontol Scand 2003;61:278–282.
3. deBurgh Norman JE, Bramley P. Textbook and Color Atlas of the Temporomandibular Joint. Chicago: Year Book, 1990:83.
4. Steinbrocker O, Traeger CH, Batterman RC. Therapeutic criteria in rheumatoid arthritis. JAMA 1949;140:659–662.
5. Kent JN, Carlton DM, Zide MF. Rheumatoid disease and related arthropathies. 2. Surgical rehabilitation of the temporomandibular joint. Oral Surg Oral Med Oral Pathol 1986; 61:423–439.

6. Cohen SG, Fletcher M. Comparison of jaw mobilization regimens [abstract 514]. J Dent Res 1991;70:329.

7. Nicolakis P, Burak EC, Kollmitzer J, et al. An investigation of the effectiveness of exercise and manual therapy in treating symptoms of TMJ osteoarthritis. Cranio 2001;19:26–32.

8. Oh DW, Kim KS, Lee GW. The effect of physiotherapy on post-temporomandibular joint surgery patients. J Oral Rehabil 2002;29:441–446.

9. Salter RB, Hamilton HW, Wedge JH, et al. Clinical application of basic research on continuous passive motion for disorders of synovial joints. A preliminary report of a feasibility study. J Orthop Res 1984;1:325–342.

10. Nitzan DW, Price A. The use of arthrocentesis for the treatment of osteoarthritic temporomandibular joints. J Oral Maxillofac Surg 2001;59:1154–1159.

11. Holmlund A. Connective tissue pathology: Arthritides. In: Thomas M, Bronstein SL (eds). Arthroscopy of the Temporomandibular Joint. Philadelphia: Saunders,1991:276–281.

12. Gynther GW, Holmlund AB, Reinholt FP, Lindblad S. Temporomandibular joint involvement in generalized osteoarthritis and rheumatoid arthritis: A clinical, arthroscopic, histologic, and immunochemical study. Int J Oral Maxillofac Surg 1997;26:10–16.

13. Gynther GW, Tronje G. Comparison of arthroscopy and radiography in patients with temporomandibular joint symptoms and generalized arthritis. Dent Maxillofac Radiol 1998;27:107–112.

14. Henny FA, Baldridge OL. Condylectomy for the persistently painful temporomandibular joint. J Oral Surg 1957;15:24–31.

15. Dingman RO, Grabb WC. Intra-capsular temporomandibular joint arthroplasty. Plast Reconstr Surg 1966;38:179–185.

16. Bach DE, Waite PD, Adams RC. Autologous TMJ disk replacement. J Am Dent Assoc 1994;125:1504–1512.

17. Merrill RG. Historical perspectives and comparisons of TMJ surgery for internal disc derangements and arthropathy. Craniomandib Pract 1986;4:74–85.

18. Tong CA, Tideman H. A comparative study on meniscectomy and autogenous graft replacement of the Rhesus monkey temporomandibular joint articular disc. 1. Int J Oral Maxillofac Surg 2000;29:140–145.

19. Moriconi ES, Popowich LD, Guernsey LH. Alloplastic reconstruction of the temporomandibular joint. Dent Clin North Am 1986;30:307–325.

20. MacIntosh RB. The case for autogenous reconstruction of the adult temporomandibular joint. In: Worthington P, Evans JR (eds). Controversies in Oral and Maxillofacial Surgery. Philadelphia: Saunders, 1994:356–380.

21. Albert TW, Merrill RG. Temporalis muscle flap for reconstruction of the temporomandibular joint. Oral Maxillofac Surg Clin North Am 1989;1:341–349.

22. Brusati R, Raffaini M, Sesenna E. The temporalis muscle flap in temporomandibular joint surgery. J. Craniomaxillofac Surg 1990;18:352–358.

23. Feinberg SE, Larsen PE. The use of a pedicled temporalis muscle-pericranial flap for the replacement of the TMJ disc. J Oral Maxillofac Surg 1989;47:142–146.

24. Rowe NL. Ankylosis of the temporomandibular joint. J R Coll Surg Edinb 1982;27:67–79.

25. Tideman H, Doddridge M. Temporomandibular joint ankylosis. Aust Dent J 1987;32:171–177.

26. Pogrel MA, Kaban LB. The role of a temporalis muscle/fascia flap used for temporomandibular joint reconstruction. J Oral Maxillofac Surg 1990;48:14–19.

27. Rotskoff KS. Long-term viability of the temporalis muscle/fascia flap for temporomandibular joint reconstruction. J Oral Maxillofac Surg 1993,51:534.

28. Thyne GM, Yoon JH, Luyk NH, McMillan MD. Temporalis muscle as a disc replacement in the temporomandibular joint of sheep. J Oral Maxillofac Surg 1992;50:979–987.

29. Bradley P, Brockbank J. The temporalis muscle flap in oral reconstruction—A cadaveric, animal and clinical study. J Maxillofac Surg 1981;9:139–145.

30. Cheung LK. The vascular anatomy of the human temporalis muscle: Implications for surgical splitting techniques. Int J Oral Maxillofac Surg 1996;25:414–421.

31. Umeda H, Kaban LB, Pogrel MA, Stern M. Long-term viability of the temporalis muscle–fascia flap used for temporomandibular joint reconstruction. J Oral Maxillofac Surg 1993;51:530–533.

32. Tong CA, Tideman H. A comparative study on meniscectomy and autogenous graft replacement of the Rhesus monkey temporomandibular joint articular disc. 2. Int J Oral Maxillofac Surg 2000;29:146–154.

33. Henry CH, Wolford LM. Reconstruction of the temporomandibular joint using a temporalis graft with or without simultaneous orthognathic surgery. J Oral Maxillofac Surg 1995;53:1250–1256.

34. Yih WY, Merrill RG. Pathology of alloplastic interpositional implants in the temporomandibular joint. Oral Maxillofac Surg Clin North Am 1989;1:415–426.

35. Ryan DE. Alloplastic implants in the temporomandibular joint. Oral Maxillofac Surg Clin North Am 1989;1:427–441.

36. Henry CH, Wolford LM. Treatment outcomes for temporomandibular joint reconstruction after Proplast-Teflon implant failure. J Oral Maxillofac Surg 1993;51:352–358.

37. Bradrick JP, Indresano AT. Failure of repetitive temporomandibular joint surgical procedures [abstract]. J Oral Maxillofac Surg 1992 (suppl 3);50:145.

38. Mercuri LG. Subjective and objective outcomes in patients with a custom-fitted alloplastic temporomandibular joint prosthesis. J Oral Maxillofac Surg 1999;57:1427–1430.

39. Van der Meulen MC, Beaupre GS, Smith RL, et al. Factors influencing changes in articular cartilage following hemiarthroplasty in sheep. J Orthop Res 2002;20:669–675.

40. Cruess RI, Kwok DC, Duc PN, Lecavalier MA, Dang GT. The response of articular cartilage to weight bearing against metal: A study of hemiarthroplasty of the hip in the dog. J Bone Joint Surg Br 1984;66:592–597.

41. LaBerge M, Bobyn JD, Drouin G, Rivard CH. Evaluation of metallic personalized hemiarthroplasty: A canine patellofemoral model. J Biomed Mater Res 1999;26:239–254.

42. Breckenbaugh RD, Tressler A, Johnson EW Jr. Results of hemiarthroplasty of the hip using a cemented femoral prosthesis. A review of 109 cases with average follow-up of 36 months. Mayo Clin Proc 1977;52:349–353.

43. Petrera P, Rubash HE. Revision total hip arthroplasty: The acetabular component. J Am Acad Orthop Surg 1995;3:15–21.

44. Amstutz HC, Grigoris P, Safran MR, Grecula MJ, Campbell PA, Schmalzried TP. Precision-fit surface hemiarthroplasty for femoral head osteonecrosis. Long-term results. J Bone Joint Surg Br 1994;76:423–427.

45. Yun AG, Martin S, Zurakowski D, Scott R. Bipolar hemiarthroplasty in juvenile rheumatoid arthritis. J Arthroplasty 2002;17:978–986.

46. Boyd AD Jr, Thomas WH, Scott RD, Sledge CB, Thornhill TS. Total shoulder arthroplasty versus hemiarthroplasty: Indications for glenoid resurfacing. J Arthroplasty 1990;5:329–336.

47. Gartsman GM, Roddey TS, Hammerman SM. Shoulder arthroplasty with or without resurfacing the glenoid in patients who have arthritis. J Bone Joint Surg Am 2000;82:26–34.

48. Mercuri LG. Alloplastic temporomandibular joint reconstruction. Oral Surg Oral Med Oral Pathol Oral Radiol Endod 1998;85:631–637.

49. Park J, Keller EE, Reid KI. Surgical management of advanced degenerative arthritis of temporomandibular joint with metal fossa-eminence hemijoint replacement prosthesis: An 8-year retrospective survey pilot study. J Oral Maxillofac Surg 2004;62:320–328.

50. Wolford LM, Reiche-Fischel O, Mehra P. Changes in TMJ dysfunction after orthognathic surgery. J Oral Maxillofac Surg 2003;61:655–660.

51. Wolford LM. Concomitant temporomandibular joint and orthognathic surgery. J Oral Maxillofac Surg 2003;61:1198–1204.

52. Fuselier JC, Wolford LM, Pitta MC, Talwar M. Condylar changes after orthognathic surgery with untreated TMJ internal derangement [abstract]. J Oral Maxillofac Surg 1998(suppl 1);56:61.

53. Kerstens HC, Tuinzing DB, Golding RP, van der Kwast WA. Condylar atrophy and osteoarthrosis after bimaxillary surgery. Oral Surg Oral Med Oral Pathol Oral Radiol Endod 1990;69:274–280.

54. Moore KG, Gooris PJ, Stoelinga PJ. The contributing role of condylar resorption in orthognathic surgery: A retrospective study. J Oral Maxillofac Surg 1991;49:448–460.

55. De Clercq CA, Neyt LF, Mommaerts MY, Abeloos JV, De Mot BM. Condylar resorption in orthognathic surgery: A retrospective study. Int J Adult Orthodon Orthognath Surg 1994;9:233–240.

56. Arnett GW, Tamborello JA. Progressive class II development: Female idiopathic condylar resorption. Oral Maxillofac Surg Clin North Am 1990;2:699–716.

57. Crawford JG, Stoelinga PJ, Blijdorp PA, Brouns JJ. Stability after reoperation for progressive condylar resorption after orthognathic surgery: Report of seven cases. J Oral Maxillofac Surg 1994;52:460–466.

58. Trieger N, Hoffman CH, Rodriquez E. The effect of arthrocentesis of the temporomandibular joint in patients with rheumatoid arthritis. J Oral Maxillofac Surg 1999;57:537–540.

59. Yara S, Kurihashi K, et al. A case of rheumatoid arthritis of the temporomandibular joints: Arthroscopic findings and efficacy of arthrocentesis. Jpn J Oral Maxillofac Surg 2001; 46:46–54.

60. Quinn JH, Bazan NG. Identification of prostaglandin E_2 and leukotriene B_4 in the synovial fluid of painful, dysfunctional temporomandibular joints. J Oral Maxillofac Surg 1990;48:968–971.

61. Holmlund A, Hellsing G, Wredmark T. Arthroscopy of the temporomandibular joint: A clinical study. Int J Oral Maxillofac Surg 1986;15:715–721.

62. Gynther GW, Holmlund AB. Efficacy of arthroscopic lysis and lavage in patients with temporomandibular joint symptoms associated with generalized osteoarthritis or rheumatoid arthritis. J Oral Maxillofac Surg 1998;56:147–151.

63. Kopp S, Carlsson GE, Haraldson T, Wenneberg B. Long-term effect of intra-articular injections of sodium hyaluronate and corticosteroids on temporomandibular joint arthritis. J Oral Maxillofac Surg 1987;45:929–935.

64. Vallon D, Akerman S, Nilner M, Petersson A. Long-term follow-up of intra-articular injections into the temporomandibular joint in patients with rheumatoid arthritis. Swed Dent J 2002;26:149–158.

65. Bjornland T, Larheim TA. Synovectomy and diskectomy of the temporomandibular joint in patients with arthritic disease compared with diskectomy in patients with internal derangement. A 3-year follow-up study. Eur J Oral Sci 1995; 103:2–7.

66. Heffez LB. Arthroscopy. In: Kaplan AS, Assael LA (eds). Temporomandibular Disorders: Diagnosis and Treatment, Philadelphia: Saunders, 1991:628–662.

67. Murakami K. Arthroscopy of the temporomandibular joint. In: Bell WH (ed). Modern Practice in Orthognathic and Reconstructive Surgery, vol 1. Philadelphia: Saunders, 1992: 608–616.

68. Hollingsworth J. Management of Rheumatoid Arthritis and its Complications, Chicago: Yearbook, 1978.

69. Millender L, Nalebuff E. Preventive surgery—Tenosynovectomy and synovectomy. Orthop Clin North Am 1975;6:765–792.

70. Efskind L. Experimentelle Untersuchungen uber die Anatomie und Physilogie der Gelenkkapsel. Acta Orthop Scand 1941; 12:214–220.

71. Fassbinder HG. Pathologie Rheumatisher Erkrankugen. Berlin: Springer, 1975:217.

72. Moberg E. Cartilage lesions. In: Hijimans W, Paul WD, Hershel H (eds). Early Synovectomy in Rheumatoid Arthritis. Amsterdam: Excerpta Medica, 1969:173–177.

73. Haanæs HR, Larheim TA, Nickerson JW, Pahle JA. Discectomy and synovectomy of the temporomandibular joint in the treatment of rheumatoid arthritis: Case report with a three-year follow-up study. J Oral Maxillofac Surg 1986; 44:905–910.

74. Bjornland T, Larheim TA, Haanæs HR. Surgical treatment of temporomandibular joints in patients with chronic arthritic disease: Preoperative findings and one-year follow-up. Cranio 1992;10:205–210.

75. Wolford LM, Cottrell DA, Henry C. Sternoclavicular grafts for temporomandibular joint reconstruction. J Oral Maxillofac Surg 1994;52:119–128.

76. Lindqvist C, Jokinen J, Paukku P, Tasanen A. Adaptation of autogenous costochondral grafts used for temporomandibular joint reconstruction: A long-term clinical and radiologic follow-up. J Oral Maxillofac Surg 1988;46:465–470.

77. Lindqvist C, Pihakari A, Tasanen A, Hampf G. Autogenous costochondral grafts in temporomandibular joint arthroplasty. A survey of 66 arthroplasties in 60 patients. J Maxillofac Surg 1986;14:143–149.

78. MacIntosh RB. Current spectrum of costochondral and dermal grafting. In: Bell WH (ed). Modern Practice in Orthognathic and Reconstructive Surgery, vol 2. Philadelphia: Saunders, 1992:904–949.

79. MacIntosh RB. The use of autogenous tissue in temporomandibular joint reconstruction. J Oral Maxillofac Surg 2000;58:63–69.

80. Perrott DH, Umeda H, Kaban LB. Costochondral graft construction/reconstruction of the ramus/condyle unit: Long-term follow-up. Int J Oral Maxillofac Surg 1994;23:321–328.

81. Freitas RZ, Mehra P, Wolford LM. Autogenous versus alloplastic TMJ reconstruction in rheumatoid-induced TMJ disease [abstract]. J Oral Maxillofac Surg 2002;58(suppl 1):43.

82. Mehra P, Wolford LM. Custom-made TMJ reconstruction and simultaneous mandibular advancement in autoimmune/connective tissue diseases [abstract]. J Oral Maxillofac Surg 2000;58(suppl 1):95.

83. Saeed NR, Kent JN. A retrospective study of the costochondral graft in TMJ reconstruction. Int J Oral Maxillofac Surg 2003;32:606–609.

84. Brewer EJ Jr, Bass J, Baum J, et al. Current proposed revision of JRA criteria. JRA Criteria Subcommittee of the Diagnostic and Therapeutic Criteria Committee of the American Rheumatism Section of The Arthritis Foundation. Arthritis Rheum 1977;20(suppl 2):195–199.

85. Wood PH. Nomenclature and classification of arthritis in children. In: Munthe E (ed). The Care of Rheumatic Children. Basel: Eular, 1978:47–50.

86. Svensson B, Feldmann G, Rinder A. Early surgical-orthodontic treatment of mandibular hypoplasia in juvenile chronic arthritis. J Craniomaxillofac Surg 1993;21:67–75.

87. Charnley J. Low Friction Arthroplasty of the Hip: Theory and Practice. Berlin: Springer, 1979.

88. McBride KL. Total temporomandibular joint reconstruction. In: Worthington P, Evans JR (eds). Controversies in Oral and Maxillofacial Surgery. Philadelphia: Saunders, 1994:381–396.

89. Kent JN, Misiek DJ. Controversies in disc condyle replacement for partial and total temporomandibular joint reconstruction. In: Worthington P, Evans JR (eds). Controversies in Oral and Maxillofacial Surgery. Philadelphia: Saunders, 1994:397–435.

90. Mercuri LG. Considering total temporomandibular joint replacement. Cranio 1999;17:44–48.

91. Mercuri LG. The use of alloplastic prostheses for temporomandibular joint reconstruction. J Oral Maxillofac Surg 2000;58:70–75.

92. Donlon WC (ed). Total Temporomandibular Joint Reconstruction. Oral and Maxillofacial Surgery Clinics of North America, vol 12. Philadelphia: Saunders, 2000.

93. Zide MF, Carlton DM, Kent JN. Rheumatoid disease and related arthropathies. 1. Systemic findings, medical therapy, and peripheral joint surgery. Oral Surg Oral Med Oral Pathol 1986;61:119–125.

94. Kent JN, Block MS, Homsy CA, Prewitt JM 3rd, Reid R. Experience with polymer glenoid fossa prosthesis for partial or total temporomandibular joint reconstruction. J Oral Maxillofac Surg 1986;44:520–533.

95. Speculand B, Hensher R, Powell D. Total prosthetic replacement of the TMJ: Experience with two systems 1988–1997. Br J Oral Maxillofac Surg 2000;38:360–369.

96. Saeed NR, McLeod NMH, Hensher R. Temporomandibular joint replacement in rheumatoid-induced disease. Br J Oral Maxillofac Surg 2001;39:71–75.

97. Mishima K, Yamada T, Sugahara T. Evaluation of respiratory status and mandibular movement after total temporomandibular joint replacement in patients with rheumatoid arthritis. Int J Oral Maxillofac Surg 2003;32:275–279.

98. Chase DC, Hudson JW, Gerard DA. The Christensen prosthesis. A retrospective clinical study. Oral Surg Oral Med Oral Pathol Oral Radiol Endod 1995;80:273–278.

99. Mercuri LG, Wolford LM, Sanders B, White RD, Hurder A, Henderson W. Custom CAD/CAM total temporomandibular joint reconstruction system: Preliminary multicenter report. J Oral Maxillofac Surg 1995;53:106–115.

100. Wolford LM, Pitta MC, Reiche-Fischel O, Franco PF. TMJ Concepts/Techmedica custom-made TMJ total joint prosthesis: 5-year follow-up study. Int J Oral Maxillofac Surg 2003;32:268–274.

101. Mercuri LG, Wolford LM, Sanders B, White RD, Giobbie Hurder. Long-term follow-up of the CAD/CAM patient fitted total temporomandibular joint reconstruction system. J Oral Maxillofac Surg 2002;60:1440–1448.

102. Scott AS, Frew AL Jr. Bilateral enlargement of the mandibular coronoid processes in a patient with rheumatoid arthritis of the temporomandibular joints. J Oral Surg 1975;33:787–789.

Surgical Management of Internal Derangements

Daniel M. Laskin

There is extensive literature on the surgical management of internal derangements of the temporomandibular joint (TMJ). However, the variety of operations that have been described for treatment of these conditions attests to the difficulty that is still being encountered in the successful surgical management of such problems. A number of factors could account for this situation. In some instances, it may be related to an inaccurate preoperative diagnosis. In other instances, it may be due to selection of the wrong operation or incorrect performance of the appropriate operation. Even when the diagnosis is correct and the operation is performed properly, however, poor results can occur because the treatment was directed only toward relief of the symptoms, without considering management of the etiologic factors.

The etiology and diagnosis of internal derangements have been presented in previous chapters (see chapters 8 and 16.) The purposes of this chapter are to describe the various operations that have been proposed for the treatment of internal derangements of the TMJ, to discuss their proper indications, and to review the available evidence supporting their use.

Arthrocentesis

Arthrocentesis was developed as a modification of TMJ arthroscopy when it was discovered that the mechanical lysis of adhesions and lavage of the joint, which is the basis of all TMJ arthroscopy, was just as successful in treating internal derangements as when additional intra-articular manipulations were also included.[1] Furthermore, it was found that disc repositioning usually was not essential to achieve pain relief and eliminate the restriction of mouth opening. Therefore, it was generally no longer considered necessary to visualize the joint to accomplish these objectives.

Arthrocentesis, a relatively noninvasive procedure with no significant complications, involves the placement of two hypodermic needles into the upper joint space, which allows irrigation with lactated Ringer solution to remove inflammatory cytokines and hydraulic distension of the joint. When used in conjunction with manual manipulation of the jaw, this procedure breaks up any adhesions and increases the range of motion. The latter results in redistribution of the forces within the joint, eliminating their concentration in one area, and allows healing and adaptation of the retrodiscal tissue into a pseudodisc (Fig 32-1).

Indications

Arthrocentesis is most commonly used to treat patients with anteriorly displaced, nonreducing discs (closed lock) or those with disc adhesion (stuck disc). However, it can also be used as a palliative procedure for patients with acute episodes of degenerative[2] or rheumatoid arthritis[3] and to relieve the pain in patients who have painful clicking in the TMJ that does not respond to medical management. However, in these patients, joint manipulation is usually not performed.

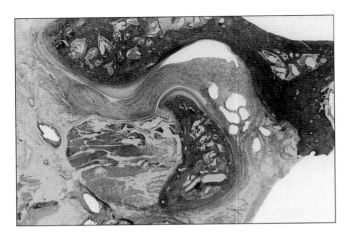

Fig 32-1 Histologic section of a human TMJ with an anteriorly displaced intra-articular disc. The retrodiscal tissue that now occupies the articular zone has adapted into an avascular, fibrous pseudo-disc that no longer resembles the characteristic retrodiscal tissue located posterior to the condyle. (Hematoxylin-eosin stain.)

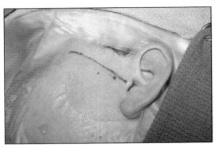

Fig 32-2 Canthotragal line and the standard marks indicating placement of the needles in the anterior and posterior recesses of the TMJ.

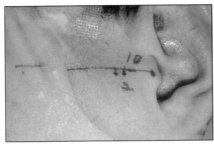

Fig 32-3 Marks indicating points of needle insertion in the posterior recess using the modified technique.

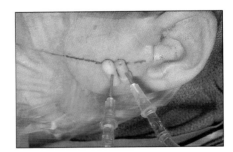

Fig 32-4 Placement of needles in the modified technique.

Technique

The procedure can be done while the patient is under local anesthesia plus intravenous sedation or under general anesthesia. The latter option is preferable, because the patient is more relaxed and this permits more effective jaw manipulation.

The landmarks originally recommended for determining the sites of needle placement are the same as those used for insertion of the cannulas for TMJ arthroscopy. After a line connecting the lateral canthus of the eye with the midpoint of the tragus is drawn, the location where the needle is inserted in the posterior recess is marked at a point 10 mm forward on and 2 mm below the canthotragal line. The location where the needle is inserted in the anterior recess is marked at a point 20 mm forward on and 8 mm below the canthotragal line (Fig 32-2). However, because access to the anterior recess is not necessary, as it is when the entire joint must be visualized during arthroscopy, it is easier merely to insert the anterior needle 2 to 3 mm in front of the posterior needle (Figs 32-3 and 32-4).

After the points of insertion for the two needles have been marked, an 18-gauge needle on a 10-mL syringe filled with 2% lidocaine containing a 1:200,000 concentration of epinephrine is inserted in the posterior recess of the upper joint space (Fig 32-5) while an assistant holds the mandible in the wide-open position. When proper location in the joint space is confirmed by injection and aspiration of the local anesthetic, 1 mL of the solution is injected to distend the joint space and the syringe is detached. A 20-gauge needle on a 10-mL syringe containing lactated Ringer solution is then inserted in front of the first needle. Proper positioning in the joint is confirmed when injection of the solution results in its exit from the posterior needle (Fig 32-6).

The 20-gauge needle is then connected to a 50-mL syringe containing lactated Ringer solution via a short intravenous tubing, and a similar tubing is attached to the 18-gauge needle to allow the effluent to be collected in a basin (Fig 32-7). The joint is then irrigated with 200 to 400 mL of lactated Ringer solution. Ideally, this amount of solution should be used because it is the amount required to remove all of the inflammatory cytokines from the joint[4];

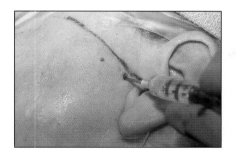

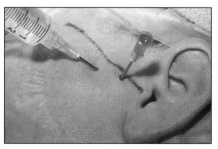

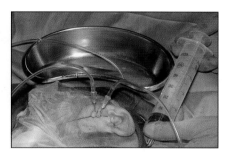

Fig 32-5 Injection of local anesthetic solution in the posterior recess through an 18-gauge needle.

Fig 32-6 Placement of the second needle in the anterior recess using the standard technique. When the needle is placed correctly in the joint space, the lactated Ringer solution will exit from the posterior needle.

Fig 32-7 Injection of lactated Ringer solution into the 20-gauge needle and exiting through the 18-gauge needle and the intravenous tubing to the basin. In this patient, both needles have been placed in the posterior recess.

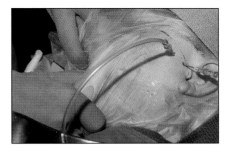

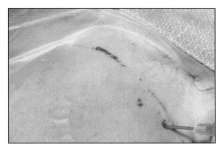

Fig 32-8 Manipulation of the mandible during the procedure to achieve an increased range of mouth opening.

Fig 32-9 Injection of the betamethasone solution in the superior joint space.

when this is not accomplished, there is less chance that the procedure will be successful.[5]

During lavage of the joint, an assistant repeatedly stretches the mouth as far open as possible to break any adhesions and improve joint mobility in patients with anteriorly displaced, nonreducing discs (Fig 32-8), but this generally is not done in patients with disc reduction or with degenerative or rheumatoid arthritis.

When the procedure is completed, the anterior needle is removed. In patients with an internal derangement or in those with rheumatoid arthritis, 6 mg of a short- and long-acting betamethasone combination (Celestone, Schering-Plough) is injected through the posterior needle (Fig 32-9). This has an anti-inflammatory action and reduces postsurgical discomfort. However, in patients with degenerative joint disease, it is preferable to inject sodium hyaluronate.[6]

The key to success of arthrocentesis in patients with anteriorly displaced, nonreducing discs is the ability of the patient to maintain the additional amount of mouth opening achieved by the procedure (40 mm or more). This is accomplished by placing no restrictions on diet

and by having patients exercise by stretching the mouth open as widely as possible for 20 repetitions at least 4 times a day until their range of motion remains stable.

Tissue distention from diffusion of the irrigating solution when a needle is improperly placed, or when the joint capsule has been multiply perforated during attempts to correctly place a needle, is the main complication that can occur during arthrocentesis. The only other complication reported is a single case of an extradural hematoma.[7]

Analysis of Clinical Data

No prospective, randomized, double-blind clinical trials have evaluated the effectiveness of arthrocentesis for the treatment of any of the conditions for which it has been used. Those studies that have been done are mainly retrospective case series that sometimes fail to distinguish the type of internal derangement being treated, are not observer blinded, frequently have only a short follow-up period, do not have a control group for comparison, and have involved the use of differing intra-articular irrigation

Table 32-1	**Arthrocentesis for internal derangements of the TMJ***			

Study	Type of study	Diagnosis	Patients/ joints	Procedure
Nitzan et al[8]	R: NC	ADDwoR	17/17	Arthrocentesis and betamethasone
Dimitroulis et al[9]	R: NC	ADDwoR	46/60	Arthrocentesis
Murakami et al[10]	R: NC	ADDwoR	20/20	Arthrocentesis and betamethasone
Fridrich et al[11]	R: NC	ADDwR: 2 ADDwoR: 6	8/11	Arthrocentesis and betamethasone
Hosaka et al[12]	R: NC	ADDwoR	20/20	Arthrocentesis
Nitzan et al[13]	R: NC	ADDwoR	39/40	Arthrocentesis
Carvajal and Laskin[14]	R: NC	ADDwoR	32 jts	Arthrocentesis and betamethasone
Sakamoto et al[15]	R: NC	ADDwoR	18/18	Arthrocentesis
Alpaslan and Alpaslan[16]	P: C	1. ADDwR 2. ADDwoR	16/19 15/22	1. Arthrocentesis: 4/6 1. Arthrocentesis and SH: 12/13 2. Arthrocentesis: 4/9 2. Arthrocentesis and SH: 11/13
Nishimura et al[17]	R: NC	ADDwoR	100/103	Arthrocentesis and betamethasone
Ishimara et al[18]	R: NC	Severe TMD (16: ID)	26 pts	Arthrocentesis and etodolac (oral)
Kunjur et al[19]	R: NC	Refractory pain	298/405	Arthrocentesis and morphine
Alpaslan et al[20]	R: NC	ID	34/48	Arthrocentesis and betamethasone

*VAS = visual analog scale; R: NC = retrospective, no control; P: C = prospective, control; ADDwoR = anterior disc displacement without reduction; ADDwR = anterior disc displacement with reduction; ID = internal derangement; SH = sodium hyaluronate; succ = successful; unsucc = unsuccessful; jts = joints; pts = patients; NA = not applicable; TMD = temporomandibular disorder.

solutions and postarthrocentesis medications (Table 32-1). Thus, a direct comparison among these studies is difficult.

However, the one meta-analysis that was done using the existing literature, but with an estimated historical control group, concluded that arthrocentesis was effective for patients with nonreducing disc displacement at all of the assumed control group improvement rates.[21] Moreover, those clinical studies that have been published (see Table 32-1) generally seem to show that arthrocentesis does reduce pain and improve function in a significant number of patients with anteriorly displaced, nonreducing discs. Although this also appears to be true when arthrocentesis is used for the other suggested indications (painful clicking, degenerative joint disease, and rheumatoid arthritis), there are no controlled studies and only a few retrospective clinical series that have evaluated such treatment, and therefore there is insufficient evidence to make positive statements about its effectiveness in these situations.

Arthroscopic Surgery

Arthroscopic surgery of the TMJ was first introduced by Ohnishi in 1975.[22] Prior to that time, internal derangements were managed by open surgical procedures involving either discoplasty or discectomy. This modality opened a new era in the diagnosis and treatment of such conditions. Initially, arthroscopic surgery involved merely lavage of the joint and the use of a probe to break up adhesions, but the field rapidly advanced with the introduction of improved instrumentation and imaging techniques so that ultimately oral and maxillofacial surgeons were able to perform essentially all of the intra-articular manipulations performed by the orthopedic surgeon in the knee joint. As a result, arthroscopic surgery became the initial treatment of choice for internal derangements of the TMJ.

Follow-up	Pre- and posttreatment mouth opening (mm)	Pre- and posttreatment pain score (VAS)	Pre- and posttreatment function score (VAS)
4–14 mo	24.1–42.7	8.75–2.31	10.24–2.16
6–30 mo	24.6–42.3	NA	10.0–2.7
6 mo	30.6–42.5	6.9–2.4	7.2–1.9
Mean: 13.3 mo	33–41	66–23	79–37.5
36 mo	30.6–44.5	6.9–1.1	7.2–1.5
6–37 mo	23.1–44.2	9.2–1.4	9.3–2.7
10–96 mo	25.3–43.8	8.5–1.8	8.5–1.7
3 mo	36.8–41.6	63.7–36.1	NA
24 mo	41.8–44.8	NA	NA
	40.2–45.2		
	24.0–31.0		
	28.4–39.0		
1 wk–6 mo	33–47 (succ)	None (68%)	NA
	30–36 (unsucc)	No change (93%)	
2 wk	32–36	65–35	59–40
12 mo	NA	6+ (288 pts)	NA
		0 (144 pts)	
		< 5 (88 pts)	
3–60 mo	32.5–38.7	5.6–3.0	5.4–2.7

Indications

Arthroscopic surgery has been used to treat anteriorly displaced, nonreducing discs by various techniques: lysis of intra-articular adhesions and joint lavage[1]; lateral capsular release[23]; anterior disc release; and disc repositioning and fixation by methods such as retrodiscotomy and posterolateral release,[24] scarification of the retrodiscal region with electrocautery,[25] injection of a sclerosing solution, or a laser,[26] and stabilization of the disc by the use of a suture.[27]

Arthroscopic lysis and lavage can also be used to treat pain in those patients with painful clicking or popping in the TMJ that does not respond to medical management. However, the joint sounds are not eliminated by the procedure unless disc repositioning and stabilization are also performed.

Technique

Although various arthroscopic approaches to the TMJ have been described,[28] the one most commonly used is the posterolateral approach to the upper joint space. The inferior joint space is seldom entered because the limited area makes it difficult to insert the trocar without damaging the surface of the condyle. The posterior landmark for insertion of the trocar into the upper joint space is 10 mm forward on and 2 mm inferior to the canthotragal line (see Fig 32-2). The mandible is distracted downward and forward, and the superior joint space is distended by the injection of approximately 3 mL of 1% lidocaine containing 1:200,000 epinephrine. The solution is injected from a 5-mL syringe with a 27-gauge needle, which is aimed in a medial and slightly anterosuperior direction until there is contact with the glenoid fossa.

A 2- to 3-mm vertical skin incision is made at the injection site, and the lateral capsule is punctured with a sharp trocar in an arthroscopic sheath inserted in the same direction as the previous injection needle. Once this has been accomplished, the sharp trocar is exchanged for a blunt trocar, and the arthroscopic sheath is advanced further into the upper joint space. The mean puncture depth is about 27 mm,[29] and the use of a graded trocar sheath is helpful in preventing too deep a penetration.

McCain[30] has described an alternative technique for penetrating the upper joint space. A sharp trocar in the arthroscopic sheath is placed through the skin at the site previously described and advanced with an axially rotating motion toward the inferior border of the zygomatic arch. Once the arch is contacted, the trocar is stepped inferiorly until it drops off the bone and the lateral capsule is encountered. The blunt trocar is then substituted for the sharp trocar and advanced into the upper joint space.

When the upper joint space has been entered, the blunt trocar is removed and the arthroscope is inserted to verify correct positioning. A second arthroscopic cannula is then inserted to allow triangulation of the surgical instruments. This puncture site is located on the canthotragal line 10 mm anterior and 8 mm inferior to the first puncture site, and the trocar is inserted in a posterosuperior direction under arthroscopic guidance. Once both cannulas have been properly placed, the entire upper joint space can be visualized and the arthroscope and the surgical instruments can be interchanged as necessary.

Ohnishi[22] described an endaural approach to the superior joint space that has been modified by Moses,[28] who recommended that the upper joint space be penetrated first using the previously described posterolateral approach. Then the arthroscope is rotated and angled superiorly, posteriorly, and laterally so that the light shines through the anterior wall of the external auditory meatus. The mandible is then distracted downward and forward, and the anterior wall of the meatus is penetrated with a sharp trocar in a 30-degree arthroscopic cannula. Entrance into the joint is monitored via the arthroscope. When proper placement has been confirmed, the arthroscope is placed in the endaural cannula and the other cannula can be used as the working portal. It is claimed that the endaural approach provides better visualization than the lateral approaches and improved access for instrumentation.[28]

Analysis of Clinical Data

Although numerous authors have reported good to excellent results with arthroscopic surgery for the treatment of internal derangements of the TMJ, no randomized, controlled clinical studies have been performed to confirm these findings. Moreover, many of the studies have not distinguished between patients with reducing and nonreducing anteriorly displaced discs, have varied in the types of surgical procedures done, and have lacked long-term follow-up. A review of the literature by White[31] has shown that there does not appear to be any difference between the results obtained when only lysis of adhesions and lavage of the joint are performed and those obtained when more advanced surgical techniques are also included.

Because arthroscopy and arthrocentesis are both used to treat internal derangements of the TMJ, it raises the question of whether they are equally effective. To answer this question it is necessary to compare the results obtained when each procedure was evaluated in different studies as well as the results obtained when both procedures were used in the same study. Moreover, it is necessary to compare arthrocentesis not only with arthroscopic lavage of the joint and lysis of adhesions but also with arthroscopic lavage combined with other intra-articular procedures such as lateral capsular release, anterior lateral pterygoid release, retrodiscal cauterization or sclerosis, and disc repositioning and suturing.

Although it is difficult to make direct comparisons among the studies on arthroscopic management of internal derangements because of the variability in the patient selection and the methods of data collection, the mean success rate appears to be about 84%. However, similar results have also been reported for arthrocentesis.[14,32] Moreover, although direct-comparison studies by Fridrich et al[11] and Murakami et al[10] showed arthroscopy to be slightly more effective, studies by Goudot et al,[33] Sanroman,[34] and Kropmans et al[35] found no significant difference.

It has been argued that, even if both procedures are therapeutically equal, arthroscopy has the advantage of allowing any intra-articular pathologic conditions to be observed and treated. However, in the management of most internal derangements, direct observation is seldom necessary. Moreover, arthroscopy has a number of disadvantages: It is more invasive than arthrocentesis; there is greater postoperative morbidity; it is a more expensive procedure; and it has greater potential for complications. Serious complications such as arteriovenous fistula[36,37]; facial, trigeminal, and auditory nerve injury[38-41]; otitis media[42]; perforation of the glenoid fossa[30]; extradural hematoma[43]; broken instruments[44]; and perforation of the tympanic membrane and middle ear[41,45] have been reported with arthroscopic surgery. In contrast, the only complication reported with arthrocentesis has been one case of extradural hematoma.[7] These advantages of arthrocentesis support the contention that it should be the initial treatment of choice for internal derangements that are unresponsive to medical management.

Discoplasty

Although some patients with internal derangements are successfully treated by nonsurgical means or by arthrocentesis or arthroscopic surgery, there is still a group of patients who do not respond to these procedures and for whom an arthrotomy and disc surgery are necessary. In such circumstances, every attempt should be made to salvage the disc with a discoplasty.

Indications

There are two main indications for discoplasty. First, it is used to treat painful clicking or popping in the TMJ (anterior disc displacement with reduction) that has not responded to nonsurgical management and when less invasive procedures such as arthrocentesis or arthroscopic surgery have failed to eliminate the pain. Patients with painless clicking are not treated surgically except in the few instances where the joint sounds are so loud as to be socially unacceptable to the patient. The second indication for discoplasty is in patients with anteriorly displaced, nonreducing discs who continue to have pain and limited mouth opening despite treatment by either arthrocentesis or arthroscopic surgery.

Technique

A preauricular approach is generally used to gain access to the TMJ for a discoplasty. This approach is described in chapter 28. Once the joint capsule is exposed, the upper joint space is distended with a local anesthetic solution and is opened with a No. 11 scalpel blade. The incision is started anteriorly and proceeds posteriorly to avoid cutting into the retrodiscal tissues and causing excessive bleeding. The incision is kept close to the contour of the glenoid fossa to prevent cutting of the disc and is facilitated by downward distraction of the condyle with a large towel clamp placed at the mandibular angle.

Once the upper joint space is opened, any adhesions are lysed and a Freer elevator is placed in the posterior recess and pushed distally to reposition the disc. When it is determined that the disc can be adequately repositioned, the lower joint space is opened via a parallel incision in the lateral capsular sulcus, which then allows free movement of the disc. The surface of the condyle is inspected and, if any irregularities exist, they are removed with a bone file. A high condylar shave should not be performed, because this removes any residual cartilage and cortical bone on the surface of the condyle and predisposes to further degenerative changes. Any open bite that results from repositioning of the disc is temporary and will self-correct as the disc adapts to the condylar contour.

A sufficient wedge of retrodiscal tissue is now removed so that when the incisions are closed with a continuous 4-0 Mersilene suture (Ethicon) the disc remains in its normal anatomic position. The use of a continuous suture rather than interrupted sutures for this purpose makes suturing of the retrodiscal tissue much easier and avoids irritating knots. Special attention should be paid to suturing the disc tightly to the capsule, because this provides a stronger incision line than that in the retrodiscal tissue and helps to assure that the disc stays in proper position. Any excessive capsular tissue should be excised before the disc is sutured to the capsule laterally.

When suturing of the disc is completed, the upper joint space is closed, and the remaining deep layers are successively reapproximated. The skin incision is closed with a running 5-0 nylon subcuticular suture. A pressure dressing is applied for 48 hours.

Analysis of Clinical Data

All of the studies that have evaluated the effectiveness of discoplasty have been retrospective clinical series without control or comparison groups (Table 32-2). Moreover, many of the studies combined patients with both anteriorly displaced reducing and nonreducing discs without identifying the number of each. More favorable results would be expected for the former type of internal derangement, because such patients generally have fewer pathologic conditions of the joint; thus, combination of the two types of derangement in the study could have a positive effect on the final results that would be misleading if a disproportionate number of reducing discs were included. In addition, in many of the reported studies, the surgery included not only a discoplasty but also a high condylar shave and/or an eminectomy. Because the data revealed no significant difference in the success rates between discoplasty alone and discoplasty performed with the latter procedures, most surgeons no longer include them.

Despite the inadequacies in the reported case series (see Table 32-2), they do generally show that more than 75% of the reported cases benefited from disc repositioning. Therefore, discoplasty may be indicated as a second-

Table 32-2	Discoplasty for internal derangements of the TMJ*					
Study	**Type of study**	**Condition**	**Procedure**	**Patients/ joints**	**Follow-up**	**Results**
McCarty and Farrar[46]	R: NC	ID	Reconstructive arthroplasty and disc repositioning	327 jts	6 y	94% success
Mercuri et al[47]	R: NC	ID	Disc repair and arthroplasty and eminectomy	21 pts	Not stated	91.3% felt better
Hall[48]	R: NC	ADDwR ADDwoR	Discoplasty and eminectomy	20 jts	Mean: 18.1 mo	65% pain-free; 35% mild pain
Dolwick[49]	R: NC	ADDwoR	Discoplasty	50 pts/54 jts	Mean: 24 mo (12–60 mo)	94% success
Weinberg[50]	R: NC	ID	Discorrhaphy	33 pts/40 jts	44 mo	88.8% better
Dolwick and Sanders[51]	R: NC	ID	Discoplasty and eminectomy	68 pts/78 jts	Mean: 36 mo (18–60 mo)	55% excellent; 35% good
Benson and Keith[52]	R: NC	ID	Discoplasty and high condylectomy	60 pts	Mean: 23.7 mo (6–48 mo)	88.3% improved
Weinberg and Cousens[53]	R: NC	ID	Meniscocondylar plication	89 jts	6–24 mo	90.7% considerable improvement
Walker and Kalamchi[54]	R: NC	ID	Discoplasty and high condylotomy	50 pts/65 jts	4–24 mo	100% success
Anderson et al[55]	R: NC	ID	Discoplasty	33 pts	Mean: 18.5 mo	77% pain-free
Montgomery et al[56]	R: NC	ID	Discoplasty	51 pts/74 jts	6 mo–6 y	89% decreased pain
Kerstens et al[57]	R: NC	ID	Discoplasty and eminectomy	17 jts	Mean: 19.7 mo (14–29 mo)	86.8% felt better
Dolwick and Nitzan[58]	R: NC	ID	Discoplasty	152 pts/155 jts	6 mo–8 y	90% had 70%–80% improvement
Baldwin and Cooper[59]	R: NC	ID	Discoplasty and eminectomy	92 pts/119 jts	Mean: 44 mo	49% asymptomatic; 19% improved
Vazquez-Delgado et al[60]	R: NC	ID	Meniscocondylar plication	20 pts/29 jts	Mean: 51.2 mo	VAS (pain) reduced in 92.3%

*R: NC = retrospective, no control; ID = internal derangement; ADDwR = anterior displacement with reduction; ADDwoR = anterior displacement without reduction; VAS = visual analog scale; pts = patients; jts = joints.

ary procedure in those patients in whom arthrocentesis or arthroscopic surgery has been unsuccessful.

Discectomy

Although ideally every effort should be made to retain the intra-articular disc by performing a discoplasty, this is not always possible. In such cases it is necessary to remove the disc by performing a discectomy.

Indications

Removal of the intra-articular disc is indicated when there is a large, irreparable perforation or if it is so misshaped, shortened, or rigid that it cannot be properly repositioned.

Technique

When a discectomy is to be performed, the surgical exposure of the joint is the same as for a discoplasty until the disc is isolated. The medial disc attachment is then severed with a small, curved scissors. This is facilitated by approaching the area via the lower joint space rather than the upper joint space. Next, the disc is detached from the capsule and the lateral pterygoid fibers anteriorly. Finally, it is separated from the retrodiscal tissue.

The retrodiscal separation is performed last because this is the most vascular region, and earlier detachment will result in bleeding that is difficult to control because of the poor access. If excessive bleeding does occur, it can usually be controlled by seating the condyle firmly in the fossa for a few minutes. This act compresses the retrodiscal tissue and eliminates the bleeding or reduces it sufficiently to allow the source to be identified and coagulated. When a discectomy is performed, the synovial tissue should be allowed to remain so that the patient is not left with a poorly lubricated joint.

Once a discectomy has been performed, the surgeon is faced with a decision regarding whether disc replacement is necessary. As the operation was originally described, no replacement was used.[61] However, because of the radiographic changes that generally occurred in the condyle after such a procedure, and the fact that some patients still had incomplete pain relief and decreased joint mobility, many surgeons believed that disc replacement was necessary. Silicone rubber (Silastic, Dow Corning) was one of the first materials to be used as a permanent disc replacement.[62] However, because of its unfavorable wear properties, and the resultant foreign-body reaction that developed in some patients,[63,64] it was eventually abandoned as a permanent interpositional material. As an alternative, temporary Silastic sheeting was advocated to prevent adhesions and to form a connective tissue capsule that would serve as a pseudodisc when the Silastic was subsequently removed.[65] However, this too was found to produce destructive condylar lesions.[66]

The Proplast-Teflon (Vitek) interpositional implant was introduced in 1985 as an alternative to the use of silicone rubber. Although the early reports described near 90% success,[67,68] ultimately it was discovered that implant wear debris caused a foreign-body reaction that resulted in severe destruction of the TMJ and surrounding tissues.[69] Marketing was suspended in 1988, and the product was recalled in 1990.[70]

Because of the poor results obtained with the alloplastic materials, surgeons turned to autogenous tissues as a source for disc replacement; auricular cartilage,[71,72] dermis,[73] and temporalis muscle[74] have all been used for this purpose. However, because of the inconsistent results with these tissues, many surgeons are now returning to the original operation and not providing any disc replacement.[75–77]

Most studies on discectomy indicate that the patients will show postoperative radiographic evidence of condylar change, consisting of flattening and subchondral sclerosis.[75] Because these changes are generally not associated with symptoms other than crepitation, and similar changes are often observed in the contralateral joint that has not been surgically treated, it has been concluded that in most instances they are adaptive changes to altered joint loading rather than a degenerative process.

Analysis of Clinical Data

Although there are retrospective clinical reports to support the use of each of the autogenous tissues that have been recommended to replace the intra-articular disc, the tremendous variation in the way these studies were conducted, the way the data were collected and reported, and the differing follow-up periods make comparisons among studies in a given group, as well as comparisons among groups, very difficult, if not impossible.

In the one meta-analysis that was done, involving an exhaustive Medline search of the literature from 1965 to 2001,[78] there were only four studies (n = 432; mean follow-up of 5.7 years) involving discectomy without disc replacement, two studies on use of the temporalis flap (n = 35; mean follow-up of 2.2 years), and one study on the use of a dermal graft (n = 17; mean follow-up of 3 years) that met the minimal inclusion criteria. These criteria were (1) the inclusion of at least 10 subjects, (2) the completion of documented follow-up, (3) the use of objective tests for preoperative and postoperative assessment of pain and jaw function, and (4) the application of established criteria for therapeutic success (absence of joint pain and maximum interincisal opening greater than 35 mm).

The authors calculated the mean success rate for each type of disc replacement. They found mean success rates of 91.4% for the temporalis flap, 82.4% for the auricular cartilage graft, and 87.9% for the dermal graft. In a similar analysis of discectomy without disc replacement, they found a mean success rate of 86.5%.[78] These similar findings seem to indicate that disc replacement is not necessary.

Condylotomy

Condylotomy for the surgical treatment of internal derangements has been used in Europe for many years[79] but has gained only limited popularity in the United States.[80] Although referred to as a *condylotomy*, the technique actually involves a vertical ramus osteotomy similar to that used for orthognathic surgery. Thus, it is an extra-articular operation that does not directly involve the intra-articular disc. Rather, the procedure is supposed to increase the joint space by producing a downward and forward movement of the condylar segment and thereby decrease the load on the retrodiscal tissue and relieve pain and dysfunction. It is claimed that the operation also can result in a more normal disc-condyle relationship in patients with minimally displaced discs.[81]

Indications

The chief indications for the condylotomy procedure are painful clicking in the TMJ that has not responded to nonsurgical therapy and the management of nonreducing discs (closed lock). However, it is contraindicated in patients in whom it is difficult to control the occlusion, such as edentulous patients or those with poor intercuspation of the teeth.

Technique

The operation is performed intraorally through a vertical incision made over the external oblique ridge of the mandible, starting just above the level of the occlusion and extending forward in the vestibule approximately 3 to 4 cm.[82] The periosteum and overlying masseter muscle are reflected, exposing the lateral aspect of the ramus from the sigmoid notch to the angle of the mandible. A Bauer retractor is then placed in the sigmoid notch to provide good access and visibility.

A vertical osteotomy, extending from the sigmoid notch to the region of the mandibular angle, posterior to the antelingula, is made with an oscillating saw. When the osteotomy is completed, the patient is placed in maxillomandibular fixation, and the amount of condylar sag is determined by measuring the distance between the inferior aspect of the condylar segment and the inferior border of the mandible. Generally 2 to 3 mm of condylar sag is sufficient. If a greater amount is desired, some of the medial pterygoid muscle can be removed. Finally, the condylar segment is either trimmed to fit lateral to the ramus or the anterior edge is trimmed to create a butt joint.[80]

The patient is kept in complete maxillomandibular fixation for 8 to 10 days. Afterward, only a single, light orthodontic elastic is placed in the canine region bilaterally so that there is anterior traction on the mandible. These are worn continuously for 6 weeks, except when the patient is brushing the teeth and eating a soft, nonchewy diet.

Analysis of Clinical Data

The data supporting the use of condylotomy have been reviewed by Upton.[83] As with other operations involving the TMJ, the retrospective nature of the studies, the lack of controls, and the variations in technique make it impossible to make direct comparisons of the results. Generally, a 72% to 85% reduction in symptoms was reported. On the other hand, Banks,[84] an early proponent of the procedure, more recently indicated that he had abandoned use of the procedure because of the unpredictability of the results.

The stated intent of this operation is to unload the joint by increasing the intra-articular space and to produce an improved relationship between the condyle and the disc.[81] Because the TMJ is a pressure-bearing joint, and thus there must be contact between the articulating components, unloading the joint appears to be an unattainable goal. Moreover, it is not possible to accurately image the joint space on transcranial, transpharyngeal, or panoramic radiographs. Therefore, any preoperative diagnosis of joint space narrowing and postoperative diagnosis of joint space enlargement are subject to question, particularly when a standardized radiographic technique has not been used; unfortunately this has been the situation in the published reports.

Any success that this operation may have in relieving pain in the joint is probably due to the change in the disc-condyle relationship, which shifts the load to a less traumatized area of retrodiscal tissue or to the disc itself. However, if the goal is to correct the disc-condyle relationship, this can always be accomplished with a discoplasty but is not always possible with a condylotomy. Moreover, discoplasty has the added advantage of placing the disc back in its normal anatomic relationship with the condyle rather than trying to fit the condyle to an abnormally positioned disc as occurs with a condylotomy. Discoplasty also has the advantage of not requiring maxillomandibular fixation or the use of training elastics postoperatively.

Conclusion

Although there have been no good prospective, randomized, double-blinded clinical trials to substantiate the effectiveness of any of the procedures recommended for surgical management of internal derangements of the TMJ, case series and clinical experience indicate that procedures such as arthrocentesis, arthroscopic surgery, discoplasty, and discectomy can be used with reasonably good success in properly selected cases.

When an operation is unsuccessful, it is usually not the result of a failure to correct the anatomic derangement but rather the result of a failure to eliminate or control causative factors, such as chronic parafunction. Unfortunately, few of the reported case series have indicated whether a nonrecurring etiology, such as a traumatic episode, or a persistent behavior, such as chronic tooth clenching and grinding, was a factor in causing or perpetuating the internal derangements, whether or not the parafunction was controlled, and what effect this had on the final outcome.

Several studies have shown that each time a patient has an additional operation on the TMJ, the success rate decreases significantly.[85] This supports the contention that, if surgery is indicated, the surgeon should first use the least invasive procedure that can be effective. Thus, arthrocentesis should be the initial operation of choice for most internal derangements that are not manageable nonsurgically. If this is unsuccessful, then arthroscopic surgery or discoplasty should be considered. Discectomy should never be performed if the disc is salvageable, because there is no sound clinical evidence to support the use of any of the currently known disc substitutes.

References

1. Sanders B. Arthroscopic management of internal derangements of the temporomandibular joint. Oral Maxillofac Surg Clin North Am 1994;6:259–269.
2. Nitzan DW, Price A. The use of arthrocentesis for the treatment of osteoarthritis of the temporomandibular joints. J Oral Maxillofac Surg 2001;59:1154–1159; discussion 1160.
3. Trieger N, Hoffman CH, Rodriguez E. The effect of arthrocentesis of the temporomandibular joint in patients with rheumatoid arthritis. J Oral Maxillofac Surg 1999;57: 537–540; discussion 540–541.
4. Kaneyama K, Segami N, Nishimura M, Sato J, Fujimura K, Yoshimura H. The ideal lavage volume for removing bradykinin, interleukin-6 and protein from the temporomandibular joint by arthrocentesis. J Oral Maxillofac Surg 2004; 62:657–66l.
5. Nishimura M, Segami N, Kaneyama K, Sato J, Fujimura K. Comparison of cytokine level in synovial fluid between successful and unsuccessful cases in arthrocentesis of the temporomandibular joint. J Oral Maxillofac Surg 2004;62: 284–287; discussion 287–288.
6. Guarda-Nardini L, Tito R, Staffieri A, Beltrame A. Treatment of patients with arthrosis of the temporomandibular joint by infiltration of sodium hyaluronate: A preliminary study. Eur Arch Otorhinolaryngol 2002;259:279–284.
7. Carroll TA, Smith K, Jakubowski J. Extradural haematoma following temporomandibular joint arthrocentesis and lavage. Br J Neurosurg 2000;14:152–154.
8. Nitzan DW, Dolwick MF, Martinez GA. Temporomandibular joint arthrocentesis: A simplified treatment for severe, limited mouth opening. J Oral Maxillofac Surg 1991;49: 1163–1167; discussion 1168–1170.
9. Dimitroulis G, Dolwick MF, Martinez A. Temporomandibular joint arthrocentesis and lavage for the treatment of closed lock: A follow-up study. Br J Oral Maxillofac Surg l995;33:23–26; discussion 26–27.
10. Murakami KI, Hosaka H Moriya Y, Segami N, Iizuka T. Short-term treatment outcome study for the management of temporomandibular joint closed lock. A comparison of arthrocentesis to nonsurgical treatment and arthroscopic lysis and lavage. Oral Surg Oral Med Oral Pathol Oral Radiol Endod 1995;80:253–257.
11. Fridrich KL, Wise JM, Zeitler DL. Prospective comparison of arthroscopy and arthrocentesis for temporomandibular joint disorders. J Oral Maxillofac Surg 1996;54:816–820; discussion 821.
12. Hosaka H, Murakami K, Goto K, Iizuka T. Outcome of arthrocentesis for temporomandibular joint with closed lock at 3 years follow-up. Oral Surg Oral Med Oral Pathol Oral Radiol Endod 1996;82:501–504.
13. Nitzan DW, Samson B, Better H. Long-term outcome of arthrocentesis for sudden-onset, persistent, severe closed lock of the temporomandibular joint. J Oral Maxillofac Surg 1997;55:151–157; discussion 157–158.
14. Carvajal WA, Laskin DM. Long-term evaluation of arthrocentesis for the treatment of internal derangements of the temporomandibular joint. J Oral Maxillofac Surg 2000;58: 852–855; discussion 856–857.
15. Sakamoto I, Yoda T, Tsukahara H, Imai H, Enomoto S. Comparison of the effectiveness of arthrocentesis in acute and chronic closed lock: Analysis of clinical arthroscopic findings. Cranio 2000;18:264–271.
16. Alpaslan GH, Alpaslan C. Efficacy of temporomandibular joint arthrocentesis with and without injection of sodium hyaluronate in treatment of internal derangements. J Oral Maxillofac Surg 2001;59:613–618; discussion 618–619.
17. Nishimura M, Segami N, Kaneyama K, Suzuki T. Prognostic factors in arthrocentesis of the temporomandibular joint: Evaluation of 100 patients with internal derangement. J Oral Maxillofac Surg 2001;59:874–877; discussion 878.
18. Ishimaru JI, Ogi N, Mizui T, Miyamoto K, Shibata T, Kurita K. Effects of a single arthrocentesis and a COX-2 inhibitor on disorders of temporomandibular joints. A preliminary clinical study. Br J Oral Maxillofac Surg 2003;41:323–328.
19. Kunjur J, Anand R, Brennan PA, Ilankovan V. An audit of 405 temporomandibular joint arthrocentesis with intra-articular morphine infusion. Br J Oral Maxillofac Surg 2003; 41:29–31.
20. Alpaslan C, Dolwick MF, Heft MW. Five-year retrospective evaluation of temporomandibular joint arthrocentesis. Int J Oral Maxillofac Surg 2003;32:263–267.
21. Reston JT, Turkelson CM. Meta-analysis of surgical treatments for temporomandibular articular disorders. J Oral Maxillofac Surg 2003;61:3–10; discussion 10–12.

22. Ohnishi M. Arthroscopy of the temporomandibular joint [in Japanese]. Kokubyo Gakkai Zasshi 1975;42:207–213.

23. Moses JJ, Poker ID. TMJ arthroscopic surgery: An analysis of 237 patients. J Oral Maxillofac Surg 1989;47:790–794.

24. Heffez LB. Arthroscopy. In: Kaplan AS, Assael LA (eds). Temporomandibular Disorders. Philadelphia: Saunders, 1992: 656.

25. Torro AW. TMJ Arthroscopy: A Diagnostic and Surgical Atlas. Philadelphia: Lippincott, 1993:119–134.

26. Kondoh T, Norihiko T, Yutaka S, Kanichi S. Arthroscopic laser surgery for persistent closed-lock of the TMJ accompanied with intracapsular adhesion. Educational Summaries and Outlines. Presented at the American Association of Oral and Maxillofacial Surgeons, 71st Annual Meeting and Scientific Sessions, San Francisco, CA, 20–24 September 1989.

27. Tarro AW. Arthroscopic treatment of anterior disc displacement: A preliminary report. J Oral Maxillofac Surg 1989;47: 353–358.

28. Moses JJ. Endaural arthroscopic approach. In: Thomas M, Bronstein SL (eds). Arthroscopy of the Temporomandibular Joint. Philadelphia: Saunders, 1991:192–198.

29. Holmlund A, Hellsing G. Arthroscopy of the temporomandibular joint. An autopsy study. Int J Oral Surg 1985;14: 169–175.

30. McCain JP. Arthroscopy of the human temporomandibular joint. J Oral Maxillofac Surg 1988;46:648–655.

31. White RD. Arthroscopic lysis and lavage as the preferred treatment for internal derangement of the temporomandibular joint. J Oral Maxillofac Surg 2001;59:313–316.

32. Nitzan DW. Arthrocentesis for management of severe closed lock of the temporomandibular joint. Oral Maxillofac Surg Clin North Am 1994;6:245–257.

33. Goudot P, Jaquinet AR, Hugonnet S, Haefliger W, Richter M. Improvement of pain and function after arthroscopy and arthrocentesis of the temporomandibular joint: A comparative study. J Craniomaxillofac Surg 2000;28:39–43.

34. Sanroman JF. Closed lock (MRI fixed disc): A comparison of arthrocentesis and arthroscopy. Int J Oral Maxillofac Surg 2004;33:344–348.

35. Kropmans TJ, Dijkstra PU, Stegenga B, de Bont LG. Therapeutic outcome assessment in permanent temporomandibular joint disc displacement. J Oral Rehabil 1999;26:357–363.

36. Moses JJ, Topper DC. Arteriovenous fistula: An unusual complication associated with arthroscopic temporomandibular joint surgery. J Oral Maxillofac Surg 1990;48:1220–1222.

37. Preisler SA, Koorbusch GF, Olson RA. An acquired arteriovenous fistula secondary to temporomandibular joint arthroscopy: Report of a case. J Oral Maxillofac Surg 1991;49: 187–190.

38. Carter JB. Complications of temporomandibular joint arthroscopy. In: Thomas M, Bronstein SL (eds). Arthroscopy of the Temporomandibular Joint. Philadelphia: Saunders, 1991:310–322.

39. Greene MW, Van Sickels JE. Survey of TMJ arthroscopy in oral and maxillofacial surgery residency programs. J Oral Maxillofac Surg 1989;47:574–576.

40. Applebaum EL, Berg LF, Kumar A, Mafee MF. Otologic complications following temporomandibular joint arthroscopy. Ann Otol Rhinol Laryngol 1988;97:675–679.

41. Tsuyama M, Kondoh T, Seto K, Fukuda J. Complications of temporomandibular arthroscopy: A retrospective analysis of 301 lysis and lavage procedures performed using the triangulation technique. J Oral Maxillofac Surg 2000;58: 500–505; discussion 505–506.

42. Sanders B. Arthroscopic surgery of the temporomandibular joint: Treatment of internal derangement with persistent closed lock. Oral Surg Oral Med Oral Pathol 1986;62: 361–372.

43. Murphy MA, Silvester KC, Chan TY. Extradural haematoma after temporomandibular joint arthroscopy. A case report. Int J Oral Maxillofac Surg 1993;22:332–335.

44. Tarro AW. Instrument breakage associated with arthroscopy of the temporomandibular joint: Report of a case. J Oral Maxillofac Surg 1989;47:1226–1228; discussion 1228–1229.

45. Van Sickels JEA Nishioka GJ, Hegewald MD, Neal GD. Middle ear injury resulting from temporomandibular joint arthroscopy. J Oral Maxillofac Surg 1987;45:962–965.

46. McCarty WL, Farrar WB. Surgery for internal derangements of the temporomandibular joint. J Prosthet Dent 1979;42: 191–196.

47. Mercuri LG, Campbell RL, Shamaskin RG. Intra-articular meniscus dysfunction surgery. A preliminary report. Oral Surg Oral Med Oral Pathol 1982;54:613–621.

48. Hall MB. Meniscoplasty of the displaced temporomandibular joint meniscus without violating the inferior joint space. J Oral Maxillofac Surg 1984;42:788–792.

49. Dolwick MF. Surgical management. In: Helms CA, Katzberg RW, Dolwick MF (eds). Internal Derangements of the Temporomandibular Joint. San Francisco: Radiology Research and Education Foundation, 1983:167–191.

50. Weinberg S. Eminectomy and meniscorhaphy for internal derangements of the temporomandibular joint. Rationale and operative technique. Oral Surg Oral Med Oral Pathol 1984;57:241–249.

51. Dolwick MF, Sanders B. TMJ Internal Derangement and Arthrosis Surgical Atlas. St Louis: Mosby, 1985.

52. Benson BJ, Keith DA. Patient response to surgical and nonsurgical treatment for internal derangement of the temporomandibular joint. J Oral Maxillofac Surg 1985;43:770–777.

53. Weinberg S, Cousens G. Meniscocondylar plication: A modified operation for surgical repositioning of the ectopic temporomandibular joint meniscus. Oral Surg Oral Med Oral Pathol 1987;63:393–402.

54. Walker RV, Kalamchi S. A surgical technique for management of internal derangement of the temporomandibular joint. J Oral Maxillofac Surg 1987;45:299–305.

55. Anderson DM, Sinclair PM, McBride KM. A clinical evaluation of temporomandibular joint disk plication surgery. Am J Orthod Dentofacial Orthop 1991;100:156–162.

56. Montgomery MT, Gordon SM, Van Sickels JE, Harms SE. Changes in signs and symptoms following temporomandibular joint disc repositioning surgery. J Oral Maxillofac Surg 1992;50:320–328.

57. Kerstens HC, Tuinzing DB, Van Der Kwast WA. Eminectomy and discoplasty for correction of the displaced temporomandibular joint disc. J Oral Maxillofac Surg 1989;47:150–154.

58. Dolwick MF, Nitzan DW. TMJ disk surgery: 8-year follow-up evaluation. Fortschr Kiefer Gesichtschir l990;35:162–163.

59. Baldwin AJ, Cooper JC. Eminectomy and plication of the posterior disc attachment following arthrotomy for temporomandibular joint internal derangement. J Craniomaxillofac Surg 2004;32:354–359.

60. Vazquez-Delgado E, Valmaseda-Castellon E, Vazquez-Rodriguez E, Gay-Escoda C. Long-term results of functional open surgery for the treatment of internal derangement of the temporomandibular joint. Br J Oral Maxillofac Surg 2004;42:142–148.

61. Boman K. Temporomandibular joint arthrosis and its treatment by extirpation of the disk: A clinical study. Acta Chir Scand 1947;95:1–154.

62. Hansen WC, Deshazo BW. Silastic reconstruction of the temporomandibular joint meniscus. Plast Reconstr Surg 1969;43: 388–391.

63. Dolwick MF, Aufdemorte TB. Silicone-induced foreign body reaction and lymphadenopathy after temporomandibular joint arthroplasty. Oral Surg Oral Med Oral Pathol 1985;59: 449–452.

64. Acton C, Hoffman G, McKenna H, Moloney F. Silicone-induced foreign-body reaction after temporomandibular joint arthroplasty. Case report. Aust Dent J 1989;34:228–232.

65. Wilkes CH. Surgical treatment of internal derangements of the temporomandibular joint. A long-term study. Arch Otolaryngol Head Neck Surg 1991;117:64–72.

66. Westesson PL, Eriksson L, Lindstrom C. Destructive lesions of the mandibular condyle following diskectomy with temporary silicone implant. Oral Surg Oral Med Oral Pathol 1987;63:143–150.

67. Carter JB. Meniscectomy in the management of chronic internal derangements of the temporomandibular joint. Presented at the American Association of Oral and Maxillofacial Surgeons 65th Annual Meeting, San Diego, CA, 21–25 Sept 1983.

68. Keirsch TSA. The use of Proplast-Teflon implants for meniscectomy and disc repair in the temporomandibular joint. American Association of Oral and Maxillofacial Surgeons Clinical Congress, Jan 1984.

69. Kaplan PA, Ruskin JD, Tu HK, Knibbe MA. Erosive arthritis of the temporomandibular joint caused by Teflon-Proplast implants: Plain film features. Am J Roentgenol 1988;151: 337–339.

70. US Food and Drug Administration. TMJ Implants: A Consumer Information Update. Rockville, MD: US Food and Drug Administration, November 1990.

71. Perko M. Indications and contraindications for surgical management of the temporomandibular joint [in German]. Schweiz Monatsschr Zahnheilkd 1973;83:73–81.

72. Waite PD, Matukas VJ. Use of auricular cartilage as a disc replacement. Oral Maxillofac Surg Clin North Am 1994; 6:349–354.

73. Tucker MR. Use of autogenous dermal grafts in treating internal derangements of the temporomandibular joint. Oral Maxillofac Surg Clin North Am 1994;6:323–334.

74. Feinberg SE. Use of composite temporalis muscle flaps for disc replacement. Oral Maxillofac Surg Clin North Am 1994;6: 335–348.

75. Eriksson L, Westesson PL. The need for disc replacement after discectomy. Oral Maxillofac Surg Clin North Am 1994; 6:295–305.

76. McKenna SJ. Discectomy for the treatment of internal derangements of the temporomandibular joint. J Oral Maxillofac Surg 2001;59:1051–1056.

77. Hall HD. The role of discectomy for treating internal derangements of the temporomandibular joint. Oral Maxillofac Surg Clin North Am 1994;6:287–294.

78. Kramer A, Lee JJ, Beirne OR. Meta-analysis of TMJ discectomy with or without autogenous/alloplastic interpositional materials: Comparative analysis of function outcome [abstract]. J Oral Maxillofac Surg 2004;62(suppl 1):49.

79. Banks P, Mackenzie I. Condylotomy. A clinical and experimental appraisal of a surgical technique. J Maxillofac Surg 1975;3:170–181.

80. Nickerson JW Jr. The role of condylotomy for treating internal derangements of the temporomandibular joint. Oral Maxillofac Surg Clin North Am 1994;6:277–294.

81. Hall HD, Nickerson JW Jr, McKenna SJ. Modified condylotomy for treatment of the painful temporomandibular joint with a reducing disc. J Oral Maxillofac Surg 1993;51:133–142; discussion 143–144.

82. Hall HD. The condylotomy procedure. Atlas Oral Maxillofac Surg Clin North Am 1996;4:93–106.

83. Upton LG. The case for mandibular condylotomy in the treatment of the painful, deranged, temporomandibular joint. J Oral Maxillofac Surg 1997;55:64–69.

84. Banks P. The case against mandibular condylotomy in the treatment of the painful deranged, temporomandibular joint. J Oral Maxillofac Surg 1997;55:70–74.

85. Mercuri LG, Wolford LM, Sanders B, White RD, Hurder A, Henderson W. Custom CAD/CAM total joint reconstruction system: Preliminary multicenter report. J Oral Maxillofac Surg 1995;53:106–115; discussion 115–116.

CHAPTER 33

Treatment of Myogenous Pain and Dysfunction

Glenn T. Clark

This chapter focuses on the management of myogenous masticatory pain (MMP) and is divided into three parts. First, a practical approach to the differentiation of MMP into appropriate subcategories is proposed. It suggests separating myogenous pains according to their anatomic extent and location into local myalgia, regional craniocervical myalgia, and widespread chronic myalgia, with special emphasis on the specific historical and clinical examination criteria needed to properly use the terms *myofascial pain* and *fibromyalgia*. This classification system differs from the more formal taxonomy discussed in chapter 17, and the intention is to aid the clinician in treating various real-life clinical conditions.

The second part of this chapter discusses the probable mechanisms underlying chronic myogenous pain, including trauma, muscle hyperactivity, muscle hypoperfusion, and peripheral and central neuronal sensitization. Current concepts about the specific mechanisms underlying trigger-point phenomena also are discussed.

The third part of the chapter focuses on the evidence-based treatment of these MMP conditions, using physical medicine modalities such as thermal treatment, exercise and stretching, and needling-injection therapy, as well as several types of pharmacologic agents, including analgesics, tricyclic antidepressants, muscle relaxants, and various topical medications. In addition, the specific topic of botulinum toxin injections is included in this discussion. This chapter does not address the issue of occlusal appliance therapy, which is covered in chapter 25.

Myogenous Pain in the Masticatory System

When a patient exhibits pain and dysfunction in the masticatory musculature, this is described broadly as masticatory myalgia or MMP. Unfortunately the term *myalgia* is not highly specific, and several subcategories are needed to correctly distinguish the clinical problems with which patients present. There are at least three ways of describing the myalgia subcategories; they include differentiation by *(1)* the anatomic features, extent, and location of the pain, *(2)* the etiology, and *(3)* the underlying pain mechanism (Table 33-1). At present there is no accepted method or system of classifying muscle pain that incorporates all three categories.

The anatomic approach to MMP classification includes *(1)* focal masticatory myalgia, *(2)* regional craniocervical myalgia (involving several muscles of the jaw and neck on the same side), and *(3)* widespread chronic myalgia. For local and regional myalgia, if some additional anatomic features such as taut bands, trigger points within the taut bands, and referred pain sensations on sustained compression of the trigger point are added, then the term *myalgia* can be changed to *myofascial pain*.[1] For widespread chronic myalgia, if the appropriate criteria are satisfied, then the term *fibromyalgia* is used (see chapter 22).[2]

It is always preferable to add to this anatomic-based classification system by identifying the suspected etiology for the muscle pain. For example, local and regional

Table 33-1	Chronic myogenous pains affecting the masticatory muscles*		
Myogenous condition	**Anatomic basis**	**Etiology**	**Pain mechanism**
Localized myalgia (iatrogenic trauma)	Unilateral pain in the medial pterygoid associated with trismus	Anesthetic injection–based myositis	Cellular damage and inflammation
Localized myalgia (traumatic injury)	Unilateral pain in masseter or temporalis	Traumatic injury to side of jaw or temple	Cellular damage and inflammation
Localized myalgia (stress/parafunction)	Usually the masseters bilaterally	Sustained parafunction (clenching)–induced muscle pain	Hypoperfusion with accumulation of endogenous algesic substances
Localized myalgia (extrapyramidal)	Usually the jaw closers (masseter and temporalis muscles) bilaterally	Sustained tightening of the jaw muscles because of medications (eg, SSRIs)	Hypoperfusion with accumulation of endogenous algesic substances
Localized secondary myalgia (joint disease induced)	Usually unilateral involving the anterior temporalis and deep masseter on affected side	Secondary to local TMJ disease (either arthritis or internal derangement)	Hypoperfusion with accumulation of endogenous algesic substances
Primary regional myalgia/myofascial pain	Usually unilateral pain involving the temporalis, trapezius, splenius capitus, and SCM	Stress- and/or clenching-induced regional muscle pain (with trigger points, taut bands, and referral)	Combination of hypoperfusion and peripheral sensitization of muscle nociceptors
Secondary regional myalgia/myofascial pain	Usually unilateral pain involving the temporalis, trapezius, splenius capitus, and SCM	Secondary to local TMJ disease (either arthritis or internal derangement)	Combination of hypoperfusion and peripheral sensitization of muscle nociceptors
Widespread chronic myalgia/fibromyalgia	Bilateral jaw closers in addition to the other common fibromyalgia sites	Unknown, but clearly aggravated by stress	Peripheral and central sensitization of muscle nociceptors and pain pathways

*SSRIs = selective serotonin reuptake inhibitors; SCM = sternocleidomastoid.

masticatory myalgia may be caused by one of the following: (1) direct muscle trauma, (2) parafunction and/or stress (primary myogenous pain), or (3) association with local temporomandibular joint (TMJ) disease (secondary myogenous pain). Primary myogenous pain means that no other local pathologic entity that might be causing the muscle pain, such as TMJ osteoarthritis or internal derangement, has been identified.

Etiology is more relevant to the discussion of local and regional myalgia (whether secondary or primary) than it is to widespread chronic myalgia such as fibromyalgia. In the latter condition, the patient's pain is usually so long-standing that, by the time fibromyalgia is diagnosed, the original etiology is not discoverable.

The pathophysiologic mechanisms underlying various types of muscle pain have only recently become better understood, although many of the details still remain controversial or unknown. Muscle pain can be grouped according to one of the following mechanisms: (1) local cellular and humoral inflammation (ie, myositis) where muscle and/or fascial tissue damage has occurred, (2) accumulation of endogenous chemicals within the contractile elements of the muscle proper or within the soft tissues in and around the muscles, (3) altered neurogenic tissues within the muscle (eg, sensitized muscle nociceptors) that have a lowered threshold and even spontaneous activation, and (4) central sensitization and plasticity of the pain pathways from the trigeminal nucleus or spinal cord to the cortex. Certainly, knowledge about the underlying mechanism of a specific patient's muscle pain would influence or even dictate treatment choice. More information about how endogenous chemicals may accumulate, what they are, what nociceptors they excite, and when and how these nociceptors become sensitized will be addressed later, in the section on mechanisms of chronic muscle pain (also see chapters 4 and 5).

Local Myalgia Resulting from Direct Trauma

Local myalgia can develop as a result of muscle injury that causes histologically evident changes in the muscle called *myositis*.[3,4] Such injuries are not common in the masticatory system, but when they occur they are quite dramatic. Patients typically exhibit strong focal pain and severely limited mouth opening because of secondary trismus.[5]

The most common traumatic cause of myositis in the masticatory system is an inadvertent intramuscular injection of a local anesthetic during dental treatment. In these cases, the nature of the injury is influenced by the amount of injected solution, the type of anesthetic used, and, more importantly, whether a vasoconstrictor such as epinephrine was including in the anesthetic solution. Several authors have described and documented the effect of an inadvertent anesthetic injection into muscle tissue.[6–9]

The neck musculature can be injured during a low-velocity rear-end collision, but current data suggest that the jaw-opening and jaw-closing muscles themselves are not stretched or torn during this type of motor vehicle accident (see chapter 18).

Finally, it has been claimed that tearing-type damage and tissue inflammation can occur in the masticatory muscles of some patients as a result of high levels of sustained clenching and eccentric bruxism-like contraction. Several researchers have tried to induce this type of muscle pain in volunteers by having them perform prolonged sustained centric and eccentric exercises of the jaw.[10–13] The data from these experiments show that some acute pain is inducible during and shortly after the exercise task, and some mildly increased muscle tenderness can be demonstrated, but overall the masticatory motor system is actually quite resistant to this form of muscle injury.

When direct muscle trauma is suspected as the etiology, the traumatic event is usually easily identified in the history. The standard treatment for traumatic myalgia is rest of the jaw, ice, nonsteroidal anti-inflammatory drugs (NSAIDs), and later frequent daily active mobilization of the jaw until a normal range of movement is restored.[14] The last step is important because traumatic myositis frequently induces a substantial trismus. This trismus is a logical and appropriate acute response but, if prolonged, it can lead to chronic loss of jaw motion because of muscle contracture.[15] Most healthy patients manage to overcome these injuries and achieve normal function with a minimal amount of disruption, but poorly treated patients often end up with significant long-term limitation of jaw opening.

Primary Myalgia Resulting from Stress and/or Parafunction

Often local and regional myalgias are not strongly associated with a traumatic event or any other local pathologic problems in the masticatory system. In these cases, the clinician should ask about medications, stress, and/or parafunction (both during waking and sleeping) in a search for the cause of the pain. When a patient admits to these behaviors, the clinician will typically diagnose a primary myalgia arising from stress and/or parafunction. Oral parafunctions include both waking and sleeping tooth clenching and grinding as well as other oral habits such as chronic gum chewing.[16]

Several studies have reported that there is a moderately strong positive association between self-reported clenching and chronic masticatory myofascial pain.[17–19] Unfortunately, these studies do not specify whether the clenching occurred during waking or sleeping periods, because to do so accurately requires an actual recording of the jaw motor behaviors over moderately long periods of time (2 weeks minimum). However, parafunction during sleep should be suspected in patients who report increased pain and jaw limitation on awakening in the morning.

One recent study has used the Symptom Checklist-90 revised questionnaire to examine various potential contributing factors, such as sociodemographic characteristics, clenching, grinding, head-neck trauma, and psychological factors, for their effect on chronic masticatory myofascial pain.[20] This was a case-control study with 83 patients with MMP, selected from the dental clinics of the Jewish General Hospital and Montreal General Hospital, Montreal, Canada, and 100 concurrent controls. Using unconditional logistic regression analysis, the researchers found that self-reported tooth clenching and grinding was significantly associated with either an elevated anxiety score (odds ratio = 8.48) or an elevated depression score (odds ratio = 8.13) in the patients with chronic MMP. They concluded that tooth clenching, trauma, and female gender strongly contributed to the presence of chronic MMP, even when other psychological symptoms were similar between subjects.

Grinding-only behavior, age, household income, and education were not related to chronic MMP,[20] but this lack of association between tooth grinding and chronic muscle pain is in conflict with other studies. For example, one group of researchers performed a questionnaire-based epidemiologic cross-sectional study and another used a clinically based case-control design.[21,22] These two studies found a positive relationship between self-reported nocturnal tooth grinding and self-reported jaw pain. To resolve this conflict will require additional data.

With regard to stress, psychological factors have been associated with chronic facial and jaw pain, but current research cannot determine if the chronic pain is influencing the psychological factors or vice versa.

If stress or parafunction is suspected as the etiology, and these behaviors are persistent, a behavioral modification approach to treatment is more logical. The standard methods of modifying parafunction include oral appliances and avoidance training. The management of stress, which can be accomplished pharmacologically and/or behaviorally, will be reviewed later in this chapter (also see chapter 26).

Secondary Myalgia Resulting from Active Local Pathologic Conditions

Sometimes local and even regional myalgia will develop in response to a local painful pathologic process such as an acute arthritis affecting the TMJ. In these cases, the muscle pain develops unilaterally (on the side of the pathologic condition, assuming it is one-sided). The pain in the muscle tissue is secondary, but it may generate an equal or greater degree of tenderness to palpation as the joint. The fact that the nociceptors inside a joint or even inside a tooth can induce a secondary motor reaction in the anatomically adjacent muscle has been clearly demonstrated in the literature.[23,24]

The most common form of secondary jaw and cervical motor activation occurs with a painful arthritis or internal derangement of the TMJ.[25] However, these reactions are also likely to occur with acute pulpal pain, osteomyelitis, or other mandibular bone or soft tissue infections. When a patient presents with one-sided muscle pain in the absence of trauma, strong stress, or a history of parafunction, the clinician should carefully examine the TMJ for local disease or dysfunction.

When a patient presents with both a local pathologic process and muscle pain that seems to have developed after the pathologic condition began, it is logical and appropriate to manage or minimize the local pathosis first and then reevaluate the secondary myogenous pain for resolution or persistence. In some cases, acute traumatic trismus can convert to chronic contracture of the involved muscle.[26]

Myofascial Pain (Local or Regional)

The International Association for the Study of Pain, Subcommittee on Taxonomy, has classified myofascial pain as pain in any muscle with trigger points that are very painful to compression during palpation and cause referred pain.[27] Essentially the term *myofascial pain* is used only when specific criteria are satisfied. These criteria are both subjective (history based) and objective (examination based) in nature. The three subjective criteria that patients should exhibit include *(1)* spontaneous, dull, aching pain and localized tenderness in the involved muscles, *(2)* stiffness in the involved body area, and *(3)* easily induced fatigability with sustained function. The four objective criteria are *(1)* a hyperirritable spot in a palpably taut band of skeletal muscle or muscle fascia, *(2)* a patient-reported new or increased dull, aching pain in a nearby site on sustained compression of this hyperirritable spot, *(3)* a decreased range of unassisted movement of the involved body area, and *(4)* weakness without atrophy and the absence of a neurologic deficit to explain this weakness.

Many have included the presence of referred autonomic phenomena on compression of the hyperirritable spot and/or a twitch response to snapping palpation of the taut bands as additional diagnostic criteria.[28–32] However, the inclusion of these criteria is not endorsed by some because they are not reliably present physical findings.[1] The most interesting aspect of the latter study[1] was that taut muscle bands and muscle twitches were common and noted equally in all three diagnostic groups (fibromyalgia, regional myofascial pain, and healthy control subjects). This finding suggests that the clinical examination–based criteria for myofascial pain alone are not reliable and therefore that myofascial pain patients are best identified through a combination of historical and clinical criteria. Finally, the results of this research report suggest that additional work is needed to establish a reliable set of diagnostic criteria for this disorder.

Myofascial pain appears to be a completely different entity than localized traumatic myalgia, in that the former is not associated with any histologically evident tissue damage or inflammation. Several investigators have attempted to biopsy the muscles of patients who have myofascial pain but have found no unique tissue-based evidence of inflammatory disease. In recent years, a number of explanations have been offered for this puzzling pain phenomenon.[33–37]

However, the more interesting question may be, "What are trigger points and how do they develop?" Several studies based on needle electromyography (EMG) have reported that sustained, spontaneous EMG activity can be found within 1 to 2 mm of a hyperirritable or trigger point in a muscle but not in the control nonpainful sites or from the surface above the muscle.[38] The fact that this activity is influenced (increased) by the sympathetic nervous system was recently demonstrated when a Valsalva maneuver was used to induce a transient sympathetic activation.[38] This research suggests that sympathetic neural outflow increases painful-area motor nerve activity and this may be contributing to a focal muscle contraction (palpable taut band) at the painful trigger-point site.

After reviewing the literature on myofascial trigger points, Hong and Simons[39] concluded that the electrical activity characteristics of trigger points are similar to those described from needle EMG recording in and around motor endplates. They speculated that the spontaneous activity recorded from trigger points is probably related to excessive release of acetylcholine (ACh) at the endplate. They also speculated that these endplates were abnormal because the sensory nerves fibers that surround them are sensitized and are spontaneously active or active during stressful periods of the day; in turn, this causes local pain and more focal motor nerve activity in the endplate.

Additional study of this issue is needed, but in another recent review it was proposed that several responses occur when a motor endplate becomes dysfunctional.[40] First, the release of ACh produces a muscle contraction that, among other things, causes a compression of local vasculature in the area and produces a reduction in the local supply of oxygen. This impaired circulation, combined with the increased metabolic demands generated by contracted muscles, results in a rapid depletion of local adenosine triphosphate (ATP). Specifically, one study showed that ATP directly inhibits ACh release, so depletion of ATP increases ACh release.[41] In the muscle cell, ATP powers the calcium pump that returns calcium to the sarcoplasmic reticulum. Hence, loss of ATP also impairs the reuptake of calcium, which increases contractile activity.[42] Finally, the ATP energy crisis causes a local release of a variety of chemicals, peptides, and cytokines (ie, bradykinins, cytokines, serotonin, histamine, potassium, prostaglandins, leukotrienes, somatostatin, and substance P) that have the potential to activate and sensitize nociceptive nerves in the region.

In those cases where trigger points and taut bands are evident in a muscle, several therapeutic methods are suggested, including stretching of the taut bands and direct stimulation of the trigger point via needling or injection of a local anesthetic.[43] These methods are reviewed in detail in the section on treatment. If sympathetic neural activity is a factor in aggravating trigger points, behavioral or pharmacologic methods to reduce stress also seem indicated.

Fibromyalgia

Based on epidemiologic studies, syndromes of widespread chronic musculoskeletal pain are reported to occur in 4% to 13% of the general population.[44–46] Fibromyalgia, a specific disorder with published criteria, is less common, with a prevalence of about 2% in the community (see chapter 22). Widespread diffuse musculoskeletal pain syndromes, in particular fibromyalgia, often occur in concert with several additional diseases, most notably chronic fatigue syndrome, irritable bowel syndrome, temporomandibular disorders, and headaches. In general, fibromyalgia is treated using multimodal approaches that simultaneously target the biologic, psychological, environmental, and social factors that maintain the pain.

The American College of Rheumatology has set forth criteria for the diagnosis of fibromyalgia,[47] and these criteria include specific duration, location, and examination findings that must be satisfied. The duration criteria specify that a history of widespread pain has to be present for at least 3 months. Moreover, for pain to be considered widespread, it must involve both sides of the body and be located above and below the waist. The location criteria state that the pain must involve multiple areas of the axial skeleton, including the cervical spine, anterior chest, and thoracic spine or lower back regions. If the patient has lower back pain, this will satisfy the criteria for pain below the waist. Finally the examination findings criteria specify that a "painful" response must be elicited in 11 of 18 tender point sites on digital palpation. The criteria specify the exact location of these tender point sites, and they also specify that a manual finger palpation force of approximately 4 kg is to be used during the examination. Responses to palpation are categorized as no pain, tender, and painful.[47]

With regard to the underlying differences between fibromyalgia and local myalgia, regional myalgia, or myofascial pain, there is substantial evidence that fibromyalgia sufferers have central neuronal changes in their pain-processing system. For example, fibromyalgia patients show clear-cut altered sensory processing compared to normal subjects. Normal subjects show an increase in their pain threshold with repeated skin stimulation, but this does not occur in patients with fibromyalgia, which suggests a reduced descending inhibitory pain suppression system.[44] Moreover, functional CNS changes in individuals with fibromyalgia can be demonstrated by several different imaging techniques. For example, one study reported that fibromyalgia patients exhibit a decreased thalamic and caudate blood flow compared to healthy controls on single photon emission computed tomography imaging.[48] Finally, patients with fibromyalgia show substantially elevated levels of substance P in their cerebrospinal fluid, which would enhance the likelihood of sensitization of second-order spinal neurons.[49,50] More information on neural sensitization is provided in chapters 3 and 5.

Mechanisms of Nontraumatic, Primary Myogenous Pain

Muscle Hyperactivity

For many years, when a patient presented with a nontraumatic, chronic primary myogenous pain disorder in the masticatory system, it was hypothesized that stress was causing the condition. The key factor in this concept was that stress produced an elevated level of waking, resting, or background muscle hyperactivity in jaw and/or neck muscles, and this in turn caused chronic pain in the hyperactive muscle. For example, the previously cited studies that concluded that self-reported tooth clenching by patients is a moderate risk factor for chronic masticatory myalgia support this concept.[17–19]

The stress–muscle hyperactivity–pain theory was also used to explain episodic headache, and the term *muscle contraction headache* was used for many years. This term was eventually replaced with the current term, *tension-type headache*, in the headache lexicon.[51] This change was necessitated because data started accumulating that muscle contractions were not highly correlated with the pain experienced in episodic nonmigraine headache. Nevertheless, in the field of temporomandibular disorders, this concept initially developed and persisted because some electromyographic data showed that patients with masticatory muscle pain often had greater resting muscle activity in their painful muscles than did nonpain subjects.[52,53]

Associations do not prove causality, and sometimes the cause-effect relationship is the opposite of what was expected. In the case of chronic muscle pain, the best current evidence now suggests that elevated daytime levels of resting muscle activity are not the cause of the myogenous pain or tension-headache pain; instead, the pain itself causes a predictable elevation in daytime muscle activity. Moreover, when pain-inducing substances are directly injected into the muscles of healthy subjects, only a small elevation in masticatory muscle activity is produced.[54–56]

Laboratory-based studies that examine background or resting muscle activity do not necessarily capture or mimic the full range of motor activities and behaviors, such as tooth clenching, that might be exhibited in the natural environment (outside of the laboratory). For this reason, several researchers have investigated the effect of pain on muscle activity (and vice versa) in the natural

environment. These data are mixed, depending on the methods used and the disease being studied. For example, two studies examined whether temporalis muscle activity is greater in subjects prone to episodic tension-type headache (n = 36) than in matched nonheadache controls (n = 36).[57,58] Subjects recorded their cumulative temporalis muscle activity with a portable EMG recorder every 30 minutes for 3 days and nights. The subjects also recorded their pain and stress levels every 30 minutes in a diary.

The results demonstrated that patients with episodic tension headache pain had some clear EMG elevations compared with normal controls, but these elevations happened primarily during function (chewing and talking) and the EMG patterns were not correlated with the general rise and fall of the headache pain. The analysis did show that the highest correlation coefficient values occurred between pain and stress ($r = .33$) in the headache group. It also showed that headache subjects seemed to use their temporalis muscles with less efficiency, or that they had more reactive splinting-guarding muscle activity than did nonheadache subjects during function.[57,58] In other words, this elevated EMG level is more likely a consequence of the pain rather than a cause of it in tension-type headache sufferers.

The previously cited question-based data on the association of clenching and masticatory muscle pain[21] is interesting but not conclusive. One problem is that no good, objective data on the habitual behavior of clenching are available. This may be because clenching, which is assumed to be around 10% to 15% of the maximum voluntary contraction force level, is occurring below the commonly recorded threshold in most long-term EMG analyses performed on the jaw-closing muscles. One study examined the masseter muscle activity during the whole day in children and young adults.[59] However, it reported only on masseter muscle activity, which was 25% higher than the maximum voluntary contraction levels. Moreover, the process of recording subjects with EMG during the daytime may interfere with the behavior of interest.

At this time, there are no conclusive data that show whether low levels of abnormal daytime muscle behavior contribute to local or regional myalgia or myofascial pain in the masticatory system. Such data is difficult to gather because of the moderate behavioral invasiveness of such studies, namely, wearing an EMG recorder continuously for several days while recording pain and stress information in a daily diary every 30 minutes. Therefore, the issue of daytime clenching patterns as an etiology or mechanism for masticatory myalgia pain is still unsettled.

With regard to sleeping levels of temporalis muscle activity, one study found no statistical differences between headache and nonheadache sufferers.[58] It may also be that sleep bruxism is not highly related to masticatory muscle pain, but additional data are needed in this population. In summary, while the aforementioned data are applicable primarily to tension-type headache and even may generalize to local or regional myalgia, these data do not support the concept that stress causes elevated nonfunctional muscle hyperactivity that then causes masticatory muscle pain or even episodic tension-headache pain.

Muscle Hypoperfusion

Another proposed mechanism underlying nontraumatic primary myogenous pain is that it could be the result of intramuscular hypoperfusion. This hypothesis was reviewed in detail recently.[60] More than 30 years ago, Fassbender and Wegner[61] first hypothesized that intramuscular hypoxia was a possible cause of localized myalgia, based on biopsy specimens collected from the trapezius muscle in patients with primary fibromyalgia patients.

More recently, a study examined the role of blood supply and oxidative metabolism via muscle biopsies from 25 female workers with trapezius myalgia and 21 healthy female teachers.[62] It was reported that the number of capillaries per fiber area was significantly lower in the subjects suffering from myalgia than in those without trapezius myalgia. The authors concluded that the capillary supply of the trapezius muscle was affected in work-related trapezius myalgia but that more studies are needed to understand possible mechanisms that would explain the occurrence of these muscle fiber and vascular changes.

Dynamic muscle blood flow in fibromyalgia has been studied by numerous researchers using a variety of methods. The xenon 133–based studies showed that blood flow differences in fibromyalgia patients are not evident in a resting condition but become so only during and after physical activity.[63,64] Bilateral laser-Doppler blood flow assessment also showed that an impaired regulation of the microcirculation in the muscle is of central importance in chronic trapezius myalgia, causing nociceptive pain.

Of course, the changes in a more chronic widespread disease such as fibromyalgia may not generalize to local and regional myalgia disorders. For this reason, several researchers have looked at local masticatory myalgia and blood flow. Using the method of near infrared (NIR) spectroscopy, one study found that patients with local myalgia have a reduced postcontraction hyperemic response, suggesting altered perfusion.[65]

Unfortunately, contraction-based experiments are subject to error because of differences in the contraction abilities of pain and nonpain subjects. Another study compared local myalgia and nonmyalgia patients through the technique of cold-pressor stimulation of a hand or foot (where no muscular contraction was induced) to produce vasodilatation. This study found that intramuscular perfusion is significantly reduced in the subjects with local myalgia. The authors hypothesized that the differences in vasodilative response in the subjects with focal myalgia might be related to desensitization of β-adrenergic receptors, which occurs with long-term exposure to the stress-associated neurotransmitter, epinephrine.[66] The roles of long-term pain and chronic stress and their effect on the response patterns in the microvasculature need additional study.

Although not all of the aforementioned studies used controlled conditions, and the bias control measures could have been improved in every study, the data are largely objective (measures of blood flow) and consistent. Moreover, these studies were performed by various researchers at different sites using at least three different methods to monitor blood flow (laser-Doppler, xenon 133, and NIR spectroscopy). Overall, these studies suggest that there are demonstrable changes in intramuscular perfusion of the masseter and trapezius muscles in patients with chronic regional myalgia. This hypoperfusion occurs both during and after muscle activity.

Finally, the issue of stress, pain, and blood flow in the jaw system recently was examined in a study that reported on healthy adult female volunteers performing a 2-hour mental stress task.[67] These researchers monitored cardiac rates using electrocardiography (ECG), as well as muscle activity using EMG, recording from the anterior temporalis and superficial masseteric muscles bilaterally. They also recorded intramuscular blood flow in the masseter with an NIR spectroscopy method. They found that the EMG activity of the temporalis muscle, but not the masseter muscle, was increased during the stress task. This finding is reasonable because the anterior temporalis muscle is the primary postural muscle of the jaw, so it would more likely be influenced by stress than would the superficial masseter.

These authors also used the ECG-based R-R interval analysis to assay for changes in the sympathetic nervous system, and they found the temporalis EMG elevations to be consistent with elevated sympathetic activity.[67] In the masseter muscle, despite little change in integrated electromyographic activity, there were notable changes in the hemodynamic parameters; there was also a decrease in total hemoglobin in the muscle during the stressful period. These results suggest that stress produces a reactive vasoconstrictive effect on the masseter muscle.

This vasoconstrictive response is somewhat paradoxic, because normally acute stress causes an increase in heart rate resulting from a release of endogenous epinephrine, and this substance then also causes intramuscular vasodilatation. Because these authors did not demonstrate any strong change in heart rate (the ECG only showed a change from 72 to 74 beats per minute during the stress task), and it was a prolonged stress response, it is possible that the expected initial vasodilative effect of endogenous epinephrine release would be transient and then a longer lasting vasoconstrictive effect would predominate. Overall, these authors concluded that the hemodynamic properties of the jaw muscles are susceptible to prolonged mental stress, and the response is a vasoconstrictive one.[67] Whether a long-term period of environmental stress could and does cause intramuscular vasoconstriction will require additional study by other researchers, and possibly even studies conducted in the natural environment with combined portable EMG, ECG, and intramuscular blood flow–monitoring equipment. Unfortunately, such equipment does not exist currently.

Muscle Pain Location and Nociceptor Sensitization

Nontraumatic primary myogenous pain occurs in roughly the same anatomic locations from patient to patient. For example, in the masticatory and craniocervical systems, the painful muscles are the trapezius, the sternocleidomastoid, the splenius capitus, the anterior temporalis, and the masseter. These muscles contain a moderately high level of type 1 (slow twitch) muscle fibers. A scientific finding of importance related to this topic was described in a recent study.[68] The authors looked at which muscles are more sensitive to ischemic damage; specifically, they examined fast- and slow-contracting motor units sampled from the first dorsal interosseous muscle in human volunteers. The experimental subjects were asked to hold an abduction force for approximately 10 minutes under normal conditions. This task was repeated under ischemic conditions after sufficient rest of 4 to 5 minutes. The slow time-to-peak motor units, which are presumably the slow twitch type 1 fibers, were clearly more sensitive to ischemia than were the fast time-to-peak group.[68]

This finding has been reported in other muscles as well, and it appears clear that the type 1 muscle fibers are more susceptible to ischemic injury. This would explain why postural muscles, which have a much higher proportion of slow twitch (type 1 fibers), are much more likely to exhibit diminished perfusion and show ischemic injury sites.[68]

Proof that a hypoxic environment can induce muscle pain comes from several authors.[69,70] For example, in humans, intramuscular injections of acidic solutions have been shown to elicit muscle pain.[71] Moreover, nuclear magnetic resonance studies on the pH inside human muscle cells have shown that pH values of 6 or

lower can be reached during the ischemia associated with sustained contractions or exhaustive exercise.[72,73]

The next issue to consider is how local and regional myalgia can convert to a myofascial pain disorder with trigger points or to a widespread pain condition such as fibromyalgia. Understanding how and to what degree localized muscle pain can turn into chronic muscle pain requires knowledge about the topic of neuronal sensitization, as discussed in chapters 3 and 5 on neuropathic pain mechanisms. Current knowledge about muscle pain mechanisms, and specifically about jaw muscle activity, intramuscular blood flow, and the effect of prolonged stress on masticatory muscle blood flow, suggests the following hypothesis to explain the development of chronic muscular pain:

1. Prolonged stress may cause local intramuscular hypoperfusion, which seems to selectively target muscles with higher proportions of type 1 (slow twitch) fibers that are involved in postural maintenance.
2. This focal hypoperfusion induces an ischemic condition and local muscle pain.
3. Once the pain develops to a sufficient level in the muscle or fascial tissues, it causes a reactive muscle activation (taut bands and even whole muscle splinting or trismus) that is most evident when the patient actually attempts to function.
4. If the right type and amount of algesic chemicals are released, then the local muscle pain area can produce a peripheral nociceptor sensitization and even a more central pain pathway sensitization.
5. When this occurs, myofascial pain trigger points are likely to develop and some susceptible patients will develop more widespread pain.

This hypothesis is probably a far more viable theory for explaining local primary nontraumatic myalgia than previous concepts, such as lactic acid buildup or muscle hyperactivity arising from occlusal interferences.

One study has examined whether patients with primary fibromyalgia also have serologic markers of ischemic injury.[74] The researchers compared 85 female patients with primary fibromyalgia and 80 age-, height-, and weight-matched healthy women for serologic evidence of oxidative distress. They reported that levels of malondialdehyde (a toxic metabolite of lipid peroxidation and a marker of free radical damage) were significantly higher and levels of superoxide dismutase (an intracellular antioxidant enzyme) were significantly lower in fibromyalgia patients than in the controls. The authors concluded that these findings supported the hypothesis that fibromyalgia is, at least in part, an oxidative disorder.

Table 33-2	Top 12 patient-rated treatments for fibromyalgia*		
Type of therapy		**Rank**	**n**
Hydrotherapy/spa therapy		8.9	21
List making		8.4	49
Sleep (mattresses)		8.4	25
Rest		8.3	79
Bodywork therapies (trigger-point/myofascial therapy)		8.1	20
Bodywork therapies (therapeutic massage)		8.0	68
Duragesic (Janssen), etc (transdermal fentanyl)		7.9	27
Vicodin (Abbott), etc (hydrocodone and acetaminophen)		7.9	25
Klonopin (Roche), etc (clonazepam)		7.8	29
Soma (Wallace), etc (carisoprodol)		7.6	31
Ultram (Ortho-McNeil), etc (tramadol)		7.5	30
OxyContin (Purdue Pharma) (controlled-release oxycodone hydrochloride)		7.4	84

*Data from RemedyFind.[75]

Evidence-Based Treatment

The scientific evidence on treatment efficacy for chronic myogenous pain of all types is of various levels of quality. Therefore, rather than limit the discussion only to data from randomized blinded and controlled studies, it is best to look at this issue from several different perspectives. Three types of data will be discussed. First, the review will focus on how individual consumers of healthcare (the patients themselves) have rated various treatment methods for fibromyalgia. Although similar information from patients about local and regional myalgia treatment preferences would also be of interest, fibromyalgia is the only condition for which a moderate amount of patient-based rating is available for review. Second, the information that the various medical professional societies (those whose members deal routinely with chronic muscle pain) provide to the public about treatment on their websites will be evaluated. Third, and at the top of the scientific hierarchy, are data tabulated from various systematic review articles on chronic myogenous pain disorders. The emphasis will be on those review articles that specifically deal with local or regional myogenous pain in the craniocervical or temporomandibular region. However, when such information is not available, outcome reviews of treatment for lower back pain will be considered, with generalization of the data on this regional musculoskeletal disorder to masticatory myogenous pain. Finally, systematic reviews on the treatment of fibromyalgia or other chronic pain disorders will be considered when no systematic reviews were available for myogenous pain. Although the collection of such diverse information has it disadvantages, it is hoped that the advantages and overall conclusions outweigh the limitations of this approach.

Patient-Based Rating of Treatments

One method of deciding on the most efficacious treatment is to ask the patients who have been suffering with their chronic illness which treatments worked best for them. Such data must be judged as less than stringent in the scientific world of evidence ranking, because such opinions are fraught with bias. Nevertheless, patient rankings of treatments are interesting and their preferences, taken from a nonprofit website,[75] have been included. This website allows patients to log on and rate what they find works best for them on a scale of 0 to 10 (0 = poorest; 10 = best treatment), although voters are unscreened and their diagnosis is unconfirmed by the website.

On December 22, 2004, a number of contemporary treatments for fibromyalgia were rated (Table 33-2). The interesting aspect of this ranking is that the top 4 were self-administered treatments; hydrotherapy or "spa therapy" was the highest ranked treatment. It is also interesting to note that the top 6 therapies were either behavioral or physical medicine in nature, while the bottom 6 therapies in this list of the top 12 were opioid, benzodiazepine, or muscle relaxant medications. The one category of medications that was endorsed by two of the three medical specialty organizations reviewed in this chapter, namely antidepressants (see the next section), was not listed among the top 12 treatments.

Several articles in the medical literature have examined the effect of thermal and spa type therapy on widespread musculoskeletal pain, and most of them have reported that patients experienced substantial improvement with moderately long-lasting benefits.[76] If indeed the disorder of chronic nontraumatic myalgia is an oxidative, stress-induced, and maintained pain, then any modality such as spa therapy, which induces moderate vasodilatation, might be as highly therapeutic, as the patients responding to the website indicated.[75]

Expert Opinions About Treatment

The second level of scientific data reviewed for this chapter includes statements about appropriate chronic muscle pain treatment gathered from the websites of professional societies (Table 33-3). First, information was collected from one major nonprofit patient organization, the National Fibromyalgia Association.[77] This group is primarily organized by patients and their advocates, although the association has a medical advisory board. In addition, the statements on muscle pain treatment from three professional medical societies in the United States were evaluated. These societies were the American Academy of Physical Medicine and Rehabilitation,[78] the American College of Rheumatology,[79] and the American Academy of Family Physicians.[80] The nonprofit association and each medical academy had an area on its website that either posted information or presented an expert opinion article regarding treatment of fibromyalgia (see Table 33-3).

Treatments were organized under four categories, which included self-treatment procedures, medications, physical medicine procedures, and behavioral treatment. The patient-run organization lists multiple forms of treatment but does not rank or judge the relative efficacy of these treatments. The three professional medical societies endorse fewer forms of treatment. The only two that are endorsed by all three medical societies are exercise-based treatment and medications. The medications endorsed by two of the professional societies include a low dose of a tricyclic antidepressant and/or a selective serotonin reuptake inhibitor. Only one medical group suggested that opioids are appropriate. Finally, two of the medical societies suggested that behavioral therapy would be appropriate. It is likely that the recommendations of the medical societies are based on the scientific literature.

Published Analytic Reviews on Treatment

The third and final level of data analyzed was taken from the published systematic reviews of the literature on the different treatments that have been recommended for the various types of chronic muscle pain (Table 33-4). The reviews considered most valuable were those that qualified for inclusion in the Cochrane Library database, an international collaboration that promotes evidence-based reviews of the literature.[81] The search only produced major review articles on eight treatment categories, although Table 33-3 identifies 20 different categories of therapy. Table 33-4 lists the final recommendation of these reviews in a simplified form (yes or no).

Those treatment methods that have not been subjected to systematic reviews are not discussed in this chapter, with the exception of botulinum toxin injections for myofascial pain. Because this therapy is new and has fairly widespread media and public attention, it was included although a systematic review of its effect on musculoskeletal pain is not available.

Self-directed treatment

The National Fibromyalgia Association recommends strongly that fibromyalgia sufferers make many lifestyle accommodations. The specific self-directed treatments (which in this context means treatments that are not medical office–based) that the association endorses are nonspecific nutritional supplements, relaxation-meditation techniques (eg, yoga, relaxation exercises, breathing techniques, and aromatherapy), daily exercise (eg, gentle aerobic exercise and stretching); avoidance of stimulants (caffeine, sugar, and alcohol), participation in a local fibromyalgia support group, and thermal therapy for pain relief. The extent to which patients incorporate these self-directed treatments into their life will largely depend on the severity of their problem. Fortunately patients with local and even regional myalgia or myofascial pain will have far less disability and life interference than will patients with fibromyalgia and other forms of widespread chronic pain.

The only self-directed treatments in the aforementioned list that have a substantial body of literature worthy of review are exercise therapy and thermal therapy. Exercise therapy is the one treatment endorsed by all three of the medical societies reviewed. The two systematic reviews available also offer a consistent point of view. One is a Cochrane Library review that examined 16 clinical trials that included a total of 724 participants.[82] Seven studies were judged high-quality training studies: four on aerobic training; one on a mixture of aerobic, strength,

Table 33-3	Patient organization and medical society recommendations for treatment of fibromyalgia*			
Suggested treatment approach	**National Fibromyalgia Association**[77]	**American Academy of Physical Medicine and Rehabilitation**[78]	**American College of Rheumatology**[79]	**American Academy of Family Physicians**[80]
Self-treatment approaches				
Lifestyle adaptation	Yes	NS	NS	NS
Nutrition (eg, herbs and nutritional supplements)	Yes	NS	NS	NS
Relaxation-meditation techniques (eg, yoga, relaxation exercises, breathing techniques, and aromatherapy)	Yes	NS	NS	Yes
Exercise (eg, gentle exercise and stretching)	Yes	Yes	Yes	Yes
Avoidance of stimulants (caffeine, sugar, and alcohol)	Yes	NS	NS	NS
Fibromyalgia support groups	Yes	NS	NS	Yes
Thermal therapy	Yes	NS	NS	NS
Medications	Yes	Yes (but medication NS)	Yes (TCAs and SSRIs)	Yes (TCAs, SSRIs, and opioids, but not NSAIDs)
NSAIDs and nonopioid analgesics	Yes	NS	NS	Not recommended
Opioid pain medications	Yes	NS	NS	Yes
Antidepressants (eg, TCAs and SSRIs)	Yes	NS	Yes	Yes
Muscle relaxants (various types)	Yes	NS	NS	NS
Sleep medications	Yes	NS	NS	NS
Physical medicine treatments				
Local trigger-point injections	Yes	NS	NS	NS
Botulinum toxin injections	NS	NS	NS	NS
Stimulation therapy (eg, acupuncture)	Yes	NS	NS	Yes
Physical therapy (eg, therapeutic massage, myofascial release therapy, and acupressure)	Yes	NS	NS	Yes
Manual therapy (eg, osteopathic or chiropractic manipulation)	Yes	NS	NS	Yes
Behavioral treatments				
Behavior management of sleep	Yes	NS	NS	NS
Psychological treatment (eg, cognitive therapy and biofeedback)	Yes	NS	Yes	Yes

*NS = not specified; TCAs = tricyclic antidepressants; SSRIs = selective serotonin reuptake inhibitors; NSAIDs = nonsteroidal anti-inflammatory drugs.

Table 33-4	Systematic reviews of myogenous pain treatment*			
	No. of reviews available	Cochrane Library review[81]	Disease reviewed	Recommendation
Lifestyle adaptation	0	0	NA	NA
Nutrition (eg, herbs and nutritional supplements)	0	0	NA	NA
Relaxation-meditation techniques (eg, yoga and others)	0	0	NA	NA
Exercise (eg, aerobic exercise and stretching)	2	2	Fibromyalgia	Yes (aerobic exercise); no (stretching)
Avoidance of stimulants (caffeine, sugar, and alcohol)	0	0	NA	NA
Fibromyalgia support groups	0	0	NA	NA
Thermal therapy	1	0	Mixed rheumatic disease	Yes (but data is limited because of quality of studies
NSAIDs and nonopioid analgesic medications	4 (topical only)	3 0	Acute/chronic musculoskeletal pain	Yes (when applied in a topical cream)
Opioid pain medications	0	0	NA	NA
Antidepressants (eg, TCAs and SSRIs)	1	0	Fibromyalgia	Yes (for fibromyalgia)
Muscle relaxants (various types)	3	0	Lower back pain and fibromyalgia	Yes (but short-term effect and some medications are subject to abuse)
Sleep medications	0	0	NA	NA
Local triggerpoint injections or dry needling	1	0	Myofacial pain	Yes (but needling of triggerpoint is more important than substance injected)
Botulinum toxin injections	0	0	NA	NA
Stimulation therapy (eg, acupuncture)	3	0	Fibromyalgia Chronic pain Lower back pain	Yes (for fibromyalgia, but data on lower back pain is not conclusive)
Physical therapy (eg, therapeutic massage, myofascial release therapy, and acupressure)	0	0	NA	NA
Manual therapies	0	0	NA	NA
Behavior management of sleep (all forms)	0	0	NA	NA
Psychological treatment (eg, cognitive therapy and biofeedback)	3	0	NA	Yes (but overall weak effect and not good for pain relief)

*TCAs = tricyclic antidepressants; SSRIs = selective serotonin reuptake inhibitors; NSAIDs = nonsteroidal anti-inflammatory drugs.

and flexibility training; one on strength training; and two with exercise training as part of a composite treatment. The other study was not in the Cochrane Library and examined 17 clinical trials of exercise treatment in a fibromyalgia population.[83] Both studies endorsed aerobic exercise as a beneficial evidence-based treatment for fibromyalgia. Both also suggested that supervised low-intensity aerobics has sufficient, although weak, evidence to recommend it.

The review data on thermal therapy are not in the Cochrane Library. The review examined 15 published articles that evaluated thermal and spa therapy in a mixed group of rheumatic disease patients.[76] The results of this systematic review suggest that this form of treatment produces a consistent positive result. This review, along with the fact that that it is also the highest patient-rated treatment approach, makes thermal therapy worthy of consideration as an evidence-based treatment, although caution must be used by those patients who are hypotensive and heat intolerant.

Physical medicine

Many physical medicine methods are recommended for treatment of local and regional myalgia and myofascial pain as well as fibromyalgia. These treatments include local trigger-point injection therapy and manual physical therapy procedures, including therapeutic massage, myofascial release therapy, acupressure, acupuncture, and osteopathic or chiropractic manipulation. As with self-directed therapies, the extent to which a patient pursues these treatments will depend on the severity of the problem. In attempting to decide how much and which physical medicine treatments should be used, the clinician may find it interesting that bodywork therapies, namely triggerpoint therapy, myofascial therapy, and therapeutic massage, were the fifth and sixth highest ranking therapies, according to patients; these techniques were ranked higher than all of the pharmacologic therapies. Neither the National Fibromyalgia Association nor the medical societies have endorsed botulinum toxin injections at this time.

The literature reviews on physical medicine for myogenous pain include one study on triggerpoint injections and needling[43] and three on acupuncture.[84–86] The review on triggerpoint therapy does offer an endorsement of this method and suggests that dry needling is a viable therapy; injection of a local anesthetic or corticosteroid solution into the triggerpoint is not needed for improved efficacy. However, it suggests that the needling effect may not be more than a powerful placebo treatment.

The three systematic reviews on acupuncture examined different disease entities and reached different conclusions. The review that focused on fibromyalgia was not a Cochrane Library review.[84] It endorsed acupuncture as better than sham acupuncture. The second review on acupuncture and chronic pain (of all types) was also not a Cochrane Library review.[85] It stated that the available studies were not of sufficient methodologic quality to offer an endorsement. The third review, on acupuncture for management of acute and chronic lower back pain, was a Cochrane Library review.[86] It examined 11 clinical trials but stated that only 2 were of high quality. It also concluded that the available studies were not of sufficient methodologic quality to offer an endorsement.

Although no systematic, multiple-study literature review has yet been performed, botulinum toxin was examined in a randomized double-blind study on 33 patients with refractory myofascial pain (11 patients in each group).[87] One group received normal saline and the other two groups received injections of either 50 or 100 units of botulinum toxin into triggerpoints in the cervicothoracic paraspinal muscle area. The researchers were not able to demonstrate statistically significant differences in improvement between the groups, and botulinim toxin cannot be endorsed as evidence-supported treatment for triggerpoints based on current research.

Pharmacologic-based treatment

Many pharmacologic agents have been suggested for treatment of local and regional myalgia and myofascial pain as well as fibromyalgia. These treatments include NSAIDs, opioid pain medications, antidepressant medications (eg, tricyclic antidepressants and selective serotonin reuptake inhibitors), benzodiazepines and other muscle relaxants, and sleep-modifying medications (see chapter 23).

Deciding which medication and how much to use is difficult, especially because many of the medications suggested are being used for an indication not approved by the US Food and Drug Administration. Medications with enough literature to permit a systematic review are the topical pain medications, the muscle relaxants, and the antidepressants. Of these, most of the reviews are based on treatment of chronic nonspecific musculoskeletal pain disorders and not masticatory-specific myalgia. None demonstrate high efficacy, but all show some promise. Two reviews in the Cochrane Library database examined topical medications for the treatment of either chronic musculoskeletal pain (containing NSAIDs) or acute and chronic pain of all types (rubefacient with salicylate).[88,89]

Neither disease group in these reviews specifically involved chronic myogenous pain. The review concluded that topical medications containing NSAIDs were effective and safe in treating chronic musculoskeletal conditions for 2 weeks.[88] The review of topically applied rubefacients containing salicylates concluded that these medications may be efficacious in the treatment of acute pain but that they have moderate to poor efficacy for chronic musculoskeletal and arthritic pain.[89] A review of the use of topical capsaicin for chronic musculoskeletal and/or neuropathic pain concluded that it has not been shown to be an effective stand-alone topical treatment.[90]

There have been four systematic reviews on the use of muscle relaxants for musculoskeletal pain. Two were focused on acute and nonspecific lower back pain, and both were in the Cochrane Library database.[91,92] These reviews examined randomized, placebo-controlled studies that used cyclobenzaprine, benzodiazepines, carisoprodol, or metaxalone. They concluded that all of these medications provided positive short-term benefits for this population but cautioned that the medications, especially carisoprodol and the benzodiazepines, had to be used with great caution because of their potential to be abused. One systematic review in the Cochrane Library examined the effect of cyclobenzaprine on fibromyalgia patients.[93] Cyclobenzaprine-treated patients were three times as likely to report overall improvement and to experience a moderate reduction in individual symptoms, particularly sleep problems, the first few days of use. The authors suggested that this medication did not produce any change in tender point palpation and the effect might be short lived; nevertheless, with these cautions, cyclobenzaprine was recommended as being an evidence-based treatment for fibromyalgia. In contrast, cyclobenzaprine was not rated in the top 12 treatments by the patients who participated in the poll on the RemedyFind website (see Table 33-2).[75]

A non–Cochrane Library review of muscle relaxants for myofascial face pain was published recently.[94] This systematic review concluded that the use of muscle relaxants in patients with myofascial pain involving the masticatory muscles seems to be justified but that current research can only be judged as weak. Therefore, the risk-benefit ratio of these medications must be considered before use.

One review on the use of various antidepressants for the treatment of fibromyalgia has been published.[95] This study indicated that there is enough evidence to support their use. The medical societies also all endorsed the use of medications for fibromyalgia, and two specifically suggested antidepressant medications as appropriate therapy. The efficacy of nonopioid analgesics (over-the-counter or pre-scription) and opioid analgesics for chronic musculoskeletal pain or fibromyalgia were not reviewed.

Behavioral management

Many behavioral therapies have been suggested for treatment of local and regional myalgia and myofascial pain as well as fibromyalgia (see chapter 26). Moreover, two of the three medical societies endorsed this form of therapy as justified and efficacious. These treatments include various forms of therapy with a psychologist, the most common being cognitive behavioral therapy. Sometimes these methods are a component of a combined multidisciplinary program and sometimes they are stand-alone treatments. One area of behavioral therapy that is recommended by the National Fibromyalgia Association is behavioral therapy dealing with sleep disturbance.

Two reviews have covered the use of behavioral therapy for both fibromyalgia and chronic musculoskeletal pain.[96,97] The results suggested that stand-alone behavioral therapy is not a powerful treatment and, in fact, that exercise therapy is equal or better in efficacy.[96] The use of a multidisciplinary approach for fibromyalgia was reviewed and found not to be highly efficacious either.[97] The third review in this area concluded that nonpharmacologic treatments (mostly behavioral in nature) are better than pharmacologic treatment when the two methods are compared directly.[98]

Final Recommendations

The decision of which treatment is appropriate for myogenous pain of the masticatory system begins with a correct diagnosis. In addition, it is very helpful if both the etiology and mechanism underlying the pain can be determined. If the correct etiologic and mechanism-based diagnosis is made, then the appropriate treatment choice should logically follow. Unfortunately, more than 20 types of therapy have been identified in this chapter, and systematic reviews of the published data have only been conducted for 8 of these therapies. Given these limitations, the best recommendations that can be made are as follows:

1. For the patient with traumatic-onset local myalgia with secondary trismus, the commonsense recommendations for treatment are rest, ice, and NSAIDs. As the symptoms subside, frequent daily active mobilization of the jaw is recommended, until normal motion is achieved.
2. For the patient with secondary local or regional myalgia, it is appropriate to manage or minimize the local

pathologic condition first and then reevaluate the myogenous pain to determine if it has resolved or persists.

3. For the patient with local myalgia that appears secondary to self-reported parafunction, the use of an occlusal appliance is indicated (see chapter 25).

4. For the patient with any form of nontraumatic chronic myogenous pain, regardless of whether it is local, regional, or widespread myalgia (or with myofascial triggerpoints and/or fibromyalgia), if daily stress is suspected to be an important etiologic factor, it is likely that several of the following treatments are appropriate:

a. Daily aerobic exercise is beneficial; this exercise program can be supervised or self-directed.

b. Hot packs should be applied to the painful local or regional areas. Whole body thermal therapy (spa therapy or even hot baths daily) should also be considered for those patients who can tolerate the heat without other medical consequences.

c. Low doses of a tricyclic antidepressant (eg, amitriptyline or nortriptyline) may be helpful both as an adjunctive pain medication and to improve sleep. One review even suggested that the evidence is sufficient to recommend combining a low-dose tricyclic antidepressant with a low-dose selective serotonin reuptake inhibitor.[79]

d. Muscle relaxants, such as cyclobenzaprine or one of the various benzodiazepines, appear to be a logical choice for managing acute myogenous pain, but the long-term effects of these treatments for chronic myogenous pain are questionable.

e. For the patient with myofascial pain and local triggerpoints that generate referred pain when compressed, the use of a local anesthetic injection or dry needling of the most hyperirritable spots appears better than no treatment but may not be better than a credible placebo.

f. For the patient with myofascial pain, the data on the effectiveness of botulinum toxin injections into triggerpoints are not sufficient to make a recommendation.

g. For the patient with fibromyalgia, acupuncture treatments have been found to be better than sham acupuncture, but the data are limited.

h. For the high-stress–reporting patient with chronic myogenous pain that is associated with anxiety and/or depression, the evidence suggests that psychologically based treatments may be helpful, especially when the patient is resistant to medications or intolerant of their side effects.

References

1. Wolfe F, Simons DG, Fricton J, et al. The fibromyalgia and myofascial pain syndromes: A preliminary study of tender points and trigger points in persons with fibromyalgia, myofascial pain syndrome and no disease. J Rheumatol 1992;19:944–951.
2. Yunus MB, Kalyan-Raman UP, Kalyan-Raman K. Primary fibromyalgia syndrome and myofascial pain syndrome: Clinical features and muscle pathology. Arch Phys Med Rehabil 1988;69:451–454.
3. Aoki T, Naito H, Ota Y, Shiiki K. Myositis ossificans traumatica of the masticatory muscles: Review of the literature and report of a case. J Oral Maxillofac Surg 2002;60:1083–1088.
4. Steiner M, Gould AR, Kushner GM, Lutchka B, Flint R. Myositis ossificans traumatica of the masseter muscle: Review of the literature and report of two additional cases. Oral Surg Oral Med Oral Pathol Oral Radiol Endod 1997;84:703–707.
5. Reiter S, Winocur E, Gavish A, Eli I. Severe limitation of mouth opening [in Hebrew]. Refuat Hapeh Vehashinayim 2004;21:36–46, 95.
6. Haas DA. Localized complications from local anesthesia. J Calif Dent Assoc 1998;26:677–682.
7. Stone J, Kaban LB. Trismus after injection of local anesthetic. Oral Surg Oral Med Oral Pathol 1979;48:29–32.
8. Luchetti W, Cohen RB, Hahn GV, et al. Severe restriction in jaw movement after routine injection of local anesthetic in patients who have fibrodysplasia ossificans progressiva. Oral Surg Oral Med Oral Pathol Oral Radiol Endod 1996;81:21–25.
9. Yagiela JA, Benoit PW, Buoncristiani RD, Peters MP, Fort NF. Comparison of myotoxic effects of lidocaine with epinephrine in rats and humans. Anesth Analg 1981;60:471–480.
10. van Steenberghe D, De Vries JH, Hollander AP. Resistance of jaw-closing muscles to fatigue during repetitive maximal voluntary clenching efforts in man. Arch Oral Biol 1978;23:697–701.
11. Clark GT, Adler RC, Lee JJ. Jaw pain and tenderness levels during and after repeated sustained maximum voluntary protrusion. Pain 1991;45:17–22.
12. Clark GT, Jow RW, Lee JJ. Jaw pain and stiffness levels after repeated maximum voluntary clenching. J Dent Res 1989;68:69–71.
13. Arima T, Svensson P, Arendt-Nielsen L. Experimental grinding in healthy subjects: A model for postexercise jaw muscle soreness? J Orofac Pain 1999;13:104–114.
14. Wheeler AH. Myofascial pain disorders: Theory to therapy. Drugs 2004;64:45–62.
15. Yano H, Yamamoto H, Hirata R, Hirano A. Post-traumatic severe trismus caused by impairment of the masticatory muscle. J Craniofac Surg 2005;16:277–280.
16. Christensen LV, Tran KT, Mohamed SE. Gum chewing and jaw muscle fatigue and pains. J Oral Rehabil 1996;23:424–437.
17. Widmalm SE, Christiansen RL, Gunn SM. Oral parafunctions as temporomandibular disorder risk factors in children. Cranio 1995;13:242–246.

18. Schiffman EL, Fricton JR, Haley D. The relationship of occlusion, parafunctional habits and recent life events to mandibular dysfunction in a non-patient population. J Oral Rehabil 1992;19:201–223.

19. Carlsson GE, Egermark I, Magnusson T. Predictors of bruxism, other oral parafunctions, and tooth wear over a 20-year follow-up period. J Orofac Pain 2003;17:50–57.

20. Velly AM, Gornitsky M, Philippe P. Contributing factors to chronic myofascial pain: A case-control study. Pain 2003; 104:491–499.

21. Goulet JP, Lavigne GJ, Lund JP. Jaw pain prevalence among French-speaking Canadians in Quebec and related symptoms of temporomandibular disorders. J Dent Res 1995;74: 1738–1744.

22. Molina OF, dos Santos J Jr, Nelson SJ, Grossman E. Prevalence of modalities of headaches and bruxism among patients with craniomandibular disorder. Cranio 1997;15:314–325.

23. Sunakawa M, Chiang CY, Sessle BJ, Hu JW. Jaw electromyographic activity induced by the application of algesic chemicals to the rat tooth pulp. Pain 1999;80:493–501.

24. Cairns BE, Sessle BJ, Hu JW. Evidence that excitatory amino acid receptors within the temporomandibular joint region are involved in the reflex activation of the jaw muscles. J Neurosci 1998;18:8056–8064.

25. Clark GT, Choi JK, Browne PA. The efficacy of physical medicine treatment, including occlusal appliances, for a temporomandibular disorder population. In: Sessle BJ, Bryant PS, Dionne RA (eds). Temporomandibular Disorders and Related Pain Conditions. Seattle: IASP Press, 1995:375–397.

26. Yamaguchi T, Satoh K, Komatsu K, et al. Electromyographic activity of the jaw-closing muscles during jaw opening—Comparison of cases of masseter muscle contracture and TMJ closed lock. J Oral Rehabil 2002;29:1063–1068.

27. Classification of chronic pain. Descriptions of chronic pain syndromes and definitions of pain terms. Prepared by the International Association for the Study of Pain. Subcommittee on Taxonomy: Pain 1986;3(suppl):S1–S225.

28. Travell JG. Myofascial trigger points: Clinical view. In: Bonica JJ, Albe-Fessard D (eds). Advances in Pain Research and Therapy. New York: Raven Press, 1976:919–926.

29. Travell JG, Simons DG. Myofascial Pain and Dysfunction: The Trigger Point Manual. Baltimore: Williams & Wilkins, 1983.

30. Simons DG. Muscle pain syndromes. 1. Am J Phys Med 1975;54:289–311.

31. Simons DG. Muscle pain syndromes. 2. Am J Phys Med 1976;55:15–42.

32. Kellgren JH. Observations on referred pain arising from muscle. Clin Sci 1938;3:175–190.

33. Mense S. Considerations concerning the neurobiologic basis of muscle pain. Can J Physiol Pharmacol 1991;9:610–616.

34. Mense S. Nociception from skeletal muscle in relation to clinical muscle pain. Pain 1993;54:241–289.

35. Mense S. Referral of muscle pain new aspects. Pain Forum 1994;3:1–9.

36. Simons DG. Neurophysiologic basis of pain caused by trigger points. APS J 1994;3:17–19.

37. Fields HL. Brainstem modulation of nociceptor-driven withdrawal reflexes. Ann NY Acad Sci 1989;563:34–44.

38. Chung JW, Ohrbach R, McCall WD Jr. Effect of increased sympathetic activity on electrical activity from myofascial painful areas. Am J Phys Med Rehabil 2004;83:842–850.

39. Hong CZ, Simons DG. Pathophysiologic and electrophysiologic mechanisms of myofascial trigger points. Arch Phys Med Rehabil 1998;79:863–872.

40. McPartland JM. Travell trigger points—Molecular and osteopathic perspectives. J Am Osteopath Assoc 2004;104: 244–249.

41. Giniatullin RA, Sokolova EM. ATP and adenosine inhibit transmitter release at the frog neuromuscular junction through distinct presynaptic receptors. Br J Pharmacol 1998; 124:839–844.

42. Mense S, Simons DG. Muscle Pain: Understanding its Nature, Diagnosis, and Treatment. Philadelphia: Lippincott Williams & Wilkins, 2001.

43. Cummings TM, White AR. Needling therapies in the management of myofascial trigger point pain: A systematic review. Arch Phys Med Rehabil 2001;82:986–992.

44. Wolfe F, Ross K, Anderson J, et al. The prevalence and characteristics of fibromyalgia in the general population. Arthritis Rheum 1995;8:19–28.

45. Croft P, Rigby AS, Boswell R, et al. The prevalence of chronic widespread pain in the general population. J Rheumatol 1993;20:710–713.

46. Lindell L, Bergman S, Petersson IF, et al. Prevalence of fibromyalgia and chronic widespread pain. Scand J Primary Health Care 2000;18:149–153.

47. Wolfe F, Smythe HA, Yunus MB, et al. The American College of Rheumatology 1990 criteria for the classification of fibromyalgia: Report of the multicenter criteria committee. Arthritis Rheum 1990;30:160–172.

48. Mountz JM, Bradley LA, Alarcon GS. Abnormal functional activity of the central nervous system in fibromyalgia syndrome. Am J Med Sci 1998;315:385–396.

49. Vaeroy H, Helle R, Forre O, Kass E, Terenius L. Elevated CSF levels of substance P and high incidence of Raynaud phenomenon in patients with fibromyalgia: New features for diagnosis. Pain 1988;32:21–26.

50. Russell IJ, Orr MD, Littman B, et al. Elevated cerebrospinal fluid levels of substance P in patients with the fibromyalgia syndrome. Arthritis Rheum 1994;37:1593–1601.

51. Classification and diagnostic criteria for headache disorders, cranial neuralgias, and facial pain. Headache Classification Committee of the International Headache Society. Cephalalgia 1988;8(suppl 7):1–96.

52. Sohn MK, Graven-Nielsen T, Arendt-Nielsen L, Svensson P. Effects of experimental muscle pain on mechanical properties of single motor units in human masseter. Clin Neurophysiol 2004;115:76–84.

53. Clark GT, Beemsterboer PL, Rugh JD. Nocturnal masseter muscle activity and the symptoms of masticatory dysfunction. J Oral Rehabil 1981;8:279–286.

54. Ashton-Miller JA, McGlashen KM, Herzenberg JE, Stohler CS. Cervical muscle myoelectric response to acute experimental sternocleidomastoid pain. Spine 1990;15:1006–1012.

55. Stohler CS, Zhang X, Lund JP. The effect of experimental jaw muscle pain on postural muscle activity. Pain 1996;66:215–221.

56. Svensson P, Houe L, Arendt-Nielsen L. Bilateral experimental muscle pain changes electromyographic activity of human jaw-closing muscles during mastication. Exp Brain Res 1997;116:182–185.

57. Clark GT, Sakai S, Merrill RL, Flack VF, McCreary CP. Cross correlation between stress, pain, physical activity, and temporalis muscle EMG in tension-type headache. Cephalalgia 1995;15:511–518, discussion 451.

58. Clark GT, Sakai S, Merrill R, Flack VF, McArthur D, McCreary C. Waking and sleeping temporalis EMG levels in tension-type headache patients. J Orofac Pain 1997 Fall;11:298–306.

59. Miyamoto K, Ishizuka Y, Ueda HM, Saifuddin M, Shikata N, Tanne K. Masseter muscle activity during the whole day in children and young adults. J Oral Rehabil 1999;26:858–864.

60. Maekawa K, Clark GT, Kuboki T. Intramuscular hypoperfusion, adrenergic receptors, and chronic muscle pain. J Pain 2002;3:251–260.

61. Fassbender HG, Wegner K. Morphology and pathogenesis of soft-tissue rheumatism [in German]. Z Rheumaforsch 1973;32:355–374.

62. Larsson B, Bjork J, Kadi F, Lindman R, Gerdle B. Blood supply and oxidative metabolism in muscle biopsies of female cleaners with and without myalgia. Clin J Pain 2004;20:440–446.

63. Lund N, Bengtsson A, Thorborg P. Muscle tissue oxygen pressure in primary fibromyalgia. Scand J Rheumatol 1986;15:165–173.

64. Klemp P, Nielsen HV, Korsgard J, Crone P. Blood flow in fibromyotic muscles. Scand J Rehabil Med 1982;14:81–82.

65. Delcanho RE, Kim YJ, Clark GT. Haemodynamic changes induced by submaximal isometric contraction in painful and non-painful human masseter using near–infra-red spectroscopy. Arch Oral Biol 1996;41:585–596.

66. Acero CO Jr, Kuboki T, Maekawa K, Yamashita A, Clark GT. Haemodynamic responses in chronically painful, human trapezius muscle to cold pressor stimulation. Arch Oral Biol 1999;44:805–812.

67. Hidaka O, Yanagi M, Takada K. Mental stress–induced physiological changes in the human masseter muscle. J Dent Res 2004;83:227–231.

68. Gossen ER, Ivanova TD, Garland SJ. Ischemia sensitivity and motoneuron after hyperpolarization in human motor units. Muscle Nerve 2004;30:195–201.

69. Graven-Nielsen T, Jansson Y, Segerdahl M, et al. Experimental pain by ischaemic contractions compared with pain by intramuscular infusions of adenosine and hypertonic saline. Eur J Pain 2003;7:93–102.

70. Issberner U, Reeh PW, Steen KH. Pain due to tissue acidosis: A mechanism for inflammatory and ischemic myalgia? Neurosci Lett 1996;208:191–194.

71. Steen AE, Reeh PW, Geisslinger G, Steen KH. Plasma levels after per oral and topical ibuprofen and effects upon low pH-induced cutaneous and muscle pain. Eur J Pain 2000;4:195–209.

72. Pan JW, Hamm JR, Rothman DL, Shulman RG. Intracellular pH in human skeletal muscle by 1H NMR. Proc Natl Acad Sci U S A 1988;85:7836–7839.

73. Zatina MA, Berkowitz HD, Gross GM, Maris JM, Chance B. 31P nuclear magnetic resonance spectroscopy: Noninvasive biochemical analysis of the ischemic extremity. J Vasc Surg 1986;3:411–420.

74. Bagis S, Tamer L, Sahin G, et al. Free radicals and antioxidants in primary fibromyalgia: An oxidative stress disorder? Rheumatol Int 2005;25:188–190.

75. RemedyFind [website]. Available at: http://www.remedyfind.com. Accessed 16 Sept 2005.

76. Karagulle MZ, Karagulle M. Balneotherapy and spa therapy of rheumatic diseases in Turkey: A systematic review [in German]. Forsch Komplementarmed Klass Naturheilkd 2004;11:33–41.

77. The National Fibromyalgia Association [website]. Available at: http://www.fmaware.org. Accessed 16 Sept 2005.

78. American Academy of Physical Medicine and Rehabilitation [website]. Available at: http://www.aapmr.org. Accessed 16 Sept 2005.

79. American College of Rheumatology [website]. Available at: http://www.rheumatology.org. Accessed 16 Sept 2005.

80. American Academy of Family Physicians [website]. Available at: http://www.aafp.org. Accessed 16 Sept 2005.

81. The Cochrane Collaboration [website]. Available at http://www.cochrane.org. Accessed 16 Sept 2005.

82. Busch A, Schachter CL, Peloso PM, Bombardier C. Exercise for treating fibromyalgia syndrome. The Cochrane Database of Systemic Reviews [website]. In: The Cochrane Library, Issue 4, 2004. Oxford, England: Update Software. Available at: http://www.mrw.interscience.wiley.com/cochrane/clsysrev/articles/CD003786/frame.html. Accessed 16 Sept 2005.

83. Kurtze N. Fibromyalgia—Effect of exercise [in Norwegian]. Tidsskr Nor Laegeforen 2004;124:2475–2478.

84. Berman BM, Ezzo J, Hadhazy V, Swyers JP. Is acupuncture effective in the treatment of fibromyalgia? J Fam Pract 1999;48:213–218.

85. Lee TL. Acupuncture and chronic pain management. Ann Acad Med Singapore 2000;29:17–21.

86. van Tulder MW, Cherkin DC, Berman B, Lao L, Koes B. The effectiveness of acupuncture in the management of acute and chronic low back pain. A systematic review within the framework of the Cochrane Collaboration Back Review Group. Spine 1999;24:1113–1123.

87. Wheeler AH, Goolkasian P, Gretz SS. A randomized, double-blind, prospective pilot study of botulinum toxin injection for refractory, unilateral, cervicothoracic, paraspinal, myofascial pain syndrome. Spine 1998;23:1662–1666.

88. Mason L, Moore RA, Edwards JE, Derry S, McQuay HJ. Topical NSAIDs for chronic musculoskeletal pain: Systematic review and meta-analysis. BMC Musculoskelet Disord 2004;5:28.

89. Mason L, Moore RA, Edwards JE, McQuay HJ, Derry S, Wiffen PJ. Systematic review of efficacy of topical rubefacients containing salicylates for the treatment of acute and chronic pain. BMJ 2004;328:995; comment 998.

90. Mason L, Moore RA, Derry S, Edwards JE, McQuay HJ. Systematic review of topical capsaicin for the treatment of chronic pain. BMJ 2004;328:991; comment 998.

91. van Tulder MW, Touray T, Furlan AD, Solway S, Bouter LM. Cochrane Back Review Group. Muscle relaxants for nonspecific low back pain: A systematic review within the framework of the Cochrane collaboration. Spine 2003;28:1978–1992.

92. Toth PP, Urtis J. Commonly used muscle relaxant therapies for acute low back pain: A review of carisoprodol, cyclobenzaprine hydrochloride, and metaxalone. Clin Ther 2004;26:1355–1367.

93. Tofferi JK, Jackson JL, O'Malley PG. Treatment of fibromyalgia with cyclobenzaprine: A meta-analysis. Arthritis Rheum 2004;51:9–13.

94. Manfredini D, Landi N, Tognini F, Orlando B, Bosco M. Muscle relaxants in the treatment of myofascial face pain. A literature review. Minerva Stomatol 2004;53:305–313.

95. O'Malley PG, Balden E, Tomkins G, Santoro J, Kroenke K, Jackson JL. Treatment of fibromyalgia with antidepressants: A meta-analysis. J Gen Intern Med 2000;15:659–666.

96. Hadhazy VA, Ezzo J, Creamer P, Berman BM. Mind-body therapies for the treatment of fibromyalgia. A systematic review. J Rheumatol 2000;27:2911–2918.

97. Karjalainen K, Malmivaara A, van Tulder M, et al. Multidisciplinary rehabilitation for fibromyalgia and musculoskeletal pain in working age adults. The Cochrane Database of Systemic Reviews [website]. In: The Cochrane Library, Issue 3, 1999. Oxford, England: Update Software. Available at: http://www.mrw.interscience.wiley.com/cochrane/clsysrev/articles/CD001984/frame.html. Accessed 16 Sept 2005.

98. Rossy LA, Buckelew SP, Dorr N, et al. A meta-analysis of fibromyalgia treatment interventions Ann Behav Med 1999;21:180–191.

Treatment of Maxillofacial Movement Disorders

Leon A. Assael

Treatment of maxillofacial movement disorders has historically been based on attempts to mitigate the expressed symptoms (eg, alteration of normal functional movements) rather than to address the underlying etiologic pathosis in the basal ganglia. Treatments designed to address only the expression of abnormal movement are often similar for many diseases. For example, the use of botulinum toxin for the management of oromandibular dystonia is the same as that for treatment of blepharospasm or essential tremor, although the etiologies of these disorders differ. On the other hand, treatment directed at the underlying pathologic condition, such as administration of levodopa for Parkinson disease, is disease specific but not symptom specific. The dopaminergic effect of levodopa acts directly on the etiologic site in the basal ganglia.

To organize discussion of these issues, this chapter is arranged according to treatment for symptoms common to many diseases rather than in terms of disease-specific treatment. However, the management of maxillofacial movement disorders is often performed via multiple approaches involving concomitant treatment for the peripheral expression of movement disorders and the associated central nervous system dysfunction. Although treatment specific to maxillofacial movement disorders can be useful in some patients, a global approach to these disorders also focuses on other aspects of treatment strategy. This global approach includes improvement of the patient's quality of life and care that meets the individual patient's desires and needs.

Symptom-Based Treatment

Hypokinesia, Akinesia, and Rigidity

Hypokinesia, often associated with parkinsonian syndromes, is a failure of initiation and appropriate temporal sequence of movement. In the maxillofacial region, difficulties with facial expression, speech, chewing, and swallowing become apparent. One of the most basic therapies for hypokinesia is the practice of sequential movement in a repetitive and prescribed fashion. Modest, but not progressive, improvement in upper extremity function has been noted in one study of practice exercises for hypokinesia.[1]

Hypokinesia-affected Parkinson disease patients undergo physical and occupational therapy exercises involving both passive and active purposeful movements. Practice movements are often focused on improving activities of daily living, such as communicating or grooming. However, a combination of head, neck, and facial muscle practice movements for hypokinesia may also be used.

Looking into a mirror while the facial muscles are being exercised can give the patient helpful visual feedback to encourage appropriate movement. In addition to visual cues, the use of interactive verbal prompts, mimicking, and memory cues may be helpful in the therapy for facial hypokinesia. However, when hypokinesia is associated with a cognitive decline, practice movements will likely be less effective.

Hypokinesia associated with dementia and Alzheimer disease or resulting from a cerebrovascular accident, head injury, HIV encephalitis, brain tumor, or multiple sclerosis causes progressive loss of function that may hasten death. Relief of rigidity, a "locked-in" hypokinesia state, may provide significant improvement in patients with these diseases. Passive motion of akinetic muscle groups can offset some of the muscle wasting associated with disuse. Drug therapy is mostly directed toward the basal ganglia pathosis; the leading drug is levodopa. In addition, the use of lorazepam has occasionally produced significant improvement in patients in these locked-in akinetic states.[2]

Akinesia and rigidity are also associated with patient falls.[3] Rigidity of the facial muscles and muscles of mastication can result in dental injury or, rarely, fracture of facial bones when falls occur, because the facial akinesia leaves the patient unable to protect the face from impact. Strategies to prevent falls and maxillofacial and orthopedic injury resulting from rigidity should be part of the treatment of these patients.

Oral appliances to protect against dental injury may be of value in a limited number of patients. However, patients with akinesia may be unable to prevent displacement of appliances or prostheses into the airway. Therefore, judicious assessment of the patient must be completed before an oral prosthesis is used in the rigid or akinetic patient.

Bradykinesia

Slow motor performance (bradykinesia) is associated with diseases of the basal ganglia but is also a universal progressive finding in aging, where there is loss of dorsolateral brain function.[4] Speech, swallowing, mastication, and facial expression are affected in the head and neck. Decreased range of motion, decreased strength, delayed initiation of movement, and decreased velocity may require treatment.

The most obvious treatment for bradykinesia in the maxillofacial region is alteration of the diet to improve chewing and swallowing. Progression to a soft or liquid diet may also result in the need for assistance with feeding from a health aide. In addition, patients must be allowed sufficient meal time to obtain adequate nourishment.

Patients with bradykinesia often need assistance with oral hygiene. In such instances, a mechanical toothbrush and other oral hygiene aides are useful. Substantial safety, social, and community support systems are necessary for patients with bradykinesia.

Levodopa is the established mainstay of pharmacologic therapy for akinesia and bradykinesia associated with loss of dopaminergic function of the basal ganglia.

Hypotonia

Hypotonia, in which muscles are flaccid and weak, produces a classic facial appearance and functional abnormalities in mastication, breathing, and speech. Speech therapy and physical therapy are methods of strengthening the affected muscles and improving their tone. Growth hormone has also been effective in improving muscle strength in patients with Prader-Willi syndrome and other congenital hypotonias.[5]

Children with hypotonia can also suffer from upper airway obstruction, especially obstructive sleep apnea. Distraction osteogenesis has been successfully used in such children to improve the upper airway and relieve the sleep apnea.[6] Hypotonia may be associated with cleft lip and palate, as in Kabuki syndrome, or it may occur in isolation.[7] In the former group, problems of speech, swallowing, and dental occlusion can be severe.

Palatopharyngoplasty is a surgical procedure that can be used to mitigate velopharyngeal insufficiency and thus improve speech and swallowing in patients with hypotonia.[8] Orthodontic therapy and subsequent orthognathic surgery during adolescence are often necessary because of the growth and development problems associated with congenital hypotonias.

Stimulation of normal function may promote improved oral facial development in the hypotonic child. Devices to promote sucking, feeding, and dentofacial development are broadly used.[9] Although their efficacy has not been established in clinical trials, oral appliances may serve to encourage facial growth and possibly to improve dental occlusion.

Hyperkinesia

The most common form of maxillofacial hyperkinesia is bruxism. Although bruxism has been presumed to be related to increased emotional stress or occlusal abnormality, it can also be associated with alcoholism, head injury, and medications such as levodopa and serotonin reuptake inhibitors.[10,11] Whereas there is evidence that severe emotional stress can affect the course of both diurnal and nocturnal bruxism, the role of occlusion in initiating bruxism has been minimized by recent research.[12] Hence, alteration of the dental occlusion by irreversible means is not recommended for the treatment of bruxism.

Treatment of bruxism ideally should be focused on elimination of the underlying cause. However, when the specific etiology cannot be determined, oral appliances can be helpful in preventing the dental and muscular consequences of sleep bruxism (see chapter 25). On a short-term basis, a low dose of the tricyclic antidepressant amitriptyline (10 to 20 mg at bedtime) also can be used to alter the sleep cycle and decrease bruxing activity.

Choreic hyperkinesias occur in Huntington disease and tardive dyskinesia and in the elderly. Although therapy directed at the cause of the underlying condition is necessary, protective oral appliances are often an important adjunct.

Dyskinesia

Oral dyskinesias are characterized by abnormal movements of facial and jaw muscles that cause patients distress. Although they are often of unclear etiology, they can be related to the use of certain psychotropic drugs (tardive dyskinesia), which cause hypersensitivity of the dopamine receptors. Elimination of the drug or a reduction of the dose may resolve the problem, but sometimes the condition can be permanent.

New oral prostheses also have been associated with the onset of oral dyskinesia. Altered occlusion or a bolus effect caused by the prosthesis may induce hypersalivation and dyskinesia. Adjustment or alteration of the prosthesis may play a role in alleviating such oral dyskinesias.[13]

Tremor

Oral facial tremor may be the result of Parkinson disease, or it may be an essential tremor. So far, no therapy directed at the specific aspects of essential oral facial tremor has been reported, so the clinician must rely on commonsense approaches to the management of these patients. The tremor is always worsened by fatigue and anxiety. Establishing the dental occlusion in a functional position for prosthetic or restorative dentistry may be problematic in such patients. The use of mouth props and decreasing the anxiety associated with treatment will often reduce the impact that an oral facial tremor has on dental treatment.

Dystonia

Dystonias can produce rotation and contracture of the limbs, spine, head, and neck. Skeletofacial asymmetry and malocclusion may result from dystonia. Treatment of dys-

tonia focuses on symptomatic management with physical therapy, supportive therapy, and pharmacologic therapy.

Orthopedic braces can be useful in improving the patient's posture and cervical spine position. They may also prevent muscle shortening and the resulting fixed rotation of the spine. Because dystonias can respond to a geste antagoniste (sensory trick), orthopedic braces designed to relieve dystonia can be built with pressure points that correspond to these sites, thus generating muscle release.[14] Transcutaneous electrical neurostimulation has been used for dystonia as well.

Various strategies for drug therapy for dystonia are currently in use. These drug categories include:

1. *Dopaminergic drugs.* At least one form of dystonia, dopa-responsive dystonia, improves with levodopa therapy.
2. *Antidopaminergic drugs.* Earlier-generation antipsychotic drugs are not effective in the treatment of dystonia. Newer agents such as clozapine, which affects dopamine-induced activity by binding to dopamine receptors, are useful in the treatment of oromandibular dystonias.[15]
3. *Anticholinergic drugs.* Trihexyphenidyl and diphenhydramine are two drugs with an anticholinergic effect that are useful for the treatment of some dystonias, such as blepharospasm. Dry mouth, dental caries, and drowsiness are debilitating side effects in some patients who undergo chronic anticholinergic treatment for dystonia.
4. *Benzodiazepines.* Diazepam and lorazepam historically have been used for craniocervical dystonia. Although still in common use, their efficacy does not compare to that of other, more directed therapies for dystonia.
5. *γ-Aminobutyric acid autoreceptor agonist drugs.* Baclofen may be of greater utility in oromandibular dystonia and cranial dystonia than in more generalized dystonias.
6. *Local anesthetics.* Injection of lidocaine can offer temporary relief of dystonia. Repeated injections are sometimes used. Although alcohol blocks have been used in the past, this therapy has now been supplanted by use of botulinum toxin. Local anesthesia might best serve today as a means of preassessing the value of botulinum toxin for specific sites of dystonia.
7. *Botulinum toxin.* Type A botulinum toxin has been shown to be effective in many patients with dystonia. In the first randomized clinical trial, more than twice as many patients treated with botulinum toxin experienced improvement compared with those who received a placebo.[16] Injections into the belly of the affected muscles are effective for 10 to 24 weeks. After repeated injections, the dystonia may have more sustained abatement, possibly because of atrophy of the affected mus-

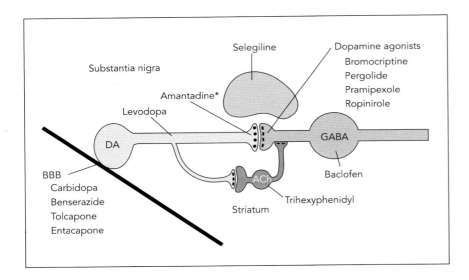

Fig 34-1 Sites of action of common drugs used in Parkinson disease. (BBB) Blood-brain barrier; (DA) dopamine; (ACh) acetylcholine; (GABA) γ-aminobutyric acid autoreceptor. *Site of action not known. (Adapted from *Parkinson Disease: Etiology, Diagnosis and Management.*[19])

cle. The dose of type A botulinum toxin is dependent on the size of the muscle (usual range, 5 to 50 units). This agent must be used carefully, because there is a potential for the solution to spread to sites that may produce undesirable results, such as in the soft palate, where displacement of the solution may result in hypotonia and a consequent swallowing disorder.

8. *Antiepileptic drugs.* Paroxysmal dystonias are treated with a variety of antiepileptic agents, such as phenytoin.

Direct deep brain stimulation of the internal globus pallidus via a neurosurgically placed probe is a reversible means of ameliorating dystonia. A prospective controlled clinical trial of direct deep brain stimulation has demonstrated marked improvement in patients with dystonia that is not responsive to medications.[17]

Disease-Specific Treatment

Parkinson Disease

In Parkinson disease, the degenerating cells in the substantia nigra are the dopaminergic cells. Dopamine depletion of greater than 90% results in parkinsonian symptoms.

Also, dopamine receptors in the substantia nigra and striatum (D1 and D2 dopamine receptors) are depleted in the early phase of the disease, resulting in loss of dopamine production.[18] Drug strategies for treatment of the symptoms of Parkinson disease fall into the following categories:

1. Direct replacement of dopamine
2. Dopamine agonists
3. Drugs to prevent metabolism of levodopa
4. Monoamine oxidase B inhibitors to prevent the breakdown of dopamine in the brain
5. Anticholinergic drugs to diminish tremor and rigidity
6. Amantadine, an antiviral drug with presynaptic and postsynaptic modulation qualities

These agents act in various sites involved in the production and use of dopamine. Their action may be presynaptic or postsynaptic (Fig 34-1). Levodopa is administered orally and acts to directly replace depleted sites of dopamine production in the substantia nigra. Stimulation of D1 and D2 receptors with dopamine agonists is a hallmark of pharmacotherapy of Parkinson disease.

The neuroprotection strategy in the treatment of Parkinson disease is designed to inhibit the further destruction of nigral cells. Although various agents such as vitamin E and selegiline have been used for neuroprotection, their efficacy has not yet been proven. Recently, attention has been directed toward the use of minocycline, an antibiotic, for its potential neuroprotective qualities.[20]

Surgical treatment of Parkinson disease has included thalamotomy and pallidotomy performed with stereotactic and other minimally invasive approaches. These procedures have afforded a modicum of benefit to a majority of patients.[21] Of particular interest is the use of fetal dopaminergic tissue transplanted into the brain of patients with Parkinson disease. The first randomized clinical trial of this method produced measurable improvement in the young patient with Parkinson disease.[22]

Essential Tremor

Essential tremor remains a common but often untreated or self-treated movement disorder. The most time-honored method to reduce essential tremor is consumption of ethyl alcohol. Even small doses of alcohol at mealtime have produced sustained improvement, but the risk of alcohol abuse remains, because progressively larger doses may be necessary.[23]

β-Adrenergic blockers, especially propranolol and more recently arotinolol, are effective in obtaining objective improvement of essential tremor.[24] Antiepileptics such as primidone and phenobarbital are utilized with varying success.[25] Many other drugs widely used in other movement disorders, such as benzodiazepines and antiparkinsonian drugs, are also used. Thalamic surgery, either involving stimulation or thalamotomy, has been used as well.

Orobuccolingual Tardive Dyskinesia

Chronic treatment with antipsychotic drugs that block central nervous system dopamine receptors can produce a variety of maxillofacial movement problems, including unpredictable lip smacking, cheek and lip biting, tongue projecting, and generalized facial restlessness. Limiting the use of neuroleptic drugs to doses necessary to control psychoses and drug selection that limits risk are the hallmarks of prevention or mitigation of tardive dyskinesia. The severity of orobuccolingual tardive dyskinesia may relate to the dental status of some patients. In one study, unrestored edentulous patients were found to have more severe symptoms than dentate patients.[26]

Myotonic Dystrophy

Oculogyric crisis

Oculogyric crisis is characterized by its sudden onset and startling feature of upwardly directed eyes, extended neck, and thrusting tongue. Attention to the underlying precipitating cause is key to the treatment of an oculogyric crisis. Although psychotropic drugs are often the precipitating factor, other prescription drugs, for example

cetirizine, a common drug for treating seasonal allergies, can induce this condition in a self-limiting way.[27] Withdrawal of the drug and waiting for the effect to abate generally result in a reversal of the symptoms.

Spontaneous Oral Dyskinesias

Craniocervical dystonia (oromandibular dystonia or Brueghel syndrome)

This focal dystonia includes muscle spasm and altered jaw position, such as laterognathia. Cases temporally associated with lengthy dental treatment have been reported.[28] Limiting the extent of uncomfortable jaw positioning during treatment is likely a useful preventive measure.

Blepharospasm

This condition can occur in isolation or involve a complete hemifacial spasm. It is treated with a botulinum toxin A injection of 5 to 10 units, anticholinergics, benzodiazepines, or a combination of these drugs.

Torticollis

In general, torticollis is a movement disorder most frequently occurring in infants and children. Therapy with oral medication for such movement disorders in children involves special consideration with regard to growth and mental development.[29] Orthopedic splints generally will not prevent facial growth asymmetry. In fact, chin pressure from orthopedic devices can adversely impact maxillomandibular growth.

Huntington Disease

Therapeutic advances in the treatment of Huntington disease have been slow, in spite of an enhanced understanding of the genetic loci for this disease. Treatment for this neuropsychiatric disorder, which is characterized by dementia, paranoia, and choreas, is directed at the movement disorder as well as the psychosis and altered behavior.

Riluzole, olanzapine, and amantadine are used for the movement disorders of Huntington disease. Selective serotonin reuptake inhibitors and mirtazapine are of value for the treatment of anxiety and depression. Antipsychotic drugs may also be necessary.[30]

An understanding of the molecular biology of Huntington disease may lead to effective treatment in the future. It is a polyglutamine (polyQ) disorder in which proteins in the central nervous system produce polyQ-encoding repeats within otherwise unrelated gene products. This accumulation of polyQ causes death of the affected neurons. Drugs are being developed to prevent the accumulation of polyglutamine and thus prevent such loss of neurons.[31]

Because of the long prodrome of Huntington disease (sometimes decades in length), neuroprotective treatment strategies are also being considered. Ciliary neurotrophic factor is known to be protective of striatum neurons. Phase I clinical studies involving its placement into the brain of subjects with Huntington disease are now underway.[32]

Tics

Tourette syndrome

The vocal and motor tics of Tourette syndrome can cause oral injury.[33] Such patients require special attention during dental treatment because of the sudden unanticipated and uncontrolled movements that may occur. Restraining the patient is not a workable approach because it may produce a greater dystonia. Judicious control of dental instruments is recommended.

Myoclonus

Palatal myoclonus is a sudden clicking of the palate and pharynx that may also involve the ears (tinnitus or tympanic myoclonus) or eyes (oculopalatal myoclonus) Imaging of the brain, especially the brainstem, may reveal that the underlying cause is a stroke, neoplasm, or vascular malformation. In the absence of a treatable underlying cause, 5 units of botulinum toxin injected in the soft palate muscles has been shown to temporarily eliminate the myoclonic contractions.[34]

Summary

The ideal treatment of maxillofacial movement disorders relies on proper diagnosis and intervention directed at the underlying pathologic condition. It is preferable to direct treatment toward the etiologic factors but, when it is not possible to address these factors, symptomatic treatment also can be used. Often, dental procedures, medical therapies, and surgical intervention can be combined to offer patients with maxillofacial movement disorders substantial improvement in their condition.

References

1. Agostino R, Curra A, Soldati G, et al. Prolonged practice is of scarce benefit in improving motor performance in Parkinson's disease. Mov Disord 2004;19:1285–1293.
2. Alisky JM. Is the immobility of advanced dementia a form of lorazepam-responsive catatonia? Am J Alzheimers Dis Other Demen 2004;19:213–214.
3. Syrjala P, Luukinen H, Pyhtinen J, Tolonen U. Neurological diseases and accidental falls of the aged. J Neurol 2003;250:1063–1069.
4. Ross GW, Petrovitch H, Abbott RD, et al. Parkinsonian signs and substantia nigra neuron density in descendants elders without PD. Ann Neurol 2004;56:532–539.
5. Allen DB, Carrel AL. Growth hormone therapy for Prader-Willi syndrome: A critical appraisal. J Pediatr Endocrinol Metab 2004;17(suppl 4):1297–1306.
6. Preciado DA, Sidman JD, Sampson DE, Rimell FL. Mandibular distraction to relieve airway obstruction in children with cerebral palsy. Arch Otolaryngol Head Neck Surg 2004;130:741–745.
7. Schrander-Stumpel CT, Spruyt L, Curfs LM, Defloor T, Schrander JJ. Kabuki syndrome: Clinical data in 20 patients, literature review, and further guidelines for preventive management. Am J Med Genet A 2005;132:234–243.
8. Brondsted K, Liisberg WB, Orsted A, Prytz S, Fogh-Andersen P. Surgical and speech results following palatopharyngoplasty operations in Denmark 1959–1977. Cleft Palate J 1984;21:170–179.
9. Korbmacher H, Limbrock J, Kahl-Nieke B. Orofacial development in children with Down's syndrome 12 years after early intervention with a stimulating plate. J Orofac Orthop 2004;65(1):60–73.
10. Hartmann E. Alcohol and bruxism. N Engl J Med 1979;301:333–334.
11. Ellison J, Stanziani P. SSRI-associated nocturnal bruxism in four patients. J Clin Psychiatry 1993;54:432–434.
12. Manfredini D, Landi N, Romagnoli M, Bosco M. Psychic and occlusal factors in bruxers. Aust Dent J 2004;49:84–89.
13. Blanchet PJ, Rompre PH, Lavigne GJ, Lamarche C. Oral dyskinesia: A clinical overview. Int J Prosthodont 2005;18:10–19.
14. Jankovic J. Treatment of dystonia. In: Watts R, Koller W (eds). Movement Disorders: Neurologic Principles and Practice. New York: McGraw-Hill, 1997:443.
15. Hanagasi HA, Bilgic B, Gurvit H, Emre M. Clozapine treatment in oromandibular dystonia. Clin Neuropharmacol 2004;27:84–86.
16. Truong D, Duane DD, Jankovic J, et al. Efficacy and safety of botulinum type A toxin (Dysport) in cervical dystonia: Results of the first US randomized, double-blind, placebo-controlled study. Mov Disord 2005;20:783–791.
17. Vidailhet M, Vercueil L, Houeto JL, et al. Bilateral deep-brain stimulation of the globus pallidus in primary generalized dystonia. New Engl J Med 2005;352:459–467.

18. Poewe W, Granata R. Pharmacological treatment of Parkinson's disease. In: Watts R, Koller W (eds). Movement Disorders: Neurologic Principles and Practice. New York: McGraw-Hill, 1997:201.

19. Parkinson Disease: Etiology, Diagnosis and Management [teaching slide set]. New York: WE MOVE (Worldwide Education and Awareness of Movement Disorders), 2000.

20. Zemke D, Majid A. The potential of minocycline for neuroprotection in human neurologic disease. Clin Neuropharmacol 2004;27:293–298.

21. Sidiskis J. Indications for surgical treatment of Parkinson's disease and outcome [in Lithuanian]. Medicina (Kaunas) 2003;39:990–995.

22. Greene P, Fahn S. Status of fetal tissue transplantation for the treatment of advanced Parkinson's disease. Neurosurg Focus 2002;13(5):e3.

23. Koller W, Busenbark K. Essential tremor. In: Watts R, Koller W (eds). Movement Disorders: Neurologic Principles and Practice. New York: McGraw-Hill, 1997:376.

24. Lee KS, Kim JS, Kim JW, Lee WY, Jeon BS, Kim D. A multicenter randomized crossover multiple-dose comparison study of arotinolol and propranolol in essential tremor. Parkinsonism Relat Disord 2003;9:341–347.

25. Serrano-Duenas M. Use of primidone in low doses (250 mg/day) versus high doses (750 mg/day) in the management of essential tremor. Double-blind comparative study with one-year follow-up. Parkinsonism Relat Disord 2003; 10:29–33.

26. Sandyk R, Kay SR. Edentulousness and neuroleptic-induced neck and trunk dyskinesia. Funct Neurol 1990;5:361–363.

27. Fraunfelder FW, Fraunfelder FT. Oculogyric crisis in patients taking cetirizine. Am J Ophthalmol 2004;137:355–357.

28. Schrag A, Bhatia KP, Quinn NP, Marsden CD. Atypical and typical cranial dystonia following dental procedures. Mov Disord 1999;14:492–496; comment 2000;15:366.

29. Edgar TS. Oral pharmacotherapy of childhood movement disorders. J Child Neurol 2003;18(suppl 1):S40–S49.

30. Bonelli RM, Wenning GK, Kapfhammer HP. Huntington's disease: Present treatments and future therapeutic modalities. Int Clin Psychopharmacol 2004;19:51–62.

31. Zhang X, Smith DL, Meriin AB, et al. A potent small molecule inhibits polyglutamine aggregation in Huntington's disease neurons and suppresses neurodegeneration in vivo. Proc Natl Acad Sci U S A 2005;102:892–897.

32. Bloch J, Bachoud-Levi AC, Deglon N, et al. Neuroprotective gene therapy for Huntington's disease, using polymer-encapsulated cells engineered to secrete human ciliary neurotrophic factor: Results of a phase I study. Hum Gene Ther 2004;15:968–975.

33. Friedlander AH, Cummings JL. Dental treatment of patients with Gilles de la Tourette's syndrome. Oral Surg Oral Med Oral Pathol 1992;73:299–303.

34. Jero J, Salmi T. Palatal myoclonus and clicking tinnitus in a 12-year-old girl—Case report. Acta Otolaryngol Suppl 2000;543: 61–62.

Surgical Management of Benign and Malignant Neoplasms

Lewis Clayman

Neoplasia of the mandibular condyle is uncommon and has unique clinical features; consequently, it presents both diagnostic and treatment dilemmas because of the overlap of symptoms with the more commonly occurring temporomandibular disorders (TMDs). Some of these lesions are unusual enough to be considered curiosities, and even the most commonly occurring tumorlike disorder, synovial chondromatosis, has been represented in the worldwide literature by fewer than 100 cases. Because of the overlap in signs and symptoms between condylar and synovial neoplasia and various TMDs, it is unlikely that a clinician would ordinarily include a tumor originating from the condyle or the synovium as a very good possibility in the differential diagnosis. Hence, the frequently encountered delay in the diagnosis of temporomandibular joint (TMJ) neoplasms is the result of a very low index of suspicion on the part of the examining clinician.

Selection of a course of treatment for entities that rarely occur is also difficult because of the lack of reliable data related to treatment outcomes. The evidence on which treatment decisions are generally based is far from adequate at this time. Moreover, data on long-term surveillance are generally lacking. Most reports either provide follow-up results of less than 2 years or do not report these data at all. Thus, the clinician often must make judgments about the treatment of patients with TMJ neoplasms using available data viewed through the prism of personal experience in treating neoplastic disease in other maxillofacial sites.

The TMJ contains bone, synovium, blood vessels, connective tissue, peripheral nerve fibers, and cartilage, and it is in close proximity to the superior head of the lateral pterygoid muscle. Consequently, neoplasms can arise from any one or combination of these tissues. Because

the condyle is cartilaginous in origin, osteochondromas, osteomas, and chondromas would be expected, and, in fact, these are among the more commonly occurring tumors in this site. Giant cell lesions would also be expected, because these are also known to occur preferentially in bone of cartilaginous origin and are found in bones subject to trauma associated with intraosseous hemorrhage. In addition, some tumorlike swellings that are not truly neoplastic, such as synovial chondromatosis, require consideration in the evaluation of masses in the TMJ.[1,2]

Secondary involvement of the joint also can occur by direct invasion from pathologic conditions arising adjacent to it or from metastasis. In fact, the most commonly reported neoplastic disease in the TMJ has been either an isolated metastasis or a direct extension from metastatic disease in the ramus. In the largest such series, 33 of the 40 reported cases of malignant disease within the condyle developed through one of these mechanisms.[3] This is in contradistinction to benign neoplasia, where extension to the condyle from such lesions in the ramus of the mandible is distinctly uncommon.[1,4]

The general rarity of condylar tumors is clarified by the detailed review by Nwoku and Koch[5] of 3,200 head and neck tumors treated in the Clinic for Maxillofacial and Plastic Surgery in Dusseldorf over a period of 20 years. They found only seven tumors of the mandibular condyle. Three of these were osteoma or osteochondroma and three were giant cell tumors, confirming the expectation that most of these tumors would be bone, cartilage, or giant cell lesions. In another, more recent comprehensive review of head and neck tumors from a major referral center in Toulouse, only six lesions of the TMJ were found.[6] These consisted of three cases of synovial chondromatosis, two cases of crystal dep-

Table 35-1	Classification of condylar tumors*	
Cell type	**Benign**	**Malignant**
Cartilage	Chondroblastoma Chondromyxoid fibroma Osteochondroma Chondroma	Chondrosarcoma
Bone	Osteoma Osteoid osteoma Osteoblastoma	Osteosarcoma Sarcoma: Paget disease, radiation
Marrow elements Hematopoietic		Plasmacytoma Myeloma Ewing sarcoma Lymphoma
Fat		Liposarcoma
Fibrous connective tissue	Desmoplastic fibroma Fibromyxoma Ossifying fibroma Nonossifying fibroma	Fibrosarcoma Malignant fibrous histiocytoma
Synovium	Proliferations: synovial chondromatosis, pigmented villonodular synovitis, ganglion, synovial cyst	Synovial sarcoma
Odontogenic	Myxoma Ossifying myxoma Ameloblastoma	
Uncertain etiology	Giant cell tumor Langerhans histiocytosis	Giant cell tumor
Vascular elements blood vessels	Hemangioma Glomus tumor	Angiosarcoma Hemangioendothelioma Hemangiopericytoma
Lymph vessels	Lymphangioma	Lymphangiosarcoma
Nerve tissue	Neurilemoma Neurofibroma Ganglioneuroma	

*Adapted from Spujt et al[9] and Batsakis.[10]

osition disease presenting as a pseudotumor and one case of synovial sarcoma.

The list of benign tumors and pseudoneoplastic diseases occurring in the joint includes synovial chondromatosis, pigmented villonodular synovitis, osteochondroma, chondroblastoma, osteoma, osteoid osteoma, "benign" osteoblastoma, giant cell tumor, Langerhans histiocytosis, ganglion, hemangioma, neurofibroma, neurilemoma, fibro-osseous lesions, nonossifying fibroma, myxoma and ossifying myxoma, and ameloblastoma (see chapter 21). The malignant lesions include the various sarcomas (osteogenic, chondrogenic, and fibrogenic), plasmacytoma and multiple myeloma, lymphoma, and metastasis and direct extension of malignancy from the nasopharynx or the parotid gland[3,7,8] (Table 35-1).

Among the signs and symptoms commonly associated with benign neoplasia of the mandibular condyle are a new-onset malocclusion, in particular unilateral apertognathia; trismus; mandibular deviation on mouth opening; reduction in maximum interincisal opening (MIO); joint noise; painless swelling, particularly in the preauricular region; and mandibular or facial asymmetry.[11,12] The preauricular location of a mass has led many clinicians to the mistaken consideration of primary parotid disease as the most likely entity for consideration in the differential diagnosis. For example, a case has been reported in which a neurofibroma of the joint was misdiagnosed as a parotid tumor.[13] Parotidectomies have also been performed on normal glands, after which the correct diagnosis of a TMJ tumor was made.[14]

With malignant lesions, most of the same signs and symptoms would be expected. In addition, the patient would be more likely to experience pain increased by jaw function, paresthesias, and altered hearing on the affected side.[3]

There has been little change in the treatment of benign bony TMJ lesions over the past 40 years, except that in some cases the condyle may be preserved rather than automatically resected, as was commonly done. In addition, efforts to use arthroscopic surgery in selected cases have been reported.[15] In general, small benign tumors of the condyle require a subperiosteal resection through a preauricular approach; larger ones, in which the periosteum has been breached, require a condylectomy. Occasionally, a conservative parotidectomy may also be required.[16] In addition, some slow-growing benign lesions with a very low recurrence potential, in particular the osteochondroma, may be removed in segments, preserving most of the condyle.[17,18]

In the treatment of malignant lesions, expectations of their probable behavior should be based on the known characteristics of the specific tumor in other maxillofacial sites, because there is invariably inadequate information to differentiate treatment options based on their behavior in the TMJ. In general, malignant lesions require wider access, usually by a temporal extension of the preauricular incision, and a willingness to remove adjacent structures en bloc if possible. This would include the parotid gland, facial nerve branches, and the skull base in the middle cranial fossa.[19–21]

Benign Neoplasms

Synovial Chondromatosis

This is the most common lesion of the TMJ that presents with characteristics of a tumor. However, it really is a pseudotumor with unique properties. The nomenclature has been imprecise, and this entity has been referred to variably as *synovialoma, synovial chondromatosis, synovial metaplasia, articular chondrosis, synovial chondrometaplasia, osteochondromatosis, periarticular tenosynovial chondrometaplasia*, and *diffuse enchondroma of the joint capsule*. However, the generally accepted term is *synovial chondromatosis*.[22,23]

The lesion maintains a particular resonance in the collective consciousness of oral and maxillofacial surgeons because of its colloquial name, *joint mice*. This combines an imaginative name and an unusual problem, where the name mimics one of the characteristics of the disorder. The joint is noisy, the crepitation calling to mind the nibbling of mice, and the fragments created within the joint are suggestive of the small fragments left behind after the mice have completed their work of destroying the joint.

Synovial chondromatosis represents a metaplastic process, the formation of nodules of cartilage within the synovial membrane.[24] During the early phase, some of these particles separate and some become loose bodies. Later in the process, nearly all become loose bodies, ranging in size from less than 1 mm to about 4 mm. They can number in the hundreds.[8,12] It is a benign, chronic, and progressive condition without any tendency to resolve spontaneously.[25] Conservative treatment consists of removal of the loose bodies and synovium, combined with arthroplasty. This usually suffices and the tendency to recur is low. Long-term follow-up data are poor; few patients have been observed beyond 2 years, and many reports fail to provide any follow-up information. Progression to malignancy in joints other than the TMJ has been reported in only two instances.[26,27]

Patients generally present with symptoms of vague pain in the preauricular area that may be associated with a lateral shift of the mandible. Swelling also may be present. An initial snap on opening is often heard, and there may be crepitation within the joint. The latter finding is more common later in the disease, when the degree of joint destruction is more pronounced. Pain may occur on palpation, and a mass may be present.[12,28,29] Some patients may have difficulty in closing the mouth. This finding may occur periodically as the loose bodies change position and alter the joint mechanics.

Synovial chondromatosis in the TMJ has only been reported as a monoarticular problem, and it is more common in the right than the left joint.[30] In the largest review, by Warner et al,[8] 82% of the patients had pain, 65% had swelling, and 50% had both. The MIO is usually normal,[24] although von Arx et al[23] found that 24% of their patients had a reduced MIO.

Because the signs and symptoms were so similar to those of some of the other TMDs, diagnosis is usually delayed, often for a period of years. The presence of a preauricular mass may be misinterpreted as a benign neoplasia of the parotid gland.[31] In some cases, the correct diagnosis was not made until after a parotidectomy was performed.[32] This lesion might occur in concert with other joint pathology; cases of chondromatosis have been reported concurrent with villonodular synovitis[33] and condylar hyperplasia.[34]

The first case of synovial chondromatosis was reported by the great German surgeon, Georg Axhausen,[28] in 1933. Since then the number of cases reported has reached 84, but no individual author has reported more than six cases.[8] These 84 patients have included 31 men and 53 women with an age range of 18 to 75 years. The average age at onset was 46.5 years for the males and 45.2 years for the females. The collective average age at onset was 45.7 years. In the group younger than 20 years there was 1 man and no women. Among those aged 21 to 40 years, there were 9 men and 23 women; from 41 to 60 years there were 16 men and 24 women, and from 60 to 75 years there were 5 men and 6 women. Among the 4 patients older than 70 years, there were 3 men and 1 woman. Overall the ratio of women to men was 1.7:1. The exception was in the age group older than 70 years, in which the ratio of women to men was 1:3. In other joints, it is more common in men than in women for all age groups.

The radiographic appearance of synovial chondromatosis is nonspecific. In a review of 42 cases by deBont et al,[34] 15 were interpreted as showing signs of osteoarthritis and 22, barely more than half, demonstrated loose bodies. Only 8 showed both loose bodies and signs of osteoarthritis. Other conditions also can create loose bodies in the TMJ. These include osteoarthritis, osteochondritis dissecans, intracapsular fractures of the condyle, and pyogenic and rheumatoid arthritis.[35,36]

However, most of these diseases are associated with only a small number of loose bodies. The singularity of synovial chondromatosis resides in the number of loose bodies, which vary from 1 to 480; only 15 of 42 patients in the review by deBont et al[34] had 10 or fewer loose bodies. The other diseases in the differential diagnosis were not associated with more than 10 loose bodies. In fact, in 5 of the 8 patients who had both loose bodies and signs of osteoarthritis, there were fewer than 10 loose bodies and only 3 had more than 10. Therefore, in only 5 (12%) of 42 cases of synovial chondromatosis were both loose bodies and signs of osteoarthritis found. Although these two findings are also associated with the other entities just mentioned, their occurrence is very low and, therefore, the presence of loose bodies should immediately force consideration of a diagnosis of synovial chondromatosis.

The loose bodies are found most often in the upper joint space. Only a few cases have been reported in the lower compartment. They are usually white or grayish white, firm or hard, and generally shaped like grains of rice, although occasionally they are more round. Their surface is usually smooth and the larger particles are sometimes lobulated. Occasionally their surface is rough. Sometimes the particles are loosely attached to the synovium and can be readily detached with an instrument. Rarely the bodies are found as a conglomerated mass.

Sometimes the nodules are embedded in the surface of the disc and are associated with perforations. Cases have been reported in which the disc was completely destroyed. Most of the time the condyle appears smooth, but rarely erosions or arthritic spurring are found. In some cases, the surface of the glenoid fossa may be roughened. Occasionally, a thickened joint capsule can be noted. Often the joint is distended and contains viscous, straw-colored fluid.[22,24,30]

Although nonsurgical treatment involving aspiration of joint fluid and injection of hyaluronic acid has been tried,[37] surgery is the most effective therapy. It has been suggested that the type of surgery should be based on the natural history of the disease. The metaplastic process passes through three stages: *(1)* active synovial disease without loose bodies, *(2)* synovial nodules plus loose bodies, and *(3)* multiple loose bodies associated with inactive synovial disease.[38–40] Therefore, whereas the first two stages require synovectomy plus removal of the nodules, the third stage should only require removal of the loose bodies. However, because the remaining synovium could still possess the potential for producing new loose bodies, most surgeons also recommend synovectomy in stage 3.

Discectomy is usually reserved for those patients in whom the disc has been perforated. Condylectomy is generally not required except in the rare instance when a large mass is located medial to the condyle and it cannot be removed without first removing the condyle.[22,24,30] Although arthroscopic surgery has been used in a few cases,[15] the most effective treatment is open surgery. Partial or complete synovectomy with removal of all loose bodies is the preferred treatment.[41]

It has been claimed that recurrence is rare; however, the follow-up period in all reported series has been short. Although the occasional patient has been disease free for more than a decade, the majority of reported cases have not been observed for more than 1 year and some of the surveillance periods have been as short as 2 months. Therefore, the evidence for effectiveness of treatment may be suspect. However, the best indication that treatment has been effective is the lack of reports of recurrence. Even in cases with incomplete removal of the synovium, recurrence has not been reported.[8,12,22,24,30] A rapid return to normal mastication after several weeks of a soft diet, supportive analgesics, and range of motion exercises is the usual result of treatment.

Malignant transformation of synovial chondromatosis in other joints is rare. There are only two case reports of this finding.[26,27] However, the nuclear abnormalities and multinucleated cells often observed histologically in synovial chondromatosis can be easily misinterpreted by the pathologist as signs of malignancy.[25,41] Nevertheless, malignant transformation has not been reported in the TMJ.

Osteochondroma

Osteochondroma, sometimes called *osteocartilaginous exostosis*, is the most common benign tumor of bone. It represents 35% of all benign bone tumors and 8.5% of all bone tumors.[42] However, it occurs rarely in the facial bones, where it is most commonly found in the condylar and coronoid processes.[43–45] Forty-eight cases have been reported in the mandibular condyle, and there has been only one incident of recurrence (2%), which is the same rate as that reported for osteochondroma of the long bones.[43–46] The average age at presentation is 40 years (range, 11 to 69 years), in contrast to osteochondroma of the long bones, for which the typical age of patients is younger than 20 years. Unlike in long bones, where there is a male predominance (1.8:1), in the TMJ, the ratio is reversed (1:1.8).[47] Vezeau et al[46] reported a predominance of involvement of the left condyle.

With the exception of a series of six cases reported by Wolford et al,[18] the information about the behavior and treatment of these lesions comes from reports of one or two cases accompanied by a review of the literature. The accuracy of the data supporting the diagnosis is questionable in some of the earlier reports.[48] Follow-up data are inadequate because the length of observation either was not reported or was less than 2 years in nearly half of the cases. The case series of Wolford et al[18] was the most reliable in regard to surveillance. Their retrospective review consisted of four female and two male patients with an average age of 22.3 years (range, 13 to 32 years) who were followed for an average of 51 months (range, 22 to 108 months), a mode of 34 months, and a median of 33.5 months.[18]

Most commonly, osteochondromas arise from the anteromedial aspect of the condylar neck and extend to the condylar head (see figs 21-7 and 35-1). It has been presumed that this is related to the insertion of the lateral pterygoid muscle. However, other reported sites of origin include the anterior and the posteromedial aspects of the condyle.[49]

Osteochondromas of the peripheral skeleton have been reported to originate in the planes of tendon insertion. It has been suggested that this is related to the focal accumulation of embryonic connective tissue–containing precursor cells in these sites, which may differentiate into chondroblasts. Ongoing functional stress induces hyperplasia of these cells,[42] which then become activated to form the osteochondroma.

On the other hand, experimental evidence from rabbits suggests that the lesion develops as a result of herniation of cartilage through a periosteal defect. The creation of periosteal defects in the proximal metaphysis of rabbit tibias resulted in the development of osteochondromas at the site of injury in 13 of 20 animals.[50]

Other theories consider that these lesions are derived from the peripheral displacement of undifferentiated cells from the growth cartilage[51] or that neoplastic cells arising from the periosteum form metaplastic cartilage.[52] In the TMJ, there is the consideration that residues from the cartilaginous cranium and Meckel cartilage that have not been replaced by mandibular bone persist and become activated.[53] Some reports have implicated trauma in the etiology of these lesions, but there are inadequate data to support a strong case for this hypothesis.[1,19,48,49]

The osteochondroma is readily detectable as a radiopaque mass on panoramic radiography and is well delineated on computerized tomography (CT). Scintigraphy usually shows a focal area of positive uptake.[44] The tumors occur in two forms: solitary or as part of the syndrome of osteochondromatosis, a genetic disease. There has long been debate as to whether these lesions are truly neoplastic or developmental. Recent findings from genetic analysis of isolated cases and cases of hereditary multiple osteochondromas have established the neoplastic nature of these lesions.

Aydin[45] reviewed the literature on this subject, and the summary explains the pathogenesis as follows. Deletions of q24 from chromosome 8 and p11 to p13 from chromosome 11 have been found in both the isolated sporadic and the hereditary multiple cases. These loci, called *EXT 1 (8q24, 1)* and *EXT 2 (11P11.2-12)*, may be involved in the generation of the lesions in both forms of the disease. The term *preneoplasm* has been used to describe those osteochondromas that regress at the end of skeletal growth, with *neoplasm* being reserved for those tumors that continue to grow beyond puberty. It was postulated that a solitary preneoplastic osteochondroma occurs after two successive somatic mutations on both copies of an *EXT* gene. The stepwise process of carcinogenesis continues as additional genetic abnormalities and mutations accumulate, forming first the neoplastic osteochondroma and then a chondrosarcoma. The somatic mutations may be the result of radiation damage, but this would not explain the more common occurrence of chondrosarcoma in non–radiation damaged tissue. The neoplastic cell of origin remains a matter of conjecture, possible sources being the periosteum, cartilage, and the perichondrial groove of Ranvier (in axial skeletal lesions).[45]

The risk of malignant transformation of these tumors in their more common location in nonmaxillofacial skeletal sites is less than 1% for the solitary lesions but up to 13% for the syndrome-related tumors.[54] No cases of malignant transformation of a mandibular condylar osteochondroma have been reported.[18]

The clinical signs and symptoms do not distinguish this tumor from other slow-growing tumors or tumorlike

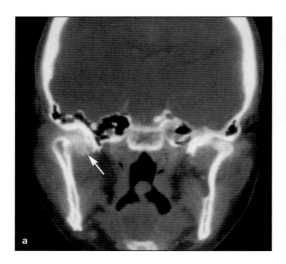
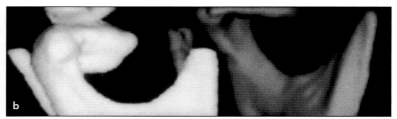

Fig 35-1 Osteochondroma. *(a)* Computerized tomographic scan, illustrating the most common position of an osteochondroma, anterior and medial to the condyle *(arrow)*. *(b)* Reconstructed tomographic scan. (Courtesy of Dr R. B. MacIntosh.)

masses of the condyle. In particular, it is difficult to distinguish from condylar hyperplasia. Radiographically, the osteochondroma usually shows a globular pattern with distorted condylar morphology (Fig 35-1), whereas in hyperplasia the condylar head is simply symmetrically enlarged and the condylar neck is usually lengthened. A slowly developing asymmetry associated with ipsilateral deviation of the chin, bowing of the mandibular body, and a unilateral posterior open bite are the most common clinical signs of condylar osteochondroma (Fig 35-2). A contralateral crossbite also may develop.

Pain, most often dull in quality, may occur when the lesion grows rapidly, and there may be tenderness on palpation over the joint. Sometimes a slight restriction both in MIO and in ipsilateral excursive movements may occur.[48] Joint noises associated with disc displacement may develop, and late in the disease process crepitation may occur.[18] If the lesion is very large, a preauricular mass may be visible and palpable, although this may not happen because many of these lesions arise from the medial anterior aspect of the condyle.[18,43,45] One case of hearing loss associated with a large condylar osteochondroma has been reported.[49] In the comprehensive review by Vezeau et al,[46] the presenting symptoms were asymmetry in 76%, pain in 52%, joint noise in 31%, and hypomobility in 28% of cases.

Histologically, the tumor contains trabecular bone with a rim of cartilage. The chondrocytes can form rows that are perpendicular to the surface of the lesion, and they may overlie a zone of endochondral ossification. This results in fusion of the cancellous bone with the normal underlying bone. There is an orderly progression within the columns of cartilage, and they show calcification and conversion to bone. The cellular features are generally normal, but there may be instances of nuclear atypia. In older lesions, the rim of cartilage may be very thin, having been largely replaced by bone.[43]

Presence of a thick, nonossified rim of cartilage in adults should initiate an intense search for the presence of a sarcoma.[46,55] If growth renews later in life, sarcomatous transformation also should be suspected.[54]

Complete excision of the lesion is necessary (Fig 35-3). In the only known case of recurrence, incomplete excision was the cause.[46] Although the disc is most often not involved, it may be stretched or completely destroyed by large lesions.[45] Frequently the condyle will be normal except for the area in contact with the lesion. Therefore, the ideal treatment is to remove the lesion, smooth the condyle, and plicate the disc.[17,18, 44,45] In their careful analysis of a subset of 30 of the reported cases of osteochondroma, Vezeau et al[46] noted that condylectomy was the most frequently performed procedure, used in 77% of the cases. Excision of the lesion with salvage of the condyle was the next most common treatment, at 23%. Discectomy was reported in 13% and discoplasty in 10%.

Minor occlusal abnormalities may require correction by orthodontics, while major ones require corrective orthognathic surgery. Sacrifice of the condyle and subcondylar process may require reconstruction with a costochondral graft, ramus osteotomy, or a joint prosthesis.

Surgical approaches start with a preauricular dissection (see chapter 28); this has been the standard procedure in recent years. Adjunctive approaches to increase access include a temporal extension, a bicoronal flap, sectioning of the zygomatic arch, a submandibular incision, or even an intraoral approach to expose the medial side of the ramus (7%).[46]

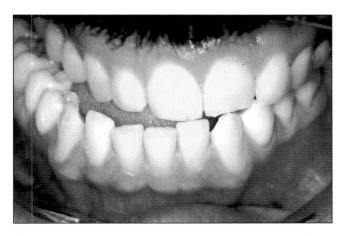

Fig 35-2 Laterognathia and open bite associated with an osteochondroma. (Courtesy of Dr R. B. MacIntosh.)

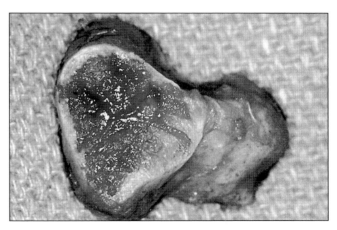

Fig 35-3 Specimen of osteochondroma, including condyle. (Courtesy of Dr R. B. MacIntosh.)

The rationale for the more conservative approach is to save the condyle and perform arthroplasty with bone files or abraders, thereby maintaining as much undamaged articulating surface as possible. The surgical problem has been to achieve adequate visual access to safely remove the entire tumor. Because most osteochondromas arise from the anteromedial aspect of the condyle, this also requires that absolute control be maintained over the medial aspect of the dissection to prevent inadvertent transection of the internal maxillary or masseteric artery, either of which has the capability of causing bleeding that is difficult to control. The solution has been to remove the osteochondroma in pieces. As each section is removed, progressively better visualization for removal of the remaining tumor develops. This way, piece by piece, the lesion is removed without needlessly sacrificing the condyle.

When the condyle has been damaged or has been extensively remodeled, it can be reshaped and/or repositioned in the glenoid fossa with a ramus osteotomy. Additional orthognathic surgery may be used as required to correct any asymmetry. This includes sagittal osteotomy of the ramus, ipsilateral inferior border ostectomy, or segmental Le Fort I osteotomy.[18] When the condyle must be removed in its entirety, costochondral grafting is required. In one case of a large osteochondroma that involved the condyle and the skull base, an alloplastic total joint prosthesis was used successfully.[43]

Thus, the available data suggest a conservative approach to the removal of the osteochondroma that allows preservation of the condyle and disc when possible. However, when this is not possible, conservative condylectomy is recommended.

Chondroma and Chondroblastoma

Despite the expectation that tumors originating from cartilage ought to be relatively common in the TMJ because a thin rim of hyaline cartilage is located just below the articulating surface of the condyle, these tumors are extremely rare. The diagnostic separation of chondroblastoma from giant cell tumors[56] and chondrosarcoma has only been consistently reliable for the past 40 years.[10] The most reliable information available about these rare lesions comes from the literature after 1970.

Chondroma

There have been 70 reported cases of chondroma, of which 80% occurred in the metaphysis of the femur, tibia, or humerus. Only six cases have been reported in facial bones, and surveillance data are insufficient to make a definitive statement about treatment.[57–63] Consequently, treatment recommendations have been based on an understanding of the behavior of these benign cartilaginous lesions in other parts of the facial skeleton. The known behavioral pattern of chondromas of the jaws includes slow growth, local invasion, expected difficulty in removal, and a subsequent clinical course beset by recurrence. In the mandible, these lesions have been reported both in the condyle and the coronoid process.[64]

The usual symptoms reported are mild preauricular pain and diminished mouth opening. With more extensive tumors, asymmetry and malocclusion, along with ipsilateral open bite and contralateral crossbite, can develop. A radiolytic lesion of the condylar head, frequently with calcifications, is visible on imaging, and the inferior joint space is enlarged.

A major problem has been obtaining tissue for a diagnostic biopsy. Because the lesion is not readily accessible to fine needle biopsy by virtue of its location and its consistency, excision has usually been performed. Because of the likelihood of some uncertainty in histologic diagnosis as a result of possible confusion with a low-grade chondrosarcoma[65] and the tendency of these tumors to recur, wide excision is generally recommended and curettage should be avoided. Some form of immediate reconstruction is also suggested whenever an adequate amount of condyle cannot be preserved.

The surgeon must have a very high degree of wariness when treating chondrogenic lesions because of the difficulty in discriminating benign from malignant ones and the knowledge that such chondrogenic lesions are more likely to be malignant than benign.[59] They are not responsive to radiation treatment, and such treatment has been associated with a risk of inducing sarcomatous transformation.[66,67] There is not enough evidence based on long-term surveillance of these few lesions after treatment to make a strong comment about their long-term behavior.[57,61–63,66]

It is presumed that these neoplasms arise from the articular cartilage, cartilage precursors located within periosteum, or from vestigial cartilage rests.[68] In one reported case, the lesion did not appear to originate from the condyle, but it filled the joint space, deforming and destroying the condyle by pressure effects.[69]

Treatment must be individualized, depending on the operative findings, the extent of destruction of the condyle and glenoid fossa, and the age and health of the patient as well as the surgeon's experience with joint reconstruction. The primary objective is to excise the lesion along with the condyle and to reconstruct the joint, restore the occlusion, and correct any facial asymmetry. However, with small lesions, much of the condyle tends to be unaffected and therefore preservation of the articulation may be possible.[58]

When the condyle is excised, appropriate reconstructive techniques include replacement by a costochondral graft or a vertical ramus osteotomy with superior repositioning of the reshaped subcondylar bone to resemble a condyle. If the disc has been destroyed, replacement with a temporalis flap or a dermal graft may be considered. With extremely large lesions, alloplastic total joint replacement may be appropriate.[43]

Chondroblastoma

There have only been four reported cases in which chondroblastomas occurred in the mandibular condyle. As with most of the rare primary tumors of bone, the surmised behavior of chondroblastomas is learned from their behavior in other parts of the skeleton. Chondroblastomas are rare, representing fewer than 1% of all bone tumors. Nine cases in the facial bones have been reported from the Mayo Clinic bone registry, and four other sporadic cases have been reported.[56,70,71] Three of the nine cases were in the condyle. All age groups may be affected, but teenagers are the most frequently affected subset.[71,72]

Chondroblastomas of the peripheral skeleton are treated by curettage; resection is reserved for recurrence. A statement about the risk of recurrence of condylar chondroblastomas cannot be made, because of lack of a sufficient number of cases with adequate long-term surveillance. However, in the long bones, recurrence usually develops within 2 years and is cured by resection.[73] A similar behavior pattern was reported for a mandibular condylar tumor that recurred 2 years after curettage and then required en bloc resection.[74] However, those cases treated initially by block resection have not recurred.[69] There has been one report of metastasis after biopsy.[74]

Osteoma

There is an indistinct boundary among an osteoma, an exostosis, and a torus. Attempts to define the differences histologically extend back to the work of Fetissof[75] in the 1920s. On a clinical basis, the exostosis, of which the torus is an example, usually occupies a specific location in the jaws, grows during puberty, and then stops growing. They are more properly considered to be hamartomas.[76] Exostoses may be multiple and are more likely to be found in the maxilla. They also may be found at the insertion of muscles or tendons. They present as hard, well-demarcated, submucosal masses. On imaging they appear as well-circumscribed opaque masses.

Endosteal exostoses (enostoses) are localized growths of dense bone that grow into the medullary space instead of away from it. The mandible is a more likely site for endosteal growth than the maxilla. Of the two forms, the exostotic is more common.

The most common sites for solitary mandibular osteomas are the lingual and lateral aspects of the mandibular ramus. The condyle rarely is affected. Only 15 cases involving the condyle have been reported. The ages of the patients in these cases have ranged from 26 to 74 years. Most cases occur in the fourth decade. Because various forms of dense bone formation are common in the jaws, it is likely that cases of osteoma are underreported in the literature.[8,77]

The lesion consists of mature bone, frequently connected to the bone from which it originates by a slender stalk. However, the point of attachment may also be sessile.[1,8,78–80] The tumor occurs most frequently on the bones of the cranium and face, most commonly in the nose and paranasal sinuses. An association with a previous traumatic incident has been suggested for more than half a century in case reports documenting prior trauma to the side of the face on which the lesion later develops.[1,81] On the other hand, sinus and nasal lesions, which are much more common, have not been associated with trauma.

Histologically there are two variants of the osteoma. A compact osteoma is composed of dense, mature lamellar bone with few marrow spaces. The cancellous variety has trabeculae of mature lamellar bone with intervening fatty or fibrous marrow. The bony trabeculae are wide and irregularly distributed, and few osteoblasts are present in the inner structure of the osteoma.[82,83] The haversian canals are normal. Therefore, in the gross state, the compact form looks like dense cortical bone with a cut surface that is white-yellow and homogeneous. In the older literature, this was referred to as the *ivory form*. The cancellous variety has the appearance of spongy bone. Both are likely to be globular.[79,84]

If multiple osteomas are present, Gardner syndrome, an inherited autosomal disease characterized by osteomas, fibromas, epidermal inclusion cysts, and intestinal polyps, should be considered (see fig 21-11). Because the intestinal polyps have a 100% probability of becoming malignant with time, recognition of the link between multiple osteomas and the syndrome can be lifesaving.[8,85]

Treatment of osteoma is excision, and no recurrences or malignant transformations have been reported.

Osteoid Osteoma and Osteoblastoma

These two entities are extremely rare in the TMJ. The literature includes one reported case of osteoid osteoma of the condyle,[86] one case of osteoid osteoma of the articular eminence,[87] and three cases of osteoblastoma of the condyle.[88–90] Only 11 cases of osteoid osteoma have been reported in the jaws, with a male to female ratio of 2.3:10 and an age range of 7 to 20 years. For the condylar lesions, the age range was 14 to 20 years.[8,86]

Osteoblastomas rarely occur in the jaw, and the most comprehensive report lists only 24 gnathic cases. In this series, the ratio of male to female patients was 2:1, with an average age of 17.2 years and a range of 5 to 37 years. The lesions were randomly distributed throughout the jaws; 15 occurred in the mandible and 8 in the maxilla. In 1 case, the site was not specified. In this series, none were reported in the condyle and only 3 cases have been reported in the literature.[88–90] In extragnathic sites, the

age ratio is the same, averaging 17 years and ranging from 3 to 78 years. Almost 90% of the patients were younger than 30 years, and the lesions most commonly occurred in the vertebral column and the appendicular skeleton.[91]

These two rare lesions are benign and probably represent variants of a basic osteoblastic tumor. The histologic parameters do not completely permit their separation, so the size and clinical presentation are used to aid in diagnosis. Histologically, the trabeculae of woven bone and osteoid are regular and lie in a vascular fibrous tissue. The degree of mineralization varies, but is usually greatest in the central aspect of the lesion, presenting as a calcified nidus. Variations occur in regard to the amount of bone deposition and cellularity of the fibrous tissue. The trabeculae in the osteoblastoma tend to be broader, more widely separated, and more vascular than those in the osteoid osteoma.

The major distinction is made on a clinical basis. The osteoid osteoma has limited growth potential and is rarely larger than 1 cm in greatest diameter, while the osteoblastoma is usually larger and keeps growing[10] and therefore has the capability of deforming or destroying the condyle.[8]

In the jaws, the clinical presentation of these lesions varies by site. Pain is a common symptom, and swelling occurs in most of the cases. There are no reports of sensory change induced by the lesion. There may be expansion of the cortices, which are, however, usually still intact. The area of swelling may be very tender to palpation. Teeth may become sensitive to percussion or mobile or may show signs of resorption.[91] Recently a classification based on behavioral parameters has been suggested by Dorfman and Czerniak,[92] who reserve the term *osteoid osteoma* for lesions smaller than 1.5 cm in diameter, *osteoblastoma* for those between 1.5 and 4.0 cm, and *aggressive osteoblastoma* for lesions larger than 4.0 cm.

The periphery of the osteoid osteoma generally shows sclerotic bone, but the degree of sclerosis does not correlate with the age of the lesion. However, the presence of sclerotic borders is more likely to be accepted as part of the diagnosis of osteoid osteoma even if the lesion is larger than 1 cm.[93]

The few cases of osteoid osteoma and osteoblastoma reported do not permit any definitive statements about their management. However, wide and complete excision seems to be associated with successful treatment. In the review of osteoblastomas of the jaws, the longest period of follow-up surveillance was 9 years.[88] However, among the 24 cases reported, 2 patients experienced 3 recurrences (at 6 months and "twice within 2 years"). There were no reports of follow-up for 5 patients and less than 1 year for 8 of the remaining 19 patients. Of the remaining 11 patients, 7 had surveillance for 2 years or less, and only 3 patients were observed for more than 3 years.

Because there are no reliable long-term data about recurrence, it cannot be definitively stated that the biologic behavior of the osteoblastoma is clearly one of low aggressiveness. However, if it is not, reports of either recurrence or metastatic osteosarcoma (confirming a missed diagnosis) probably would have appeared in the literature after a period of years. Alternatively, local recurrence would have called into question the histologic diagnosis, and this has not been reported.

As previously noted, the clinical and histologic characteristics of osteoid osteoma and osteoblastoma overlap significantly, and adequate surgical resection will be more or less challenging depending on the size of the lesion and whether it extends beyond the joint structures.

Nonossifying Fibroma, Odontogenic Fibroma, Desmoplastic Fibroma, and Myxofibroma

There are three variants of nonossifying fibroma of intraosseous origin: nonossifying fibroma, desmoplastic fibroma, and odontogenic fibroma. All three are uncommon, and the odontogenic fibroma is imperfectly separated from the others by the presence of odontogenic epithelium within the tumor.[94] The nonossifying fibromas originate from the mesenchyme of the jaw. Variable degrees of myxoid stroma change, and the distinctive vascular pattern of some lesions establish them as a fibrous variant of the myxoma, the fibromyxoma, which suggests that these lesions are part of a continuum. The desmoplastic fibroma may be only a more densely collagenized form of central nonossifying fibroma. This entity has an accepted counterpart in the long bones, unlike myxoma, which occurs only in facial bones.[10]

There have only been three reported cases of nonossifying fibroma of the mandibular condyle.[95–97] Two patients were women, aged 18 and 20 years. Radiographically, well-circumscribed radiolucencies of tshe condyles were present.[8,84,96,97] Treatment consisted of resection of the condyle. The gross specimens showed a circumscribed, encapsulated tumor with a gray-white surface that was firm on palpation.

Microscopically, the central portion of the lesion consisted of bundles of spindle-shaped fibroblasts. At the edge of the lesion, lipid-laden histiocytes or foam cells were present. Multinucleated giant cells and hemosiderin were observed occasionally throughout the tissue. The ratio between fibroblasts and collagen varied throughout the tumor. The essential histologic differential diagnosis was with well-differentiated fibrosarcoma, in which, even with a similar histologic pattern, the fibroblasts will always be plumper. Malignant fibrous histiocytoma must also be considered.

One case of a desmoplastic fibroma of the condyle has been reported.[98] This is a benign tumor of connective tissue that resembles the desmoid tumor of abdominal and extra-abdominal sites. It has been reported in the mandible but not in other facial bones. There is no sex predilection, and most of the tumors present in the second decade. Most commonly the patients complain of swelling, intermittent pain, and limitation of jaw function. Imaging shows a pattern of cortical destruction that indicates aggressive behavior of the tumor.[10] In a 1980 case review, there were 48 reported skeletal cases and 9 mandibular cases, and the condyle was affected in a 27-year-old woman.[99]

The histology of the desmoplastic fibroma shows abundant collagen and irregular, spindle-shaped fibroblasts following the long axis of the collagen fibers. There are slight nuclear atypia, no mitoses, and nearly normal nuclear chromatin. No foam cells, giant cells, or ossification is present. The histologic differential diagnosis is between low-grade fibrosarcoma, aggressive fibromatosis, and malignant fibrous histiocytosis. Other considerations are aneurysmal bone cyst, giant cell tumor, monostotic fibrous dysplasia, and nonossifying fibroma.[98]

Based on experience with other skeletal sites, the recommended treatment for desmoplastic fibroma is resection. However, a recent report of using aggressive curettage for five desmoplastic fibromas occurring outside of the head and neck region demonstrated success at follow-up periods ranging from 5.5 to 9 years.[99]

Fibrous Dysplasia

Fibrous dysplasia is more common in the maxilla than the mandible and manifests similar growth characteristics as in other parts of the skeleton, where it is more common. There is gradual replacement of normal bone without clear radiographic or pathologic demarcation between abnormal and normal bone. In children, fibrous dysplasia may exhibit a more aggressive pattern of destruction.[100]

The customary findings of a slow-growing tumor that caused disturbances in the occlusion were reported in a very rare case of condylar fibrous dysplasia.[1] This 28-year-old woman noticed a slowly developing asymmetry of the face with a left crossbite. The radiograph showed a radiolytic lesion with a diffuse pattern that caused elongation and expansion of the condyle neck. She had another lesion of the body of the mandible with a similar radiographic appearance. Treatment results were not reported.

Because of the paucity of cases of fibrous dysplasia involving only the TMJ, there are no specific guidelines regarding treatment in this area. Although the condition tends to be self-limiting, usually by the third decade of life, waiting for a lesion of the condyle to stop growing would incur the risk of impaired mandibular function as well as the development of a severe malocclusion and possible facial deformity. Thus, following diagnosis by biopsy, condylectomy would appear to be a logical choice.

In cases involving the region surrounding the glenoid fossa as part of more generalized craniofacial fibrous dysplasia, treatment may not be indicated if there is no interference with function. However, if function is impaired, partial or complete resection and reconstruction of the articulation may be necessary, depending on the extent of the condition.

Although transformation of fibrous dysplasia into a sarcoma has been reported in the craniofacial region, it is a rarity and has never been reported in the jaws. Radiation therapy is never indicated, because malignant transformation has been noted following such treatment.

Myxoma

The odontogenic myxoma is a neoplasm originating from mesenchyme within the jaw bones, presumably from the mesodermal portion of the tooth germ[68] or from primitive nonodontogenic mesenchymal rests.[101] In the largest bone registry, no cases were found in bones other than the jaw.[42] In other skeletal sites, similar tumors are most likely fibromas with an unusually high amount of mucoid material.[102] In the jaws, it most commonly occurs in the mandible, especially in the posterior region; the descending order of frequency is in the angle, the ramus, and molar area, although what was probably the first report of a jaw myxoma was in the condyle and its histologic diagnosis was fibromyxoma.[103]

Usually these lesions are associated with teeth, including impacted teeth. Most of the patients are young—67% are between the ages of 10 and 19 years—although all ages can be affected. However, occurrence of myxomas in persons older than 50 years in all jaw sites is unusual. There is no sex predilection.

It was suggested in one of the earliest complete reviews that the myxoma is locally aggressive with a high potential for recurrence after conservative treatment.[104] By the mid-1960s, many respected authorities were advocating resection in recognition of the aggressive behavior of these tumors.[105,106] A study from Memorial–Sloan Kettering Cancer Center reported on 10 patients with six mandibular myxomas. The average age was 23 years, and all patients were treated by radical surgery except for one. The only lesion that recurred was the one that was treated conservatively. This recurrence was discovered after 5 years. After follow-up periods ranging from 9 to 28 years, there were no recurrences in the group receiving radical surgery.

Similar results were reported in a series of nine cases by White et al,[107] and it is now generally accepted that these lesions should receive aggressive resection. The presumption, based on the literature, is that early recurrence, within 2 years, represents a persistent tumor that was not adequately removed.[108] However, there is a case report in which a recurrence developed 30 years after the initial surgery.[109] For those lesions treated by curettage, there were a few failures among patients generally followed for fewer than 18 months.[107] However, there was one case reported of recurrence developing 15 years after enucleation and curettage.[110] With mandibular myxomas, recurrence has even been reported after marginal resection of the mandible, but not after hemimandibulectomy.[111]

The most common complaints of patients with a myxoma of the TMJ are related to reduced mouth opening and pain, although these are not invariable findings. Growth of the lesions is reported to be slow, and they are generally asymptomatic until they became large enough to interfere with jaw function. The patients are most likely to be diagnosed as having a TMD until pain, crepitation, swelling, and mandibular asymmetry develop, initiating aggressive investigation. Occasionally malocclusion and the presence of a mass are noted.[112,113]

In a series of mandibular myxomas, two occurred in the condyle.[107] Moreover, only six cases of condylar myxoma have been reported since 1947.[1,103] Nevertheless, it would be prudent to apply the recommendations for other sites in the mandible to the treatment of condylar myxomas.

The radiographic assessment generally shows multilocular radiolucencies, sometimes with a honeycombed, soap bubble, or mottled appearance but with a generally well-defined periphery or even a sclerotic border. The radiographic differential diagnosis includes ameloblastoma, giant cell lesion, cyst, or fibrous dysplasia.[113,114]

Histologically, the cells are triangular, round, ellipsoid, or stellate with long, delicate anastomosing cytoplasmic processes in an extracellular matrix of loose mucoid material. The cytoplasm is finely granular, and the nuclei are ovoid, densely staining, and have few mitoses. If a large amount of collagen is present, this variant is designated as fibromyxoma, but the aggressive nature of the tumor does not change. Nuclear pleomorphism may also be present, but this does not correlate with an increase in recurrence rate.[42] Nests of odontogenic epithelium may be present but are not required to make the diagnosis.[110] Positive staining for the mesenchymal marker vimentin

Table 35-2				Case studies: Myoxoma of the condyle*			
Sex/age (y)	Pain	Mass	Trismus	Treatment	Recurrence	Follow-up (mo)	Study
F/27	–	+	–	Curettage/phenol Condylectomy	+ –	No data 24	Halfpenny et al[114]
F/48	+	+	+	Condylectomy/ vertical osteotomy Tumor removed piecemeal	–	0.2	Slootweg and Wittkamp[110]
M/16	–	+	–	Condylectomy/ vertical osteotomy	–	20	Halfpenny et al[114]
F/62	?	+	?	Curettage	–	18	Warner et al[8]
M/37	–	+	?	Condylectomy/ en bloc resection	–	60	Warner et al[8]
F/57	+	–	+	Condylectomy/ rib graft	Not reported	36	Lo Muzio et al[115]

*F= female; M = male; – = absent; + = present; ? = unknown.

establishes the cell of origin as being derived from odontogenic mesenchyme.[115] The histologic differential diagnosis includes myxoid liposarcoma with secondary invasion of the jaws, fibrosarcoma with myxoid changes, and primary liposarcoma of bone.[111]

In the gross specimen, the cut surface is gray or yellow-white and has a slimy appearance. There is no true capsule, but the apparent presence of a pseudocapsule might fool the surgeon into believing that this is truly an encapsulated tumor.[85,114]

Surgical treatment of the condylar tumor requires resection, including condylectomy and en bloc removal of the tumor. Adjacent vital structures should be preserved whenever possible. Although cases treated by curettage have, in fact, not recurred, the lowest recurrence rate is associated with more radical resection. If necessary the lesion may have to be removed in pieces to safely access its medial extent.

Restoration of condylar function may be achieved with a costochondral graft or by reshaping the subcondylar region, creating a vertical ramus osteotomy, and repositioning the ramal segment upward until the neocondyle seats in the glenoid fossa.[113] There is no role for radiation therapy.

The six reports cited in Table 35-2 are the only ones of myxoma of the mandibular condyle. The period of follow-up was at least 18 months in all but one case, with a range of 4 days to 5 years and an average of 26 months. The two cases in which curettage was used resulted in recurrence in one; the time to recurrence was not specified. The other patient treated by curettage was only followed for 18 months. It is generally recommended that observation extend beyond 2 years, because most lesions recur within 2 years of treatment. Three of the four patients treated by resection were observed for at least 2 years, with a range of 20 to 60 months, and there were no recurrences. These cases, although their number is limited, had adequate long-term surveillance to support resection as the treatment of choice.

Giant Cell Lesions

True giant cell tumors of the facial bones are extremely rare, and most of those originally reported as such during the first half of the 20th century were later reclassified as other bone lesions that happened to contain giant cells. The giant cell granuloma almost always occurs in relation to the tooth-bearing parts of the jaws, and giant cell tumors have been reported in all areas of the jaws. Two cases of giant cell granuloma were reported by Thoma[1] in 1954; he cited an article by Hofer[116] that reported two other condylar cases. One was in a 23-year-old man with a prior traumatic injury to the ipsilateral temporal area and another was in a 20-year-old woman with preauricular swelling present for 3 months. No other additional details were reported.[116]

The true giant cell tumor of bone is extremely rare in the facial bones and particularly in the condyle. Histologically it differs from the giant cell granuloma by the rare presence of osteoid in the tumor, minimal hemosiderin deposition or inflammatory infiltrate, and giant cells that are different from osteoclasts. The tumor contains an abundance of giant cells that are larger than those in the granulomas, and they dominate the histologic pattern. However, even with the advent of immunocytochemistry, it is still not possible to separate the giant cells in the tumor from those in the granuloma. Staining for α-1-trypsin is positive both for the giant cells in the giant cell tumor and in other lesions containing giant cells.[118]

The main points of differentiation in terms of clinical presentation are that the giant cell tumor occurs most commonly in individuals aged 20 to 24 years and rarely in persons younger than 20 years and that these lesions are usually smaller than 5 cm. Giant cell granulomas are more common in younger patients. Because the giant cell tumor of the long bones is known to be aggressive and even to metastasize, aggressive resection is recommended for giant cell tumors of the condyle.[68,84]

Aneurysmal Bone Cyst

There have been only a few case reports of an aneurysmal bone cyst of the mandibular condyle.[118] It is really a pseudocyst with no epithelial lining, which is filled by sinusoids containing blood and a liberal number of giant cells. Definitive treatment requires resection or aggressive curettage and possible adjunctive cryotherapy because simple curettage is associated with a high recurrence rate.[8]

Langerhans Cell Granulomatosis

This neoplasm was known as *histiocytosis* when described by Lichtenstein[119] in his 1953 classification of the triad of diseases consisting of eosinophilic granuloma, Hand-Schüller-Christian disease, and Letterer-Siwe disease; the current term is *Langerhans cell granulomatosis*. It is theorized that these lesions represent an immunologic neoplasm consisting of Langerhans cells.[120–122] Histologically, sheets of these cells predominate and the number of eosinophils vary. Giant cells and zones of necrosis may coexist, and fibrosis becomes more prominent as the lesion ages. The Langerhans cell that contains rod-shaped Birbeck granules has been identified by immunocytochemistry as the marker that confirms the true immunologic nature of this disorder (see fig 21-22b).

Thirteen cases of Langerhans cell granulomatosis occurring in the mandibular condyle have been reported, in patients ranging from 6 to 44 years of age. These patients may be asymptomatic, but, more frequently, they have localized preauricular pain and swelling. Radiographically, the bony lesion is well demarcated and osteolytic. Histologically, the dominant feature is sheets of benign Langerhans cells admixed with eosinophils.

Treatment is by surgical curettage, and there is a low expectation of recurrence. In a case report of a child with Langerhans cell granulomatosis, the condyle-ramus unit was restored with a costochondral graft 2.5 years after curettage. Seven years later, he was disease free and had a MIO of 35 mm.

Low-dose irradiation has been used in extragnathic sites for extensive lesions in inoperable sites or where pathologic fracture of a weight-bearing region might occur.[100] Intralesional steroid injections have been partially successful as well.[123]

Hemangioma

Hemangioma of the TMJ is extremely rare; only five cases of condylar origin[124–126] and one whose origin was the synovium (synovial hemangioma)[127] have been reported. Hemangiomas of the jaws have a peak occurrence in the second decade of life,[128] whereas all central hemangiomas of bone have a peak occurrence in the fourth decade of life.[129] They are also extremely rare lesions; intraosseous hemangiomas account for only 0.7% of all osseous neoplasms.

Most craniofacial hemangiomas occur in the mandible, and two thirds involve the ramus or body.[10] They are slow-growing, expansile masses that radiographically usually demonstrate a honeycomb, sun ray, or spoked wheel appearance. Preoperative assessment with contrast enhanced CT may show increased blood flow, but the usefulness of angiography may be questioned because most of these are low-flow lesions. Fine needle aspiration may not be productive.[128] The differential diagnosis includes ameloblastoma, odontogenic keratocyst, central giant cell lesion or tumor, aneurysmal bone cyst, and a metastasis.

The patients with TMJ hemangiomas generally presented with typical complaints of facial pain and jaw dysfunction, and some had been treated with bite appliances. Restriction of jaw motion had occurred as the lesions enlarged. The patients ranged in age from 27 to 44 years.

The three condylar cases were treated by resection. The single case of synovial hemangioma was successfully treated by removal of the synovium and the disc, from which the lesion originated. Because bleeding during the operation is a major concern, ligation of the external carotid artery was performed in one case but was found to be of no value in reducing bleeding.[130] Treatment was successful in all four patients, but long-term follow-up information was lacking in three case reports, and one case report did not include any postoperative information.

Other treatment possibilities for hemangioma include those for any central hemangioma of bone, which include embolization, cryotherapy, injection of a sclerosing solution, radiation therapy, and possibly interferon.

Neurilemoma (Schwannoma)

The neurilemoma is a slow-growing benign neoplasm that originates from the Schwann cells that deposit myelin around nerve fibers. They are encapsulated lesions found most commonly in the head and neck region. The histologic points of interest regarding the cellular schwannoma are that cellularity is increased, nuclear pleomorphism and hyperchromatism exist, mitotic activity is high, and no Verocay bodies are present. Microscopically, the pattern is suggestive of malignancy, but these lesions have do not metastasize and few have recurred.[131,132] The benign variety stains positively for S-100, and the malignant type does not.

Most patients are middle aged. There have been two reported cases involving the mandible.[131,132] Neither involved the condyle directly, but in one the epicenter was the posterior body of the mandible, and there was secondary involvement of the condyle. Treatment was by curettage, but no follow-up information was reported.

Neurofibroma

There has only been one case report of a neurofibroma of the TMJ,[13] and therefore it represents a surgical curiosity. The lesion arose from the articular disc and was treated by wide local excision.

Isolated neurofibromas in other areas have been associated with a lower recurrence rate than the multiple lesions occurring in von Recklinghausen neurofibromatosis. In addition, the chance of malignant degeneration has been reported to be lower for the isolated neurofibroma.[133]

Pseudotumors and Cysts

Pigmented villonodular synovitis

Pigmented villonodular synovitis is usually found in the knee. There have been 22 TMJ cases reported in the English-language literature, and the first report was published in 1973.[134] Patients of any age may be affected; reported cases have ranged from 10 to 70 years. However, there is a modal peak during the fourth decade, in which one third of the cases occur. After this peak age there is a gradual decline in the number of cases, so that most of the patients develop this disorder after the age of 30 years and before the age of 50 years. Females predominate by a factor of 1.4.

The presenting clinical symptom is swelling and pain. Other symptoms suggestive of a TMD were present in 15 of 22 cases, and radiographic signs of a destructive lesion of the joint were present in 18 of 22 cases. However, unlike the usual case of a neoplasm masquerading as a TMD, several cases of pigmented villonodular synovitis appeared as masses in the parotid gland associated with otologic signs, particularly obstruction of the external auditory canal and diminished hearing.[6]

The natural history of pigmented villonodular synovitis is that of a slowly growing, locally destructive benign lesion. Two forms occur: localized and aggressive. The more discrete localized variant is also called *giant cell tumor of the tendon sheath*.[8] Microscopically, the amount of tissue proliferation depends on the age of the tumor. As aging occurs, the predominantly histiocytic infiltrate, with inflammatory cells and multinucleated giant cells, diminishes and the tumor becomes more fibrous. Usually hemosiderin is present, along with dilated blood vessels and giant cells, calling to mind the pattern of an aneurysmal bone cyst.

Treatment is by complete excision, which may be difficult if the lesion is extensively infiltrating. When the tumor presents as a more circumscribed mass, it is more easily removed. Complete excision is required to prevent recurrence.

Ganglion and synovial cysts

There are 18 cases in the English-language literature described as a ganglion or synovial cyst of the TMJ.[8,135] The difference between these two lesions is not always accurately presented, and sometimes the terms are used synonymously. A ganglion is a pseudocyst with a fibrous connective tissue wall, resulting when myxoid degeneration softens the joint capsule. There is no synovial cell lining. A synovial cyst is a true cyst arising from displacement or herniation of synovial tissue (Fig 35-4).

The patient is generally a woman (by a margin of 2:1) and ranges in age from 22 to 64 years. Two thirds of patients present with pain. As expected, most of these lesions arise from the synovium; only two cases actually arose from the mandibular condyle. It was recommended that the lesion be excised. For smaller lesions, this meant removal with preservation of as much synovium as possible.[135]

Little information about long-term surveillance is available, but there are no reports of recurrence.[8] The general principle of removing the condyle when it is largely replaced by abnormal tissue, both for completeness of extirpation and for proper microscopic examination, should be followed. There are few data to guide therapy, but the reasonable approach has been to remove this slow-growing and noninvasive lesion with minimal disturbance to joint structures except in the case of destruction of the condyle, where condylectomy is required.[135]

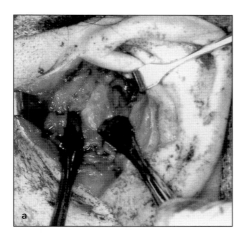 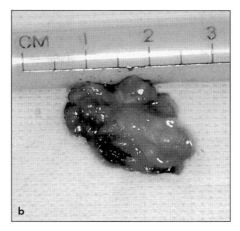

Fig 35-4 Synovial cyst. *(a)* Cyst protruding through the temporomandibular ligament. *(b)* Specimen of synovial cyst and disc after removal.

Synovial chondromatosis

Synovial chondromatosis, despite its most striking characteristic of abundant small particles of cartilage within the joint space, really is a disease of the synovium and should be included in the differential diagnosis when diseases of synovial origin are being considered (see the benign neoplasms section in this chapter, as well as chapter 21).

Primary Malignancies of the TMJ

Primary malignancies of the TMJ are very rare, but the most common are sarcomas, particularly chondrosarcoma and synovial chondrosarcoma. Thawley et al[136] consider malignant bone tumors to originate from the osteogenic mesenchymal matrix cells that produce osteoid, bone, cartilage, or fibrous tissue. This leads to subclassification of the tumors as osteoblastic, chondroblastic, fibroblastic, and telangiectatic varieties of sarcoma.[136] There have also been reports of synovial sarcoma, fibrosarcoma, malignant fibrous histiocytoma, osteosarcoma, leiomyosarcoma, and epithelioid sarcoma.

Every cartilage-producing head and neck tumor in an adult should be considered to be potentially malignant, because underdiagnosis has been reported to be as high as 20%.[59] The English-language literature was comprehensively reviewed by Warner et al[8] in 2000, and they found that 11 of 23 cases of sarcoma of the TMJ produced cartilage. Of these, 9 were chondrosarcomas and 2 were synovial chondrosarcomas. The remaining 12 cases were mainly distributed between synovial sarcomas and malig-

nant fibrous tumors (4 in each group). Only 1 case of osteosarcoma and 1 case of epithelioid carcinoma were reported. Since that review, 3 additional cases of osteosarcoma have been reported in the literature.[137,138]

The typical presentation of a malignant tumor of the mandibular condyle usually includes a painful mass associated with variable degrees of reduced jaw movement. The differential diagnosis of a painful mass of the TMJ must also include benign bony neoplasia–like chondromyxoid fibroma and giant osteoid osteoma, as has been noted earlier in this chapter.

These malignant tumors are often slow-growing lesions that are associated with a progressive increase in pain, particularly during function, and they usually do not cause trismus until later in the course of the disease, when they have reached a large size. Two cases of sarcoma of the TMJ have also resulted in hearing loss, one because of eustachian tube obstruction[139] and one because of actual obstruction of the external auditory canal.[140] The duration of symptoms prior to presentation for medical care has been reported to range from 6 months to 6 years.[140,141]

Chondrosarcoma

Chondrosarcoma of the head and neck is rare, although it constitutes 40% of the reported TMJ sarcomas, which themselves are very uncommon. In terms of the bony skeleton, head and neck lesions account for only 1% of all chondrosarcomas.[123] Retrospective reviews have shown that chondrosarcoma of the skeleton is more common in men and that there is an average age at presentation of 33 years.[65] However, in a small series of nine cases, the TMJ tumor was more common in women by a 2:1 ratio, with an average age at presentation of 48.5 (range, 29 to 75 years).[8,141] In contrast, osteosarcoma is more common in the skeleton, but there have been only four reported cases of osteosarcoma of the mandibular condyle.[137,138,142]

The production of malignant cartilage along with cellular pleomorphism are the hallmarks of the chondrosarcoma and the synovial chondrosarcoma. Cellularity is increased, and the cartilage cells tend to be large, may contain multiple nuclei or one large nucleus, and reside in a myxomatous matrix. Mitoses are uncommon except in high-grade lesions but, when present, may take bizarre forms. Grossly, chondrosarcomas are pseudoencapsulated lesions, whitish or slightly grayish in color.[139]

Based on the small number of cases in the facial bones in general and in the TMJ in particular, it is difficult to make definitive treatment recommendations. Failure of local control was the cause of death for most patients, and the lung was the most common site for distant spread.[143] In one study, all of the patients with positive margins died of local and distant disease.[144] Disease-free survival in several studies ranged from 30% to 40%, with follow-up periods ranging from a few months to several years.[144,145] Unless cervical lymphadenopathy is present, there is no indication for radical neck dissection.[140]

There have been 14 reported cases of chondrosarcoma of the TMJ.[139–141,146–150] Treatment has been individualized according to the extent of spread of the tumor beyond the condyle. Superficial parotidectomy, removal of the zygomatic arch and/or the temporal bone, and other skull base resections were performed as required. One patient with an extensive tumor received postoperative radiotherapy and eight cycles of methotrexate. None of the patients in these retrospective case reports relapsed with locoregional disease, despite direct invasion of the tumor into adjacent structures.[139–141,146–150]

Chondrosarcoma was originally held not to be sensitive to radiation, but more recently radiation has been advocated as appropriate adjuvant therapy for patients who have unresectable tumors, high-grade lesions, or positive margins.[151–154] However, because follow-up information was missing for one patient and ranged from 4 months to 7 years for the others, and only 3 patients were observed for more than 2 years, a definitive statement cannot be made regarding such treatment. Moreover, although the chondrosarcoma is sensitive to radiation, the response is slow.[154]

Condylar chondrosarcoma seems to have a less aggressive course than chondrosarcoma of the rest of the mandible, other head and neck sites, or the remainder of the body.[140] Chondrosarcoma also has been held to have a better prognosis than osteosarcoma in isolated reports,[155] but others have not discerned any difference.[156,157] Individualization of treatment based on the principles of achieving clear margins, and consideration of adjuvant radiotherapy or chemotherapy for those with positive margins or high-grade histologic findings, would seem reasonable.

Osteosarcoma

Osteosarcoma is common in skeletal sites. However, only 6% to 9% of these lesions occur in the jaws, and only four cases have been reported in the TMJ. In the skeleton, the average age of presentation of the first symptom is in the teenage years, whereas the mean age for presentation of jaw osteosarcoma is 27 to 33 years.[68,158–160] Other diseases that have been implicated as risk factors for the development of osteosarcoma include Paget disease, fibrous dysplasia, and retinoblastoma.[161,162] Radiation therapy of the head and neck is another risk factor; sarcomas reportedly have developed 5 to 45 years after such treatment.[163]

There are two major patterns of hard tissue formation in this type of sarcoma, the osteoblastic and the chondroblastic, but the prognosis is not related to the cell type except for those lesions affecting the axial skeleton, where the chondroblastic type may have a better prognosis.[164] More than 10% of lesions do not fall into any single definable category. Either type may range from low to high grades of differentiation and survival may well relate to grading.

The histologic grade is assessed based on the degree of atypia and tumor cellularity. Low-grade lesions are most likely to have minimal atypia, produce a mature extracellular matrix, and may be hard to diagnose as malignant. It is these low-grade lesions that account for the difficulty noted with the diagnosis of osteoblastomas, so that most of them, on careful review of their histologic appearance, are reclassified as osteosarcomas. High-grade lesions tend to exhibit tumor necrosis, abundant mitoses, and little matrix between cells and contain highly pleomorphic cells that are usually larger than normal osteoblasts. The malignant osteoid may vary from focal, delicate, lacelike calcified osteoid to thick lamina with broad, interconnecting trabeculae that may be nearly normal. The chondrosarcoma may produce both malignant cartilage and malignant osteoid.

Preoperative assessment of tumor behavior cannot be based only on the cell type in the biopsy, because any tumor may show areas evidencing different patterns. Final analysis cannot be completed until the entire resection specimen has been evaluated. Postoperative assessment of margins is crucial, because longer survival has been associated with negative margins. In fact, 30-month survival for patients with jaw osteosarcoma has been reported as being 70% for those with negative margins, but this rate falls to only 10% for those with positive margins.[165]

It has also been observed for several decades that the rate of survival for patients with osteosarcoma of the jaws is better than that for patients with osteosarcoma affecting other bones.[160] Kassir et al[166] performed a meta-analysis of nonrandomized studies of osteosarcoma of the head and neck in 1997. Their findings support the generally held conviction that osteosarcoma of the jaw bones has a better prognosis than that in extragnathic sites ($P < .001$). They found that the overall 5-year survival for head and neck osteosarcoma was 37%, with equal outcomes for maxilla and mandible. Treatment by surgery alone resulted in better survival statistics than did surgery with adjuvant therapy ($P < .03$). A problematic issue in the study was that margin status was not available in the majority of cases.

Their conclusion supports the general consensus about surgical treatment for all of the malignant bone tumors; the role for radiation and chemotherapy in the management of head and neck osteosarcoma remains unproven. Nevertheless, they recommend that adjuvant therapy be considered because of the poor prognosis for osteosarcoma of the head and neck.[166]

The clinical presentation in the four reported TMJ cases has varied.[137,138,142] However, the patients all had either painful altered joint function or a mass that was diagnosed after a significant delay. Imaging was helpful in assessing the extent and the general pattern of invasion. Surgery involved wide excision. The frozen section diagnosis was unreliable, and re-resection after permanent sections became available was the more common treatment. The lesions that were extensive were treated with adjuvant radiation therapy and/or chemotherapy, but no information was provided about the long-term results. Radical neck dissection was reserved for positive cervical lymphadenopathy.[156,158,159,167,168] Management of tumors that invaded the skull base required craniofacial resection and immediate reconstruction with bone, soft tissue, or both, with particular emphasis on maintaining separation between the dura and the infratemporal fossa.[169]

The use of preoperative and postoperative chemotherapy in association with adequate radical resection in cases of long bone osteosarcoma has been shown to increase survival through improvement in local control.[170] Goepfert et al[163] reported that chemotherapy in combination with surgery for head and neck osteosarcoma improved 5-year survival to 55% from 42% for surgery alone ($P < .25$). For several patients in whom preoperative chemotherapy was used, the definitive resections showed that no viable tumor was present, and in these patients the disease-free interval was increased. There are no good prospective data to support this policy, but extrapolation from the treatment data on osteosarcoma in other sites in the head and neck suggests that combination therapy improves survival.

The observation has also been made that mandibular osteosarcoma is more likely to be associated with tumor-free margins at resection and this creates a survival advantage over those of the maxilla.[144,171] Moreover, young patients have better survival statistics than do older ones.[172]

Synovial Sarcoma

Synovial sarcoma constitutes about 10% of all soft tissues sarcomas,[173] but it is not common in the jaws. Only 32 cases have been reported in the head and neck regions, and the most common site among these was the tongue.[6,174,175] Only four cases were primary to the TMJ.[6,14,173–175]

This tumor originates from spindle cells arising from undifferentiated primitive mesenchyme[173] in either a monophasic or a biphasic pattern; a majority of the cases are biphasic. However, there is no clear difference in behavior between the two types, although one report suggested that the monophasic type was more aggressive.[160] The histologic differential diagnosis for the more common monophasic type is with fibrosarcoma, leiomyosarcoma, malignant schwannoma, and hemangiopericytoma. The most frequent problem is its differentiation from fibrosarcoma. Although there are subtle histologic distinctions, the diagnosis is generally made by immunohistochemistry. The synovial sarcoma stains positively for periodic acid–Schiff, cytokeratin A, and epithelial membrane antigen. It also stains positively for vimentin, as does fibrosarcoma.[174]

Metastasis from head and neck synovial sarcomas has been reported in 50% of the cases. The lungs, cervical nodes, and bone are the usual sites of spread. Consequently, chemotherapy has been advocated as part of the treatment program to minimize metastases. Recurrence rates have varied from 30% to 50%, and survival at 5 years has averaged 30% to 50%. However, by 10 years, the survival rate had fallen to 10% to 30%.[174]

The four patients with synovial sarcoma of the TMJ[6,14,175,176] were all men ranging in age from 22 to 57 years. The most common findings were the presence of pain, altered occlusion, and a mass. Pain had been present from 5 to 24 months before treatment was sought, although one patient had chronic joint discomfort for 22 years that was not caused by the tumor. Preoperatively, incorrect diagnoses included lipoma, parotid tumor, and "TMJ syndrome." As is usual, those patients presenting with a mass were generally considered to have a lesion of the superficial lobe of the parotid gland and those without a mass were diagnosed as having a TMD, usually myofascial pain secondary to bruxism. Both pain and occlusal changes worsened with growth of the mass.

Imaging or surgical exploration demonstrated a destructive, aggressive lesion that extended beyond the limits of the joint to involve either the adjacent musculature or the glenoid fossa. Treatment was by block excision. When the glenoid fossa was involved, in one patient the bone was left in place to avoid entering the middle cranial fossa[14] and in another a formal craniofacial resection was performed with skull base resection.[176] Three of the four patients received postoperative radiation therapy and two also received chemotherapy. In one of these patients, metastasis to the ilium occurred during treatment.[176] There was no follow-up information in one case, one patient died at 15 months, and two patients were alive and disease free at 5 and 9 months.

There is inadequate information on which to form a strong recommendation regarding treatment. However, the general principles of adequate tumor clearance through en bloc or wide local excision, including complete synovectomy, seem appropriate. Radical neck dissection was used in one patient without palpable lymphadenopathy, but in whom the CT scan was "suspicious" of nodes along the spinal accessory chain. There is no clearly established role for chemotherapy. However, for a patient with a large tumor showing destruction of adjacent tissues, the use of an aggressive soft tissue sarcoma chemotherapy protocol in an adjunctive role would be worthy of consideration.

Fibrosarcoma

Fibrosarcoma of the TMJ is very rare; only three cases have been reported between 1947 and 1998. Its presentation is similar to the cases of synovial cell sarcoma previously reviewed. One patient whose case has not been reported in the literature was also treated at our institution. She was a 27-year-old white woman who presented with a preauricular mass, joint noise, and a malocclusion (Fig 35-5a). A CT scan showed the lesion to originate from the joint and extend medially and inferiorly (Fig 35-5b). The condyle and a soft tissue mass were resected through a preauricular approach with a temporal extension. The zygomatic arch was removed to permit access to the tumor and was then replaced as a free bone graft (Figs 35-5c and 35-5d). She has been disease free for 16 years. Treatment by wide local resection has been adequate and should be considered to be the treatment of choice for this type of tumor.

Multiple Myeloma and Plasmacytoma

Multiple myeloma and its unifocal equivalent, the plasmacytoma, have been reported in the mandibular condyle. Although multiple myeloma is the most common primary malignancy of bone, it has only been reported in the mandibular condyle seven times, in patients ranging in age from 41 to 70 years.[177] Two patients presented with a pathologic fracture of the mandible.

The lesions consist of plasma cells of varying maturity and extracellular amyloid deposition. The classic radiographic appearance involves punched-out radiolucent areas without a sclerotic border. Laboratory studies often confirm the presence of an abnormal M (myeloma) protein in blood and urine. The patients may also have a monoclonal gammopathy.[8] The plasmacytoma is a solitary lesion containing plasma cells. It is generally accepted that it represents an early stage of multiple myeloma.

Multiple myeloma is treated with systemic chemotherapy. The prognosis is poor, with a 5-year survival rate of 25%. Patients with plasmacytoma are more fortunate; only 25% of them develop multiple myeloma within 3 years and another one third do not develop the disseminated form for up to 10 years.[65] Treatment of the solitary plasmacytoma is simple curettage.

Metastatic Tumors of the TMJ

The most common malignant tumor of the TMJ is one that has metastasized to the region. Thoma,[1] in 1954, described a case of adenocarcinoma, arising from an unknown primary site, that presented as an osteomyelitis of the condyle and was later resected by condylectomy. In the same article, he also made reference to an earlier case of a metastatic malignant tumor that destroyed the condyle and the glenoid fossa in a 53-year-old patient, but no additional details were given. Reference was also made to a case report of a metastatic melanosarcoma of the big toe that produced an osteolytic lesion of the condyle, but there was no information about the age or gender of the patient. The article included a new case report of a 51-year-old woman presenting with pain and swelling in the TMJ who was treated with vitamin injections, immobilization of the jaw, a bite appliance, and heat. The difficulty with this case was that the radiograph did not show any sign of destruction of the joint, and the diagnosis of neoplasia was not made

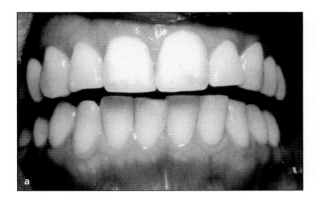

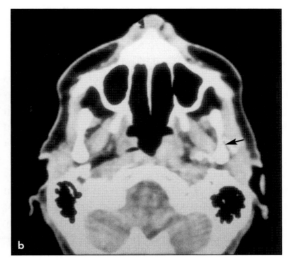

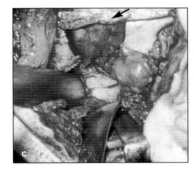

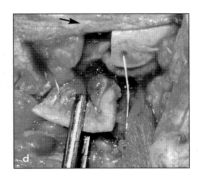

Fig 35-5 Fibrosarcoma of the joint. *(a)* Malocclusion induced by the tumor. *(b)* Computerized tomographic scan, revealing extension of the fibrosarcoma into the medial aspect of the TMJ and ramus *(arrow)*. *(c)* Surgical access, improved by removal of the zygomatic arch *(arrow)*. *(d)* Reconstruction of the arch as a free bone graft after removal of the tumor. *(arrow)* Zygomatic arch. (Courtesy of Dr R. B. MacIntosh.)

until an exploratory arthrotomy was performed. A condylectomy was performed and postoperative radiotherapy (dose unspecified) was given with the new machine located at the Massachusetts Institute of Technology. The patient's tumor was osteoblastic, containing osteoid and osseous tissue with infrequent mitotic figures, and was diagnosed as a transitional-cell carcinoma. The primary tumor was never found.[1]

In a more recent report, a complete accounting of metastatic tumors to the jaws confirmed their frequency at about 3%.[178] The most common was adenocarcinoma originating from the female breast; lung and prostate were other common primary sites. In the most recent review, Nortje et al[179] reviewed 37 cases from the literature and added their own patient, a 43-year-old man with metastatic melanoma to the condyle. There have also been 5 additional cases reported: a third case of metastatic rectal adenocarcinoma[180] and unique cases of hepatocellular carcinoma,[181] chordoma,[182] retinoblastoma,[183] and rectal carcinoma.[175] Of the 43 cases reported, 9 (21%) were from the female breast (3 intraductal carcinomas, 1 carcinoma,

and 5 adenocarcinomas) and 8 (19%) were from the lung (either bronchogenic carcinoma or squamous cell carcinoma except for two, which were adenocarcinomas). The next most common site was actually "unknown" in 6 cases (14%), and the prostate accounted for 5 cases (12%).

The diagnostic dilemma with metastatic tumors is the same as with primary malignancies of the joint: The symptoms bear great commonality to those of certain TMDs. Another confounding factor is confusion with an infection, because a metastasis may cause pain in the joint or involve a preauricular mass that may be associated with lymphadenopathy. Moreover, pain, limited mouth opening, limited lateral excursions, and deviation on mouth opening are nonspecific findings.

In addition to metastasis to the condyle or TMJ, there can be secondary involvement of the joint by direct extension of malignant neoplasms from the skin, ear, parotid, nasopharynx,[184] or the parapharyngeal space. Such situations are more likely to occur than a primary or metastatic malignancy.[185]

Conclusion

Most of the data in this chapter are based on single case reports or small case series. This is expected with lesions of such rarity. Therefore, treatment considerations generally must be based on the behavior of these neoplasms in other facial bones. These principles can then be applied to the condylar cases, with modification to account for management of the disc and the cranial base.

Unless they are aggressive, benign tumors are treated by curettage and simple excision, along with recontouring of the condyle. If they are aggressive, condylectomy with or without discectomy becomes the treatment of choice. Disc replacement with a dermal graft or temporalis flap may be considered. Reconstruction can be done either with a costochondral graft, sliding ramus osteotomy after contouring the condylar neck to function as a condyle, or alloplastic joint replacement.

Primary malignant disease requires an en bloc resection. This means at least a condylectomy and discectomy or, if the lesion is extensive, a hemimandibulectomy with disarticulation. Extension into the glenoid fossa or temporal bone requires craniofacial resection and immediate reconstruction. Lateral extension beyond the joint may require parotidectomy. Postoperative radiotherapy should be considered for patients with extensive disease and when the tumor has close or positive margins. Preoperative and postoperative chemotherapy according to one of the sarcoma protocols may be helpful, particularly for osteosarcoma, but its use is generally based on individual judgment rather than supporting data.

Direct extension of malignant disease into the joint has been reported, primarily from index lesions in the nasopharynx[184] or parotid gland.[185] Treatment of the disease within the joint is part of the general process of securing an adequate margin of resection of the primary process. This requires extensive tissue sacrifice, often including skin. Immediate reconstruction may require free tissue transfer.

It is always important to maintain a high level of suspicion that a TMD that does not respond in the customary and expected way to treatment may not be a TMD. A careful review of the history and physical findings may reveal previously unappreciated details that suggest alternative diagnosis. At that point, the clinician needs to obtain sophisticated imaging, followed by fine needle, arthroscopic, or open biopsy, when possible, in order to establish the correct diagnosis. Ultimately, surgical procedures will be required, both to treat the problem and to establish the final histologic diagnosis.

References

1. Thoma KH. Tumors of the condyle and temporomandibular joint. Oral Surg Oral Med Oral Pathol 1954;7;1091–1107.
2. Ramon Y, Lerner MA, Leventon G. Osteochondroma of the mandibular condyle: Report of a case. Oral Surg Oral Med Oral Pathol 1964;17;16–21.
3. Bavitz B, Chewning C. Malignant disease as temporomandibular joint dysfunction: Review of the literature and report of case. J Am Dent Assoc 1990;120:163–166.
4. Carlson E. Disarticulation resections of the mandible: A prospective review of 16 cases. J Oral Maxillofac Surg 2002; 60:176–181.
5. Nwoku ALN, Koch H. The temporomandibular joint: A rare localization for bone tumours. J Maxillofac Surg 1975;2: 113–119.
6. Allias-Montmayeur F, Durroux R, Dodart L, Combelles R. Tumours and pseudotumorous lesions of the temporomandibular joint: A diagnostic challenge. J Laryngol Otol 1997;3:776–781.
7. Thoma KH. Tumors of the mandibular joint. J Oral Surg Anesth Hosp D Serv 1964;22;61–67.
8. Warner BF, Luna MA, Newland JR. Temporomandibular joint neoplasms and pseudotumors. Adv Anat Pathol 2000;7: 365–381.
9. Spjut HJ, Dorman HD, Fechner RE, Ackerman LV. Atlas of Tumor Pathology. Fascicle 5. Tumors of Bone and Cartilage. Washington, DC: Armed Forces Institute of Pathology, 1971.
10. Batsakis JG. Tumors of the Head and Neck, ed 2. Baltimore: Williams & Wilkins, 1979.
11. Tveteras K, Kristensen S. The aetiology and pathogenesis of trismus. Clin Otolaryngol 1986;11:383–387.
12. Kusen GJ. Chondromatosis: Report of case. J Oral Surg 1969; 27:735–738.
13. Van Damme PA, Freihofer HPM, DeWilde PCM. Neurofibroma in the articular disc of the temporomandibular joint: A case report. J Craniomaxillofac Surg 1996;24:310–313.
14. DelBalso AM, Pyatt RS, Busch RF, Hirokawa R, Fink CS. Synovial cell sarcoma of the temporomandibular joint. Computed tomographic findings. Arch Otolaryngol 1982;108: 520–522.
15. Carls FR, Hochstetter AV, Engelke W, Sailer HF. Loose bodies in the temporomandibular joint: The advantages of arthroscopy. J Craniomaxillofac Surg 1995;23:215–221.
16. Steinhardt LG. Surgery of the temporo-mandibular joint. Int Dent J 1968;18:59–78.
17. Rivera H, Bastidas R, Acevedo AM. A conservative surgical approach of osteochondroma affecting the mandibular condyle. Invest Clin 1998;29:117–124.
18. Wolford LM, Mehra P, Franco P. Use of conservative condylectomy for treatment of osteochondroma of the mandibular condyle. J Oral Maxillofac Surg 2002;60:262–268.
19. Melarky WD, Roffinella JP, Kaplan H. Osteo-cartilaginous exostosis (osteochondroma) of the mandibular condyle. J Oral Surg 1966;24:271–275.

20. Sesenna E, Tullio, Ferrari S. Chondrosarcoma of the temporomandibular joint: A case report and review of the literature. J Oral Maxillofac Surg 1997;55:1348–1352.

21. Gobetti JP, Turp JC. Fibrosarcoma misdiagnosed as a temporomandibular disorder: A cautionary tale. Oral Surg Oral Med Oral Pathol Oral Radiol Endod 1998;85:404–409.

22. Lustman J, Zeltser R. Synovial chondromatosis of the temporomandibular joint. Review of the literature and case report. Int J Oral Maxillofac Surg 1989;18:90–94.

23. Von Arx DP, Simpson MT, Batman P. Synovial chondromatosis of the temporomandibular joint. Br J Oral Maxillofac Surg 1988;26:297–305.

24. Norman JE, Stevenson RL, Painter DM, Sykes DG, Feain LA. Synovial osteochondromatosis of the temporomandibular joint. An historical review with presentation of three cases. J Craniomaxillofac Surg 1988;16:212–220.

25. Ballard R, Weiland LH. Synovial chondromatosis of the temporomandibular joint. Cancer 1972;30:791–795.

26. Mullins F, Berard CW, Eisenberg SH. Chondrosarcoma following synovial chondromatosis: A case study. Cancer 1965;18:1180–1188.

27. Hamilton A, Davis RI, Hayes CD, Mollam RAB. Chondrosarcoma developing in synovial chondromatosis. J Bone Joint Surg Br 1987;69:137–140.

28. Axhausen G. Pathologie und therapie des Kiefergelenkes. Fortschr Zanheilkd 1933;9:171–186.

29. Schulte WC, Rhyne RR. Synovial chondromatosis of the temporomandibular joint: Report of a case. Oral Surg Oral Med Oral Pathol 1969;28:906–913.

30. Forssell K, Happonen RP, Forssell H. Synovial chondromatosis of the temporomandibular joint. Report of a case and review of the literature. Int J Oral Maxillofac Surg 1988;17:237–241.

31. Thompson K, Schwartz HC, Miles JW. Synovial chondromatosis of the temporomandibular joint presenting as a parotid mass: Possibility of confusion with benign mixed tumor. Oral Surg Oral Med Oral Pathol 1986;62:377–380.

32. Akhtar M, Mahajan S, Kott E. Synovial chondromatosis of the temporomandibular joint. J Bone Joint Surg Am 1977;59:266–267.

33. Tagaki M, Ishikawa G. Simultaneous villonodular synovitis and synovial chondromatosis of the temporomandibular joint. Report of a case. J Oral Surg 1981;39:699–701.

34. deBont LGM, Blankestijn J, Panders AK, Vermey A. Unilateral condylar hyperplasia combined with synovial chondromatosis of the temporomandibular joint. Report of a case. J Maxillofac Surg 1985;13:32–36.

35. Innovay J. A rare case of benign synovialoma of the mandibular joint. Oral Surg 1962;15:775–780.

36. Blenkinsopp PT. Loose bodies of the temporomandibular joint, synovial chondromatosis or osteoarthritis. Br J Oral Surg 1978;16:12–20.

37. Iacopino AM, Wathen WF. Craniomandibular disorders in the geriatric patient. J Orofac Pain 1993;7:38–52.

38. Milgram JW. The classification of loose bodies in human joints. Clin Orthop Relat Res 1977;124:282–291.

39. Milgram JW. The development of loose bodies in human joints. Clin Orthop Relat Res 1977;124:292–303.

40. Milgram JW. Synovial osteochondromatosis: A histopathological study of thirty cases. J Bone Joint Surg Am 1977;59:792–801.

41. Dahlin DC. Bone Tumors: General Aspects and Data on 6,221 Cases, ed 3. Springfield, IL: Thomas, 1981:405.

42. Unni KK. Dahlin's Bone Tumors. General Aspects and Data on 11,087 Cases, ed 5. Philadelphia: Lippincott-Raven, 1996:11–23.

43. Karras SC, Wolford LM, Cottrell DA. Concurrent osteochondroma of the mandibular condyle and ipsilateral cranial base resulting in temporomandibular joint ankylosis: Report of case and review of the literature. J Oral Maxillofac Surg 1996;54:640–646.

44. Saito T, Utsunomiya T, Furutani M, Yamamoto H. Osteochondroma of the mandibular condyle; a case report and review of the literature. J Oral Sci 2001;43:293–297.

45. Aydin MA. Osteochondroma of the mandibular condyle: Report of 2 cases treated with conservative surgery. J Oral Maxillofac Surg 2001;59:1082–1089.

46. Vezeau PJ, Fridrich KL, Vincent SD. Osteochondroma of the mandibular condyle: Literature review and report of two atypical cases. J Oral Maxillofac Surg 1995;53:954–956.

47. Schajowicz F. Tumors and Tumorlike Lesions of Bone: Pathology, Radiology and Treatment. New York: Springer, 1994.

48. Iizuka T, Schroth G, Laeng RH, Ladrach K. Osteochondroma of the mandibular condyle. J Oral Maxillofac Surg 1996;54:495–501.

49. Seki H, Fukuda M, Takahashi T, Mitsuyoshi I. Condylar osteochondroma with complete hearing loss: Report of a case. J Oral Maxillofac Surg 2003;61:131–133.

50. Hwang SK, Park BM. Induction of osteochondromas by periosteal resection. Orthopedics 1991;14: 809–812.

51. Langenskiold A. The stages of development of the cartilaginous foci in dyschondroplasia (Ollier's disease). Acta Orthop Scand 1967;38:174–180.

52. Lichtenstein L. Bone Tumors, ed 5. St Louis: Mosby, 1977.

53. Kermer C, Rasse M, Undt G, Lang S. Cartilaginous exostosis of the mandible. Int J Oral Maxillofac Surg 1996;25:373–375.

54. Jaffe HL. Tumors and Tumorous Conditions of the Bones and Joints. Philadelphia: Lea & Febiger, 1961:143–168.

55. Vigorita VJ. Orthopaedic Pathology. Philadelphia: Lippincott-Williams & Wilkins, 1999.

56. Dahlin DC, Ivins JC. Benign chondroblastoma: A study of 125 cases. Cancer 1972;30:401–413.

57. Van Hemelryck T, Richard L, Cartier S, Rives JM, Cantaloube D. Periosteal or juxtacortical chondroma of the mandibular condyle [in French]. Rev Stomatol Chir Maxillofac 1993;94:267–270.

58. Brocheriou C, Payen J. Tumeurs cartilagineuses des maxillaries: A propos de 11 observations. Ann Anat Pathol 1975;20:23–34.

59. Chaudhry AP, Rabinovitch MR, Mitchell DF, Vickers RA. Chondrogenic tumors of the jaws. Am J Surg 1961;102:403–411.

60. Villemey JM. Tumeurs du Condyle Maxillaire Revelatrices de Myeloma Multiple [thesis]. Lyon, France, 1979.

61. Lurie R. Solitary enchondroma of the mandibular condyle: A review and case report. J Dent Assoc S Afr 1975;30:589–593.

62. Jokinen K Stenback F, Palva A, Sutinen S. Benign cartilaginous tumour of the TMJ. J Laryngol Otol 1976;90:299–303.

63. Deboise A, Compere JF, Peron JM, et al. Primary mandibular condyle tumors [in French]. Rev Stomatol Chir Maxillofac 1981;82:93–97.

64. Batsakis JG, Dito WR. Chondrosarcoma of the maxilla. Arch Otolaryngol 1962;75:55–61.

65. Neville BW, Damm DD, Allen CM, Bouquot JE. Oral and Maxillofacial Pathology. Philadelphia: Saunders, 1995.

66. Huvos AG. Bone Tumors: Diagnosis, Treatment and Prognosis, ed 2. Philadelphia: Saunders, 1991:276–279, 295–313.

67. Lazow SK, Pihlstrom RT, Solomon MP, Berger JR. Condylar chondroma: Report of a case. J Oral Maxillofac Surg 1998;56: 373–378.

68. Shafer WG, Hine MK, Levy BM. Textbook of Oral Pathology, ed 4. Philadelphia: Saunders, 1983.

69. Spahr J, Elzay RP, Kay S, Frable WJ. Chondroblastoma of the temporomandibular joint arising from articular cartilage: A previously unreported presentation of an uncommon neoplasm. Oral Surg Oral Med Oral Pathol 1982;54:420–435.

70. Kondoh T, Hamada Y, Kamei K, Seto K. Chondroblastoma of the mandibular condyle; Report of a case. J Oral Maxillofac Surg 2002;60:198–203.

71. Goodsell JO, Hubinger HL, Mich S. Benign chondroblastoma of mandibular condyle: report of case. J Oral Surg 1964;22:355–363.

72. Unni KK. Dahlin's Bone Tumors: General Aspects and Data on 11,087 Cases. Philadelphia: Lippincott-Raven, 1996:47–57.

73. Fechner RE, Mills SE. Chondroblastoma. In: Rosai J (ed). Atlas of Tumor Pathology, 3rd Series. Fascicle 5. Tumor of Bone and Cartilage. Washington, DC: Armed Forces Institute of Pathology, 1993:91–95.

74. Kyriakos M, Land VH, Penning HL, Parker SG. Metastatic chondroblastoma: Report of a fatal case with a review of literature on atypical, aggressive, and malignant chondroblastoma. Cancer 1985;55:1770–1789.

75. Fetissof AG. Pathogenesis of osteomas of the nasal and accessory sinuses. Ann Otol Rhinol Laryngol 1929;38:404–420.

76. Richards HE, Strider JW Jr, Short SG, Theisen FC, Larson WJ. Large peripheral osteoma arising from the genial tubercle area. Oral Surg Oral Med Oral Pathol 1986;61:268–271.

77. Schneider LC, Dolinsky HB, Grodjesk JE. Solitary peripheral osteoma of the jaws: Report of case and review of the literature. J Oral Surg 1980;38:452–255.

78. Green AE, Bowerman JE. An osteoma of the mandible. Br J Oral Surg 1974;12:225–228.

79. Nelson DF, Gross RD, Miller FE. Osteoma of the mandibular condyle: Report of case. J Oral Surg 1972;30:761–766.

80. Swanson KS, Guttu RL, Miller ME. Gigantic osteoma of the mandible: Report of a case. J Oral Maxillofac Surg 1992;50: 635–638.

81. Graham MD. Osteomas and exostosis of the external auditory canal. A clinical, histopathologic and scanning electron microscopic study. Ann Otol 1979;88:566–672.

82. Kazuhisha B, Murakama K, Iizuka T, Ono T. Osteoma of the mandibular condyle. Int J Oral Maxillofac Surg 1987;16: 372–375.

83. Miyachi T. Clinical Histopathology. Tokyo: Kyorin Shoin, 1976:706.

84. Lucas RB. Pathology of Tumours of the Oral Tissues, ed 3. Edinburgh: Churchill Livingstone, 1976.

85. Gardner EJ, Richards RG. Multiple cutaneous and subcutaneous lesions occurring simultaneously with hereditary polyposis and osteomatosis. Am J Hum Genet 1953;5:139–147.

86. Lind PO, Hillerstrom K. Osteoid osteoma in the mandibular condyle. Acta Otolaryngol 1964;75:467–474.

87. Yang C, Qiu WL. Osteoid osteoma of the eminence of the temporomandibular joint. Br J Oral Maxillofac Surg 2001;39: 404–406.

88. Weinberg S, Katsikeris N, Pharoah M. Osteoblastoma of the mandibular condyle; review of the literature and report of a case. J Oral Maxillofac Surg 1987;45:350–355.

89. Svennson B, Isacsson G. Benign osteoblastoma associated with an aneurysmal bone cyst of the mandibular ramus and condyle. Oral Surg Oral Med Oral Pathol 1993;76:433–436.

90. Asada Y, Suzuki I, Suzuki M, Fukushima M. Atypical multiple benign osteoblastomas accompanied by simple bone cysts. J Oral Maxillofac Surg 1991;18:166–171.

91. Smith RA, Hansen LS, Resnick D, Chan W. Comparison of the osteoblastoma in gnathic and extragnathic sites. Oral Surg Oral Med Oral Pathol 1982;54:285–298.

92. Dorfman HD, Czerniak B. Bone Tumors. St Louis: Mosby, 1998.

93. Lichtenstein L, Sawyer WR. Benign osteoblastoma: Further observations and report of twenty additional cases. J Bone Joint Surg Am 1964;46:755–765.

94. Walker DG. Benign nonodontogenic tumors of the jaws. J Oral Surg 1970;28:39–57.

95. Makek M. Non-ossifying fibroma of the mandible: A common lesion with unusual location. Arch Orthop Trauma Surg 1980;96:225–227.

96. Aldred MJ, Breckon JJW, Holland CS. Non-osteogenic fibroma of the mandibular condyle. Br J Oral Maxillofac Surg 1989;27:412–416.

97. Tom BM, Rao VM, Farole A. Nondiscogenic causes of temporomandibular joint pain. Cranio 1991;9:220–227.

98. Nishida J, Tajima K, Abe M, et al. Desmoplastic fibroma. Aggressive curettage as a surgical alternative for treatment. Clin Orthop Relat Res 1995;320:142–148.

99. Taguchi N, Kaneda T. Desmoplastic fibroma of the mandible; report of case. J Oral Surg 1980;38:440–444.

100. Moenning JE, Williams KL, McBride JS, Rafetto LK. Resorption of the mandibular condyle in a 6-year-old child. J Oral Maxillofac Surg 1998;56:477–482.

101. Harrison JD. Odontogenic myxoma: Ultrastructural and histochemical studies. J Clin Pathol 1973;26:570–582.

102. McClure DK, Dahlin DC. Myxoma of bone. Report of 3 cases. Mayo Clin Proc 1977;52:249–253.

103. Thoma KH, Holland DJ, Rounds CE. Tumors of the mandibular condyle; report of two cases. Clin Mass Gen Hosp 1947: 344–350.

104. Zimmerman DC, Dahlin DC. Myxomatous tumors of the jaws. Oral Surg 1958;11:1069–1080.

105. Gorlin RJ, Chaudhry AP, Pindborg JJ. Odontogenic tumors; classification, histopathology and clinical behavior in man and domesticated animals. Cancer 1961;14:73–101.

106. Killey HC, Kay LW. Fibromyxomata of the jaws. Br J Oral Surg 1965;2:124–130.

107. White DK, Chen SY, Mohnac AM, Miller AS. Odontogenic myxoma. A clinical and ultrastructural study. Oral Surg 1975;39:901–917.

108. Bucci E. Odontogenic myxoma: Report of a case with peculiar features. J Oral Maxillofac Surg 1991;49:91–94.

109. Lund V, Harrison J (eds). Tumors of the Upper Jaw. New York: Churchill Livingstone, 1993.

110. Slootweg PJ, Wittkamp RM. Myxoma of the jaws. An analysis of 15 cases. J Maxillofac Surg 1986;14:46–52.

111. Ghosh BC, Huvos AG, Gerold FP, Miller TR. Myxoma of the jaw bones. Cancer 1973;31:237–240.

112. Thoma KH. Oral Surgery, ed 5. St Louis: Mosby, 1969.

113. Colburn JF, Epker BN. Myxoma of the mandibular condyle-surgical excision with immediate reconstruction. J Oral Surg 1975;33:351–355.

114. Halfpenny W, Verey A, Bardsley MA. Myxoma of the mandibular condyle. A case report and review of the literature. Oral Surg Oral Med Oral Pathol Oral Radiol Endod 2000; 90:348–353.

115. Lo Muzio L, Nocini P, Favia G, Procaccini M, Mignogna MD. Odontogenic myxoma of the jaws. Oral Surg Oral Med Oral Pathol Oral Radiol Endod 1996;82:426–33.

116. Hofer O. Diagnosis and therapy of the giant cell granuloma of the jaws [in German]. Zeitschr Stomatol 1952;49:324–328.

117. Ling L, Klein MJ, Sissons HA, Steiner GC. Lysozyme and alpha 1-antitrypsin in giant-cell tumor of bone and in other lesions that contain giant cells. Arch Pathol Lab Med 1986; 110:713–718.

118. Motamedi MHK. Destructive aneurysmal bone cyst of the mandibular condyle: Report of a case and review of the literature. J Oral Maxillofac Surg 2003;60:1357–1361.

119. Lichtenstein L. Histocystosis X. Arch Pathol 1953;56:84–102.

120. Osband ME, Lipton JM, Lavin P, et al. Histiocytosis X: Demonstration of abnormal immunity. T-cell histamine-H$_2$-receptor deficiency and successful treatment with thymic extract. N Engl J Med 1981;304:146–153.

121. Harrist TJ, Bhan AK, Murphy GF, et al. Histiocytosis X: In situ characterization of cutaneous infiltrates with monoclonal antibodies. AM J Clin Pathol 1983;79;294–300.

122. Murphy GF. Monoclonal anti-T6 antibody and Langerhans cells. Br J Dermatol 1982;107:487–489.

123. Cohen M, Zornoza J, Cangir A, Murray JA, Wallace S. Direct injection of methylprednisolone sodium succinate in the treatment of solitary eosinophilic granuloma of bone: A report of 9 cases. Radiology 1980;136:289–293.

124. Del Balso AM, Banyas JB, Wild L. Hemangioma of the mandibular condyle and ramus. AJNR Am J Neuroradiol 1994; 15:1703–1705.

125. Uotila E, Westerholm N. Hemangioma of the temporomandibular joint. Odontol Tidskr 1996;74:202–206.

126. Whear NM. Condylar hemangioma—A case report and review of the literature. Br J Oral Maxillofac Surg 1991;29:44–47.

127. Atkinson TJ, Wolf S, Anavi Y, Wesley R. Synovial hemangioma of the temporomandibular joint; report of a case and review of the literature. J Oral Maxillofac Surg 1988;46:804–808.

128. Regezi JA, Sciubba JJ. Oral Pathology: Clinical Pathologic Correlations, ed 3. Philadelphia: Saunders,1999.

129. Greenspan A, Remagene W. Differential Diagnosis of Tumors and Tumor-like Lesions of Bones and Joints. Philadelphia: Lippincott-Raven, 1998.

130. Schindel J, Matz S, Edlan A, Abraham A. Central cavernous hemangioma of the jaws. J Oral Surg 1978;36:803–807.

131. Redman RS, Guccion JG, Spector CJ, Keegan BP. Cellular schwannoma of the mandible: A case report with ultrastructural and immunohistochemical observations.. J Oral Maxillofac Surg 1996;54:339–344.

132. White W, Shiu MH, Rosenblum MK, Erlandson RA, Woodruff JM. Cellular schwannoma. A clinicopathologic study of 57 patients and 58 tumors. Cancer 1990;66:1266–1275.

133. Sordillo PP, Helson L, Najdu SI, et al. Malignant schwannoma—Clinical characteristics, survival and response to therapy. Cancer 1981;47:2503–2509.

134. Lapayowker MS, Miller WT, Levy WM, Harwick RD. Pigmented villonodular synovitis of the temporomandibular joint. Radiology 1973;108:313–316.

135. Copeland M, Douglas B. Ganglions of the temporomandibular joint: Case report and review of the literature. Plast Reconstr Surg 1988;81:775–776.

136. Thawley SE, Panje WR, Batsakis JG, et al (eds). Comprehensive Management of Head and Neck Tumors. Philadelphia: Saunders, 1987:1518.

137. Abubaker AO, Braun TW, Sotereanos GC, Erickson ER. Osteosarcoma of the mandibular condyle. J Oral Maxillofac Surg 1986;44:126–131.

138. Zorzan G, Tulio A, Bertolini F, Sesenna E. Osteosarcoma of the mandibular condyle: Case report. J Oral Maxillofacial Surg 2001;59:574–577.

139. Richter KJ, Freeman NS, Quick DA. Chondrosarcoma of the temporomandibular joint: Report of case. J Oral Surg 1974; 32:777–781.

140. Batra PS, Estrem SA, Zitsch RP. Chondrosarcoma of the temporomandibular joint. Otolaryngol Head Neck Surg 1999; 120:951–954.

141. Nitzan DW, Marmary Y, Hassan O, Elidan J. Chondrosarcoma arising in the temporomandibular joint: A case report and literature review. J Oral Maxillofac Surg 1993;51:312–315.

142. Dos Santos DT, Cavalcanti MGP. Osteosarcoma of the temporomandibular joint: Report of 2 cases. Oral Surg Oral Med Oral Pathol Oral Radiol Endod 2002;94:641–647.

143. Arlen M, Tollefsen HR, Huvos AG, Marcove RC. Chondrosarcoma of the head and neck. Am J Surg 1970;120: 456–460.

144. Venner J, Rice DH, Newman AN. Osteosarcoma and chondrosarcoma of the head and neck. Laryngoscope 1984;94: 240–242.

145. Murayama S, Suzuki I, Nagase M, et al. Chondrosarcoma of the mandible. Report of case and a survey of 23 cases in the Japanese literature. J Craniomaxillofac Surg 1988;16:287–292.

146. Gingrass PP. Chondrosarcoma of the mandibular joint: Report of case. J Oral Surg 1954;12:61–63.

147. Lanier VC, Rosenfeld L, Wilkinson HA. Chondrosarcoma of the mandible. South Med J 1971;64:711–714.

148. Nortje CJ, Farman AG, Grotepass FW, Van Zyl JA. Chondrosarcoma of the mandibular condyle. Report of a case with special reference to radiographic features. Br J Oral Surg 1976;14:101–111.

149. Morris MR, Clark SK, Porter BA. Chondrosarcoma of the temporomandibular joint: Case report. Head Neck Surg 1987;10:113–117.

150. Sessana E, Tullio A, Ferrani S. Chondrosarcoma of the temporomandibular joint: A case report and review of the literature. J Oral Maxillofac Surg 1997;55:1348–1352.

151. Burkey BB, Hoffman HT, Baker SR, Thornton AF, McClatchey KD. Chondrosarcoma of the head and neck. Laryngoscope 1990;100:1301–1305.

152. Finn DG, Goepfert H, Batsakis JG. Chondrosarcoma of the head and neck. Laryngoscope 1984;94:1539–1544.

153. Harwood AR, Drajbach JL, Fornasier VL. Radiotherapy of chondrosarcoma of bone. Cancer 1980;45:2769–2777.

154. Kim RY, Salter MM, Brascho DJ. High-energy irradiation in the management of chondrosarcoma. South Med J 1983;76:729–735.

155. Doval DC, Kumar RV, Kannan V, et al. Osteosarcoma of the jawbones. Br J Oral Maxillofac Surg 1997;35:357–362.

156. Garrington GE, Scofield HH, Cornyn J, Hooker SP. Osteosarcoma of the jaws. Analysis of 56 cases. Cancer 1967;20:377–391.

157. Batsakis JG, Solomon AR, Rice DH. The pathology of head and neck tumors: Neoplasms and cysts of bone and notochord. 7. Head Neck Surg 1980;3:43–47.

158. Clark JL, Unni KK, Dahlin DC, Devine KD. Osteosarcoma of the jaw. Cancer 1983;51:2311–2316.

159. Forteza G, Comenero B, Lopez-Barea F. Osteogenic sarcoma of the maxilla and mandible. Oral Surg Oral Med Oral Pathol 1986;62:169–184.

160. Kragh LV, Dahlin DC, Erich JB. Cartilaginous tumors of the jaws and facial regions. Am J Surg 1960;99:852–936.

161. Mark RJ, Sercarz JA, Tran L, Dodd LG, Selch M, Calcaterra TC. Osteosarcoma of the head and neck. The UCLA experience. Arch Otolaryngol Head Neck Surg 1991;117:761–766.

162. Lahti A, Sundell B. Reconstruction of the mandibular bone and the condyle after tumour surgery. Ann Chir Gynaecol Fenn 1973;62:155–160.

163. Goepfert H, Raymond AK, Spires JR, et al. Osteosarcoma of the head and neck. Cancer Bull 1990;42:342–354.

164. Lewis M, Perl A, Som PM, Urken ML, Brandwein MS. Osteogenic sarcoma of the jaw: A clinicopathologic review of 12 patients. Arch Otolaryngol Head Neck Surg 1997;123:169–174.

165. Delgado R, Maafs E, Alfeiran A, et al. Osteosarcoma of the jaw. Head Neck 1994;16:246–252.

166. Kassir RR, Rassekh CH, Kinsella JB, Segas J, Carrau RL, Hokanson JA. Osteosarcoma of the head and neck: Meta-analysis of nonrandomized studies. Laryngoscope 1997;107:56–61.

167. Pease GL, Maisel RH, Cantrell RW. Surgical management of osteogenic sarcoma of the mandible. Arch Otolaryngol 1975;101:761–762.

168. Russ JE, Jesse RH. Management of osteosarcoma of the maxilla. Am J Surg 1980; 140:572–576.

169. Kuppersmith RB, Disher MJ, Deveikis JP, et al. Management of an osteogenic sarcoma of the maxilla. Ann Otol Rhinol Laryngol 1994;103:408–412.

170. Rosen G, Caparros B, Huvos AG, et al. Preoperative chemotherapy for osteogenic sarcoma: Selection of postoperative adjuvant chemotherapy based on the response of the primary tumor to preoperative chemotherapy. Cancer 1982;49:1221–1230.

171. Bertoni F, Dallera P, Bacchini P. Marchetti, Campobassi A. The Istituto Rizzoli-Beretta experience with osteosarcoma of the jaw. Cancer 1991;68:1555–1563.

172. Huvos AG. Bone Tumors: Diagnosis, Treatment and Prognosis, ed 2. Philadelphia: Saunders 1991:85–156.

173. Enzinger FM, Weiss SW. Soft Tissue Tumors. St Louis: Mosby, 1988:659–688.

174. Miloro M, Quinn PD, Stewart JCB. Monophasic spindle cell synovial sarcoma of the head and neck: Report of two cases and review of the literature. J Oral Maxillofac Surg 1994;52:309–313.

175. Stadelman WK, Cruse CW, Messina J. Synovial cell sarcoma of the temporomandibular joint. Ann Plast Surg 1995;35:664–668.

176. White RD, Makar J, Steckler RM. Synovial sarcoma of the temporomandibular joint. J Oral Maxillofac Surg 1992;50:1227–1230.

177. Gonazalez J, Elondo J, Trull JM, Del Torres I. Plasma cell tumours of the condyle. Br J Oral Maxillofac Surg 1991;29:274–276.

178. Stypulkowsda J, Bartkowski S, Panas M, Zaleska M. Metastatic tumors of the jaws and oral cavity. J Oral Surg 1979;37:805–89.

179. Nortje CJ, van Rensburg LJ, Thompson IOC. Case report. Magnetic resonance features of metastatic melanoma of the temporomandibular joint and mandible. Dentomaxillofac Radiol 1996;25:292–297.

180. Balestreri L, Canzonieri V, Innocente R, Cattelan A, Perin T. Temporomandibular joint metastasis from rectal carcinoma; CT findings before and after radiotherapy. A case report. Tumori 1997;83:718–720.

181. Yoshimura Y, Matsuda S, Naitoh SI. Hepatocellular carcinoma metastatic to the mandibular ramus and condyle: Report of a case and review of the literature. J Oral Maxillofac Surg 1997;55:287–306.

182. Meneghini F, Castellani A, Camelin N, Zanetti U. Metastatic chordoma to the mandibular condyle: An anterior surgical approach. J Oral Maxillofac Surg 2002;60:1489–1493.

183. King DL, Shapiro SD, Beall JC. Metastatic retinoblastoma of the maxilla and mandible: Report of case. J Dent Child 1976;43:347–349.

184. Epstein JB, Jones CK. Presenting signs and symptoms of nasopharyngeal carcinoma. Oral Surg Oral Med Oral Pathol Oral Radiol Endod 1993;75:31–36.

185. Owen GO, Stelling CB. Condylar metastasis with initial presentation of TMJ syndrome. J Oral Med 1985;40:198–201.

Management of Idiopathic Condylar Resorption

M. Anthony Pogrel and Radhika Chigurupati

Condylar resorption can be defined as a progressive alteration in the condyle shape and a decrease in condyle mass. Although patients may develop temporomandibular joint (TMJ) symptoms in association with this process, in many patients such symptoms are absent, and the first indication of the condition is that patients exhibit a decrease in posterior facial height, retrognathism, and a progressive anterior open bite with clockwise rotation of the mandible (Fig 36-1).[1]

The exact etiology of the condition is unknown, although it has been associated with a number of systemic medical conditions including rheumatoid arthritis, systemic lupus erythematosus, scleroderma, and neoplasia. It has also been attributed to forces generated during trauma, orthodontic and orthopedic treatment (Fig 36-2), and orthognathic surgery.[2–11] Steroid use also has been suspected to be a predisposing factor. In most cases, however, there is no identifiable precipitating event, and hence the term *idiopathic condylar resorption* is used.[12] The condition is poorly understood but appears to have a predilection for females who have preexisting TMJ dysfunction, a high mandibular plane angle, and small condyles on long, slender condylar necks and who are usually in the age range of 15 to 35 years[13,14] (Fig 36-3). The condition is almost always bilateral.

Some authorities believe that the underlying cause may be abnormal joint loading and subsequent pressure resorption. This theory seems most prevalent in cases

that occur following orthognathic surgery and has been investigated in detail by Arnett et al.[15,16] Following orthognathic surgery, and in particular sagittal split osteotomy, the condyles may be torqued during placement of rigid fixation, placing excessive pressure on either the medial or lateral pole of the condyle and causing a subsequent resorption and clinical relapse that, in susceptible patients, can progress to outright idiopathic condylar resorption (Fig 36-4). Such cases can be quite dramatic (Fig 36-5). Virtually all have involved young females with preexisting long, slender condylar processes. Scheerlinck et al[17] reported an incidence of 7.7% following sagittal split osteotomy in 103 patients, and it has been suggested that when patients fulfill all of the at-risk criteria their chance of developing postoperative idiopathic condylar resorption following this operation may be as high as 12.5%. Susceptible patients with mandibular advancements of 10 mm or more may be particularly prone to postoperative condylar resorption.[18]

Condylar bone changes caused by alterations in joint loading and subsequent remodeling probably occur after most mandibular osteotomies, but the reason they become so extensive in some patients is unknown, although Milam has suggested that idiopathic condylar resorption is an extreme form of osteoarthritis (see chapter 7). The predominance of this condition in females in their second and third decades certainly suggests a hormonal connection, and estrogen receptors have been identified in the TMJ.[19,20]

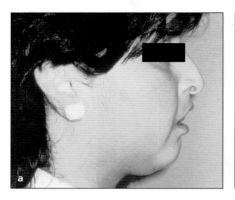

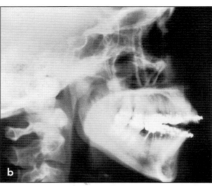

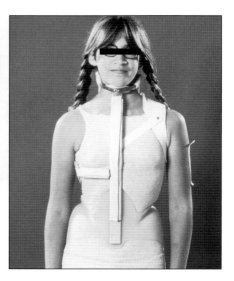

Fig 36-1 *(a)* Typical appearance of a patient with condylar resorption. Note the retrognathism, clockwise rotation of the mandible, and lip incompetence secondary to the open bite. In this patient, the condition is secondary to scleroderma. *(b)* Lateral cephalometric radiograph of the patient in Fig 36-1a. Note the shortening of the condyles, clockwise rotation of the mandible, retrognathism, and anterior open bite.

Fig 36-2 Orthopedic frame used for spinal support of patients with scoliosis and kyphosis. If wrongly adjusted, it can put pressure on the mandible and condyles and induce resorption.

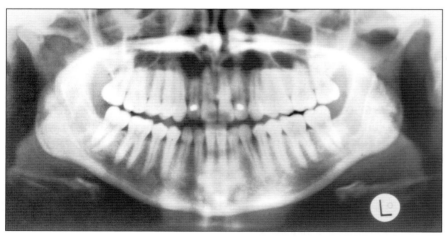

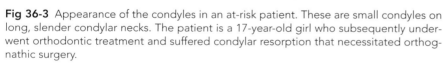

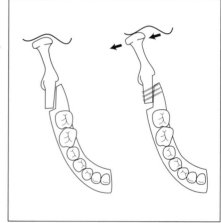

Fig 36-3 Appearance of the condyles in an at-risk patient. These are small condyles on long, slender condylar necks. The patient is a 17-year-old girl who subsequently underwent orthodontic treatment and suffered condylar resorption that necessitated orthognathic surgery.

Fig 36-4 Condylar torquing caused by rigid screw fixation following sagittal split osteotomy when the fragments do not line up anatomically *(arrows)*. Correct treatment in such cases is either nonrigid fixation or the use of shims of some type to hold the bone ends apart and the condyles in their anatomic position.

An alternative theory is that the etiology may be a form of osteonecrosis in which the blood supply to the mandibular condyles is diminished, and a condition similar to osteonecrosis of the hip can occur, resulting in joint collapse and resorption[21] (Figs 36-6 and 36-7). It has been suggested that the mandibular condyle is supplied by an end artery, which can be occluded by a displaced disc, thus interrupting the arterial blood supply, although others have argued that this is anatomically incorrect. The proponents of this theory recommend revascularization of the condyle by drilling holes in it through the cortical plate until bleeding is obtained[22] (Fig 36-8).

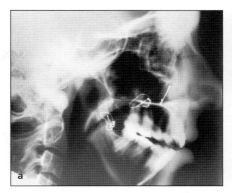
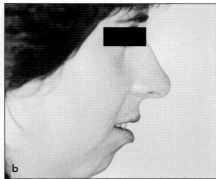
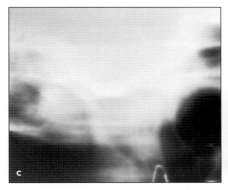
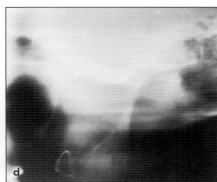

Fig 36-5 *(a)* Lateral cephalometric radiograph showing condylar resorption following maxillary and mandibular orthognathic surgery carried out with nonrigid fixation. *(b)* Clinical appearance of the patient after condylar resorption. Note the mandibular retrognathism, microgenia, and lip incompetence. *(c and d)* Tomograms of the condyles of the patient in Figs 36-5a and 36-5b. Note the almost total resorption of the condyles.

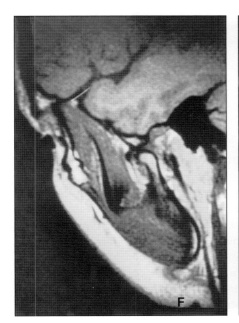
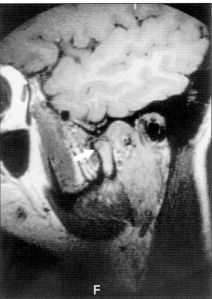
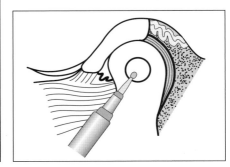

Fig 36-6 Magnetic resonance image of a normal left condyle. Note the high consistent marrow signal *(white)* and regular cortical bone outline *(black)*.

Fig 36-7 Magnetic resonance image of a condyle undergoing collapse. Note the irregular and inconsistent marrow signal *(arrow)* and irregular cortical outline *(black)*.

Fig 36-8 Revascularization of the condyle by lateral decortication and encouragement of bleeding.

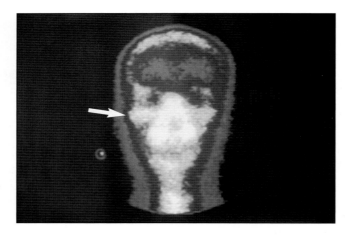

Fig 36-9 Anteroposterior bone scan showing activity in both condyles. The activity is higher on the right side *(arrow)*.

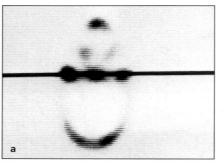
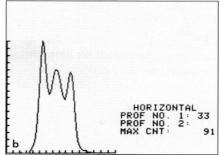

Fig 36-10 Single photon emission computerized tomography scan. *(a)* Axial slice that includes both condyles and the clivus. *(b)* Relative activity in both condyles and clivus activity in the middle. The activity in the condyle on the right is the same as that in the clivus, whereas the condyle on the left shows greater activity.

Diagnosis

The investigation of idiopathic condylar resorption includes both systemic and local examinations. Systemically, the patient should be evaluated for rheumatoid arthritis, scleroderma, and other autoimmune diseases that can cause bone resorption. Appropriate laboratory tests include measurement of the erythrocyte sedimentation rate and C-reactive protein level (which would be raised) and serologic tests for specific antigens, including rheumatoid factor (positive in 80% of patients with rheumatoid arthritis and 33% with scleroderma) and antinuclear antibodies (present in 40% to 60% of patients with rheumatoid arthritis).

A history of steroid use should be elicited, because this could cause bone resorption. Any history of use of orthodontic or orthopedic devices should also be investigated, because this could also cause increased loading on the condyles. The latter would include some types of orthopedic braces for the management of scoliosis and kyphosis and orthodontic appliances such as chin cups and mandibular extraoral traction devices that cause distalization of the condyles.[1]

Local investigations include a panoramic radiograph and tomograms or a computerized tomographic scan for evaluation of the condylar size and architecture. Particular attention should be paid to the mass of the condyles, because they are generally small and slender in patients suffering from idiopathic resorption. Attention should also be paid to the cortical outline of the condyle, because this is generally lost during the active phase. However, once the resorption has been inactive for a year or longer, the condyle usually becomes recorticated. A lateral cephalometric radiograph will also reveal some shortening of the ascending ramus of the mandible, clockwise mandibular rotation, and varying degrees of open bite.

Radioisotope uptake studies will indicate if any active metabolic activity is occurring in the mandibular condyles. These studies are normally carried out with a bone-seeking phosphate isotope such as technetium 99m polyphosphate, pyrophosphate, or methylene diphosphonate. These isotopes are injected intravenously and are taken up by areas of active bone formation and incorporated into actively forming bone matrix.[23] Therefore, pure bone resorption may not produce a positive bone scan, but any new bone formation will.

The scan normally involves three phases. The first phase, known as the *blood flow phase*, shows the degree of uptake of the isotope, which is dependent on blood flow to the region. In the second phase, the isotope is taken up by the actively forming bone matrix, and in the third (excretion) phase, the isotope is eliminated and found mainly in the kidneys, ureter, or bladder. The stage of interest in patients with suspected idiopathic condylar resorption is the uptake phase in the bone matrix, and this normally occurs between 2 and 4 hours after injection of the isotope (Fig 36-9).

A more sophisticated technique than an ordinary bone scan involves single photon emission computerized tomography, in which 6.5-mm slices can be made in any plane. An axial slice taken through both condyles will also include the clivus of the skull, which is a very inactive area metabolically.[24] In this way, condylar activity can be compared with clivus activity, and the ratio between them can be calculated. This ratio can be used to define the amount of activity in the condyle (Fig 36-10). An alternative technique compares activity in the condyles with activity in the fourth lumbar vertebra, which in most patients is also a fairly inactive area and can be used as a control.[25]

On bone scans, most mandibular condyles normally show some activity until subjects are in their late teens, when growth in the condyle ceases; however, it is symmetric activity. Activity beyond the normal age or asymmetric activity may be of significance. Repeated bone scans can be used to assess when either growth or resorption has ceased and to determine when definitive or interventional surgery could or should be carried out.

Management

Because idiopathic condylar resorption remains a poorly defined condition, there are relatively few guidelines for its management. In theory it could be corrected either by orthognathic surgery to reposition the mandible, leaving the condyles in their current position, or by mandibular repositioning and replacement of the condyles into their premorbid anatomic position. Before orthognathic surgery is attempted, it is essential that the disease process has ceased; this can usually be ascertained by serial radiographs, serial models of the occlusion, or bone scans of the condyles. If progress has ceased, then theoretically orthognathic surgery should be possible. However, the results of this type of surgery have been unpredictable.

Crawford et al[26] reviewed a group of seven patients with progressive condylar resorption following orthognathic surgery that included a sagittal split osteotomy to advance the mandible. They were all treated by repeated orthognathic surgery, which included a sagittal split osteotomy. Five patients showed further skeletal evidence of relapse postoperatively, and one of these again showed relapse after a third sagittal split osteotomy.

Merkx and Van Damme[27] treated eight patients who developed condylar resorption after sagittal split osteotomy and noted unsatisfactory results in four patients treated with repeated orthognathic surgery. More stable results were achieved in four patients treated by an occlusal appliance and either orthodontic or prosthodontic management.

Arnett and Tamborello[28] described six patients with progressive condylar resorption treated by orthognathic surgery. Five patients had further resorption postoperatively. The only stable patient was the one who had preoperative occlusal appliance therapy to stabilize the TMJ. A second group of eight patients received preoperative stabilization therapy with appliances and anti-inflammatory medications before orthognathic surgery, and in seven of these patients the results were stable over the long term.

Huang et al[1] reported that, of 13 patients undergoing orthognathic surgery for the management of idiopathic condylar resorption, only 5 had a stable, asymptomatic end result. Four patients were stable but had postoperative TMJ symptoms, while 4 underwent recurrent, progressive condylar resorption.

These reports indicate that if orthognathic surgery is to be attempted as the treatment for condylar resorption, the resorptive process must have ceased, as confirmed by tomographs, occlusal casts, or an isotope bone scan. The joint should also be stabilized by means of an occlusal

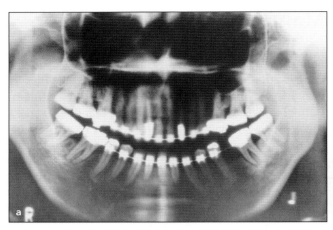
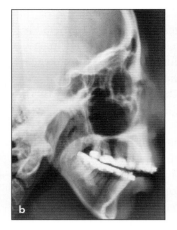
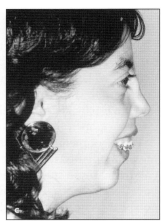
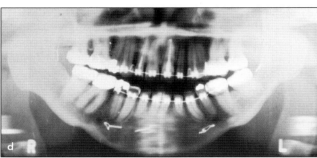
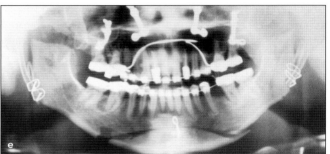

Fig 36-11 *(a)* Appearance of the condyles in a 26-year-old woman who had bilateral condylar resorption, possibly because of orthodontic forces on the condyle. *(b)* Lateral cephalometric radiograph of the patient at the completion of orthodontic treatment. There was no retrognathism or open bite at the commencement of orthodontic treatment. *(c)* Clinical appearance of the patient. Note the retrognathism, microgenia, and lip incompetence. *(d)* Patient following treatment with sagittal split osteotomies of the mandible and a genioplasty. This treatment caused further condylar resorption down to the sigmoid notch. *(e)* Patient after Le Fort I level maxillary osteotomy, bilateral costochondral graft replacement of the condyle, and a repeated genioplasty. Coronectomies were also performed. The ribs were placed posterior to the ramus and secured with wires.

appliance and anti-inflammatory medications and perhaps an anticollagenase agent, such as a tetracycline, should be used in an attempt to reduce the possibility of an adverse outcome. Even so, it appears that mandibular orthognathic surgery (particularly sagittal split–type surgery) has the potential to reactivate condylar resorption, presumably by altering the vascular or loading dynamics. For this reason it has been suggested that orthognathic surgery for this condition be restricted to the maxilla only.[28]

An alternative treatment consists of replacement of the affected joints by means of an autologous costochondral graft or an alloplastic total joint. This treatment can be carried out whether the resorptive process is active or quiescent. Costochondral grafting for the management of idiopathic condylar resorption has been reported by Huang et al,[1] who described five patients treated in this

way, all of whom had a stable end result and no continued resorption (Fig 36-11). The reason that resorption does not affect the costochondral graft is unknown.

There is little literature available on the management of this condition with alloplastic joint replacement, but it would seem that the result would be equivalent to that with alloplastic joint replacement in general (see chapter 31). At this time, two alloplastic joints approved by the US Food and Drug Administration are commercially available.[29–31]

Synovectomy and arthroplasty have been recommended to arrest unilateral condylar hyperplasia.[32,33] Using a similar logic, Wolford and Cardenas[34] have reported success with synovectomy, disc repositioning, ligament repair, and orthognathic surgery performed simultaneously to arrest the resorptive process and correct the consequent deformity.

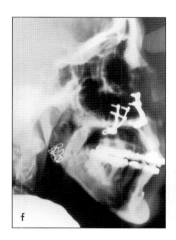

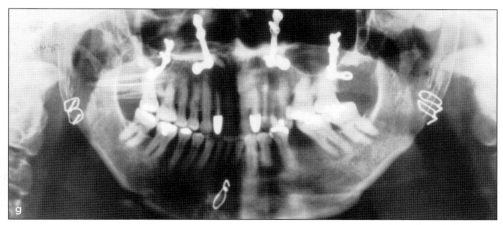

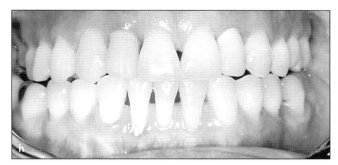

Fig 36-11 *(continued)* *(f)* Postoperative lateral cephalometric radiograph revealing good occlusion and profile. *(g)* Panoramic radiograph of the patient 15 years after orthognathic surgery and costochondral grafts. Note the remodeling of the costochondral grafts to resemble condyles more closely. The occlusion is stable and the patient can open her mouth more than 40 mm. *(h)* Occlusion of the patient 15 years after orthognathic surgery and costochondral grafts. There has been no occlusal relapse.

Summary

At the present time, there are no evidence-based studies on the management of condylar resorption, and further research is needed in the areas of etiology and management. Prospective studies, which would probably have to be multicentered to generate sufficient numbers with long-term follow-up, are urgently required.

The present state of knowledge indicates that inactive condylar resorption requiring relatively small corrective jaw movements should be treated by maxillary orthognathic surgery, if possible; mandibular orthognathic surgery (particularly a sagittal split osteotomy to advance the mandible) should be undertaken with extreme caution. When the condyles are still actively resorbing despite treatment, or the corrective jaw movements are large, condylar reconstruction with a costochondral graft is probably indicated. The reported success with this procedure, plus the avoidance of major orthognathic surgery, makes this the current treatment of choice.

References

1. Huang YL, Pogrel MA, Kaban LB. Diagnosis and management of condylar resorption. J Oral Maxillofac Surg 1997;55:114–119; discussion 119–120.
2. Ogus H. Rheumatoid arthritis of the temporomandibular joint. Br J Oral Surg 1975;12:275–284.
3. Ogden GR. Complete resorption of the mandibular condyles in rheumatoid arthritis. Br Dent J 1986;160:95–97.
4. Ramon Y, Samra H, Oberman M. Mandibular condylosis and apertognathia as presenting symptoms in progressive systemic sclerosis (scleroderma). Pattern of mandibular bony lesions and atrophy of masticatory muscles in PSS, presumably caused by affected muscular arteries. Oral Surg Oral Med Oral Pathol 1987;63:269–274.
5. Lanigan DT, Myall RW, West RA, McNeill RW. Condylysis in a patient with a mixed collagen vascular disease. Oral Surg Oral Med Oral Pathol 1979;48:198–204.
6. Osial TA Jr, Avakian A, Sassouni V, Agarwal A, Medsger TA Jr, Rodnan GP. Resorption of the mandibular condyles and coronoid processes in progressive systemic sclerosis (scleroderma). Arthritis Rheum 1981;24:729–733.

7. Iizuka T, Lindqvist C, Hallikainen D, Mikkonen P, Paukku P. Severe bone resorption and osteoarthrosis after miniplate fixation of high condylar fractures. A clinical and radiologic study of thirteen patients. Oral Surg Oral Med Oral Pathol 1991;72:400–407.

8. Lindqvist C, Soderholm AL, Hallikainen D, Sjovall L. Erosion and heterotopic bone formation after alloplastic temporomandibular joint reconstruction. J Oral Maxillofac Surg 1992;50:942–949; discussion 950.

9. Phillips RM, Bell WH. Atrophy of mandibular condyles after sagittal ramus split osteotomy: Report of case. J Oral Surg 1978;36:45–49.

10. Sesenna E, Raffaini M. Bilateral condylar atrophy after combined osteotomy for correction of mandibular retrusion. A case report. J Maxillofac Surg 1985;13:263–266.

11. Bouwman JP, Kerstens HC, Tuinzing DB. Condylar resorption in orthognathic surgery. The role of intermaxillary fixation. Oral Surg Oral Med Oral Pathol 1994;78:138–141.

12. Rabey GP. Bilateral mandibular condylysis—A morphanalytic diagnosis. Br J Oral Surg 1977;15:121–134.

13. Moore KE, Gooris PJ, Stoelinga PJ. The contributing role of condylar resorption to skeletal relapse following mandibular advancement surgery: Report of five cases. J Oral Maxillofac Surg 1991;49:448–460.

14. Kerstens HC, Tuinzing DB, Golding RP, van der Kwast WA. Condylar atrophy and osteoarthrosis after bimaxillary surgery. Oral Surg Oral Med Oral Pathol 1990;69:274–280.

15. Arnett GW, Milam SB, Gottesman L. Progressive mandibular retrusion—Idiopathic condylar resorption. 2. Am J Orthod Dentofacial Orthop 1996;110:117–127.

16. Arnett GW, Milam SB, Gottesman L. Progressive mandibular retrusion—Idiopathic condylar resorption. 1. Am J Orthod Dentofacial Orthop 1996;110:8–15.

17. Scheerlinck JP, Stoelinga PJ, Blijdorp PA, Brouns JJ, Nijs ML. Sagittal split advancement osteotomies stabilized with miniplates. A 2–5-year follow-up. Int J Oral Maxillofac Surg 1994;23:127–131.

18. Huang CS, Ross RB. Surgical advancement of the retrognathic mandible in growing children. Am J Orthod 1982;82:89–103.

19. Aufdemorte TB, Van Sickels JE, Dolwick MF, et al. Estrogen receptors in the temporomandibular joint of the baboon (*Papio cynocephalus*): An autoradiographic study. Oral Surg Oral Med Oral Pathol 1986;61:307–314.

20. Milam SB, Aufdemorte TB, Sheridan PJ, Triplett RG, Van Sickels JE, Holt GR. Sexual dimorphism in the distribution of estrogen receptors in the temporomandibular joint complex of the baboon. Oral Surg Oral Med Oral Pathol 1987;64:527–532.

21. Chuong R, Piper MA. Avascular necrosis of the mandibular condyle—Pathogenesis and concepts of management. Oral Surg Oral Med Oral Pathol 1993;75:428–432.

22. Chuong R, Piper MA, Boland TJ. Osteonecrosis of the mandibular condyle. Pathophysiology and core decompression. Oral Surg Oral Med Oral Pathol Oral Radiol Endod 1995;79:539–545.

23. Cisneros GJ. The Use of Bone Seeking Radiopharmaceuticals in the Assessment of Facial Growth [thesis]. Cambridge, MA: Harvard University, 1982.

24. Pogrel MA, Kopf J, Dodson TB, Hattner R, Kaban LB. A comparison of single-photon emission computed tomography and planar imaging for quantitative skeletal scintigraphy of the mandibular condyle. Oral Surg Oral Med Oral Pathol Oral Radiol Endod 1995;80:226–231.

25. Kaban LB, Cisneros GJ, Heyman S, Treves S. Assessment of mandibular growth by skeletal scintigraphy. J Oral Maxillofac Surg 1982;40:18–22.

26. Crawford JG, Stoelinga PJ, Blijdorp PA, Brouns JJ. Stability after reoperation for progressive condylar resorption after orthognathic surgery: Report of seven cases. J Oral Maxillofac Surg 1994;52:460–466.

27. Merkx MA, Van Damme PA. Condylar resorption after orthognathic surgery. Evaluation of treatment in 8 patients. J Craniomaxillofac Surg 1994;22:53–58.

28. Arnett GW, Tamborello JA. Progressive Class II development: Female idiopathic condylar resorption. Oral Maxillofac Surg Clin North Am 1990;2:699–716.

29. Mercuri LG, Wolford LM, Sanders B, White RD, Giobbie-Hurder A. Long-term follow-up of the CAD/CAM patient fitted total temporomandibular joint reconstruction system. J Oral Maxillofac Surg 2002;60:1440–1448.

30. Wolford LM, Dingwerth DJ, Talwar RM, Pitta MC. Comparison of 2 temporomandibular joint total joint prosthesis systems. J Oral Maxillofac Surg 2003;61:685–690; discussion 690.

31. Britton C, Christensen RW, Curry JT. Use of the Christensen TMJ fossa-eminence prosthesis system: A retrospective clinical study. Surg Technol Int 2002;10:273–281.

32. Luz JG, de Rezende JR, de Araujo VC, Chilvarquer I. Active unilateral condylar hyperplasia. Cranio 1994;12:58–62.

33. Feldmann G, Linder-Aronson S, Rindler A, Soderstrom U. Orthodontic and surgical treatment of unilateral condylar hyperplasia during growth—A case report. Eur J Orthod 1991;13:143–148.

34. Wolford LM, Cardenas L. Idiopathic condylar resorption: Diagnosis, treatment protocol, and outcomes. Am J Orthod Dentofacial Orthop 1999;116:667–677.

INDEX